Research and Statistical Methods
in Communication Sciences and Disorders

Research and Statistical Methods
in Communication Sciences and Disorders

David L. Maxwell, PhD
Professor, Communication Sciences and Disorders
Emerson College
Boston, MA

Eiki Satake, PhD
Associate Professor
Emerson College
Boston, MA

THOMSON

DELMAR LEARNING

Australia Canada Mexico Singapore Spain United Kingdom United States

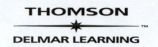

Research and Statistical Methods in Communication Sciences and Disorders
by David L. Maxwell, PhD and Eiki Satake, PhD

Vice President, Health Care Business Unit:
William Brottmiller

Editorial Director:
Cathy L. Esperti

Acquisitions Editor:
Kalen Conerly

Developmental Editor:
Juliet Steiner

Editorial Assistant:
Molly Belmont

Marketing Director:
Jennifer McAvey

Marketing Coordinator:
Chris Manion

Production Coordinator:
John Mickelbank

Project Editor:
Ruth Fisher

Art and Design Coordinator:
Christi DiNinni

Library of Congress Cataloging-in-Publication Data

Maxwell, David L.
  Research and statistical methods in communication sciences and disorders/David L. Maxwell, Eiki Satake.—1st ed.
     p. cm.
  Includes bibliographical references and index.
  ISBN 1-4018-1567-7
  1. Communicative disorders—Research—Methodology. 2. Speech theraphy—Research—Methodology. 3. Communicative disorders—Research—Statistical methods. I. Satake, Eiki. II. Title.
  RC423.M3698 2006
  616.85'5'0072—dc22

                                    2005011595

NOTICE TO THE READER

Dedication

This book is dedicated to our parents:

Minnie Marie Maxwell & William Lowell Maxwell

And

Tsunehiro Satake & Nobue Satake

Contents

Preface

When we began writing this book, our goal was to revise our previous text entitled *Research and Statistical Methods in Communication Disorders,* published in 1997, adding and subtracting from its content based on feedback from students and colleagues who had used it in their classrooms. Yet, as is often the case when taking your car in for a minor tune-up, our modest plans for revising existing chapters in the previous book turned into a major overhaul.

The book you are now reading is essentially a new book. Although sections of the previous text have been retained, this edition has grown from 9 to 13 chapters. In addition, most of the chapters of the original text have been significantly revised and updated to reflect new literature and emerging trends in the field. In our previous book, a single chapter was devoted to the topic of research design. In the current text, this material has been divided into three new chapters to focus more sharply on the advantages and limitations of experimental research designs, nonexperimental research designs, and qualitative research designs. The new chapter on qualitative research was prompted by the recommendations of colleagues and reviewers of our previous book who recognized the increasing importance and use of such methods in the field of communication sciences and disorders. In addition, we have added a new chapter devoted entirely to sampling techniques for selecting research participants and how selection bias can undermine the validity of research findings. New material has also been added pertaining to the establishment of evidence-based practice and the importance of discriminating between the power of various research studies in determining the efficacy or effectiveness of our diagnostic practices and clinical interventions. Because of these and other extensive revisions to our previous text, we view this book as sufficiently new in both structure and content to consider it to cover the essentials of research and statistical methods. This new edition reflects our belief in the importance of understanding the fundamental concepts discussed in these chapters and being able to apply them to problems encountered in everyday professional contexts—not only in the laboratory but in the clinic as well.

Philosophy and Goals

Like our previous book, the current text was written primarily for graduate students preparing for professional work in the field of communication sciences and disorders. Although the great majority of students will pursue clinical practice as opposed to research careers, this does not exempt them from the obligation of applying scientific principles in the work they will do. Whatever their professional bent, all will benefit from a working knowledge of the principles of research design and data analysis techniques, whether as intelligent consumers of scientific literature or actual producers of such literature.

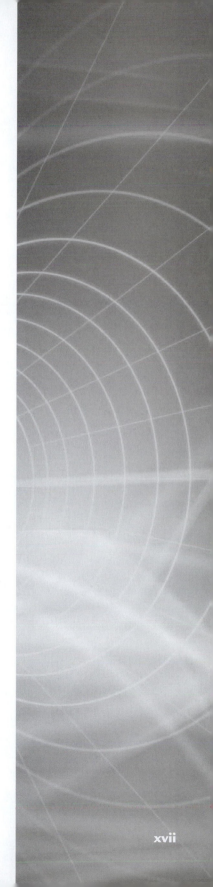

Scientific literacy is crucial for understanding research methodology as well as the statistical assumptions and techniques used for the analysis and interpretation of data. Without such literacy, it will be impossible to stay abreast of a rapidly flowing and ever-changing stream of information related to speech, language, and hearing disorders. The ability to assure quality in clinical care, to render valid diagnostic conclusions, and to discriminate factual information from fallacious reasoning is vital to the credibility and future success of our field as a scientific discipline grounded in ethical practices.

Our major goal in writing this book was for it to have sufficient breadth and depth of coverage to serve as a general introduction to the methods of research and statistics employed in the field of communication sciences and disorders. Wishing to avoid a "cookbook approach," we instead focused on writing a "user friendly" yet comprehensive text that can help students develop the kinds of analytic and critical thinking skills that will be important in maintaining and advancing their professional careers throughout a lifetime of work. Every effort has been made to meld important philosophical and theoretical concepts that underlie scientific research with practical illustrations of the methodologies that make this possible. In doing so, we have attempted to remove the mystery from scientific work by simplifying and making clear the methods that researchers as well as clinicians can use in solving problems, making decisions, and communicating knowledge to others.

Approach and Special Features

The thirteen chapters of this book are arranged in a logical sequence to illustrate both the thinking processes and action processes of scientific research as a series of interconnected steps in problem solving. As much as possible, the many research studies cited relate to problems encountered in our field. However, the scientific philosophies, concepts, and methodologies we review are universal, owing allegiance to no particular discipline.

Although students and other readers might benefit from some prior level of knowledge about the material to be presented, this is by no means a necessary condition for understanding the concepts and applications covered herein. Because students entering graduate programs in communication sciences and disorders have diverse educational experiences, we have assumed for purposes of this book that many will have little or no prior knowledge of research and statistics and, therefore, must "begin from the beginning." Although some students may have taken a course in statistics as undergraduates, we have found that few can adequately recall this subject matter or apply it to research problems as found in our professional journals. Our book is intended to integrate research methods with core statistical concepts and techniques, using clinically relevant examples while minimizing the requirements for actual calculation.

Special features of this book include:

- A topic outline at the beginning of each chapter.
- A list of learning objectives at the beginning of each chapter.

- Key terms highlighted in bold print as they first appear in each chapter to emphasize their importance and a list of such terms at the end of each chapter.
- Richly cited references to classic and present day literature that help to clarify the basis of scientific thinking and problem solving.
- Use of numerous tables, figures, and boxes to enliven the discussion of concepts and illustration of problems.
- A summary of chapter content at the end of each chapter.
- Self-learning exercises arranged in the form of completion questions at the end of each chapter to consolidate learning. The accuracy of responses may be checked against correct answers provided in an appendix (see Appendix E).
- Questions and exercises for classroom discussion are also provided at the end of each chapter to stimulate critical thinking about chapter content and its application to practical problems.
- Computer applications from Minitab and Statistical Packages for the Social Sciences (SPSS) are demonstrated in Chapter 12.
- A research article questionnaire to assist readers in evaluating research articles (see Chapter 13).
- A research proposal outline to assist readers in preparing a research proposal (see Chapter 13).
- A comprehensive glossary of key terms at the end of the book.
- A wide array of fully developed problem exercises and step-by-step illustrations of statistical applications (see Appendix A-2 to A-6). At the discretion of the instructor, one or more of these statistical applications may either be assigned to mathematically inclined students or omitted.
- An example of an NIH grant application (see Appendix C).
- An example of a poster session presentation (see Appendix D).

Electronic Classroom Manager (ECM) to Accompany Research and Statistical Methods in Communication Sciences and Disorders

In addition to the learning aids noted above, an electronic classroom manager (ECM) is available to instructors to assist them in achieving their instructional goals. The ECM contains:

- A fully developed syllabus written for the core text.
- A large bank of objective test questions to help assess factual knowledge of chapter content.
- A list of problem-based questions and exercises for each chapter to help assess integration and application of chapter content.
- Answers or suggested responses to accompany the questions and exercises for classroom discussion that conclude each chapter.

Chapter Synopses

To help readers better understand the material covered in this text, a synopsis of each of the chapters follows that can be used as a road map through the text.

Chapter 1. History and Philosophy of Science.   Provides an overview of the history, nature, and philosophy of scientific thinking, as such thought processes have evolved from the human quest to explain, predict, and control natural phenomena. Shows the linkages between logical reasoning, empiricism, theory building, operational definitions, theoretical constructs, hypothesis testing, and data collection under controlled conditions—all aspects of modern scientific problem solving. Discusses the major reasons for scientific inquiry and the relevance of scientific problem-solving skills to evidence-based clinical practice in the field of communication sciences and disorders.

Chapter 2. Getting Started: Basic Concepts of Research.   Provides a broad overview of the basic terminology and fundamental concepts underlying research. Defines and discusses the types of variables, the manner in which they are classified, and their use in scientific investigations. Introduces and distinguishes between quantitative and qualitative research; true experiments, quasi-experiments, and nonexperimental research designs; clinical, basic, and applied research; and pilot studies. Discusses the scientific method as a highly focused step-by-step process that is well represented in the various sections of a research article. Emphasizes the importance of the research process proceeding in accordance with ethical principles and practices dedicated to protecting research participants, to the greatest extent possible, from physical or emotional harm. Because much of the material in this chapter is discussed in greater detail in subsequent chapters, it may be assigned at the option of the instructor.

Chapter 3. Selecting a Research Problem.   Discusses how research questions originate and identifies issues to evaluate in selecting a problem for study. Various types of research questions are also discussed, as well as the resources available for answering them. The need for establishing rationales for investigating particular research questions and for determining the feasibility of answering them is emphasized. Ethical principles introduced in Chapter 2 are considered further in terms of specific guidelines for protecting human participants in research investigations.

Chapter 4. Reviewing the Literature and Stating Research Problems.   Discusses the purpose of a literature review as a tool for relating the findings of previous research to a problem that one wishes to investigate. The features of a well-written literature review are also discussed, using examples from a published research article, as well as the importance of such a review in establishing research questions and/or research hypotheses. How null hypotheses are used in research and their logical basis is also reviewed along with alternative approaches to null hypothesis testing.

Chapter 5. Sampling Theory and Methods.   The major theoretical principles and processes underlying the selection of a sample of subjects from a population are reviewed. The strengths and limitations of several *probability sampling* methods and *nonprobability sampling* methods are evaluated with respect to their ability to reduce selection bias and increase the validity of inferences. Several sources of selection bias and sampling errors are also discussed, together with how decisions pertaining to sample size can impact the ability of researchers to generalize statistical findings.

Chapter 6. Controlling, Measuring, and Recording Variables.   Focuses on each of these three research processes as they singly or interactively can influence the reliability and validity of a study. Makes clear how experimental control is best achieved through studies that allow for the active manipulation of one or more independent variables using methods designed to maximize systematic variance while minimizing random and systematic errors. Discusses issues to consider in selecting and specifying measurements appropriate for the dependent variable(s) of a research study and the means for calculating systematic errors (consistent errors) in relation to unsystematic errors (random errors). Defines the various types of measurement reliability and validity and provides examples of each. Identifies common response measures (frequency, latency, duration, amplitude/intensity) and several behavioral and physiological methods for recording such measurements.

Chapter 7. Causal Inferences and Threats to Their Validity.   To provide a conceptual basis for evaluating the experimental research designs discussed in Chapter 8, this chapter examines a fundamental assumption of modern day science that causal relationships exist among variables. The philosophical and methodological bases for determining causality are reviewed along with the threats to four types of validity that are typically of concern in experiments (internal validity, external validity, statistical conclusion validity, and construct validity).

Chapter 8. Experimental Designs.   A broad range of experimental designs appropriate for testing research hypotheses are reviewed. After discussing various ways to classify research studies, a classification scheme based on the ability of an investigator to achieve control over the variables under investigation, while ruling out confounding factors, is described. The most powerful of these designs in determining causality, termed *true experiments,* are first discussed, followed by an evaluation of the strengths and limitations of various quasi-experimental designs appropriate for both group and single-subject investigations. Finally, the weakest of the experimental designs, termed preexperiments, sometimes called pseudoexperiments, are described in view of their potential "fool's gold" appeal in giving the misleading impression of constituting credible approaches to scientific research.

Chapter 9. Nonexperimental Research Methods.   Although nonexperimental studies are inadequate for determining causality, they are useful for describing and categorizing variables, in exploring their associative relationships, and in determining the probability for certain outcomes in the future. Various types of nonexperimental research designs are discussed in this chapter including case studies, cohort and case-control studies, causal-comparative studies, and survey studies as exemplified in the published literature. Because of the popularity of survey research, considerable attention is given to two categories of such studies—questionnaires and interviews.

The steps involved in conducting survey studies and their relative advantages and disadvantages are discussed in considerable detail. Still another category of nonexperimental research reviewed in this chapter pertains to the evaluation of diagnostic test accuracy. Specific measures of test accuracy including test sensitivity, test specificity, and the predictive values positive and negative are defined and discussed. The methods used for calculating these indices and the probabilities for drawing correct and incorrect conclusions are also made clear.

Chapter 10. Qualitative Research Methods.   Begins by distinguishing the philosophy and methods of qualitative research from quantitative research. Proceeds by describing various qualitative research traditions including ethnography, grounded theory, phenomenology, discourse analysis, and content analysis. Examples from the literature are used to make clear how each of these traditions influences the approach taken to the collection, analysis, and interpretation of research data. What constitutes "good interpretative practices" in qualitative research is discussed in relation to various criteria that qualitative researchers use for evaluating the reliability and validity of research findings. The relevance of qualitative approaches in addressing problems in human communication that cannot be understood merely through numerical calculations is emphasized throughout the chapter.

Chapter 11. Analyzing Data: Descriptive Statistics.   Discusses the kinds of measurement scales and the types of data they yield. Presents the basic concepts underlying the application of various descriptive statistics in organizing, portraying, and analyzing data. Covers various measures of central tendency, variability, correlation, and regression. The material discussed in this chapter is discretionary given the aims of the instructor. Some students, who have completed an introductory course in statistics, may review or skip some portion of the chapter content. Others with less knowledge will benefit from the inclusion of the elementary statistical concepts that are covered.

Chapter 12. Analyzing Data: Inferential Statistics.   Presents the basic concepts of probability theory and inferential statistics as reflected in parametric and nonparametric hypothesis testing. Covers the statistical theory underlying the notion of sampling variability. Discusses the z test and Student t test and their application to one-sample and two-sample cases along with nonparametric analogs suitable for testing comparable hypotheses. Introduces the intuitive basis for the analysis of variance (ANOVA) as well as multivariate techniques and their statistical relevance. Discusses several complex statistical methods and step-by-step illustrations such as Minitab and SPSS in the analysis of statistical data. Although several advanced statistical methods are discussed, the intuitive basis of such methods should be emphasized over mathematical calculations. For the latter purpose, statistical applications of such computer programs as Minitab and SPSS for the analysis of statistical data are presented.

Chapter 13. Reading, Writing, and Presenting Research.   Discusses reading and writing skills as expressions of critical thinking and reasoning processes. Outlines the criteria for evaluating a research article and writing a research proposal. Identifies major sources of funding. Notes the steps necessary in preparing proposals for theses and dissertations and the essential requirements for "well written" proposals, whatever purpose they might serve. Comments on the opportunities for professional presentations of research and the criteria used by scholarly organizations such as ASHA in evaluating the merit of such proposals for technical papers and poster sessions.

Acknowledgments

Words of thanks are owed to several people who assisted in the preparation of this book for publication. Many graduate students at Emerson College provided valuable help by researching relevant literature for inclusion as well as providing technical assistance of various kinds. We are also grateful to Emerson College librarian Elizabeth Bezerra for her comments pertaining to a section of our book on "how to use a library." We wish to thank colleague Dr. Krista Wilkinson for information she provided about the process of applying for an NIH grant and for allowing us to include excerpts from one of her grant applications as an example of what such work entails. Another colleague, Dr. Amit Bajaj, also provided valuable assistance in editing a section of our book that pertains to recording measurements. A debt of gratitude is especially due to Dr. Vinoth Jagaroo for his valuable assistance in preparing some of the components of the electronic classroom manager.

We would like to express a special thank you to several anonymous reviewers for their incisive comments and positive suggestions that led to substantial improvements in the overall quality of this textbook and to Juliet Steiner, Developmental Editor, and Ruth Fisher, Project Editor, at Thomson Delmar Learning, who directly facilitated its completion.

To our wives, Danni and Mary, and to other family members and friends, for your patient and generous support throughout this long and time-demanding effort, we offer our heartfelt gratitude.

Finally, we wish to remember our colleague, Dr. Alan Lee Hankin, whose vital spirit lives on.

About the Authors

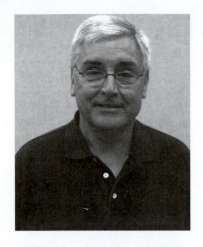

Dr. David Maxwell, Professor of Communication Sciences and Disorders, Emerson College, completed his undergraduate and graduate work in communication disorders and psychology at Southern Illinois University. Teacher, researcher, consultant, and lecturer, with expertise in orofacial malformations, stuttering, and related neurogenic disorders, he has held appointments at the Boston Naval Hospital, Boston University Medical School and Graduate School of Dentistry, Tufts New England Medical School, Eunice Kennedy Shriver Center, Massachusetts General Hospital, and the Douglas Thom Clinic for Cognitive and Behavioral Disorders. In addition to holding a tenured appointment at Emerson College, he has served as Acting Vice President of Academic Affairs and as Dean of Emerson's Academic Personnel. He has written two previous textbooks with Dr. Eiki Satake: *Research and Statistical Methods in Communication Disorders* and *Theory of Probability for Clinical Diagnostic Testing*. His personal interests include wilderness conservation, skiing, kayaking, hiking, and star gazing in the mountains of Maine. He and his wife, Danni, live in Dedham, Massachusetts.

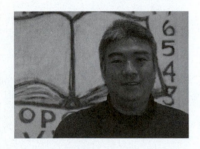

Dr. Eiki Satake is associate professor of mathematics at Emerson College in Boston, Massachusetts. He earned his B.A. in mathematics from U.C. Berkeley and M.S., Ed.M., and Ph.D. in Applied Statistics and Mathematics Education from Teachers College, Columbia University. He has published numerous articles for journals, among them *Communication Research, Educational and Psychological Measurement, International Institute of Statistics Bulletin,* and *AMATYC Review*. He has also authored and co-authored several textbooks and monographs, among them *Research and Statistical Methods in Communication Disorders, Mathematical Reasoning, Actuarial Mathematics for Finance,* and *Theory of Probability for Clinical Diagnostic Testing*. His current research interests are probability logic, an application of the Bayesian statistical methods to communication sciences and disorders, and mathematics and statistics anxiety. He is an avid squash player and lives in Framingham, Massachusetts, with his wife Mary and an exotic short-hair cat.

History and Philosophy of Science

CHAPTER 1

CHAPTER OUTLINE

LEARNING OBJECTIVES

After reading this chapter, you should be able to identify, describe, or define:

- Why and how scientific thought evolved
- Differences between the scientific method and other means of gaining knowledge
- Two types of reasoning processes underlying scientific thought: induction and deduction
- The doctrine of empiricism: its importance and limitations
- How operational definitions have advanced the work of science
- The characteristics of a "good" theory
- Why some researchers choose eclectic approaches to science instead of building theories
- Evidence-based practice

- Efficacy, effectiveness, and efficiency of treatment outcomes
- Importance of clinician-researcher partnerships
- Perspective and skills of the clinical scientist

HISTORY OF SCIENTIFIC THOUGHT

Since the time of its rudimentary beginnings, from a substrate of related disciplines including education, medicine, and psychology, the profession of communication sciences and disorders has made remarkable strides in developing a fund of knowledge firmly grounded in scientific research. The substance and relevance of our current clinical endeavors owe much to a preexisting scientific ethos that values critical thinking and objectivity in evaluating the reliability and validity of evidence and a willingness to change our theories and approaches to problems as new facts emerge. Faith in the worth of science and a commitment to its philosophy of thought and method of action has long been established.

Scientific thought began with the earliest humans whose brains had developed sufficiently to convert and elaborate raw sensory experience from a state of primitive wonderment into coherent and organized perceptions of experience. From that time onward, our evolution has been characterized by a continuous unfolding of increasingly complex mental capacities out of a quest to *explain, predict,* and *control* cause-effect relationships existing among many variables. Perhaps what we learned that was most important to the advancement of science was the way to control our environment and one another through language and the gradual emergence of powerful communication technologies.

In early history, the perceived causes for natural phenomena were attributed to the work of deities. For the Babylonians, the Bull of Heaven brought drought; the great bird Imdugud caused rain. Yet, the will of these spirits could be mediated or altered through prayer, sacrificial offerings, and related rituals. Eventually, modified forms of these early doctrines evolved into the major tenets of the world religions. These religions promulgated the belief that the superstructures of knowledge were largely impenetrable.

With the advent of numerical systems, humans began to refine their observations into quantifiable measurements. Efforts to explain the relation between causes and effects were increasingly cast as mathematical formulations of order and coherence. The secrets of the gods began to be encoded into sets of empirical definitions unified by explanatory propositions called **theories.** Such theories provided humankind with a systematic structure for thought in guiding the processes of inquiry as new facts were organized into larger units of useful knowledge.

Ancient evidence of relatively abstract theoretical thinking is found in the calculations of areas and volumes recorded on Egyptian papyrus and Babylonian tablets dating from 2000 BC. About the same time, the Chinese were beginning to formulate the first written hypotheses about the elemental composition of matter, which appeared in the *Shu-ching* or *Canonical Book of Records* (Siu, 1957). With the advent of written language, the record of the causal relations between objects and events (**variables**) forming the structure of the observable world was removed from the heavens and placed in human repositories of knowledge called libraries. From these budding scientific efforts, systematic methods have emerged spanning all fields of human knowledge that allow us to observe, investigate, and apprehend the relations between variables. As noted above, the explanation of the relations between sets of such variables generally occurs within the framework of formal propositions, or theories.

NATURE OF SCIENTIFIC THOUGHT

The work that entails the search for the answers to certain questions is called science, and the tools of such work consist of systematic research and statistical methods. For pragmatic reasons, the term *science* is almost better viewed as a verb than as a noun. Although the antecedent of the word "science" is the Latin verb *scire* (to know), to view science merely as a storehouse of knowledge belies its true character as a dynamic, fact-seeking enterprise.

Scientific knowledge does not magically spring into being but owes its existence to certain thinking and action processes. Ultimately, such processes underlie the ability to formulate a problem in terms that are empirically testable. This viewpoint is consistent with Kerlinger's (1967) notion of science as an *activity* that people do in the pursuit of valid and reliable answers to questions. While such activity often culminates in new knowledge, science is best seen as the means to this end. As we shall see, the "means" involves **hypothesis testing** under systematic, controlled, and empirical conditions. Often, according to Dewey (1922), the actual distinction between the "means" and "ends" of science is arbitrary since both involve a series of actions with the means simply occurring at an earlier stage.

Scientific versus Nonscientific Knowledge

Science is but one means of obtaining knowledge of the world. An understanding of one's experience can also be gained through subjective or personal analysis, intuition, or spiritual or religious convictions, or it can be based on what are perceived as knowledgeable statements by certain authority figures. But science, unlike such alternative approaches to knowledge, deals in *temporary* hypotheses of cause and effect relations. Scientists believe that events in the universe are interconnected and causally determined by natural factors under certain conditions of observation and measurement. Such causal relations may change under different conditions of time or space.

As made clear by modern statistical theory, nature's laws are not forged as rigid truths but exist as expressions of probability or relative chances of occurrences. Such chances are associated with certain degrees of *error* inherent in nature itself. Unlike most dogma, the language of science involves statements of **probability,** under certain conditions or proscribed limits (i.e., not statements of absolute certainty).

Logic of Science

The rational character of science is manifested in two major types of logical reasoning processes: **deduction** and **induction.** Deductive logic begins with a general premise or law, assumed to be true, which is then used to explain specific observations or behavioral occurrences. Conversely, induction involves a form of reasoning wherein a general theory or set of laws is ultimately derived from specific observations or individual cases. In actual practice, inductive reasoning, (i.e., inferences based on particular observations) is the initial starting point for most research activity from which a more general understanding or theory may be deduced.

To use a clinical example of an inductive reasoning process, as early as 1955, Sedlackova reported observing the occurrence of certain congenital anomalies (e.g., cupped ears and digital abnormalities) in association with velopharyngeal dysfunction for speech in a number of children. Subsequently, Shprintzen et al. (1978) described the presence of additional orofacial features that commonly occur in conjunction with submucous clefts or overt clefts of the secondary palate. Many of these same cases had associated cardiac defects. Still more cases documented by several clinicians in other centers revealed a spectrum of physical and functional anomalies that frequently occur in conjunction with what is now recognized as the velocardiofacial syndrome—the most common syndrome of clefting. Moreover, summarizing the results of several studies, Peterson-Falzone et al. (2001) noted that close to 75% of these cases are associated with a deletion of genetic material on the long arm of chromosome 22 (locus 22q11). Thus, beginning with specific instances (observed facts) of what were seen initially as quite distinct and unrelated anomalies, a generalization that explained the relationship of one fact to another was eventually derived (i.e., a pattern of anomalies called the velocardiofacial syndrome and a theory for its occurrence). The value of inductive reasoning is that it serves as a tool for building theories based on patterns and relationships observed in specific pieces of data.

Once a theory has been formulated, deductive reasoning can be used to explain aspects of other phenomena to which its tenets might be generalized. Drawing on our example of the velocardiofacial syndrome, the region of the genetic defect is believed to be "one of the most 'mutable' (changeable) portions of the human genome" (Peterson-Falzone et al., 2001, p. 37). Thus, as a genetic marker, it might prove to have theoretical value in *deducing* (explaining) the etiology of other syndromes with which it shares overlapping clinical features (Driscoll et al., 1992). Deductive reasoning is a process that begins with a general statement or proposition and then logically proceeds toward a specific conclusion. For instance, given the following three statements, the third statement can be logically deduced from statements one and two:

> People with features of velocardiofacial syndrome are likely to show a deletion of genetic material on the long arm of chromosome 22.
>
> *and*
>
> John is a person who demonstrates such features.
>
> *then*
>
> John is likely to show a deletion of genetic material on the long arm of chromosome 22.

As Immanuel Kant (1724–1804) aptly concluded in his *Critique of Pure Reason,* induction and deduction are not disassociated mental processes but are built-in operations of the human mind that complement and facilitate one another in problem solving. While inductive reasoning is the logical tool we use to derive general laws from separate facts, once derived, the general laws can be applied to explain new facts as they are found by means of deductive reasoning. Given this understanding, we can conclude that both inductive and deductive reasoning processes are essential for scientific progress.

Science and Empiricism

Whereas logical reasoning is important in the framework of the philosophy of science, perhaps a more significant requirement guiding actual scientific research is based on the **doctrine of empiricism,** which holds that nothing can be said to exist until it is actually *observed* to exist to some degree. Empiricism insists that the elements of the problem under investigation be observed, tested, or measured rather than left to the realm of hypothetical argument or subjective opinion. Scientists view strict reliance on logic or common sense as an untrustworthy means of gaining knowledge. According to the doctrine of empiricism, the ultimate arbiter of an issue ought to be either direct or indirect observation of the phenomenon itself.

Without the "seeing is believing" requirement of empiricism, one's approach to knowledge would have to be based largely on folklore, mysticism, speculation, hearsay, or unverified opinions expressed by people viewed as "experts" in various fields of study.

Language of Science

Despite the major premise of empiricism that "seeing is believing," the idea that "truth is within the eye of the beholder" must also be kept in mind. Different individuals may see different things through the lens of their unique personal experiences. Perhaps for this reason, Francis Bacon (1561–1626) warned scientists in 1620 to beware of four illusory idols which certain biased perspectives can impose on the reasoning process, leading to erroneous ways of "seeing" (Baird, 2000). These included:

1. Idols of the Tribe: Errors inherent in the beliefs of culture or humankind in general, (e.g., the once widely held belief that the earth is flat and the center of the universe).
2. Idols of the Cave: Errors inherent in the beliefs of a particular individual owing to private prejudices or idiosyncratic personality factors (e.g., blind or unquestioning adherence to the pronouncements of esteemed scientists, politicians, or religious figures widely perceived as "authorities" in their respective fields).
3. Idols of the Market Place: Errors arising from misleading messages or systems of thought (e.g., myths created by various media and advertising agencies that merely consuming particular products or indulging in certain behaviors significantly improves our physical, social, or emotional well-being).
4. Idols of the Theater: Errors resulting from the influence of mere words over our minds (e.g., accepting without critical evaluation aphorisms, proverbs, or slogans such as "all's well that ends well," "there are lies, damn lies, and statistics," "God bless America, land of the free").

Because of these potential pitfalls in discerning the true nature of phenomena, Bacon advocated systematizing and improving the precision of observation methods in all sciences including those concerned with the study of human behavior. No doubt, modern day science owes much to the development and refinement of such methods, although many human problems continue to arise due to people's biased perspectives about the world.

Often, the inclination of people to embrace irrational ideas and beliefs is not because the matter in question has been proved true. Instead, as Bruce Thorton (1999) succinctly noted in his book, *Plagues of the Mind,* many people today are still prone to such errors "because it is easier and more psychically gratifying than performing the hard work of reason that makes a belief well founded" (p. xvii). Stated more simply, it's easier to "eat an apple a day to keep the doctor away" than to investigate whether or not apples have medicinal value. Thorton cited the journalist Thomas Sowell, who observed that even the most respected caretakers of knowledge in our universities, the media, government, and other institutions too often use their privileged positions to advance false information or that which lacks the demands for empirical proof. Unfortunately, misinformation, half-truths, or outright lies can spread into popular culture.

Because such problems were especially prevalent during the lifetime of Francis Bacon, he, along with other philosophers and scientists, recognized the need to bolster the credibility of knowledge. Over time, this was achieved through improvements in the language used by scientists to communicate ideas and information. Increasingly, scientists adhered to the use of *objective language* in their definitions of terms or descriptions of observed objects or events. So far as possible, objective language communicates an observation according to the physical attributes of the phenomenon observed. On the other hand, the focus of *subjective language* is on what are largely the unobservable or private perceptions of an individual. Rejecting the latter approach, scientists strove to develop a new lexicon and method of operation free from such subjectivity.

Operationism

The new emphasis on objectivity in scientific work led the renowned physicist P. W. Bridgeman in 1927 to introduce a movement called **operationism,** which emphasized the importance of defining the quantitative meaning of theoretical terms in accordance with the conditions of their measurement. The movement toward operationalizing scientific language had a profound influence on not only developments in the physical sciences but the behavioral sciences as well. In order to sharpen the level of scientific discourse, the abstract and often vague meaning of various concepts began to be specified as measurable values. For example, consider the tendency among some people to evaluate another person's cognitive abilities based on what are often little more than limited interactions and informal observations of that person. As a summary of our impressions, we might conclude a person is highly intelligent, of average intelligence, or perhaps of low intelligence given our subjective opinion. Nevertheless, in the absence of objective data, such as scores obtained from standardized intelligence tests or other accepted measures, our observations would best be viewed as resulting from biased and unfounded presuppositions. Until the attributes of intelligence have been operationally defined, the notion of intelligence remains little more than a vague concept.

The process of developing operational definitions of such concepts as intelligence, language, motivation, personality, socioeconomic status, and so forth most often leads to the recognition that such factors represent a composite of attributes, all requiring specification in terms of various categories of behavior, test scores, or other outcome measures. Concepts deliberately reconstructed in this way for scientific use are called **constructs.** Constructs describe factors capable of assuming different values called variables. For research purposes, variables are typically defined *operationally* according to the manner in which they are assigned, manipulated, or measured. In addition, a variable can be defined according to whether or not it is considered to be the antecedent cause (**independent variable**) or consequent effect (**dependent variable**) under the experimental conditions. See Chapter 2 for a further discussion of variables. The conjectured relationship among such variables is usually stated in the form of a tentative **research hypothesis** formulated to be tested or evaluated under controlled circumstances termed **conditions.**

REASONS FOR SCIENTIFIC INQUIRY

Testing and Assessing Theories

Most scientific investigations begin with a problem caused by an obstacle to understanding. Such an obstacle leads to what is often a compelling motivation to describe, predict, or control behavior or circumstances. Although such motivation is a necessary ingredient of any problem-solving activity, it is not sufficient for the work of science. According to Kerlinger (1967), the majority of scientific research involves "systematic, controlled, empirical and critical investigation of natural phenomena guided by theory and hypotheses about the presumed relations among such phenomena" (p. 10). Like Kerlinger, many scientists believe that the primary reason for conducting research is to investigate hypotheses in relation to the tenets of particular theories. Such theories contain a number of statements or hypotheses about presumed relationships among classes of variables.

Three major criteria can be used in assessing the ultimate worth of any theory. First, and most important, a theory must be *empirical*—that is, it must generate hypotheses that are amenable to operational definition, objective testing, and evaluation. Unless a theory contains hypotheses that can be disproved, it has little or no scientific worth. Psychoanalytic theories of stuttering that attribute etiologic significance to repressed needs, stemming from immature sexual impulses and other unconscious urges along Freudian lines, are examples of the type for which scientific corroboration is largely lacking and is extremely difficult to achieve (Bloodstein, 1987). A second criterion for assessing the value of a theory is its relative *parsimony* in explaining the known facts about a phenomenon. According to a scientific principle based on William of Occam's rule, more commonly known as **Occam's razor,** a parsimonious theory is one that contains the fewest noncontradictory explanations. Thus, a parsimonious theory of stuttering would be one that could consistently explain the known and newly emerging facts about its origin, development, and maintenance with the fewest contradictions. A third characteristic of a "good" theory is to be found in its *heuristic quality*. In other words, is the theory fruitful in stimulating new and creative research endeavors, or does it "die on the vine" as a passing fad?

The philosopher Karl Popper (1968) noted that the main reason for scientific inquiry is to progress through a process of falsifying and refuting conjectures as to the truth of one's observations about the world. This is best accomplished by testing research hypotheses and objectively interpreting the test results in relation to the theory from which the hypotheses were originally derived. Through a process that entails sifting through "conjectures and refutations," some theories prevail, at least temporarily, as edifices of truth, while others are discarded. As noted previously, the question of whether or not a permanent truth can ever be found is debatable; therefore, the worth of a theory does not lie in its ability to discern the "absolute" truth or falsity of its propositions. Instead, the worth of a theory lies in its ability to generate *testable* propositions. For theoretical questions to have any value, the hypothesized relationships among a group of observations the theory hopes to explain must be expressed in a precise form. Because there may be multiple realities instead of a single reality underlying a particular observation, different methods for exploring and explaining its various facets are encouraged. A scientific tradition known as qualitative research, having its roots in anthropology, sociology, political science, and related fields, is especially prone to use multiple research methodologies in assessing the value of a theory. The means of enhancing the value of a theory by using multiple methods and perspectives to investigate the truth of its tenets is called **triangulation** (see Chapter 10).

Eclectic Approach to Research

Some scientists believe that there are several important justifications for research beyond testing and evaluating theories. Indeed, early advocates of strict behaviorism in the mode of B. F. Skinner argued that the tactics of hypothesis testing may blind investigators to significant bodies of knowledge that lie outside the narrow range of one's theoretical biases and problem solving. This particular philosophy was perhaps best summed up by the advice given by Skinner (1956) to study only interesting problems as they are encountered and to avoid justifying their selection based on the perceived theoretical relevance of such problems.

An often-cited strength of such a flexible research orientation is that it allows for certain potentially significant *chance* observations that sometimes turn out to be more important than the hypothesis being tested. The term **serendipity** was first used by Cannon (1945) to describe the process of accidentally discovering scientifically valuable information while exploring some unrelated problem.

A classic example of the value of serendipitous research findings is based on a study carried out at the Walter Reed Laboratories in the 1950s. In an investigation of avoidance conditioning paradigms that entailed the use of electric shock, Joseph Brady (1958) was frustrated by the inability to complete his experiments as planned because of the high mortality among the monkeys being used as subjects. During subsequent autopsy investigations, it was discovered that the animals had been subjected to a certain type of negative reinforcement schedule that had apparently resulted in a high incidence of perforated stomach ulcers. Although far from the intent of the original research, Brady and his colleagues appeared to have accidentally stumbled onto an important link between psychological stress of a certain kind and physical disease.

Sidman (1960), another well-known behaviorist, also offered several reasons for research beyond theory testing and evaluation. These included research to:

- Try out new methods or techniques
- Indulge or satisfy curiosity
- Demonstrate a new behavioral phenomenon
- Deepen understanding of the conditions influencing a behavioral phenomenon

These research rationales are especially applicable to the clinical environment wherein the needs of diverse individuals must be addressed, often by means of an **eclectic approach** that emphasizes flexibility and innovation in behavioral management. By adopting such an approach, the clinician seeks out and uses methods that seem to "work best" despite the fact that such methods may not be grounded in a particular theoretical model. In an effort to justify this practice, Kamhi (1999) has argued that there are times when *clinical pragmatism* instead of a theory driven approach should guide intervention. With respect to language, he commented in an earlier article (1993) that no single theory could possibly account for all the attributes and behaviors represented in language learning (e.g., linguistic, cognitive, affective, social, and cultural). Specifically, he noted that clinicians must work within diverse service delivery models and have knowledge of classroom management techniques, curricula, family systems, multicultural differences, psychological testing, special education and other remedial services, and so on. Because of this fact, Kamhi concluded: "No theory of language learning could possibly encompass all of these areas that impact on the provision of effective clinical services . . . providing clinical services that are theoretically coherent is not only impractical but also unrealistic" (p. 59).

In his review of philosophical debates about the importance of theory in clinical intervention, Apel (1999) cited Goldstein (1990), who suggested that efforts to force an intervention to fit within the constraints of a particular language theory could hamper creative approaches to therapy. Running counter to this view are the arguments of others that theory is essential as a framework in which to make informed decisions and to apply problem-solving skills (Johnston, 1983; Holland, 1998; Aram, 1991). Among these latter researchers, Aram (1991) goes so far as to argue that, in the absence of theory, clinicians run the risk of behaving merely as technicians.

In the field of communication sciences and disorders, applying and evaluating the efficacy of certain treatment procedures is the primary concern of most clinicians—not formal theory testing. Nevertheless, theories and hypotheses do operate either implicitly or explicitly in guiding diagnosis and therapeutic intervention (Apel, 1999). In this respect, Apel and Self (2003) commented that "clinicians should . . . provide hypotheses for the clinical phenomena they encounter rather than operating behind the thin veil of an 'it works' attitude." (p. 7). Clinical data may be collected and conclusions drawn that support existing theoretical frameworks or eventually translate into new theories and hypotheses suitable for empirical testing. As clinicians, we should remember that the richest substrate of our science is to be found in the problems we treat.

BOX 1-2 *continued*

sun-centered system explain apparent planetary motion, we choose the simpler.

5. **Scientific manipulation.** Any idea, even though it may be simple and conform to apparent observations, must usually be confirmed by work that teases out the possibility that the effects are caused by other factors.

6. **Skepticism.** Nearly all statements make assumptions of prior conditions. A scientist often reaches a dead end in research and has to go back and determine if all the assumptions made are true to how the world operates.

7. **Precision.** Scientists are impatient with vague statements: A virus causes disease? How many viruses are needed to infect? Are any hosts immune to the virus? Scientists are very exact and very "picky."

8. **Respect for paradigms.** A paradigm is our overall understanding about how the world works. Does a concept "fit" with our overall understanding or does it fail to weave in with our broad knowledge of the world? If it doesn't fit, it is "bothersome" and the scientist goes to work to find out if the new concept is flawed or if the paradigm must be altered.

9. **A respect for power of theoretical structure.** Diederich describes how a scientist is unlikely to adopt the attitude: "That is all right in theory but it won't work in practice." He notes that theory is "all right" only if it does work in practice. Indeed the rightness of the theory is in the end what the scientist is working toward; no science facts are accumulated at random. (This is an understanding that many science fair students must learn!)

10. **Willingness to change opinion.** When Harold Urey, author of one textbook theory on the origin of the moon's surface, examined the moon rocks brought back from the Apollo mission, he immediately recognized this theory did not fit the hard facts laying before him. "I've been wrong!" he proclaimed without any thought of defending the theory he had supported for decades.

11. **Loyalty to reality.** Dr. Urey above did not convert to just any new idea, but accepted a model that matched reality better. He would never have considered holding to an opinion just because it was associated with his name.

12. **Aversion to superstition and an automatic preference for scientific explanation.** No scientist can know all of the experimental evidence underlying current science concepts and therefore must adopt some views without understanding their basis. A scientist rejects superstition and prefers science paradigms out of an appreciation for the power of reality based knowledge.

13. **A thirst for knowledge, an "intellectual drive."** Scientists are addicted puzzle-solvers. The little piece of the puzzle that doesn't fit is the most interesting. However, as Diederich notes, scientists are willing to live with incompleteness rather than ". . . fill the gaps with offhand explanations."

14. **Suspended judgment.** Again Diederich describes: "A scientist tries hard not to form an opinion on a given issue until he has investigated it, because it is

continues

BOX 1-2 *continued*

so hard to give up opinions already formed, and they tend to make us find facts that support the opinions . . . There must be, however, a willingness to act on the best hypothesis that one has time or opportunity to form."

15. **Awareness of assumptions.** Diederich describes how a good scientist starts by defining terms, making all assumptions very clear, and reducing necessary assumptions to the smallest number possible. Often we want scientists to make broad statements about a complex world. But usually scientists are very specific about what they "know" or will say with certainty: "When these conditions hold true, the usual outcome is such-and-such."

16. **Ability to separate fundamental concepts from the irrelevant or unimportant.** Some young science students get bogged down in observations and data that are of little importance to the concept they want to investigate.

17. **Respect for quantification and appreciation of mathematics as a language of science.** Many of nature's relationships are best revealed by patterns and mathematical relationships when reality is counted or measured; and this beauty often remains hidden without this tool.

18. **An appreciation of probability and statistics.** Correlations do not prove cause-and-effect, but some pseudoscience arises when a chance occurrence is taken as "proof." Individuals who insist on an all-or-none world and who have little experience with statistics will have difficulty understanding the concept of an event occurring by chance.

19. **An understanding that all knowledge has tolerance limits.** All careful analyses of the world reveal values that scatter at least slightly around the average point; a human's core body temperature is about so many degrees and objects fall with a certain rate of acceleration, but there is some variation. There is no absolute certainty.

20. **Empathy for the human condition.** Contrary to popular belief, there is a value system in science, and it is based on humans being the only organisms that can "imagine" things that are not triggered by stimuli present at the immediate time in their environment; we are, therefore, the only creatures to "look" back on our past and plan our future. This is why when you read a moving book, you imagine yourself in the position of another person and you think "I know what the author meant and feels." Practices that ignore this empathy and resultant value for human life produce inaccurate science. (See Bronowski for more examples of this controversial "scientific attitude.")

Reprinted with permission from The Kansas School Naturalist, *35 (4), April 1989. Modified from Bronowski (1978), Diederich (1967), and Whaley and Surratt (1967), Emporia State University, Emporia, KS.*

SUMMARY

Scientific thinking involves several methods of reasoning that are essential to rational decision making whatever your career goals in the field of communication sciences and disorders. Before any problem can be understood, the elements that constitute it first must be carefully observed and described in operational terms. Only then can one begin to understand how one thing might relate to another. Having identified and described the independent variable (presumed cause) and dependent variable (presumed effect) of a problem in terms that can be empirically evaluated or measured, we then are in a position to study their associative and/or causative relations through an appropriate investigative technique.

As it searches for valid and reliable answers to questions, modern day science actually combines several methods including:

- Logical reasoning
- Empiricism
- Theory building
- Operational definitions of theoretical constructs
- Hypothesis testing under controlled conditions
- Data collection and analysis techniques

Through the judicious application of such methods, new facts are gained that advance our fund of knowledge in the field of communication sciences and disorders. In this chapter, we have maintained that such methods and the knowledge they generate are not confined to the laboratory but are equally vital to our work as clinicians wherever such work is performed.

KEY TERMS

theories

variables

hypothesis testing

probability

deduction

induction

doctrine of empiricism

operationism

constructs

independent variable

dependent variable

research hypothesis

conditions

Occam's razor

triangulation

serendipity

eclectic approach

extraneous variable

randomized clinical trial

ecological validity

scientific method

SELF-LEARNING REVIEW

1. Scientific thinking grew out of early human efforts to _____, _____, and _____ causal relationships.
2. Initially, the perceived causes of natural phenomena were attributed to _____ forces or spiritual _____.

3. With the advent of the numerical system, presumed causes of certain effects began to be formulated in _____ terms. _____ definitions were unified into a system of higher order definitions called _____.

4. Theories offered explanations of the _____ relations between observed objects and events termed _____.

5. Through various _____ propositions or frameworks, we apprehend the _____ between variables.

6. In essence, _____ entails the systematic search for _____ and _____ answers to questions.

7. Important tools of science include _____ and _____ methods.

8. Because science involves dynamic thought processes translated into systematic research activity, the term *science* is better viewed as a _____ than as a _____.

9. Dewey believed that the distinction between the _____ and _____ of science is arbitrary because they are simply different stages of the same process.

10. The "means" of science, which involves _____ testing, is carried out under controlled _____ or circumstances.

11. A central tenet of science is that events in the universe are _____ and _____ determined.

12. Nature's _____ are not viewed as rigid truths but express a _____ for a certain outcome having a degree of inherent _____.

13. _____ reasoning processes attest to the rational character of science. Deriving general laws or rules, based on observations of specific cases involves _____ reasoning. On the other hand, _____ entails the use of a general premise believed to be true in order to explain a specific observation.

14. Logic is first and foremost concerned with the _____ of propositions rather than their _____.

15. The edict of _____ states that "nothing can be said to exist until it is observed to exist to some degree."

16. Empiricism spurred new requirements in the language of science requiring _____ as opposed to _____ descriptions of objects and events.

17. This movement, called _____, required that _____ be intentionally reconstructed as _____ for scientific use.

18. _____ are the factors which constructs describe that are capable of assuming different values.

19. Variables may be defined _____ according to the manner in which they are assigned, manipulated, or measured.

20. Antecedent causes are defined as _____ variables, whereas those viewed as the consequent effects are called _____ variables.

21. A conjectural statement about the relationship between the dependent and independent variable is called a research _____ formulated to be tested under _____ conditions.

22. _____ reasoning is the logical tool we use to derive general laws from separate facts. Once derivved, such laws can be used to explain new facts by means of _____ reasoning.

23. Francis Bacon warned scientists to beware of four _____ that can bias the reasoning process. Idols of the _____ are beliefs of an individual owing to private prejudices or idiosyncratic personality factors. Unfortunately, as Thomas Sowell

observed, false information communicated by such idols can spread into the popular lore of _____.

24. A means of reducing subjectivity in scientific work is to insist on _____ definitions of theoretical terms in accordance with the conditions of their _____.

25. A "good theory" must be _____, _____, and _____. Ultimately, the worth of a theory lies in its ability to ask interesting _____ that lead to _____ answers.

26. _____ research that has its roots in anthropology, sociology, political science, and related fields is prone to use _____ research methodologies in assessing the value of a theory. One means of doing so is called _____.

27. Advocates of behaviorism in the mode of B. F. Skinner believe that there are several important justifications for research beyond testing and evaluating _____.

28. The behaviorist philosophy is consonant with the _____ approach or doing what seems to "work best." Others have argued that, in the absence of theory to guide one's work, clinicians run the risk of behaving merely as _____.

29. Scientific _____ means being able to read professional literature not merely in terms of its _____ but also with respect to its possible _____.

30. Support and reimbursement for health and human services is increasingly dependent on the ability of providers to demonstrate the _____ of their clinical services. ASHA has developed the National Outcome Measurement System, called _____ for short, to establish an _____ database for its professions.

31. NOMS incorporates a disorder-specific, seven-point rating scale, termed _____ _____ _____(s), for the assessment of treatment outcomes.

32. The use of any such system as NOMS should conform to sound research methods for assuring the _____ and _____ of research findings.

33. Whatever role a clinician might play, professional effectiveness can be augmented by thinking and behaving as a _____ _____. Such thinking and behaving processes characterize the so-called _____ _____.

34. The _____ of _____ requires that we maintain a high level of professional _____ and evaluate the _____ of services rendered and products dispensed.

35. Adopting a _____ _____ in our clinical work will help us achieve this goal.

QUESTIONS AND EXERCISES FOR CLASSROOM DISCUSSION

1. Write three propositions representing personal or professional beliefs that you hold to be "true."

2. Break up into small groups to discuss with your classmates how many of these propositions you can agree upon given each of your beliefs.

3. Make a list of the beliefs you hold in common along with the bases for deriving their "truth" (e.g., by means of authority figures, rationalism, intuition, or the scientific method). Were the sources of knowledge the same or did they differ in kind?

4. Make a second list of the propositions about which you disagreed. What was the basis of your disagreement (authority, rationalism, or the scientific method)?

5. Define the following terms *operationally*. Note the degree to which the variables included in your definition were assigned, manipulated, or measured based on objective as opposed to subjective criteria.

   - Motivation
   - Rapport
   - Generalization
   - Reinforcement
   - Language
   - Normality
   - Abnormality

6. Distinguish between inductive and deductive reasoning and provide an example of the use of these processes in research and theory building in the field of communication disorders.

7. According to Hewitt (2000), the profession has "... seen the rise and fall and rise again of more than one theory in the last twenty years, and this process shows no signs of coming to a halt" (p. 191). To the degree this is true, one might question the value of theory in contributing toward progress in the field. Clinicians, in particular, might question the value of theory in guiding their clinical practice. Some might opt instead to base their decisions primarily on intuition and clinical eclecticism (doing what seems to work best) instead of "wasting time" debating whether one's methods are well founded in theory. Discuss what you believe should be the role of theory and research-based approaches to clinical intervention and the implications for developing a scientifically based profession.

Getting Started: Basic Concepts of Research

CHAPTER 2

CHAPTER OUTLINE

LEARNING OBJECTIVES

This chapter is intended to provide a broad overview of the fundamental concepts and principles that underlie the research process. Much of the chapter content will be discussed in greater detail in subsequent chapters.

After reading this chapter, you should be able to identify, describe, or define:

- Types of variables as the focus of research
- Types of research
- Steps of the scientific method
- Structure and content of a research article
- Importance of ethical research principles

VARIABLES AS THE FOCUS OF RESEARCH

The major objectives of scientific research are to *describe variables,* the *hypothesized relations* among them, and the *means* of *altering* such relations through systematic forms of *manipulation or control.* For example, we might begin by describing the prevalence of certain phonological errors as observed in the speech of preschool children delayed in their expressive language development. Having classified or categorized these errors according to the type observed, we might wish to understand how they vary in association with the quantity or quality of language stimulation in the home. On this basis, parents might be instructed to interact with their children in a manner hypothesized to facilitate phonological development. The potential effect of such intervention could then be assessed.

Within this context, the rudiments of the scientific method have been described. Beginning with an observation of a particular variable, we proceed to investigate its relationship to other variables and then the manner in which these relations might be controlled through an active manipulation. A requirement for the understanding of scientific research is a basic understanding of the broad types of variables and the different roles they play in scientific inquiry.

Definitions and Types of Variables

Although describing, predicting, or controlling variables is the primary focus of most research, the meaning of the term *variable* is often ambiguous because of inconsistencies in usage. Perhaps this inconsistency is due in part to dictionary definitions of a "variable" as both an adjective (the tendency toward change) and as a noun (the thing that changes). For purposes of scientific research, the noun definition is the more common of the two; in it a variable ". . . is any attribute or property in which organisms (objects, events, people) are observed to vary" (Pedhazer & Schmelkin, 1991, p. 17). Variables can be broadly classified according to: (1) their measurement properties, (2) how they are used in various types of research, and (3) the degree to which they exert an extraneous or confounding influence on the outcome of an experiment (see Table 2-1).

Measurement Variables

From the perspective of determining what kind of measurements can be applied to them, it is useful to distinguish between variables that can only be placed into certain categories versus those upon which mathematical operations can be performed. The former of these, **qualitative variables** (i.e., categorical or grouping variables) are so named because they pertain to how people or things are placed together according to one or more attributes (e.g., gender, ethnicity, type of communication disorder, etc.). These variables can be placed into "either/or" categories of observation because people will possess at least two attributes of interest. **Dichotomous qualitative variables,** such as gender, will have two levels of assignment (i.e., male or female). **Polyotomous qualitative variables,** such as ethnicity (e.g., Caucasian,

TABLE 2-1   Classification of Variables

Type of Variable	Characteristic(s)/Definitions	Other Terms
I. Measurement Variables		
A. Qualitative Variables	Can only be placed into certain categories.	Categorical/grouping/discrete/ nominal variables
(1) Dichotomous Variables	Two level of assignment (e.g., gender)	
(2) Polyotomous Variables	More than two levels of assignment (e.g., ethnicity)	
B. Quantitative Variables	Mathematical operations can be performed and they can be ordered/ ranked according to their magnitude. Express the extent to which objects differ in degree, not in kind.	Ordinal/continuous variables
II. Research Variables		
A. Independent Variables	The antecedent factors that are manipulated, assigned, or grouped by the researcher in order to examine their affect on behavior.	Cause/treatment/factor/predictor/ nonmanipulated variables
B. Dependent Variables	The behaviors under study, the outcomes of a research study.	Observed/criterion/outcome variables
III. Extraneous Variables		
	Nuisance factors unrelated to the dependent variable or independent variable that might exert unwanted influences on the outcomes of a research study.	Confounding/nuisance variables

Asian, Hispanic), will have more than two levels of assignment. Mathematically speaking, qualitative variables are said to be discrete because the values obtained from their measurement result in finite and distinct counts. Suppose an audiologist wished to categorize the types of hearing loss seen in a particular clinic. Cases could have been coded according to the names of the hearing loss such that conductive loss = 1, sensori-neural loss = 2, mixed loss = 3. Subsequently, the audiologist further determined the relative number of cases falling into each of these categories. It makes no sense to perform arithmetical operations with such numbers. The numbers given are simply codes that specify particular categories into which a number of observations might fall. Such numbers are *discrete* in the sense that "type of hearing loss" cannot be treated numerically but only categorized into a finite set of values. Because no meaningful numerical values lie between these separate values, it makes no sense to say that any one number is "greater" or "lesser" than any other number (i.e., one type of hearing loss cannot be said to be more or less severe than another on the basis of their numerical coding). Any set of numbers could be used for such coding purposes. Thus, the numbers 9, 13, and 7 could have been arbitrarily assigned to the three types of hearing loss without altering the results. Obviously, it would make no sense to add these numbers or to subtract one from another. Beyond their coding value, such numbers are mathematically meaningless. Based on their mathematical properties, qualitative variables are termed nominal variables because they essentially exist in *name* only.

As opposed to qualitative variables, **quantitative variables** express the extent to which ". . . organisms (objects, people, events) differ in degree, not in kind." With respect to their mathematical power, quantitative variables that can be ordered according to their magnitude are at the lowest level of the "quantitative pecking order." Continuing with our previous example, as an audiologist, you might determine that the frequency of observed hearing loss was highest in the conductive category, and that sensori-neural losses exceed mixed losses. Moreover, you might assign the numbers 1, 2, and 3 to each type of hearing loss, respectively, in order to rank their prevalence. Variables that are ranked according to some characteristic are called ordinal variables. Such variables provide more information than nominal variables because categories are not only named but also ordered according to their magnitude of occurrence. Nevertheless, just as qualitative variables are said to be "discrete," so too are quantitative variables possessing ordinal properties. This is because such a ranked set of numbers cannot be broken down into smaller units than whole numbers. For example, for purposes of ranking the prevalence of various types of hearing loss, it would make no mathematical sense to assign the number .80 to a conductive loss, 1.7 to a sensori-neural loss, and so on.

Still other types of quantitative variables are called continuous variables. Such variables are called "continuous" because they theoretically exist on a continuum ranging from low to high with infinite graduations in number size. Height, weight, age, mental ability, or scores on many speech, language, or hearing tests are examples of quantitative variables. It's conceivable that the numbers representing each of these variables could be broken down into smaller and smaller units. For example, an age score could be represented as 7 years, 3 months, 2 weeks, 4 days, 12 hours, 31 minutes. In addition, an age score can be represented in decimal form such as 7.252 years, extending to an infinite array of smaller and smaller values. As represented in the population, the other continuous variables listed above possess the same properties. Quantitative variables of this kind have more statistical power and mathematical meaning than variables that can only be represented by discrete values.

In addition to possessing the mathematical property of order, continuous variables have what are known as *equal interval characteristics,* meaning that size of the intervals on a measuring scale are judged as equivalent. Thus on a test of receptive language ability such as the Peabody Picture Vocabulary Test the difference between 30 and 40 correct answers would be the same as between 60 and 70 correct answers. Although such scores would reflect different levels of language competence, the interval sizes for the two sets of numbers would be the same (i.e., 10). This permits the operations of addition, subtraction, multiplication, and division to be performed on them. For additional information about the measurement properties of variables see Chapter 11.

Research Variables

From a research perspective, two broad classes of variables that play a central role in asking and answering scientific questions are called *independent* and *dependent* variables. Through knowledge of their control and manipulation, it is possible to distinguish a well-executed experiment from one that is poorly done (Davis, 1995).

Independent variables are the antecedent factors that are manipulated, assigned, or grouped by the researcher in order to examine their effect on behavior. The behavior under study is termed the dependent variable. The term "dependent" implies that something is "dependent upon" the presence of something else. In the case of a dependent variable, it is an *observed effect* (outcome) assumed to be *associated with* or *caused by* the occurrence of the independent variable.

I. A single relationship (one independent variable (IV), one dependent
    variable (DV)).

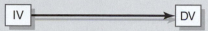

II. Multiple relationships (two independent variables, one dependent
    variable).

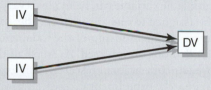

III. Multiple relationships (two independent variables, two dependent
     variables).

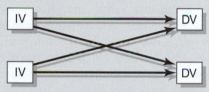

FIGURE 2-1

Various hypothesized relations between independent and dependent variables

As was noted in the previous chapter, a research hypothesis is a statement that describes the relationship between one or more dependent variables and one or more independent variables. In the simplest case, only a single relationship may be expressed by the research hypothesis. For example, I might hypothesize that recovery of linguistic ability following a stroke is related to a person's age at the time of the insult. This statement expresses a hypothesized relationship between the factor of age (independent variable) and recovery of linguistic ability (dependent variable). However, I might wish to explore the relationship of *multiple* independent variables to the dependent variable within the framework of a single experiment. In this case, the hypothesis might be expanded to include additional factors such as premorbid intelligence and educational achievement in the list of independent variables. Indeed, I might wish to expand my hypothesis still further to allow for the investigation of multiple dependent variables by including, in addition to recovery of linguistic ability, the retrieval of vocational and psychosocial skills as well. The various hypothesized relations between the independent and dependent variables just discussed are illustrated in Figure 2-1.

By applying what you learned in the preceding chapter, you should notice that the descriptions of the independent and dependent variables offered above are relatively vague and therefore would be of limited value in an actual research study. To have value, each of these variables would have to be *operationally defined* to allow for their measurement using objective criteria. For example, the participants' "age" at the time of stroke would need to be specified numerically in years and numbers of months, their "linguistic ability" according to scores on a particular test, and so forth. Furthermore, the construct of *stroke,* presumed to underlie the relationship between the independent and dependent variables, also should be operationally defined. Stroke is a generic term related to the appearance of certain neurological symptoms associated with impaired blood flow. It can result from several causes including embolism, thrombosis, hemorrhage, and the like occurring in various regions of the brain. Without a clear definition of the meaning of "stroke" according to its cause, severity, and anatomical location, the term has little value for research purposes.

Nonmanipulated versus Manipulated Independent Variables

In the example offered above, the independent variables were **nonmanipulated variables.** Age, intelligence, educational achievement, and similar physical and mental characteristics are not controllable by a researcher but preexist as states or conditions within the participants of a study. While a nonmanipulable variable can be made to vary indirectly by its *group assignment* (e.g., participants may be assigned to one group or another on the basis of age, gender, mental ability, etc.), in such cases the relationship of the independent to the dependent variable is only *observed,* not controlled or manipulated. As we shall discuss further in this chapter, such studies are best viewed as correlational research—not experimental research.

In contrast to correlational research, experimental research always involves an active manipulation of an independent variable in order to observe the effect of such a manipulation on a dependent variable. Exposing one group of participants in a study to a particular treatment, hypothesized to have therapeutic value, and then comparing the results to another unexposed group of similar participants on the same dependent variable is a classical paradigm for this type of research. Only through an active manipulation of the independent variable can an outcome be *causally related* to the influence of that manipulation. To arrive at a valid explanation of the causal nature of such an association, variations in the dependent variables resulting from sources other than the independent variable must be ruled out.

Extraneous (Confounding or Nuisance) Variables

Some variables may operate in an experiment, either known or unknown to an experimenter, that can exert an unwanted confounding influence on the dependent variable. Because of the presence of such extraneous (nuisance) variables, valid inferences about changes in the dependent variable, resulting solely from manipulations of the independent variable, may be difficult if not impossible to make. For example, suppose you wish to investigate two therapy approaches, A and B, in a downtown clinic of a large city that has no parking facilities. Participants in group A are scheduled at the clinic early in the day when metered street parking is generally available at a modest cost. On the other hand, as the consequence of being scheduled later in the day, participants in group B often must opt for more costly parking at a nearby garage. It is quite possible that the attitudes of these two groups might differ considerably and in ways that could influence their participation. Obviously, to manage what could be "the confounding influence of parking," the participants should be treated as fairly as possible. One way of neutralizing such a confounding factor would be to compensate all participants for their parking expenses.

Confounding influences due to the intrusion of extraneous variables are not always as easy to identify as in the above example. Other examples of potentially confounding influences that could have differentially impacted the performance of the two groups include possible differences in the test environment (lighting, temperature, noise levels) as well as group differences in a host of subject characteristics (age, mental ability, gender, social class, language competence, severity of the problem, etc.). As we emphasize in Chapter 6, researchers should attempt to identify as many extraneous variables as possible *prior to* an experiment in order to eliminate or control for their potential confounding effects on the dependent variable. As the adage goes, "Problems are best solved in advance instead of second-guessing what might have been."

INTRODUCTION TO THE TYPES OF RESEARCH

In a concise review of the history of the profession, Duchan (2002) noted that while some of the early treatments of communication disorders might be viewed as quackery by current standards, ". . . the pioneers, several of whom were the founding group of ASHA, set out to design diagnostic tools, concepts, and normative data for creating a more scientific base for research and practice in the field" (p. 29). An extensive list of references pertaining to the history of speech-language pathology and audiology is available on ASHA's Web site: www.asha.org. This literature makes clear that the knowledge base that underlies the daily work of clinicians has accumulated through systematic investigations, that is, the research process. Such work has entailed the contributions of professionals from diverse disciplines including medicine, psychology, education, and the social sciences, among others.

Regardless of the field of scientific inquiry, the purpose of research is to discover new knowledge by asking questions that can be answered through valid and reliable research methods. In the discussion to follow, you will be introduced to some of the terminology used by researchers to identify several of these methods along with the conceptual basis for their use. From the outset, it is important to recognize that scientific research is not a unitary approach to problem solving but includes a broad range of activities and methods that contribute toward the development or refinement of knowledge. In the field of communication sciences and disorders, perhaps the most common type of research involves the testing of relations presumed to exist among variables underlying the processes of speech, language, and hearing. Two major paradigms that guide scientific inquiry are quantitative research and qualitative research.

Quantitative Research

The traditional quantitative research paradigm used in communication sciences and disorders involves a systematic and highly disciplined approach to problem solving. *Deductive reasoning* is used initially to generate hypotheses that are then tested under tightly controlled conditions designed by the researcher to minimize bias and maximize the reliability and validity of information. In **quantitative research,** formalized tests and measuring instruments are applied to precisely and objectively specify the characteristics of data in numerical terms. Typically, such data are used to compare a group of individuals having a particular communication disorder (experimental group) with a normal group of individuals (control group). As we shall see in later chapters, comparative measures of averages and variances between such groups are considered by many to be the hallmark of valid research. Such an approach can be described as an extensive research model because it involves the aggregation and subsequent analysis of numerous individual scores as unitary indices of performance such as group mean averages. Statistical tests are then used to draw *inductive inferences* as to the probability for finding similar between-group differences in a comparable population of people tested or evaluated under similar conditions or circumstances.

The ultimate goal of most quantitative research is to prove that the hypothesis under evaluation is either true or false. Suppose that the hypothesis being tested is that children who are delayed in some aspect of language development (experimental group) will perform less well on a verbal memory task than children whose language development is normal (control group). The participants (subjects) employed in this study will be selected so as to be equivalent or closely so in all respects except for their differences in language development— that is, the sample of subjects forming the two groups will come from the same socioeconomic sector of the population, be equally represented with respect to age, gender, health status, and so on. Suppose further that we compute the scores on the verbal memory test and find that the control group achieved a relatively high verbal memory score (say, 95%) while the experimental group achieved a lower verbal memory score (say, 87%). Is this a difference that makes a difference in statistical terms? To answer the question as to whether or not our hypothesis is true or false we must ask whether or not this "sample fact," derived from a small number of observations, approximates a "true fact"—the fact that would be obtained should we repeat this study again and again.

By applying various techniques of statistical inference, we are able to determine in quantitative terms just how confident we can be in generalizing our finding to large groups or populations based on our sample results for individuals believed to represent these populations. Referring to our study of verbal memory, if our results were determined to be statistically reliable, we could expect the experimental group to have a lower mean verbal memory score than the control group almost every time the study is repeated. In the jargon of statistics, a statically reliable result is called a **significant result.** On the other hand, should the results of statistical testing suggest that the findings could have resulted from chance (accidental) factors unknown to the researcher, the results from the study would be judged as unreliable or **nonsignificant.** In passing such statistical judgments, researchers evaluate the odds for making certain types of errors (drawing wrong conclusions). The nature of such errors and the means of controlling them are discussed in Chapters 4 and 6.

Although the majority of research studies in communication sciences and disorders and related behavioral sciences have been based on what is sometimes called the extensive research approach of quantitative research, there has been a shift in recent years toward increased use of intensive approaches (single-subject research). Such methods are particularly adaptable to studying changes in one or a few individuals over an extended period of time. Such methods should not be confused with the so-called one-shot case studies. Although the latter studies often serve as a basis for a particular clinical focus, because they lack any control over extraneous variables, they have no value in establishing cause-effect relationships (see Chapter 8).

For reasons to be discussed more fully in Chapter 8, several researchers favor the use of intensive single-subject or small-N designs over extensive large-N studies for some types of problems. Single-subject studies, sometimes called **applied behavior analysis,** are aimed at the precise analysis, control, or modification of behavior. Often, data description procedures are based on the mere visual inspection of results recorded in graphic form. Furthermore, as opposed to most group designs, single-subject research emphasizes numerous *repeated measurements* of single subjects under controlled conditions.

Although there are many types of single-subject designs, the classic paradigm involves (1) establishing during a **baseline period** of recording an operant level of stable responding for a dependent variable prior to treatment; (2) introducing during a treatment period a single independent variable while recording any response changes in the dependent variable; and (3) removing the independent variable during a withdrawal period while recording any response changes in the dependent variable (see Figure 2-2). Although it is impossible to generalize results to a population based on one subject, single-subject designs may attempt to bolster the external validity of experimental findings by (1) describing the results from a number of individual subjects with similar characteristics (e.g., age, gender, IQ); (2) controlling sources of variability for each subject; and (3) demonstrating replicated findings with different subjects within the same experiment (Sidman, 1960).

The essential criterion for any study is the reliability of findings as judged by their replication in subsequent experiments. As will be discussed more fully in Chapter 8, single-subject designs typically take the form of a series of baseline–treatment trials on the same subject.

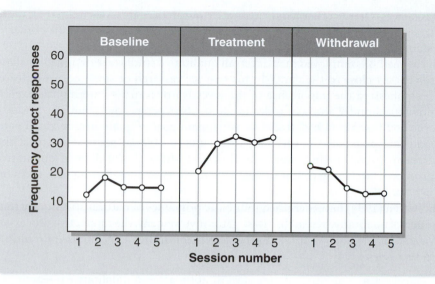

FIGURE 2-2

Basic paradigm for small-*N* designs

(*adapted from* Tactics of Scientific Research, *by M. Sidman, 1960, New York: Basic Books.*)

Differences between the baseline and treatment conditions are evaluated *within* each individual subject separately. Intensive designs are particularly applicable to many clinical studies in which generalizations about individual subjects rather than groups of subjects are sought. The "clinical situation" can provide a highly fertile source of research because human problems can be seen and intensively evaluated under controlled conditions apart from the ordinary circumstances and confounding influences of everyday life.

Qualitative Research

Some researchers hold that qualitative rather than quantitative methods are more appropriate for the study of many social and cultural aspects of human behavior. Such behavior is believed to involve a subject matter that is far more complex, dynamic, and less amenable to quantification than are the phenomena studied by biological and physical scientists. The study of patterns of family interaction in caring for a member with a terminal disease such as amyotrophic lateral sclerosis (ALS), or of the grief and coping mechanisms of parents upon learning that their child was born deaf, or the attitudes of potential employers towards persons who stutter—these and problems of a similar kind are not easily reducible to a set of numbers or measures that have meaning.

Qualitative studies involves several types of approaches that emphasize data collection in the "natural setting" such as the home, school, community, and the like. A classic example of naturalistic research is embodied in the early work of Piaget (1932), whose approach to the study of language development consisted primarily of observing and recording children's questions, reflections, and conversations. From such qualitative methods, Piaget published a number of scientific papers concerning various stages of what he termed "egocentric" and "sociocentric" speech development that in turn stimulated much additional research of a similar kind.

Unlike quantitative researchers who define as clearly as possible the concepts, variables, and hypotheses before a study begins, qualitative researchers use a variety of descriptive and interpretative methods that remain more flexible in application and that allow for the discovery of new leads to knowledge as the data emerge. As noted previously, quantitative researchers tend to emphasize relatively rigid research designs to control or eliminate bias and extraneous factors. On the other hand, qualitative researchers are likely to interact more freely with participants while trying to understand and interpret how they construct meaning from the standpoint of their own experiences.

Although the methods employed may differ, all qualitative studies are designed to allow the investigator to "get close to the data." In his seminal research of street corner culture, Liebow (1967) emphasized the importance of the investigator actually entering the experience of the individuals under study in order to adopt their perspective from the "inside." Similarly, Glesne and Peshkin (1992) stated that the main goal of qualitative research is to "understand and interpret how the various participants in a social setting construct the world around them" (p. 6). In this same vein, Kirk and Miller (1986) defined qualitative research as a process of "watching people in their own territory and interacting with them on their own terms" (p. 547).

Depoy and Gitlin (1994) have identified four basic principles of naturalistic inquiry that characterize much of qualitative research: investigator involvement, the interactive process of gathering information and analysis, prolonged engagement in the field, and use of multiple data collection strategies.

- *Investigator involvement* is an integral part of most approaches to qualitative research since the investigator is the major data-gathering tool. Instead of striving to adopt an entirely objective attitude toward the subject under investigation, as do most quantitative researchers, the central premise guiding qualitative research is that the best means of understanding the "lived experiences" of people is to become involved in their life situations or circumstances. To accomplish this goal, the investigator engages in fieldwork—that is, enters the "life field" of the people under study.
- *Gathering and analyzing information* on an ongoing basis is still another principle shared by qualitative researchers. Whereas in quantitative research data collection and analysis occurs during a defined time, qualitative researchers generally collect and evaluate information throughout the entire length of the investigation. Based on an investigator's perceptions, thoughts, and feelings about how one piece of information might link to another, the focus and methods of data gathering, shifting in accordance with "who, what, when, and where," might require further study. Through a dynamic process in which data collection and analysis becomes increasingly refined as new knowledge emerges—becomes "richer," "thicker," "more in-depth," and so forth—so too does the researcher's understanding and interpretation of reality.
- *Prolonged engagement in the field* is required in most qualitative studies. This is necessary to allow the researcher to become sufficiently immersed in the problem under investigation to obtain an in-depth understanding. However, unlike quantitative studies wherein data is typically collected on each participant during a prescribed time period, the length of the data collection period is not predetermined in qualitative studies but can vary widely depending on the researcher's judgment as to whether or not sufficient information has been obtained.
- *Multiple data collection approaches* are employed in qualitative research including observing, listening, and interacting with people in the natural contexts of their lived experiences; asking questions through the use of various interview techniques not only to obtain information from the informants but also to clarify and verify the accuracy of the information; and examining written materials such as records, diaries, charts, and progress notes in a search for reoccurring themes and patterns related to the phenomenon under study. Qualitative data are recorded in a variety of formats including field notes, diaries, photo-

graphs, audiotapes, videotapes, and so on. To facilitate the accuracy and trustworthiness of recording and reporting data, two or more data-gatherers may be used who have been trained for this purpose and who record their observations independently of one another. In addition, to assure the accuracy of information, qualitative researchers sometimes employ the method of triangulation, in which the results of several data collection strategies bearing on the same phenomenon are compared.

Qualitative research is guided by several types of research perspectives or traditions including:

- **Ethnography**—studies that seek to document the customs, social patterns, and rule-governed behavior of a culture or group of individuals. Ethnography grew out of anthropology—the science concerned with the manner in which culture influences and is influenced by how people behave, how they talk to one another, and the things they make.
- **Grounded theory**—studies that focus on the symbolic interactions among people and how they use symbols, such as language, to interpret or "make sense" of their experiences over time. Grounded theory is rooted primarily in the discipline of sociology—the science concerned with generating theories to explain social experiences. Grounded theorists do not begin a study with perceived theories or focused research questions. Instead, concepts and explanations are derived from research findings that emerge gradually in the process of collecting, coding and analyzing data—the theory that eventually evolves is "grounded" in such data.
- **Phenomenology**—studies that aim to understand how people attribute meaning to events and interactions with others during the course of daily living. As an approach to understanding the experiences of people from their own subjective viewpoint, phenomenology has a long tradition of use in the disciplines of philosophy and psychology. When adopting a phenomenological perspective, the researcher attempts to enter the world of the participants to the greatest extent possible in order to understand their thoughts, attitudes, feelings, and beliefs about various aspects of existence. The researcher gains insight through observations, in-depth interviews, and by participating in and reflecting on the lived experiences of others.
- **Discourse analysis**—studies that are concerned with the analysis of spoken and written text messages used to convey meaning or to perform particular social functions such as asking or answering questions, accusing or complimenting others, justifying actions, and the like. This approach evolved primarily from the discipline of sociolinguistics. As stated by Coyle (1995), "Discourse analysis sees language not as simply reflecting psychological and social life but as constructing it" (p. 244).

Regardless of their approach, practitioners of qualitative research are likely to eschew the use of preconceived measurements or data analysis techniques that could potentially influence or conceal the natural interaction of research subjects with their environment. When numbers are used, their primary purpose most often is to describe or represent the mere presence or absence of the quality under study rather than quantifying a specific attribute. Categories of behavior are compared, contrasted, and sorted in the search for meaningful patterns and relationships (Shaffir & Stebbins, 1991).

Although an advantage of qualitative methods may be found in their flexibility in studying a wide variety of human problems, the use of nonstandardized procedures can present many difficulties in collecting reliable and valid data. Unless attention is focused carefully on central issues, it is possible that efforts to collect, organize, and interpret data will be rendered meaningless. Another danger of qualitative research is that the interior world of the individuals or groups under study may be distorted by the mere presence of an outside observer or by whatever biases the researcher may impose based on his or her subjective views.

Despite such potential limitations, qualitative approaches of the type described above are frequently used to understand the problems of people and how they perceive these within the context of their own lived experiences. For relevant examples of such applications in the field of communication sciences and disorders, see Chapter 10.

True Experimental Research

A large number of experimental methods are available for use in scientific research that seeks to establish lawful relationships among variables. The use of all such methods goes beyond efforts to observe and describe problems to their prediction and control.

True experimental designs can be distinguished from all others on the basis of three main factors. The first of these involves the random assignment of subjects to at least two or more groups. The second requirement is for some type of active manipulation to be performed. Third, one group of subjects is treated (experimental group), and then compared with another nontreated group (control group). When compared to other research methods, true experimental designs are the most effective in controlling for sources of variance extraneous to the causal relationships under study.

For many practical and ethical reasons, it is sometimes impossible for an investigator to assign subjects randomly to treatment groups or to indiscriminately apply a particular treatment to one group while withholding it from another. This is often the case in clinical studies in which an insufficient number of appropriate subjects may preclude the use of randomization procedures. In addition, it could be argued that withholding a treatment from a target population or administering an alternative treatment with unknown effects rather than one with established benefits is an unethical if not illegal practice.

Quasi-Experimental Research

Quasi-experimental research designs are generally selected when true experimentation is impractical or impossible to perform. Typically, subjects are assigned to groups on the basis of preexisting conditions or circumstances. Suppose you work in a hospital clinic where you treat many adult patients for hoarseness accompanied by vocal nodules. Following diagnosis, the availability of therapy is on a "first-come, first-served" basis, so many patients are on a waiting list for three months or more. Although the use of randomization procedures may not be possible, you still wish to draw some conclusions about the efficacy of your treatment program.

An alternative way to estimate your program's effectiveness would be to use a **constructed control group** suitable for comparison with a treated group of patients. The two groups would be matched on a number of variables prior to treatment; these variables would possibly include such factors as degree of hoarseness, size of nodules, duration of illness, occupation, age, gender, or alcohol/tobacco consumption. Such matching would be done to rule out as many extraneous variables as possible so that any subsequent positive between-group differences could be confidently attributed to your program.

As a means of coping with extraneous variables that might invalidate an experiment, quasi-experimental methods often necessitate the use of more control procedures that do true experiments. Consequently, they are considered to be less powerful, as stated previously, and are generally recommended only when true experimentation is not possible. Yet, some investigators believe that quasi-experiments can be as effective as true experiments.

Both true experimental and quasi-experimental designs incorporate protocols that are aimed at establishing causal relations among variables. Although it is sometimes impossible in any research study to determine that an experimental manipulation has clearly produced an intended effect, designs of this type offer the greatest promise of producing unambiguous results.

Nonexperimental Research

One type of investigation in which causal relations definitely cannot be established is **nonexperimental research.** In such research, there is no attempt to achieve randomization, nor is any purposeful effort made to manipulate the variables under study. In such studies, many of which involve qualitative approaches of the type described previously, only correlational, as opposed to causal, relations can be evaluated.

Attempting to infer causal relations on the basis of the mere association between factors X, Y, or Z is risky. To illustrate why correlational designs are subject to ambiguity, consider the associative relations often found to exist between attention deficits, low IQ levels, and developmental language delays (Rutter, 1989). It might be argued that any one of these factors could give rise to the others. Alternatively, all three factors could be the common result of still another more generalized delay or abnormality in development.

Efforts to derive causative relations from correlational findings alone can lead to the kind of fallacious reasoning that is represented metaphorically as "putting the cart before the horse." Such reasoning, sometimes described as "vicious circularity," occurs when an answer is based on a question and a question on the answer. For example, one might ask: "Why do slow learners experience academic failure?" Answer: "Because of language-learning disabilities." Question: "But how do we know they are language-learning disabled?" Answer: "Because they exhibit academic failure."

Correlational studies are generally lacking in purposeful experimental manipulations that are external to or independent of the variables under study. For this reason, they are often called ex post facto studies because they search for past causes of a phenomenon that has already occurred. Efforts to derive causal relations in this manner can become hopelessly engulfed in the type of circular reasoning processes described above. As Dember and Jenkins (1970) succinctly noted, ". . . correlational designs are subject to an ambiguity of interpretation considerably greater than the normal uncertainty inherent in any research attempt" (p. 47).

Clinical Research

In evaluating and selecting a particular research design, it is important to bear in mind the purpose of the study. Particularly in the context of the clinical setting, problems are initially encountered in a qualitative form. It is often the case that numerical data are unavailable. Information must be collected from a variety of sources, including written questionnaires, client and family interviews, preexisting records, formal and informal test procedures, and the like. Ultimately, the clinician must work with whatever historical and current information about individual clients that is available. By examining the possible relations among historical factors and current conditions, an effort is made to form both a tentative hypothesis about the cause(s) of the problem and an appropriate treatment plan.

The research-oriented clinician may collect data on a number of clients with similar problems under controlled conditions of testing or treatment. It is generally the case that such a preliminary or exploratory investigation begins because of the apparent association between two or more variables. For example, the clinician might have noted during his or her work with children that weaknesses in phonological encoding and word retrieval seem to go hand in hand. Subsequently, a formal research study may be performed wherein a strong positive relationship between the two variables is demonstrated based on the strength of their statistical correlation (see Chapter 11). The next step may be to sharpen the investigative focus through the use of a true experimental or quasi-experimental design in an effort to determine whether or not the observed relationship is associative or causal in nature. To accomplish this objective, special conditions must be established to determine the extent to which an active manipulation of one factor might cause a significant change in another. Given the hypothesis that phonological encoding skills underlie word retrieval abilities, the clinician might set up a program designed to improve phonological awareness in a randomly assigned experimental group and then evaluate the effects of such training against a randomly assigned control group (true experiment). Alternatively, a comparison group matched on relevant variables might be used instead (quasi-experiment).

In choosing a particular research design, the investigator must weigh the design's relative advantages and disadvantages in view of the questions asked and the answers sought. Some designs are more appropriate at one stage of an investigation than another. Furthermore, the physical limitations imposed by certain experimental settings, the unavailability of suitable subjects and instrumentation or test materials, excessive costs, and the potential for ethical or legal violations are but some of the constraints that may influence the final selection of a specific research plan.

Applied versus Basic Research

Because the main orientation of the profession of communication sciences and disorders is to help clients solve practical problems, most scientific research focuses on solutions to problems that have immediate application. Such **applied research** is sometimes distinguished from **basic research** (pure research) that might have no presently identifiable application but is done simply to advance knowledge for its own sake. This is not to say that one type of research emphasis, applied versus basic, is better than the other. Indeed, much of the foundation of our clinical knowledge is enlightened and directed by advances in the study of "pure" or "normal" processes of speech, language, and hearing. For example, from the study of normal physiology of the inner ear, invaluable information has been gained leading to applications involving cochlea implantation. Through efforts to understand the molecular genetics of normal hearing, genetically transmitted hearing loss may be preventable in the future. Conversely, an understanding of the genetics of normal hearing may be gained by studying individuals with heritable hearing loss.

In the opinion of the present authors, the applied versus basic research distinction is somewhat irrelevant to the actual work of scientists who, regardless of the problem, engage certain thinking and action processes designed to provide better and more representative solutions to problems. Such work proceeds by what is commonly called the scientific method.

THE SCIENTIFIC METHOD AS A RESEARCH PROCESS

As noted in the previous chapter, science involves a systematic way of thinking and behaving to solve problems. Although the term "scientific method" is often used to describe an interconnected series of steps or organized activities that are uniformly followed by scientists in achieving their research goals, such a view can be erroneous or misleading. In reality, the so-called scientific method is better conceived as a **research process** that evolves though

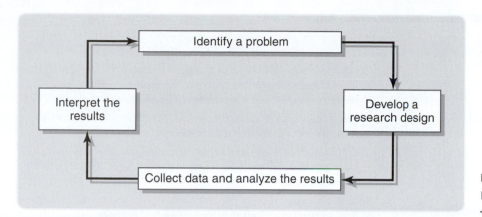

FIGURE 2-3

Research as a cyclical process

several cyclical stages. The process is sometimes depicted in the form of a loop. As shown in Figure 2-3, the major components of this process include:

- Identifying a problem that leads to an idea for a research question or hypothesis
- Developing a research design appropriate for investigating the question or hypothesis
- Collecting data and analyzing results pertinent to the question or hypothesis
- Interpreting the results in a manner that refines understanding and leads to new questions

As we are about to discuss, these components of scientific work are well reflected in the various sections of a scientific article.

Structure and Content of a Research Article

Writing up the results of a research study for publication in a professional journal within one's field is an integral part of scientific work. Why the study was done, how and to whom it was done, as well as the results and implications of the study must all be made clear. Familiarity with the structure of a research article and the kind of information contained within each section will help the reader assess the degree to which these goals have been achieved. As you read subsequent chapters in this book, you will sharpen the concepts and skills needed for the critical reading of a research article. Specific criteria for evaluating each component of a research article are covered more thoroughly in Chapter 13. Meanwhile, we will provide a brief overview of the prototypic structure and content of a research article as outlined in Table 2-2.

Abstract

Most research articles begin with an abstract or concise summary of the problem investigated, the methods used, highlights of the results and their statistical significance, and a concluding statement of implications. Key words are sometimes listed at the bottom of the abstract as cues to the specific topics covered. In essence, a good abstract provides a convenient yet accurate means of scanning the substance of the article as a whole. Its main purpose is to provide readers with just enough information to help them decide if they should read the entire article.

Introduction

The introduction section of an article, although usually not labeled as such, includes a historical overview of the theoretical foundations of the problem to be investigated based on the results of previous research. A review of relevant literature is akin to the process of scientific observation that, as noted previously, involves collecting, organizing, and interpreting available

TABLE 2-2   Structure of a Research Article

Section	Includes
Abstract	Concise summary of the research (approximately 100–150 words) that includes a description of the problem, the experimental procedures, highlights of results, and a statement of implications
Introduction	Review of relevant literature, theoretical foundations and rationale, purpose statement/research questions or hypotheses
Method	Design of study, subjects and sampling techniques, controls used, apparatus or test materials, experimental procedures, logical basis for choice of statistics
Results	Systematic presentation of relevant data, figures and tables, evaluation of data to point out significant/nonsignificant findings
Discussion	Interpretation of the meaning and importance of findings, evaluation of hypotheses and their generality, implications for future studies
References/Bibliography	Complete citations of the work of others

background information (data) related to the current problem. Such information is assembled so as to provide the basis for a logical argument or research rationale used to justify the need for additional investigation. Based on a review of preexisting knowledge and the theoretical propositions of other researchers, the introduction should lead naturally to a statement of the current problem. The researcher might state the problem by denoting the purpose of the research or posing a research question. For example:

> The purpose of this study was to examine the relative frequency of different types of phonological errors (omissions, substitutions, distortions) in the speech of children with verbal apraxia.

or

> What is the relative frequency of different types of phonological errors (omissions, substitutions, distortions) in the speech of children with verbal apraxia?

A third type of problem statement based on theoretical reasoning, prior data, or both is called a research hypothesis. As a means of defining a research problem, the use of a formal hypothesis is typically reserved for predicting associative or causal relations among the variables under study. For example:

> Verbal apraxia in children is associated with (or causative of) a significantly higher frequency of substitutions than other types of phonological errors involving omissions or distortions.

The manner in which the problem is stated in the introduction often provides some hint about the general type of statistical methods used in analyzing the data. Of the problem statements illustrated here, all three imply that measurements will be carried out to quantify the frequency of certain types of phonologic errors. In the case of the first two statements, the frequency measures will at least be totaled, averaged, converted into percentages, or statistically described in other ways. However, it is clear only in the case of the third statement, involving the research hypothesis, that sampling statistics also will be used to infer the *significance of difference* in the frequency of types.

Method

Unfortunately, the method section of a research article is frequently given the least attention by the reader because, as the *structural blueprint* for the investigation, this section often contains many tedious details. Yet, the framework of the entire investigation either stands or falls based on the strength of its methodological foundation.

Most research studies will include important information about how a study was conducted. Such information will pertain to the (1) design of the study; (2) subjects used and how they were selected; (3) apparatus or test materials employed; (4) procedures for collecting data; and (5) statistical analysis techniques. The researcher must carefully address each of these topics *prior to* conducting a study if it is to be successful. It will be too late to correct methodological errors after the study has been done. Each of these topics is discussed in greater detail below.

Design.   It is important for a researcher to provide clear and complete information about how a study was designed. From such information, the reader should learn whether the design used was primarily intended to describe the characteristics and/or associative relations among variables or was the goal to arrive at causal explanations through the use of experimental strategies. Typically, descriptive methods are chosen if an investigator wishes to observe, record, or perhaps measure certain events but has no desire to manipulate the variables of interest. The basic tool of description is systematic observation of the phenomena under investigation. *Observations* of individuals or groups in the clinical or natural setting, *surveys* of attitudes and opinions, *cohort and case-control studies,* and *prevalence and incidence studies* are examples of problems that call for nonexperimental research designs (see Chapter 9). As we noted previously, descriptive methods are often important in categorizing or classifying variables according to their physical or psychological attributes; this is a preliminary step that leads toward more definitive studies of their causal relations.

When the researcher is primarily interested in explaining the effect of one variable, the independent variable, upon another, the dependent variable, he or she selects either experimental or quasi-experimental techniques. In the field of communication sciences and disorders, such explanatory methods are frequently used to test a hypothesis about a causal relationship. Such methods are commonly employed in the search for explanations for the causes of specific disorders or to evaluate the efficacy of new diagnostic techniques or therapy procedures.

Recall that the defining feature of a true experiment versus a quasi-experiment is that the former requires random assignment of subjects to different treatment conditions, whereas the latter simply involves classifying subjects on the basis of a particular characteristic (e.g., normal hearing versus hearing impairment). Following treatment, the groups are compared on some dependent variable or performance measure. Quasi-experimental designs are weaker than true experiments because of the potential for preexisting subject differences and other extraneous variables to contaminate the results.

Subjects.   There are several types of information pertaining to how subjects were chosen that an author should provide. This information should relate to three major factors that must be considered in selecting subjects. First, the subjects should be appropriate given the goals of the study. If an investigator's intention is to study syntactical errors in Broca's aphasics, the inclusion of Wernicke's aphasics or of other types of aphasic disorders must be avoided. Ultimately, the goal of any research study is to assure the internal validity of the results, or the degree to which they can be directly attributed to the effect of a chosen independent variable as opposed to some unwanted extraneous variable. A confounding effect owing to selection can result if subject characteristics in one group differ from those in a comparison group. The old adage that "apples and oranges can't be compared" summarizes well this particular problem. In the subject section of the methods portion of the research article, the characteristics of all participants, including age, gender, intelligence, type of disorder if present, and any other relevant identifying information should be listed.

A second issue is the degree to which subjects in a study are representative of the population from which they were selected. This concern relates importantly to the establishment of external validity or the degree to which the results can be transferred to the population from which the sample was originally drawn. If a sample of subjects is not highly similar to the parent population from which it was selected, then the results will be of little or no value as they might apply to other cases under comparable conditions or circumstances. Although random selection of a sample of subjects does not assure that the sample will be representative of the population from which it was drawn, it is the best means available for accomplishing this goal (see Chapter 5).

A third issue in subject selection pertains to the number of subjects to be used. Decisions as to the number of subjects (denoted as N for the population and n for the sample) to be used in an investigation are complex. From a pragmatic perspective, the investigator will include whatever number of subjects is appropriate and available, given the particular aims of the experiment, keeping in mind that the problem of generality cannot be disposed of simply by employing large numbers of subjects. Nevertheless, it is also the case that, for purposes of detecting significant between-group differences, large samples generally lend greater power to a statistical test than do small samples. If the sample size is too small, there is a risk of failing to detect the true effect of an independent variable on a dependent variable—the main purpose of the experiment.

Apparatus and Materials.   The apparatus used in presenting stimuli and recording responses, test materials, questionnaires, and related measurement tools must also be described. All identifying information including names of manufacturers, model numbers, publishers, calibration procedures for electrical or mechanical equipment, and evidence of the reliability and validity of such instruments should likewise be included.

Procedures.   It is necessary that the procedures used in conducting an experiment be precisely delineated. This is important for at least two reasons. First, research procedures reflect the plan for the actual steps to be followed in carrying out the investigation. As far as possible, the following issues should be clarified by describing:

1. The manner in which the independent variable was administered
2. The way the dependent variable was recorded
3. The instructions given to subjects
4. The nature of the test environment

A second and equally important reason for carefully documenting research procedures is to allow for replication by other investigators. For this to occur, the essential conditions of the original experiment must be reproducible. Unfortunately, in communication disorders and other behavioral fields, replication is not yet given sufficient emphasis as a part of the scientific method as it is in many of the physical sciences. Although replication experiments in several fields, including our own, do not appear to be highly esteemed, the ability to substantiate research findings through experimental replication ought to be an integral goal of all scientific studies irrespective of the nature of the problem. Perhaps greater value will be placed on such research by future investigators and the editors of professional journals as we are increasingly required to justify, through empirical means, the efficacy of our clinical programs.

Statistical Analysis.   Often, the types of statistical analyses used and their manner of application are described toward the end of the method section. The type of statistical methods selected will vary according to the purposes they are intended to serve but will essentially consist of one or more types of three major techniques. If the aim of the statistic is only to describe the features of a set of measurable observations, descriptive statistics will be used to *summarize, condense,* and *organize* such observations into a more convenient and interpretable form of data. Tables and graphic figures may be used to display the data in a "pictorial" manner. Such descriptive statistics are also used to derive what are called **measures of central tendency** (averages), and the way in which individual scores are dispersed around such averages (**measures of variability**).

A second major type of statistic is based on investigative efforts to describe an apparent association between two or more sets of data. For example, one might wish to know the degree to which academic performance measures in children are related to various aspects of language expression and/or comprehension. Statistical tests of **correlation** may be used to describe the degree of relatedness between these or other sets of data. However, it is impossible to derive causal relationships on the basis of such comparisons alone.

A third type of statistical techniques goes beyond the mere description of variables or their association, to making **statistical inferences** about the degree to which a particular sample of subjects is representative of the population from which it was drawn. In clinical science fields, such as communication sciences and disorders, sampling or inferential statistics are commonly used to study specific disorders or diseases in a specified number of individuals. Subsequently, by means of inductive reasoning, inferences about the general nature of such conditions in the population at large may be drawn. Typically, we do not investigate specific groups of aphasic patients, people who stutter, dysarthric or hearing impaired individuals, or persons with voice disorders for their own sake but to learn more generally about how to explain or modify such problems as found in similar persons from the same population.

Essentially, we want to know the extent to which a "sample fact," derived from a small number of observations, approximates a "true fact"—the fact that would have been obtained had we examined the entire population. By applying the techniques of statistical inference, we are able to determine how confident we can be in generalizing our findings to large groups or populations based on sample results for individuals believed to represent these populations. Such confidence is based on the tolerance for making certain kinds of sampling errors owing to chance factors beyond the investigator's control.

In addition to the need for determining, prior to initiating a study, what type of statistical procedures can best be used, the **risk tolerance** for sampling errors should likewise be decided beforehand if the results are to be fairly evaluated. Such risk is conventionally preset at either a 1% (.01) or 5% (.05) chance of error (see Chapter 12). In the first case, the researcher can be at least 99% confident that no error has been made in interpreting the results. In the second case, the researcher can be at least 95% confident in his or her conclusions. Unfortunately, too many researchers are negligent in deciding such matters in advance of conducting a study. In our opinion, this practice is like waiting for the last bounce of the ball at the roulette wheel before finally placing your bets.

Perhaps the best way to conceive of statistics is as an implicit logical reasoning system made explicit in quantitative terms. Statistical probabilities are not to be confused with *certainties* in the sense that a consequent event will always follow a given antecedent cause or condition. More accurately, the "laws of statistics" can be better conceived in terms of the "likelihood" of a particular event occurring a certain percentage of time under highly defined conditions and within specified **confidence limits** (see Chapter 12). Furthermore, although a clinician may be able to predict with 95% confidence that some hypothetical number of cases similar to one's own will improve in response to treatment X under certain conditions, which particular cases might do so cannot be determined. Because statistical methods do not lead to invariant answers, they are best viewed as general guides rather than precise maps in the search for new knowledge and understanding.

Results

The main goal of the results section of a research article is to provide a straightforward presentation of the relevant data. Some research publications include not only a detailed explanation of the empirical data within this section but also a discussion of their theoretical implications. However, it is common practice within the results section to present and explain the data only in relation to the research hypotheses. *Interpretation* of findings should be avoided. The latter task is reserved for the discussion section of the research article.

Within the results section, a systemic presentation of the data should be included beginning with a precise summary of the evidence and then proceeding to a point-by-point report of each statistical analysis. Figures or graphs may be used to illustrate relevant research findings in pictorial form. Tables provide a convenient format for condensing data according to such average measures as the mean and measures of variability (the dispersion of scores around the mean) such as the standard deviation. Based on the comparison of such composite measures, which reflects differences in sets of scores *between* or *within* groups of subjects, statistical formulae can be used to calculate the significance of the results expressed as a probability value or p (see Chapter 12). For example, the notation $p < .05$ would be interpreted to mean that one could expect his or her hypothesis to be true at least 95 percent of the time with less than a 5 percent chance of error (i.e., one chance in 20 of drawing an incorrect conclusion).

As noted previously, a combination of descriptive and inferential methods, rather than a single statistical technique, is usually employed in the area of communication sciences and disorders. Although descriptive statistics permits observed variables to be specified in mathematical terms, it is only through the use of inferential statistics that generalizations are made from a selected sample of subjects to a larger population.

Discussion

After objectively presenting and explaining the results of a study in relation to the hypotheses under test, the next step is to interpret this factual information in terms of the overall issues that served as the original impetus for the investigation. In essence, the task requires looking for meaningful patterns in the data to see how they might fit within the larger framework of knowledge (i.e., preexisting theories, conceptual models, and other research findings as reviewed in the introduction).

Whereas the form of scientific reasoning leading up to the results of an experiment was largely deductive in nature, the researcher is now required to inductively draw inferences *back* to the real world based on the specific data obtained. In more specific statistical terms, the degree to which the sample data can be generalized to the population from which it was drawn is carefully evaluated. This requires a rigorous analysis of the strengths and weaknesses of the current research design with respect to such matters as the effectiveness of the sampling procedures and the adequacy of experimental controls in dealing with the unwanted effects of extraneous variables.

In a figurative sense, the discussion section of a research article requires using data not only to look backward at "things as they have been" in the past but also forward as to how "things might be" in the future. Practical recommendations for improving various aspects of the methodology may be offered. Even new hypotheses may be advanced along with suggestions about the types of experiments needed for their testing. Thus, the discussion section of a study provides a mechanism for engaging scientific reasoning processes in ways that foster continuity of knowledge and new understanding.

References

All citations of previous studies must be listed in a reference list at the end of the research article. The references used need not be exhaustive but should reflect the work of previous investigations that are clearly related to the problem under investigation. The specific manner in which references should be cited within text and in the reference list is discussed in Chapter 13.

ETHICS OF RESEARCH

We will end this chapter by briefly mentioning the importance of ethical practice in research (see Chapter 3 for a fuller discussion of ethical guidelines for protecting human subjects). In the field of communication science and disorders, researchers and clinicians might believe that questions pertaining to the ethics of research hold less importance than for professionals in other fields, such as medicine, where violating the rights of human subjects has been vividly documented. Consider, for example, the atrocious practices of Nazi Germany that used Jews, gypsies, the mentally ill, and other segregated minorities as laboratory specimens to study endurance and reaction to various diseases and untested drugs (Polit et al., 2001). More recently, in the United States, we are aware of similar violations that are equally horrifying. Beginning in the early 1930s and continuing until 1972, a study sanctioned by the U.S. Public Health Service examined the influence of syphilis on men from a black community that comprised a control group (treatment was intentionally withheld).

Although the vast majority of studies undertaken in the communication sciences and disorders do not place participants at physical risk, researchers nonetheless are often confronted with important ethical questions such as

- When a treatment is suspected but not yet proven to have value, is it ethical to assign participants to a control group, thereby denying them a potentially beneficial exposure?
- What are the ethical implications of withholding treatment information from participants (keeping them unaware as to what group they have been assigned, i.e., experimental group, placebo group, or control group)?
- Is it appropriate to publish information obtained from participants when aspects of their physical or mental state have been compromised by a disorder or disease despite having obtained permission from them or their families to do so?
- Are personal questions designed to uncover people's fears, failures, weaknesses, and so on, scientifically justifiable when it is not possible to provide therapeutic assistance?

These are but a few of the ethical dilemmas that researchers frequently encounter. To the greatest extent possible, participants in research should be protected from harm. As we shall discuss further in Chapter 3, codes of ethics have been adopted and public laws enacted to provide such protection.

SUMMARY

In this chapter, you have learned that research in the field of communication sciences and disorders is a broadly based enterprise that arises naturally out of the need to describe or explore the associative or causative relationships among variables. You also learned that various types of research are used as appropriate for the question asked or level of understanding that a researcher might wish to achieve. Fundamental to all of these approaches are the thinking processes and actions inherent to the scientific method. The importance of the scientific method is that it allows a researcher to transform hunches or questions into testable hypotheses. You learned that this is actually a highly focused step-by-step process where ideas are sharpened and subjected to investigation as reflected in the various sections of a journal article. All of this must proceed within ethical guidelines designed to protect human participants to the greatest extent possible from physical or emotional harm.

KEY TERMS

qualitative variable
dichotomous qualitative variable
polyotomous qualitative variable
quantitative variable
nonmanipulated variable
quantitative research
significant result
nonsignificant result
applied behavior analysis
baseline period
qualitative research
ethnography
grounded theory
phenomenology
discourse analysis

true experimental research design
quasi-experimental research design
constructed control group
nonexperimental research
applied research
basic research
research process
N
n
measures of central tendency
measures of variability
correlation
statistical inference
risk tolerance
confidence limits

SELF-LEARNING REVIEW

1. Major objectives of most scientific investigations are to _____ variables, the _____ relations among them, and the _____ of altering their relations.
2. Phenomena that are observed to vary are called _____.
3. _____ methods are commonly used by clinicians to _____ or _____ phenomena.
4. Relationship questions ask about the degree to which certain classes or categories of _____ change in _____ with other variables.
5. When the measure of one variable is found to be statistically related to the measure of a second variable, they are said to be _____.
6. Answering questions pertaining to differences among phenomena is generally recognized as the best means of determining _____ _____(s).
7. Two types of difference questions pertain to the search for _____ differences and _____ differences.

8. Establishing the cause(s) of variation of a phenomenon is necessary for establishing the conditions for its future _____.

9. Studies involving difference questions tend to restrict the interpretation of group differences to the systematic influence of the treatment condition, called the _____ variable, on the target of such manipulation, called the _____ variable.

10. The _____ research approach involves the study of groups, whereas the _____ research approach is best adapted to the study of single _____.

11. The primary criterion for any study is the _____ of findings based on _____.

12. A classic example of _____ research is embodied in the work of Piaget.

13. The study of customs, social patterns, and rule-governed interactions of a culture or group of individuals is termed _____ research.

14. Phenomenology is a _____ method that attempts to understand people's experiences from their own _____.

15. Qualitative studies concerned with the analysis of _____ and _____ text messages is called _____ analysis.

16. Qualitative researchers are likely to eschew the use of preconceived _____ of data analysis.

17. True experimental designs can be distinguished from all others on the basis of two major factors: (1) random _____ of subjects to at least two groups and (2) some type of active _____ to be performed on an experimental group of subjects who are then compared with a _____ group.

18. _____ -experimental designs are generally selected when true experimentation is unfeasible or impossible to perform.

19. With the exception of _____, quasi-experiments are like _____ experiments.

20. As opposed to a randomized control group, a _____ group generally requires careful _____ of subjects in order to control for the _____ influence of extraneous variables.

21. Nonexperimental research makes no effort to achieve _____ in the assignment of subjects to groups, nor are _____ procedures used in an effort to achieve _____ between groups.

22. Instead of using a randomized control group and actively manipulating an independent variable, many nonexperimental studies rely on _____ interpretations of preexisting data or observations.

23. Vicious _____ occurs when an answer is based on a question and a question on the answer.

24. A correlation _____ is used to express the degree of association between two variables.

25. The _____ method entails certain _____ and _____ processes designed to produce better and more representative solutions to problems.

26. The introductory section of a research article can be seen as the structural _____ for the investigation.

27. The rationale for a study ought to evolve naturally in the _____ section of a paper.

28. The degree to which the results of an experiment are directly attributable to the influence of an independent variable pertains to their _____ validity; _____ validity concerns the degree to which the results are _____.

29. _____ statistics are used to summarize, condense, and organize data. _____ statistics are used to draw inductive inferences from a _____ to a _____.

30. A _____ fact is derived from a sample of observations. A _____ fact would require that we examine the entire population.

31. Statistics are concerned with determining the _____ of certain observations or events within specified _____ limits.

32. The results section of a research article is generally restricted to _____ and _____ data in relation to the research _____. _____ of data is usually reserved for the discussion section.

33. To the greatest extent possible, _____ in research should be protected from _____.

QUESTIONS AND EXERCISES FOR CLASSROOM DISCUSSION

1. Identify the three major objectives of most scientific investigations. Give a clinical example of each.

2. Distinguish between qualitative and quantitative variables. Provide an example of each type as it might be investigated in a research study.

3. Distinguish between a nonmanipulated and manipulated independent variable. Provide a clinical example of each.

4. Why is quantitative group research called the extensive research model?

5. Distinguish the extensive research model from intensive single-subject designs. What are the essential features of the latter design?

6. What is ethnographic research? Give at least two examples.

7. What kinds of data recording techniques are used in qualitative research?

8. When are quasi-experimental designs selected as alternatives to true experiments? What are the two major features of this design? What common features do quasi-experiments share with true experiments given the goals of their respective protocols?

9. What kind of studies are called "ex post facto" and why? Give an example.

10. Provide an example of a clinical research question and identify the antecedent treatment conditions and consequent effects to be assessed.

11. Distinguish between applied and basic research. Is one type of research of greater value than the other? Justify your answer.

12. Describe the scientific method and evaluate its clinical utility.

13. Describe the components of a typical research article.

14. What three major elements are included in the introduction section of a research article? What type of reasoning is involved in this section?

15. Why is the method section of a research article best viewed as the "structural blueprint" for the investigation? Identify and briefly describe the four major factors to consider within the method section?

16. Distinguish between the concepts of internal validity and external validity. What is meant by a "confounding effect"?

17. Describe the importance of experimental replication. What is the essential requirement for this to occur?

18. Distinguish between descriptive statistics and inferential statistics.

19. Describe the statistical meaning of the term *probability*.
20. What is the main goal of the results section of a research article?
21. How can single-subject designs attempt to bolster external validity?
22. How does the discussion section of a research article differ from the results section?
23. How does the discussion section of an article provide a mechanism for integrating inductive and deductive reasoning?
24. Of what practical value are ethical considerations in planning a research study?
25. Based on the following examples, identify the independent and dependent variables:
    - A clinician wishes to determine the effect of speaking rate on the frequency of dysfluency in children who stutter.
    - Use of grammatical morphology was examined in two groups of children as a function of lexical diversity. One group had been diagnosed with specific language impairment (SLI) and the other group had normally developing (ND) language.
    - The ability of children with and without a hearing loss to correctly identify sequences of various types of acoustic stimuli was examined.
    - Vocabulary development was examined in two groups of children using cochlear implants in relation to two different types of educational exposures, one that had used an oral communication approach (focused on spoken language) against another that had used a total communication approach (focused on both signed and spoken language).
26. For each of the research problems in Question 25, identify a possible extraneous variable that might confound a researcher's ability to validly interpret the influence of the independent variable on the dependent variable.

Selecting a Research Problem

CHAPTER 3

CHAPTER OUTLINE

LEARNING OBJECTIVES

After reading this chapter, you should be able to identify, describe, or define:

- Three types of research questions
- How research questions originate
- Resources for researching a topic of interest
- The significance of establishing a research rationale
- Criteria for judging the feasibility of research
- The importance of evaluating ethical issues

SIGNIFICANT QUESTIONS LEAD TO SIGNIFICANT ANSWERS

A common concern among students beginning to think seriously about the importance of research and its potential relevance to their future careers is how to select and define a problem in a way suitable for systematic investigation. Certainly, we are all accustomed to asking routine questions in subjective terms that generally produce opinionated or nonscientific answers. For example, we might ask about therapy techniques that could prove useful in "motivating a client," "improving rapport," or facilitating "family intervention." Helpful colleagues may offer advice or opinions based on their own professional experience. Although many concerns of this type are quite appropriate for informal discussion and might eventually qualify as fertile areas for research, they lack the objective criteria necessary for framing a specific research question or hypothesis. Nevertheless, prior to asking a "researchable question" and developing a suitable research design for answering it, one must select a problem for study that one wishes to understand.

Before taking courses in research and statistical methods, it is understandable why students might complain of difficulties in comprehending scientific concepts and investigative processes that underlie existing fields of knowledge. Although unfamiliarity with the methods of science can impede the selection of cogent problems for research, even experienced investigators commonly encounter such difficulty. Indeed, as Hoover (1976) noted, "The hardest problem in scientific thinking occurs at the beginning of the investigation. Once you have solved it, other steps will fall into place" (p. 42).

From the outset, the primary concern in forming a research question ought to be with the likely significance of the answer. Trivial questions generally culminate in inconsequential results. As summed up by Henri Poincare (1913):

> There is a hierarchy of facts; some have no reach; they teach us nothing but themselves . . .
> There are, on the other hand, facts of great yield; each of them teaches us a new law . . . it is to these that the scientist should devote himself. (p. 554)

Although this is a lofty goal, many of the routine tasks that become ritualized in our everyday professional lives fail to stimulate the kind of creative questions that advance a field of knowledge. Nevertheless, only when faced with challenging tasks that demand solution is the imagination taxed (Merton, 1959).

Questions aimed at solving some problem are typically focused on achieving at least one of three levels of understanding. At the simplest level, researchers ask *"what"* questions that are answered through the use of various descriptive techniques designed to categorize or classify the attributes of a particular phenomenon. Often, the intended goal of such questions is to develop taxonomies of various types or subtypes of communication disorders such as stuttering, aphasia, cleft lip and palate, hearing loss, or whatever. By observing, recording, and describing the details of such disorders in the clinic or natural setting (home, school, etc.) we learn about their unique forms and features. Such knowledge is important in setting up mutually exclusive diagnostic criteria for identifying such disorders according to clusters of certain signs and symptoms. For example, by observing people who stutter, we note the behavior is typically characterized by certain primary symptoms (repetitions, prolongations, blocks) often accompanied by various secondary symptoms such as facial grimaces, circumlocutions, and other types of avoidance behavior. Before we can begin to understand any type of phenomenon, whether behavioral, physical, or biological in nature, its characteristics must be identified and described. This is the main goal and chief value of descriptive research techniques.

At the next level of complexity, *"where"* questions might be raised pertaining to the direction of associated changes in one variable in relation to another. If both variables move in the same direction, they may be positively related. On the other hand, if they move in opposite directions, they may be negatively related (see Chapter 11).

Characterizing the various features of variables and their relationship to others is frequently an essential requisite to asking *"why"* questions geared toward discerning causal relations among variables—the highest level of understanding. As noted in the previous chapter, to answer such questions, inferential statistics are often used to examine the significance of difference between two or more variables. An effort is made to explain the basis for such differences, if found.

As Merton (1959) pointed out, merely asking a question does not constitute a problem. The formulation of a problem actually consists of a three-part process involving (1) originating a question; (2) developing a rationale or statement of its importance; and (3) determining the feasibility for answering it.

ORIGINATION OF A QUESTION

Choosing a research question for investigation entails describing the broad parameters of a research area or potential field of inquiry. The decision on a subject for research typically reflects motivations and preferences having a myriad of origins based on one's personal or subjective opinions, clinical experiences, interactions with fellow students and professors, knowledge gained by attending professional conferences and workshops, as well as on the complex interplay of reading, writing, and thinking processes. Firsthand knowledge gained through one's own personal experiences is often the primary basis for deciding on a particular research topic. An article by Rachel Cohen (2003) that appeared in the *ASHA Leader* highlights how the experiences of one student led her to pursue interesting and significant research projects (see Box 3-1). Although the experiences and interests of students in communication sciences and disorders may differ widely, conducting or participating in worthy research projects of diverse kinds is often possible for those who are motivated to pursue such opportunities.

At the initial stage of research planning, students usually can express some overall interest in a particular research topic but often little more. This is frequently the case for those who are attempting to decide on a particular subject matter for a master's thesis or doctoral dissertation. When asked about the subject of their interest, most students can verbalize *what* global interest they might want to pursue: "I'm interested in the area of stuttering" (or child-language disorders, aphasia, cochlear implantation, etc.). Occasionally, the interest is more fully articulated or focused in terms of *where* they would like to direct their attention (e.g., "I'm interested in the role of anxiety in stuttering," or ". . . the influence of socioeconomic factors in child-language disorders," or ". . . gains in hearing level following cochlear implantation"). However, at such an early stage of the planning process, it is indeed rare when one can fully explain *why* a particular subject area has been selected for research.

To begin the process of selecting a topic for research, the best approach is to think about a problem that both interests and makes sense to you. For obvious reasons, researchers normally wish to identify interesting questions as opposed to dull or trivial concerns. If a compelling rationale for conducting a research study cannot be established, the results of the study are likely to be viewed by others as unimportant. The best kind of studies are those that lead to new knowledge, provide new ways of thinking about existing knowledge, or provide a basis for further research.

In thinking about the potential significance of a research problem, perhaps it is useful to recall the work of Senator William Proxmire who, in the 1980s, created the so-called Golden Fleece awards for federally sponsored projects he considered to be useless. Examples of such studies included awards given for those designed to investigate why prisoners escape from jail, why sunfish that drink tequila are more aggressive than those who don't, and the influence of scantily clad females on traffic flow. The creation and distribution of such awards was criticized by some scholars, universities, and other institutions. Nevertheless, Senator Proxmire is remembered for having stimulated considerable discussion among researchers as to the importance of establishing the *value* of research questions and the generalizability of the answers. Yet, it would be a mistake to believe that the subject matter of a particular study must have revolutionary significance to be worthy of investigation. As clinicians, we are constantly faced with asking many questions in the search for the kinds of *practical answers* that will allow

BOX 3-1

A Passion For Learning

For research speech-language pathologist Katie Ross, Alexander Pope had it right—"a little learning is a dangerous thing."

Ross' knowledge of Pope and his famous dictum predated her involvement in communication sciences and disorders—she first drew her passion for learning from an undergraduate background in psychology and English literature. Then she earned a master's degree in hearing and speech sciences at Vanderbilt University.

If a little learning is indeed dangerous, Ross was determined to gain a lot of it. After her master's degree, Ross began doctoral work at Vanderbilt University with a three-year, predoctoral fellowship to the Nashville Veterans Administration (VA) Medical Center.

"The combination of didactic, clinical, research, and professional opportunities was invaluable," she says. At Vanderbilt, Ross focused on adult neurogenic communication disorders with a minor in neurogerontology.

The VA fellowship enabled clinical education under the mentorship of clinician-scientist Terry Wertz, neurologists Howard Kirshner and Frank Freemon, and radiologist William Witt. Clinically, Ross developed and administered treatment programs for adult neurogenic clients and supervised master's-level students. She completed three independent research investigations in aphasia and normal aging under Wertz's direction and also participated in additional VA-sponsored studies of post-stroke dysphagia.

Ross' clinical experience fueled her commitment to learn more about the psychosocial aspects of normal and disordered communication in aging to improve the quality of life and rehabilitative services for veterans and the general older population. She aspired to provide students in the VA system with the clinical and research experiences they would need to become successful in speech-language pathology and to advance the field. She also strived to advance her own knowledge in both research and clinical practices so that she might incorporate her research findings into actual clinical use.

"One of the most valuable outcomes of that period was finding out how little I knew," Ross says. "The more I learned and the more clinical experience I acquired, the more questions I had. I love to learn. I love the brain. And I love the VA."

While still a doctoral student, Ross participated in workshops, scientific research meetings, and Academy of Neurologic Communication Sciences and Disorders conferences. She also presented her findings at ASHA Conventions, Clinical Aphasiology Conferences, and in peer-reviewed journals. "I was able to begin an actual clinical research career with the VA during this time." she says.

Ross has some advice for students selecting a mentor: Don't underestimate the value of human chemistry. "I was able to spend six years (master's degree, clinical fellowship year, doctorate) working with someone I truly respected as a mentor and enjoyed as a human being." she says. "Both the doctoral program and the mentoring

continues

BOX 3-1 *continued*

relationship are intense. The inevitable hurdles are much more tolerable, and the achievements much more rewarding, if you honestly love to spend time with your mentor, regardless of the task at hand."

Ross wholeheartedly recommends a research career, while also noting that the pursuit of a doctorate is certainly not for everyone. She says, "Any clinician, however, can conduct valuable research by using single-subject designs to examine the outcome of specific interventions. The rewards are real—for our patients, our profession, and ourselves."

Reprinted with permission from "A Passion for Learning" (*from* Spotlight on Students*), by Rachel Cohen, February 4, 2003,* The ASHA Leader, *pp. 17–18.*

us to better understand, predict, and interpret the results of testing procedures and treatment programs. Few would deny the importance of answering questions such as:

- Is this person's speech-language-hearing functioning within the normal range?
- Given the presence of certain signs or symptoms of abnormality, are these indicative of a particular disorder or disease process?
- How reliable and/or valid are the available diagnostic tests or strategies used for determining the specific nature of the problem?
- What etiologic factors are associated with an increased likelihood for the particular disorder or disease in question?
- How might the problem be modified through treatment?
- What intervention procedures can be expected to result in the best functional outcomes in cases of this kind?
- How can problems of this nature be prevented or their adverse consequences diminished?

These are just a few questions that can arise from clinical efforts to solve practical problems. Although some of these questions may be answered through mechanisms other than highly formalized research designs, knowledge of how to ask good questions and develop and apply scientific methods will likely improve the validity of our clinical observations and conclusions.

Important unsolved questions can also emerge from classroom discussions of research literature and the critical reading and evaluation of such literature. ASHA publishes several journals that contain original research studies and scholarly articles related to important scientific issues. These include the *Journal of Speech, Language and Hearing Research*; *Language, Speech, and Hearing Services in Schools*; *American Journal of Speech-Language Pathology*: *A Journal of Clinical Practice*; and the *American Journal of Audiology*: *A Journal of Clinical Practice*. Although each of ASHA's journals has a distinctive focus, all of them typically contain research reports that not only summarize the findings of a specific investigation but also provide an overview of other important studies relevant to the topic area. Moreover, such articles frequently contain a discussion of unresolved issues and research problems that warrant further investigation. Additional information about the scientific and clinical importance of ASHA's journals has been summarized in an article by Ellen Caswell (2004), editor and desktop publisher for ASHA. Relevant excerpts from this article are found in Box 3-2 including commentary by ASHA's vice president for research and technology and the chair of its publication board.

BOX 3-2

ASHA's Scholarly Journals: The Latest and Best Research at Your Fingertips—Literally

ASHA's four journals publish original research to meet the needs of professionals employed in a wide range of settings as well as the needs of students through the National Student Speech Language Hearing Association. The journal publication program follows:

- *JSLHR (Journal of Speech, Language and Hearing Research)* is ASHA's oldest, largest, and best-known journal and publishes research on the assessment, diagnosis, and treatment of communication disorders. A bimonthly, *JSLHR* arose from two earlier publications—*The Journal of Speech and Hearing Disorders* (1935) and *The Journal of Speech and Hearing Research* (1958).
- *LSHSS (Language, Speech, and Hearing Services in Schools)* has a strong clinical focus and publishes many continuing education products. Published quarterly, *LSHSS* began life as *Speech and Hearing Services in Schools* in 1970 to answer the need of the large number of ASHA members who work in school settings.
- *AJA (American Journal of Audiology)* publishes articles on a broad range of professional and clinical issues, including screening, assessment, and treatment techniques; supervision; administration; and case studies. Published twice a year in print and online on a rolling basis, *AJA* was created in 1991 as a clinical practice journal to meet the specific needs of practicing audiologists.
- *AJSLP (American Journal of Speech-Language Pathology)*, the most widely circulated speech-related journal, publishes clinical research and features with a clinical focus. A quarterly, *AJSLP* addresses professional issues as well as all aspects of clinical practice.

A scholarly publishing program was considered important from the Association's creation in 1925. ASHA's founders shared a common interest in improving the lives of those with communication difficulties. As a first step, they established a scholarly journal program, ensuring that the field of communication sciences and disorders would have a sound scientific base. As the knowledge base expands, the insights of research in communication disorders are integrated into the larger world of human physiology and behavior, just as research in those areas can raise new questions for researchers in our discipline.

Why We Publish

Ray D. Kent (ASHA's vice president of research and technology) considers the research base critical to the professional standing of communication disorders. "A field that builds its own research base has taken a big step toward controlling its own destiny," he says. "Our research helps authenticate our professional services. Research of high quality establishes our commitment to provide a sure foundation for clinical services."

continues

BOX 3-2 *continued*

He adds that current research has tangible—and immediate—value. "The journals feed my need to know what is happening on the research front across a variety of topics. I learn the what, the how, and the who—what are the research questions, how is the research being conducted, and who is doing the work?"

Today's journals speak to many audiences—researchers and clinicians in communication disorders, scientists in related disciplines, and in the Internet age an increasing number of consumers.

Of the journals, *JSLHR* publishes a higher proportion of basic research on both normal communication and communication disorders, but the information also has clinical value. "Even what we sometimes regard as 'basic' research can turn out to be pre-clinical research in that the discoveries can point the way to interesting and important clinical applications," Kent says.

He sees a direct clinical relevance in articles pertaining to the nature of a disorder, its assessment, and/or its treatment. "As we move toward evidence-based practice, our journals will be in the forefront in providing the information needed to consider levels of evidence. Three of our journals pertain especially to clinical practice—which a quick look at the contents will confirm."

Marc Fey, chair of the Publications Board, agrees. "There's certainly room in the clinical journals for someone to give their far-reaching views on where the basic research they're doing now will end up clinically. In fact, many studies that target the efficacy of our interventions are really designed to address basic research issues. With the current emphasis on evidence-based practice, I think we'll see more and more clinical questions being addressed with experimental methods."

The Journals Online

ASHA's Web site makes the journals more accessible, and more improvements are on the way.

Web Access

In addition to access to all titles, authors, and abstracts, members have access to HTML and PDF versions of all articles for the most recent three years. Multimedia is being added, such as including audio or video files as part of an article; and the linking to articles is increasing; for example, the <u>Literacy Gateway</u> on ASHA's Web site links members to the original journal articles they discuss.

Reprinted with permission from "The Journals on Line," by E. Caswell, September 7, 2004, The ASHA Leader, pp. 4–5, 21.

Other journal publications of research articles that are useful and relevant to the interests of speech-language pathologists and audiologists are too numerous to list completely. A partial listing, including those published by related disciplines or specialty journals that have an interdisciplinary focus, can be found in Appendix A-7.

In a field as diverse as communication sciences and disorders, it is understandable why students may have difficulty in identifying a specific research question of interest to them.

However, with minimal prompting, most can identify a broad issue or topic of concern (e.g., the diagnosis of stuttering in young children; the surgical treatment of cleft palate speech; the recovery of language in aphasic disorders; the role of language in learning disabilities). Having described the overall character of a problem, the search for a particular research topic can begin in earnest.

Specific topics pertaining to current research trends, existing controversies, and critical areas for future inquiry are often identified in special sections or issues of professional journals, monographs, and "state of the art" reports. The published proceedings of research conferences provide additional insight about current trends and potential areas of inquiry. Moreover, the policies and priorities for various research projects along with guidelines for submitting research proposals and requests for funding are published by various branches of government, foundations, and corporations. Two publications of the U.S. government, the *Federal Register* and the National Institute of Health's *NIH Guide for Grants and Contracts,* announce scientific research initiatives on a regular basis. Both publications can also be accessed online at http://www.gpoaccess.gov/fr/ and http://grants.nih.gov/grants/guide/, respectively. The National Institute on Deafness and Other Communication Disorders (NIDCD) is one of the major branches of NIH that supports biomedical and behavioral research and research training in normal and disordered processes of hearing, language, speech, and voice.

Using the Library

Despite the availability of such resources as noted, formulating a significant research question that is both personally interesting and relevant to current professional concerns can be a formidable task. Whereas journal articles and related literature generally provide rich sources of research ideas, wandering aimlessly through such material can be a frustrating and time-consuming experience. Fortunately, help is available in the form of computerized database services in libraries that allow for efficient searches of research literature.

Efficient and thorough use of library reference tools is the first step in identifying an interesting topic for research. Through PsycINFO, which is based on the print publication, *Psychological Abstracts,* concise summaries of research studies appearing in more than 17,000 national and international periodicals can be accessed. Many of these abstracts pertain to communication disorders and can be located by the use of the author or subject index. Another highly useful directory for students who are considering a research topic about which there may be little published information is *Dissertation Abstracts International*. Locating a dissertation related to your research interest can be of great help because it is likely to provide a more comprehensive literature review and related bibliographic information than that available in most journal articles. A handy online and print reference that lists all periodicals and the sources in which they are indexed is *Ulriche's Periodical Directory*.

A good means of searching for information is through the use of one or more of the computerized database services listed in Figure 3-1. With the entry of keywords that represent the essence of your subject (e.g., Parkinson's disease, dysarthria, speaking rate) the computer can quickly scan the titles and abstracts of articles in its memory and identify intersecting terms. A systematic approach to retrieving bibliographic information online is to begin the search process for articles published in the current year and work backward as far as necessary, given your particular retrieval goals. Additional useful tips for facilitating use of the library for research purposes have been offered by Judith Kuster (2003) who has written several internet columns that appear in the *ASHA Leader* and on ASHA's Web site: http://www.asha.org (see Box 3-3).

ERIC (Educational Resources Information Center)
This broad database can be used with either key words from its thesaurus or for on-line key word searches. In addition to providing a good source for searching many journal articles pertaining to children, this index typically reports on educationally relevant papers read at conventions that are not yet published in professional journals.

PsychLIT (CD-ROM) or PsychINFO (on-line)
One can search for both journal articles and book chapters on psychological topics using the database.

SSCI (Social Sciences Citation Index)
Indexes journal articles related to studies in the social sciences and related fields.

MEDLINE
One whose topic is of a medical nature can search this index, which includes the majority of citations found in Cumulated Index Medicus.

ComDisDome
Books, articles, dissertations, institutions, scholars, and Web resources related to communication disorders.

Web of Science
This site provides the most extensive multidisciplinary information from approximately 8500 of the most prestigious, high impact research journals in the world. It also allows researchers to discover who is citing their research.

FIGURE 3-1

Popular library reference indexes

Most libraries in colleges and universities have resources for searching these databases. Reference librarians can be of assistance in "honing in" on references pertinent to your topic and in teaching you to use the most efficient searching techniques.

The reference sections of recent articles will likely include references to other important studies related to the topic of interest. One way to identify an *important* research study is by noting the frequency of its citation in other investigations. After identifying the titles and authors of such studies, abstracts of those expected to prove most relevant to your own questions or information needs can be printed as desired, in addition to any other bibliographic information that you might wish to place on file for future reference. A literature review chart such as the one shown in Table 3-1 can be a useful device for summarizing the results of your search in a cogent and informative manner.

By using the techniques discussed above, you will be able to locate the majority of literature that is relevant to your problem. To conduct a more exhaustive search of literature you might have missed, you may wish to follow these suggestions of Rosnow and Rosnow (1995):

- *Contact known authors in the field* to request reprints of related research they might have conducted and for recommendations as to where you might look further. To avoid duplication, provide a bibliography listing the sources that you have already located.
- *Consult the National Technical Information Service,* a comprehensive database that should be available in your library that contains summaries of research including conference proceedings and theses.

BOX 3-3

Don't Forget The Library!

Recently I received the following: "I am a graduate student studying stuttering and wondering . . . where can I go to access the information (in text) provided in your Bibliography on Neurogenic Stuttering?"

The short (and perhaps least time consuming) answer is "Check your university library." The long answer is "There are strategies to retrieve abstracts of many research articles and even some full-text articles on the Internet although you won't find electronic versions of everything that you'll find in the library and in many cases you will have to pay for the full-text article." Here are a few strategies to try.

Free and Fee-based Databases

- **The Educational Resources Information Center's AskERIC (http://ericir. sunsite.syr.edu)** calls itself the world's largest source of education information and contains more than one million abstracts of documents and journal articles on education research and practice.
- **PubMed (http://clinical.uthscsa.edu/pubmed.htm),** an Internet interface for MEDLINE, the National Library of Medicine's bibliographic database, has over 11 million references and abstracts dating back to the mid-1960s and links to full-text articles if the publisher has a Web site that offers full text of its journals.
- **Combined Health Information Database (http://chid.nih.gov)** from the U.S. Department of Health and Human Services has health promotion and education materials and contains literature not often referenced in other databases including brochures, newsletters from patient advocacy organizations, booklets produced by federal health agencies, as well as abstracts to some peer-reviewed articles.

If you have access to an organization (e.g., a university library) that subscribes to a database such as those below you may be able to access full-text articles.

- **Ingenta (http://www.ingenta.com)** provides free access to article summaries of over 25,000 publications. Full-text articles can be ordered for a fee or, if your university subscribes to the service, are available free.
- **Cumulative Index to Nursing and Allied Health Literature (http://www. cinahl.com/prodsvcs/prodsvcs.htm)** includes slp and audiology literature, indexes articles from 1200 journals and provides full text from 17 journals online.
- **OVID (http://www.ovid.com)** has more than 300 full text journals.
- **OCLC FirstSearch (http://www.oclc.org/firstsearch)** provides access to more than 70 databases with many full-text journal articles if your library subscribes to the service.

continues

BOX 3-3 *continued*

- **Northern Light Special Collection (http://nlresearch.northernlight.com)** is an online library with over 7000 full-text journals, books, magazines, and reference works. Articles dating from January 1995 can be ordered, typically for under $4.

Professional Journals Online

Many professional journals are available on password protected sites to members. For example, ASHA Journals are available online as a member benefit **(http://professional.asha.org/resources/journals/index.cfm)**. *AJA* is available beginning with the November 1991 issue. *AJSLP, JSLHR,* and *LSHSS* are available beginning with 1999.

Some publishers provide non-subscribers abstracts of recent articles or tables of contents of journals. For example Karger **(http://content.karger.com)** provides access to *Folia Phoniatrica et Logopaedica, Phonetica, Audiology and Neuro-Otology,* and Elsevier **(http://www.elsevier.nl)** provides access to *Journal of Communication Disorders, Journal of Fluency Disorders, Journal of Phonetics* and *Journal of Pragmatics,* etc.

Several professional organizations place their full-text journals freely online 6–12 months after publication. Checking through Free Medical Journals Online **(http://www.freemedicaljournals.com)** and the Hardin Library for the Health Sciences **(http://www.lib.uiowa.edu/hardin/md/ej.html)** you'll find publications such as *British Medical Journal, Stroke, Science, American Journal of Mental Retardation* and many others.

Search Engines

Scirus.com is a specialized search engine that concentrates on scientific content and claims to find more peer-reviewed articles than other search engines. Scirus recognizes PDF and Postscript formats (most search engines just find html documents) in which scientific papers are often put online.

Sometimes authors include the full text of their articles on personal Web sites, in which case an automated search engine may uncover an article you are looking for. Since **Google.com** recognizes PDF and Postscript formats, it is a good search engine to check. For example, typing the keywords *Kuster + ASHA + Leader + column* will uncover a website with the full text of all my Internet columns since 1994 **(http://www.mnsu.edu/dept/comdis/kuster4/leader.html)**.

Reprinted with permission from "Don't Forget the Library," by J. M. Kuster, February 4, 2003, The ASHA Leader, *8(2), p. 18.*

- *Use the Internet* by providing key words including the names of authors who have done research in related areas. Useful archival resources of information as well as various discussion groups that focus on your topic might be located through this means.
- *Search for documents* related to your topic using such Government Printing Office (GPO) indexing tools as the Monthly Catalog of Government Documents and, for periodicals, the Index to United States Government Periodicals. The Government Documents

TABLE 3-1 Literature Annotation Chart

Author/Date	Source	Subjects/Age	Design	Variables	Results
Pratt et al., 1993	JSHR, 36, p. 1063	Six preschool hearing-impaired children (3:4–5:5 yrs)	Single Subject Multiple baselines Multiple levels Changing criterion	Independent variable: IBM speech viewer Dependent variable: vowel accuracy	Treatment effect demonstrated for at least one of three vowels in five subjects.

Index is an electronic index that might also prove useful. All of these U.S. government publications not only are valuable as sources of information about scientific research but also are likely to have value for clinicians in learning about amendments to Medicare laws, Public Law 94-142, laws pertaining to Americans with disabilities, and similar topics.

RATIONALE FOR A QUESTION

We noted previously that merely asking a question falls short of developing a researchable problem. Ultimately, one must ponder the significance of the question asked. Anybody who has played the game "twenty questions" is aware of the importance of asking not just any question but one that is most likely to yield the answer sought. Behind any such question, there is a **rationale** or underlying reason for asking the question in the first place. According to Merton (1959), "The requirement of a rationale curbs the flow of scientifically trivial questions and enlarges the share of consequential ones" (p. xix).

The fact of modern human existence is that we must deal with a vast amount of information. Choosing what to attend to and for what reason is necessary for the achievement of relevant and meaningful goals. Perhaps the best way to clarify the rationale for a particular question is to explain the thinking processes behind the research. As the explanation for a research study, the rationale ought to evolve naturally in the introduction section of a research article as a consequence of establishing what is known about a problem and what remains unanswered. In considering the rationale for a potential research study, some important issues to address include the following:

- Will the answer to the question help to confirm, refute, or extend previous research findings?
- Will the answer to the question be generalizable to other settings or circumstances?
- Will the answer to the question provide new information of current clinical significance or scientific importance to the profession?
- Will the answer to the question help advance the development of theory and new research?

As noted by Sidman (1960), the reasons for a question are many and ultimately reflect the subjective views of the investigator(s) about the kind of data needed by a scientific discipline. Judging the potential importance of data or the merit of what one chooses to study must rest on personal conviction and the opinions of one's colleagues. Furthermore, the history of science suggests that perceptions about the significance of certain questions can change as the result of professional trends, policy initiatives, or funding opportunities.

FEASIBILITY OF ANSWERING A QUESTION

What we undertake in research also ought to be guided by the available means of accomplishing the intended task. Although the specific details of a research investigation may be ill defined initially, there ought to be at least some tentative basis upon which to predict its successful accomplishment.

The first issue in determining the feasibility of a study is whether or not the question or hypothesis is stated in a testable form. For this determination, the constructs of an investigation and the variables selected to represent them must be defined in operational terms. Unless the independent and dependent variables can be clearly specified in accord with the empirical means of their observation and measurement, the **criterion of testability** cannot be met. Connotative or theoretical definitions fall short of satisfying this requirement. For example, some years ago it was suggested that developmental stuttering may result because of delayed myelination of critical neural pathways that underlie speech production. The testability of such a proposition would depend upon the precise specification of how and under what conditions both the dependent variable (stuttering) and independent variable (delayed myelination) would be measured. Perhaps because of difficulties involved in such specification, the theory has yet to be taken seriously as a credible etiologic explanation. Although a question that is *potentially testable* in the future may prove to have value, the better question is one that is *presently testable*.

Additional factors to consider in assessing the feasibility of answering a particular question relate to certain methodological constraints. Suppose an investigation is planned to assess hemispheric activation in autistic children in response to acoustic signals of various kinds using functional magnetic resonance imaging (FMRI). Obviously, *availability of appropriate equipment* and an *adequate number of appropriate subjects* will be necessary to achieve the goals of such a research project.

The *estimated cost* for conducting an investigation must also be weighed in determining its feasibility. Given limited resources to cover such cost, it may not be possible to accomplish the research, however great its projected value. This is not to imply that all research is costly or that only costly research has value. Indeed, some of the most groundbreaking work in various fields of science has been accomplished with relatively modest resources.

Other possible methodological constraints on answering research questions relate to the inherent *difficulty of the project* or to *time limitations*. In considering topics for a thesis or dissertation, students in particular should weigh carefully their ability not only to execute the necessary experimental procedures for completing the study but to organize, analyze and interpret the data. Lacking these technical skills, regardless of one's professional status, a study should be undertaken only with the assistance of an experienced co-investigator or consultant.

The time it will take to complete an investigation must also be considered carefully before deciding on a research topic. Longitudinal studies, designed to collect measurements on units of behavior over lengthy time periods, despite their potential merit, are often beyond the capability of an investigator. While time limitations are a significant matter for any investigator to consider in deciding a research topic, such constraints are particularly important for students to evaluate before proceeding further in their planning. No matter how interesting the research topic or how motivated students are, their primary goal should be to complete their projects successfully within the time limit as determined by their graduate programs—hopefully, to use a common adage, "before reaching retirement age."

Pilot Studies

Prior to making a commitment to the hard work, time, and expense associated with a full-scale investigation, a researcher may conduct a **pilot study.** Such a study is a smaller, preliminary version of a more extensive study that is planned. Typically, pilot studies employ only a few participants selected from the population of interest in order to check the feasibility of a research project and to make refinements as needed. During the course of the pilot study, adjustments in various aspects of the design may be made. For example, suppose you wish to compare the efficacy of two therapy interventions (independent variable A and independent variable B) in facilitating a child's correct production of a particular phoneme (dependent variable). Independent variable A might involve rewarding every correct response (continuous reinforcement) while independent variable B might entail rewarding only a certain proportion of correct productions (fixed-ratio reinforcement). The problem you wish to investigate is whether or not one of these reinforcement schedules is more effective than the other. A question that would need to be addressed in designing such a study is just how different must the two reinforcement schedules be in order to show a true difference in the outcome? If the child is rewarded, say 9 out of 10 times for a correct response under the fixed-ratio schedule, the results might not differ from those found under continuous reinforcement because of the great similarity in the two conditions. By conducting a pilot study, an investigator might have to make adjustments in the differences between the two schedules until a promising trend is seen before continuing with the final investigation (Rosenberg & Daley, 1993).

In addition to investigating appropriate values of an independent variable to be used in an investigation, pilot studies can serve such additional purposes as training researchers to accurately and reliably administer the methods and procedures of a study as planned and for testing the accuracy and reliability of various measuring instruments. By rehearsing the actual steps to be followed in a full-scale study, both small and large flaws are often revealed. A minor flaw, such as ambiguity in subjects' understanding of instructions, is often easily corrected. On the other hand, an inability to establish accurate and reliable methods for administering the independent variable and for recording the dependent variable might lead a researcher to abandon the investigation. Short of the latter circumstance, pilot studies usually can be counted on to improve the overall quality of the intended research project.

ETHICAL ISSUES AND RESEARCH PROBLEMS

Ethical issues may also hamper the feasibility of answering certain research questions. In 1974, the National Research Act was established, creating the National Commission for the Protection of Human Subjects of Biomedical and Behavioral Research. In order to qualify for research funds awarded by federal agencies, all investigators and their institutions must comply with established regulations specifically designed to protect the rights and welfare of human subjects. To do so, research institutions are required to set up **institutional review**

boards (IRB) with the charge of reviewing research proposals to determine their compliance with existing regulations. Such a board, sometimes called a human studies committee, typically consists of at least five members that include scientists and nonscientists (e.g., clergy, lawyers, nurses, social workers).

Most colleges and universities have established IRB committees charged with protecting the rights and safety of research subjects. At many institutions, research proposals may be reviewed by an appropriate committee at the departmental level before being referred to the IRB. Graduate students, like faculty and other research personnel on contract, who are planning to complete research on human subjects, must first submit a detailed research plan or protocol for review that describes the background, significance, purpose, and methods of the project as well as all risks/benefits to participants and the means of obtaining their **informed consent.** If a prospective research subject is not of legal age or deemed incompetent to make a judgment as to the risks and benefits of participating, the informed consent must be obtained from a parent or legal guardian. IRB committees have the power to approve, disapprove, or require revision of a research plan as they see fit. An outline of the procedures for preparing human investigation protocols used at Emerson College is shown in Figure 3-2.

Two issues that are weighed in the deliberations of an IRB are possible risks as compared to benefits and the means of obtaining informed consent by making clear any physical or mental risk to potential participants and those participants' rights prior to, during, and after the research investigation. Any research study entails some degree of risk if only for minor apprehension, boredom, fatigue, inconvenience, and the like. Risks that do not exceed those normally encountered in daily life or as a result of routine tests and examination procedures are typically classified as "minimal risks" by an IRB, in which case certain requirements may be waived. When the probability of discomfort or possible harm is judged to be greater than "minimal," the IRB will likely designate subjects as being "at risk." In this case, the potential for harm or injury must be weighed against the possible benefits of serving as a subject in the investigation. The resulting balance is termed the **risk/benefit ratio.**

In some investigations, the IRB might determine that even high levels of risk are tolerable if the magnitude of the probable short-term or long-term benefits is judged to be substantially greater. For example, in the medical field, patients commonly are asked to participate in testing the therapeutic benefits of new drugs with known side effects that might eventually improve the quality of the patients' lives as well as those of others with similar problems. The investigation of experimental surgical procedures for the treatment of communication disorders associated with spastic dysphonia, hypernasality, or hearing loss might be equally justifiable despite the risks from anesthesia or other complications.

In evaluating risks and potential benefits, the IRB can render a judgment only after carefully evaluating as many pros and cons as possible and recognizing that individual subjects may perceive risks and benefits quite differently given their unique needs and expectations. From an ethical perspective, researchers should attempt to reduce the degree of potential harm or discomfort associated with an investigation as much as possible while remaining consistent with the intended goals.

Ethical research practice requires that subjects be informed in writing about the general goals, specific procedures, and significance of the study; the risks of harm or discomfort; the benefits including pay or reimbursement if any; the plans for disseminating findings; and the measures such as various data-coding procedures used to safeguard confidentiality or preserve the anonymity of participants. It is also important to describe the duration of the intended study and to make clear that participation is a voluntary act than can be terminated at any time without negative consequences.

In accordance with the Emerson College Graduate Policy Manual, Section 14.0, all studies involving human subjects must be approved by the Division's and the College's Institutional Review Boards (IRB). Approval by the Division and College Committees is required even if your protocol has been approved by the agency through which you plan to recruit subjects. . . . Protocols should be approximately 5 pages in length and should conform to the following outline:

A. RESEARCH PLAN
1. Name of investigator(s)
2. Title of project
3. Background and significance of study
4. Specific aims
5. Study design
   a. Subjects
   b. Measures
   c. Procedures
   d. Confidentiality (procedures for insuring of subjects' names and records, including location and consent forms).
   e. Financial compensation (to families, subjects, or others).
6. Risks and Benefits
   a. Include risks to and potential benefits, if any, to the subject, his or her family, and/or society, as well as an analysis of risk/benefit ratio.
   b. Justification of study.

B. CONSENT FORM
The following information should be included in simple nontechnical terms, and it should be written in first person, i.e., "I understand that I am being asked to participate. . . ."
1. Title
2. Purpose of the study and why individual is being asked to participate.
3. Brief description of study procedures, especially what the subjects will be asked to do, how long it will take, and other information important from the subject's perspective.
4. Risks and benefits, including all risks and discomforts that may be associated with the procedures. Benefits should be stated clearly with distinction between personal and societal benefits expected to be derived from the study.
5. Subject's rights, including a statement of subject's/family's right to ask questions of the investigator and withdraw from the study if desired.
6. Statement of compensation where applicable.
7. Confidentiality statement
8. The name of responsible investigator and contact phone number.

FIGURE 3-2

An outline of the procedures for preparing human investigation protocols

Reprinted with permission from Emerson College Graduate Policy Manual, *September 2004, Emerson College, Boston, MA.*

Some investigators, particularly in the behavioral sciences, have argued that full disclosure of the purpose of an experiment can bias subject responses, thus distorting the outcome. Among those who argued this position was Milgram (1977). In a series of famous experiments that stirred widespread debate as to their ethics, he encouraged subjects to administer electric shocks to others whenever they made mistakes while trying to solve simple problems. Those who administered the shock were "deceived" into believing that the shocks given were real when in fact they were not. The victims in these experiments, who feigned painful reactions in response to the bogus shocks, were actually confederates of the experimenter. A startling finding was that more than half of the subjects who administered the shocks continued to obey the instructions of the experimenter (e.g., "you must continue," "you have no choice") when encouraged to increase the intensity of electricity to levels they presumed to be dangerous. In responding to the critics of these studies, Milgram (1977) said: "The central moral justification for allowing my experiment is that it was judged acceptable by those who took part in it." He went on to recommend that investigators ought to neutralize the term "deception," replacing it with more appropriate [*sic*] descriptors such as "masking" or "technical illusion."

Rosnow and Rosenthal (1996) have noted that deception is sometimes permissible in experiments as long as:

- It is necessary to the validity of the research
- The research is worth doing
- The physical and psychological risks to the participants are minimal
- Adequate debriefing will be carried out

The fourth point, pertaining to adequate "debriefing," is exemplified by the actions Milgram took to debrief his subjects following completion of the experiment. All participants were informed why it was necessary to have deceived them to assure the validity of the experiment, that their compliance with the instructions to shock others was "normal," and that they would receive a written report summarizing the results of the research. Furthermore, many participants were provided with psychiatric interviews to identify possible injurious effects resulting from their participation.

In addition to debriefing subjects through such means as described above, "dehoaxing" may be used to further convince subjects that what was told to them during a debriefing session was actually true. For example, in the case of subjects who might have suffered from injurious consequences of deception even after debriefing, Milgram might have chosen to open up the cover to the bogus electrical stimulating device to show that no wires were connected to a power outlet.

According to the American Psychological Association's ethical code of conduct (1992), researchers should ". . . never deceive participants about significant aspects that would affect their willingness to participate, such as physical risks or discomfort, or unpleasant emotional influences" (p. 1609). It goes on to say that deception or concealment should be used only when there are no acceptable alternative procedures and that subjects should be debriefed as quickly as possible. Despite the latter qualifications, some psychologists have argued forcefully that all forms of deception should be outlawed (Ortmann & Hertwig, 1997).

The authors of this text are well aware of the evidence showing that a subject's preexisting knowledge or expectations about the goals of an experiment may introduce an unwanted biasing influence (see Chapter 7). Nevertheless, in our opinion, this is no excuse for misleading subjects by supplying them with misinformation. As an alternative to such deceptive practices, subjects might be told that certain information about the treatments or conditions to be used in a study will not be disclosed until after the experiment. Provided that they agree to participate under such circumstances, it is still the responsibility of the researcher to inform them of any associated risks. In our view, studies that require the abandonment of ethical principles cannot be justified on any grounds. Researchers and clinicians alike can avoid such pitfalls by being knowledgeable about the ethical guidelines established by their profession and adhering to these as closely as possible.

Several professional organizations have published ethical standards that are useful guides to keep in mind in planning and conducting research. Among these are the American Psychological Association (APA), the American Sociological Association (ASA), the American Educational Research Association (AERA), the Society for Research in Child Development

(SRCD), and the American Speech-Language-Hearing Association (ASHA). The APA standards, first formulated in 1953, have been modified over the years but continue to be widely consulted by professionals in fields prior to conducting research with humans or laboratory animals. For the most recent version of the APA ethical guidelines for research, see http://www.apa.org/ethics/code.

ASHA's new code of ethics, approved in 2003, also addresses issues specifically related to conducting and integrating research into all aspects of professional activity. The general code was revised to address issues of research ethics pertaining to informed consent, confidentiality, human treatment of animals, and maintenance of research data (Mustain, 2003). For additional information about these revisions, see ASHA's Web site. For an informative article about ethical research and research misconduct in the field of communication sciences and disorders, see Box 3-4.

Since October 2000, the National Institutes of Health (NIH) has required that all investigators and key personnel applying for grants or contracts, whose work involves human participants, receive education in the protection of such participants. An NIH tutorial developed for this purpose is available online: http://grants.nih.gov/.

BOX 3-4

Ethics and Research

A well-known researcher, highly successful in obtaining extramural research funding and having a long list of publications, insisted that her name be included as an author on all publications emanating from her laboratory. A clinical scientist, testing the effects of an experimental treatment, compared scores from a treated group of participants to scores from a group of individuals from whom treatment was withheld. A university professor, serving as a reviewer of a manuscript submitted for publication in a research journal, provided copies of the manuscript to graduate students so that they could prepare their own critiques, as an educational exercise in peer review . . .

An ambitious graduate student, when analyzing data collected for his master's thesis, changed the numbers in two experimental conditions to make the results fit his hypothesis. A young assistant professor, eager to bolster her publication record in time for her tenure review, included published findings from another scientist in a manuscript submitted for publication and reported them as her own. A busy senior scientist, mentoring several PhD and postdoctoral students, neglected to monitor their methods of data collection.

What do these cases have in common? All of them raise questions about breaches of research ethics or of research misconduct. The latter, defined by the U.S. Department of Health and Human Services in language adhered to by the National Institutes of Health, is: "fabrication, falsification, or plagiarism, or other practices that seriously deviate from those that are commonly accepted within the scientific community for proposing, conducting, or reporting research.

continues

BOX 3-4 *continued*

Misconduct does not include honest error or honest differences in interpretations or judgments of data."

Why should I be concerned about research misconduct? The consequences of violations of research ethics can be far-reaching. On moral grounds, society expects individuals to lead their lives with honesty and the utmost respect for the well-being of others. These expectations are highest for those in positions of trust, who are responsible for the health, safety, and welfare of others—such as religious leaders, educators, and government officials. Ethical transgressions within these groups are considered especially abhorrent. And so it is with scientists, whose life's work is fundamentally about seeking truth (fact) and developing an understanding of natural and human phenomena. From the most theoretical of physicists to the most applied of clinical researchers, the underlying search for new knowledge is ultimately tied to the enhancement of human life. When those whose job it is to make discoveries and enrich our lives disregard principles of intellectual honesty, the credibility of science and those who perform that science is inestimably undermined.

What are the practical consequences of research misconduct? Recent confirmed cases of scientific misconduct are illustrative. In these cases fraudulent research activities derailed the development of a vaccine against hepatitis C, interfered with progress in understanding metastasis in prostate cancer, produced misleading data regarding auditory processing in Broca's aphasia, and misrepresented findings aimed at understanding chemical phenomena active in the edema associated with traumatic brain injury. The consequences of misconduct in one particular case, in which a graduate student falsified and fabricated data, were described as "adversely and materially affect[ing] the laboratory's ongoing research . . . by creating uncertainty about all his experimental results, necessitating verification and repetition of experiments, preventing the reporting of results for publication, and preventing the principal investigator from submitting a competitive renewal application for a NIH grant". All of these examples underscore the point that the impacts of research misconduct are serious and far-reaching.

What should be done about research misconduct? As Chris Pascal, director of the Office of Research Integrity (ORI), has written recently, an important strategy to counteract occurrences of scientific misconduct is ". . . to instill key principles of responsible research into the mission, culture, and curricula of research institutions. . . . In ORI's view, responsible research practices are critical to the quality of research. Education in these practices is necessary to develop researchers' skills and competencies not only in integrity issues, but also in the actual conduct of research."

Efforts to provide education regarding the responsible conduct of research (RCR) abound. (See the Web site of the newly formed RCR Education Consortium— http://rcrec.org—as an example.)

ASHA's Code of Ethics provides a modicum of guidance in regard to research ethics. Among the 18 statements dealing with this topic are items related to conflict

continues

BOX 3-4 *continued*

of interest, assignment of credit and acknowledgment of sources, treatment of human research participants, and truthfulness (six items!).

Perhaps as important as any of these is item IV-I: "Individuals who have reason to believe that the Code of Ethics has been violated shall inform the Board of Ethics." All members of ASHA must adhere to this "duty to report" any known, verifiable acts of scientific misconduct so that the highest moral, ethical, and research standards are upheld in our discipline. Essentially all institutions also have reporting and investigatory mechanisms in place to deal with allegations of misconduct, and it is important to become familiar with the procedure used in one's place of employment. If each of us—scientist, teacher, student, clinician—accepts this difficult but important responsibility, and if RCR education becomes a meaningful part of our curricula, our discipline will advance not only the quality of what our research discovers, but also the ethics of how we manage the discovery process. Adherence to high research ethics standards is essential if we are to trust the science that underpins all that we do.

Reprinted with permission from "Ethics and Research," by J.C. Ingham and J. Horner, March 16, 2004, The ASHA Leader, *pp. 10–11, 24–25.*

SUMMARY

We have reviewed several issues that are important to evaluate in selecting a problem for research, including the need to:

- Identify a question that you believe to be important to answer
- Understand the nature of the question to be asked, keeping in mind that
  - "what" questions seek to describe or categorize phenomena
  - "where" questions seek to examine the relationship between variables
  - "why" questions seek to determine causal relations between variables

Research questions may arise from experiences and problems that we encounter on an everyday basis in our personal and professional lives. The kinds of resources available to assist us in deciding on a particular research topic were reviewed. Finally, we emphasized the importance of carefully considering the feasibility of answering a question in view of:

- Its "testability" based on operational definitions of the independent and dependent variable
- Methodological constraints (i.e., availability of appropriate equipment, participants, financial resources, time, etc.)
- Ethical guidelines established for the protection of human subjects

KEY TERMS

rationale
criterion of testability
pilot study

institutional review boards (IRB)
informed consent
risk/benefit ratio

SELF-LEARNING REVIEW

1. "Who or what" questions are answered through the use of various _____ techniques designed to _____ or _____ phenomena.
2. Developing taxonomies of various communication disorders is important in setting up mutually exclusive _____ _____.
3. The formulation of a problem consists of: (1) originating a _____, (2) developing a _____, and (3) determining the _____ of finding the answer.
4. Asking and answering clinical questions allow us to better _____, _____, and _____ the results of testing procedures and treatment programs.
5. Two publications of the federal government that summarize scientific research initiatives on a regular basis are the _____ and the _____ Guidelines for Grants and Contracts.
6. A major branch of NIH that supports research and research training in the field of communication disorders is the _____ .
7. One way to identify an important research study is by noting the _____ of its _____ by other researchers.
8. According to Merton, the importance of a research rationale is that it ". . . curbs the flow of scientifically _____ questions and enlarges the share of _____ ones."
9. The first issue to settle in determining the feasibility of a study is whether or not the _____ or _____ is stated in a _____ form.
10. Unless the independent and dependent variables can be specified, the _____ _____ cannot be met.
11. In 1974, the National Research Act established a commission for the _____ of human subjects. Institutions are now required to set up an _____ to determine the _____ of research proposals with existing regulations.
12. Two issues of major concern in the deliberations of an IRB committee pertains to the _____ / _____ ratio and the means of obtaining _____ _____ .

QUESTIONS AND EXERCISES FOR CLASSROOM DISCUSSION

1. Scientific research always begins with some form of question about an unresolved problem.
   - Discuss the nature of "what," "where," and "why" questions as each type of question might be asked about a particular aspect of speech, language, or hearing.
   - Identify at what stage of existing knowledge one of these questions might be more appropriately asked than another.

- What are some present questions that you might have pertaining to the etiology, diagnosis, or treatment of various communication disorders?

2. As future professionals in the field of communication disorders, you will continue to confront a myriad of significant problems requiring research for their solution.
   - Identify the areas of research that presently most interest you.
   - Name some of the outstanding researchers in the field and what you believe are their major contributions.
   - Describe the types of research that these researchers have done that best fit the types of research described in this chapter.
   - Talk with a researcher in communications sciences and disorders or a related field to ascertain his/her interest in a particular area of research. Ask:
     - What led to his/her interest in the problem?
     - What does he/she find most and least interesting about the actual research process?
     - What does he/she believe to be the clinical and/or theoretical relevance of the research?
     - Given a particular research interest, what does he/she believe are the most important questions that remain to be answered?

3. Browse through several of ASHA's journals to determine what kinds of articles they publish (e.g., types of research, clinical forums, tutorials, letters to the editor). In the back pages of the journals, take note of their editorial policies with respect to:
   - Mission statements
   - Types of manuscripts accepted
   - Criteria for acceptance
   - Review policies
   - Ethical guidelines

Reviewing the Literature and Stating Research Problems

CHAPTER OUTLINE

LEARNING OBJECTIVES

After reading this chapter, you should be able to identify, describe, or define:

- How a literature review is conducted
- The characteristics of a well-written literature review
- How research questions are stated
- Two types of hypotheses
- The statistical logic and conceptual basis of hypothesis testing
- The Bayesian view of hypothesis testing
- The perspective of behaviorism

REVIEWING RESEARCH LITERATURE

Having chosen a subject matter for research, the next step in the planning process is conducting a thorough literature review relevant to the area of interest. The ways and means of organizing an efficient search as opposed to meandering aimlessly through tangential literature were discussed in the previous chapter. The goal is to read *broadly* enough to uncover present trends and controversies pertinent to the research topic but also *selectively* with the aim of discovering gaps in existing knowledge and identifying problems needing further study. Having achieved these goals, the next step is to state the research problem of interest in a manner that allows it to be investigated.

Hypothetically, suppose that one is interested in the role that early speech-language impairments might play in later occurring learning/reading disabilities. In the process of reviewing the literature, one learns that the research has consistently shown that children with speech-language impairments are at risk for reading disabilities. One wonders about the precise relationship between certain verbal disabilities and later occurring reading failure. A continued review of the literature reveals this question is highly complex. In fact, some evidence suggests that different types of speech-language impairments are related to (i.e., predict) different kinds of reading outcomes. More specifically, the results of previous research seem to suggest that standardized measures of language ability are better predictors of reading comprehension than measures of phonological awareness. On the other hand, such research also seems to indicate that measures of phonological awareness are better predictors of written word recognition than are standardized measures of language ability. As one ponders these facts, a possible therapy implication begins to emerge in the form of a tentative research question: Does phonological awareness training (e.g., sound blending, segmentation, rhyming exercises) differentially affect the skills associated with reading achievement (i.e., reading recognition versus reading comprehension)? Determining the relative influence of such training on the different components of reading competence is a question that has developed out of the framework of the selected literature review. Still other types of problems might have emerged from the interplay of reading and other variables. Indeed, sometimes a topic might change entirely as you discover new areas for investigation.

It is important to bear in mind that the purpose of a literature review done in preparation for a research study may be quite different from one connected with a term paper or similar academic project. Whereas the latter activities may be directed toward achieving a critical review and evaluation of a subject area, they seldom involve the kind of problem distillation process necessary for funneling a body of diverse facts into a well-delineated testable question or research hypothesis. Like a court attorney, increasingly one must exclude irrelevant evidence by focusing on only the facts most necessary for establishing the case for your study.

How is one to know when an adequate review of the literature has been accomplished? According to Schloss and Smith (1999), a solid literature review should allow you to:

- Verify that you have chosen an appropriate topic
- Define and refine aspects of your own study
- Begin to estimate the resources your study will require
- Establish the importance of your topic and justify the effort you will expend

We would add to this list the ideas that a good literature review should allow you to begin organizing the information you have read in a written form and in such a manner that the problem you wish to investigate will make sense to others.

Writing the Literature Review

A well-written review of the literature will make clear to the reader:

- The history of the research problem
- The theoretical and practical importance of the research problem

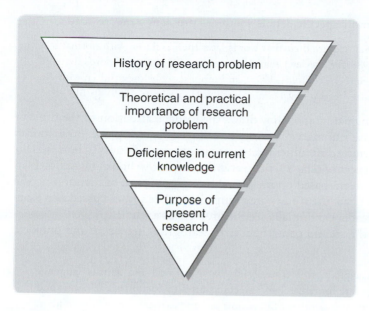

History of research problem

Theoretical and practical importance of research problem

Deficiencies in current knowledge

Purpose of present research

FIGURE 4-1

Literature review structured in the form of a four-step funnel or inverted pyramid so as to increasingly focus on the specific purpose of an investigation

- Deficiencies in current knowledge about one or more aspects of the research problem
- The purpose and direction of the present research

The beginning researcher might find viewing the structure of a literature review in metaphoric terms to be useful. The structure of such a review might be seen as analogous to a funnel or inverted pyramid in which research investigations pertaining to the broad historical elements of the problem as found in research literature are found at the top (see Figure 4-1). Such studies are reviewed first, followed by additional studies that focus increasingly on the specific problem of interest to the investigator.

As we noted above, the literature review section of a research article should start with a statement of the research problem, then proceed to make clear the importance of the problem and existing gaps in understanding. This background information should establish a compelling case, or *rationale,* for further investigation of the problem. Typically, toward the end of the literature review, the author will inform the reader as to the purpose of the current research study. To illustrate how this process unfolds in an actual research article, we will use an example from a study by Shelly Gray (2003) published in the *Journal of Speech, Language, and Hearing Research* entitled "Word-Learning by Preschoolers with Specific Language Impairment: What Predicts Success?"

The first sentence of the article states:

> There is considerable evidence that children with specific language impairment (SLI) have difficulty learning new words (Ellis, Weismer, & Nemeth, 1990; Rice, Buhr, & Oetting, 1992; Rice, Oetting, Marquis, Bode, & Pae, 1994). (p. 56)

As can be seen, at the very beginning of the article, the authors inform the reader about the broad problem to be addressed (i.e., the relationship of SLI to delays in reading acquisition). Notice that several previous studies that investigated such a relationship are cited as a general framework for a more detailed discussion to follow.

In the second sentence, more specific details about the problem were provided:

> They [children with SLI] may acquire their first words later than children with normal language (NL) (see Leonard, 1988, for a review), may produce a smaller variety of words than NL peers (e.g., Watkins, Kelly, Harbers, & Hollis, 1995), and often score below children with NL on norm referenced vocabulary tests (Gray, Plante, Vance, & Henrichsen, 1999). (p. 56)

As can be seen, in the opening paragraph, Gray draws the reader's attention to the topic of interest by providing a concise summary of research findings suggesting that preschoolers with SLI experience word learning difficulties manifested in a variety of ways. To borrow a literary term, the opening sentences of Gray's article serve as a "narrative hook" that affords an overall perspective of the problem based on previous literature. Instead of mentioning the specific details of each study cited, the studies are grouped together and discussed in a more general fashion so that the reader can initially see the problem as a whole.

In the first sentence of the second paragraph, Gray states the theoretical and practical significance of the problem:

> Because successful lexical acquisition is critically important to oral and written language development, an important task for researchers and clinicians is to document the nature and extent of word-learning difficulty within the SLI population and to determine which children are at risk for this problem. (p. 56)

In the third paragraph, the practical and theoretical significance of the problem is further refined:

> One proposed prognosticator of word-learning ability is a child's ability to hear a word once or twice and store enough information about it so that future phonological, semantic, syntactic, and non-verbal experiences elaborate its stored representation. This process is referred to as fast mapping (Carey, 1978). Without initial fast mapping, further learning cannot take place. For this reason, fast mapping has been the subject of several investigations. (p. 56)

In subsequent paragraphs, the author reviewed several additional studies that documented the nature and extent of word-learning difficulties in SLI. She concludes by stating a limitation in knowledge:

> These studies have begun to document the nature and extent of word-learning difficulty with the SLI population. SLI groups typically learn to comprehend or produce significantly fewer words than NL group, but some children with SLI perform comparably to the NL peers. . . . Comprehension of new words appears to be better than production, but the relationship between comprehension and production has not been explored. The ability to quickly store knowledge about a new word, a skill known as fast mapping, may predict later success in acquiring that word: however, the relationship between fast mapping and word learning has not been investigated. (p. 57)

By pointing out deficiencies in existing knowledge, Gray establishes a rationale for her own investigation. Such a rationale should lead naturally to a purpose statement that tells the reader what the investigator hopes to accomplish by carrying out further research.

Gray's purpose statement reads as follows:

> The purpose of this study was to compare group performance on a word-learning task designed to teach children new words in a situation similar to treatment . . . The relationship between comprehension and production of new words, as well as the relationship between

fast mapping and word learning, was investigated. Word learning success by children with SLI was evaluated to determine whether word-learning performance accurately distinguishes between children with and without SLI. (p. 58)

In theses and dissertations, the purpose statement often comprises a separate and distinct section of the paper. However, in a research article, it is most often included as an integral part of the literature review as found in the introduction. Wherever it might be found, keep in mind that the purpose statement must be clearly and concisely articulated as to convey the central intent of the study.

Here are a few tips for writing a literature review:

1. Begin by organizing the articles pertaining to the problem you wish to investigate in a chronological sequence. All of these articles should be related to a unified theme or topic you wish to investigate.
2. Use the articles at the top of your list to provide a historical context for the topic of interest. Your goal is not to *reproduce* what the author(s) said in the article(s). Instead, you should *interpret* the literature as to establish a case or rationale for what you wish to accomplish in your own research.
3. Work from an outline while making sure to establish the relationship of each article or group of articles to one another. Unless articles can be shown to be specifically related to your research problem, they should not be included.
4. Remember that the structure of a literature review should be shaped like a funnel. As you progress through the introduction section of a research paper, the articles you discuss should be increasingly relevant to the specific problem you wish to investigate, culminating in a purpose statement.
5. Perhaps the most helpful advice that we might give is to read as many literature reviews as possible in order to study the way they are structured.

STATING THE RESEARCH PROBLEM

Research Question

Merely reviewing the literature in a particular subject area and determining the need for additional inquiry falls short of establishing the criteria necessary for performing systematic research. For research to proceed, the problem must be further defined by specifying the variables of which it is constituted. After formulating a purpose statement, an investigator may elect to frame the problem in a question format before proceeding to develop specific research hypotheses. For example, in her dissertation research that examined proper name recall in younger and older adults, Barresi (1996) began by asking the following questions:

1. What effect does age have on recall of common and uncommon names and occupations?
2. What is the effect of a second learning trial on recall of common and uncommon items for each age group?
3. What effect does age have on reported use of strategies for learning common and uncommon names and occupations?
4. What is the association between reported use of strategies and recall of names and occupations in younger and older adults? (pp. 21–22)

The first three questions noted above are *difference questions* to the degree that they inquire about the effect of an independent variable (age) or treatment (second learning trial) on several dependent variables. The fourth question is a *relationship question* because it asks about the association between certain independent and dependent variables (use of certain strategies and recall abilities).

Research Hypotheses

Research questions like those noted previously should make clear the objective of the study. To refine the definition of the problem even further, investigators often transform such questions into specific research hypotheses. To be useful, hypotheses should satisfy the following four criteria:

1. The hypothesis should be formulated at the outset of a study as a declarative sentence that makes clear the predicated relationship between an independent and dependent variable.
2. The hypothesis must concisely specify the variables to be examined by defining them operationally.
3. The hypothesis must be testable by gathering specific information that is subject to statistical evaluation.
4. The hypothesis should be grounded in theory or derived from previous research.

As noted previously, questions like those used by Barresi are often preliminary to stating formal research hypotheses. In fact, some investigators may prefer the former type of format over the latter as a style for expressing problems. Such a preference might be justified on logical grounds when considerable ambiguity surrounds a problem or in cases of exploratory studies of phenomena about which few facts are known. However, in the case of Barresi's dissertation research, several previous studies related to her problem were cited which serve as a foundation for certain predictions made in the form of the following research hypotheses:

- Both younger and older subjects will recall common names (e.g., "Owens") and occupations (e.g., "surgeon") better than uncommon names (e.g., "Reisman") and occupations (e.g., "tuner") . . . Further, older adults will recall fewer items than younger adults.
- Both age groups should recall more names and occupations on the second learning trial than the first.
- Both age groups will report using similar strategies, but older adults will use them less frequently resulting in lower scores than younger adults.
- There will be a significant positive correlation between frequency of reported strategy use and recall of names and occupations for both younger and older adults. (pp. 22–23)

Note that the independent variable (i.e., age) and dependent variables (i.e., names and occupations recalled) have been made apparent in the research hypotheses along with the measure to be used (i.e., frequency) in assessing the predicted findings.

Barresi could have carried the definition of her research one step further by expressing her hypotheses in the null form as statements of **statistical equality** (i.e., no significant between-group difference). Nevertheless, the fact that hypotheses are not explicitly stated in such a manner does not mean that researchers will fail to conduct appropriate statistical tests in order to reject the implicit assumption of "no difference" if warranted. No matter how a research hypothesis is stated, if used in conjunction with inferential statistics (see Chapter 12), it must imply a null hypothesis that is subject to a probability estimate.

Unfortunately, journal editors commonly accept articles for publication when their author(s) have neglected entirely the importance of defining the problem either as a question or as a formalized research hypothesis. Some might contend that such an omission does not constitute neglect but an unspoken understanding that "seasoned researchers" will automatically understand the parameters of a problem despite the lack of its formal explication. In our opinion, while writing good research questions and research hypotheses can be a laborious and time-consuming task, there is no better means available for defining and clarifying the variables to be studied in an experiment. As an investigative tool, the well formulated question or hypothesis is to a researcher what the scalpel is in the hands of a surgeon. It creates the conditions for cutting through the vagaries of words and ill-conceived ideas to focus sharply on a scientific problem. It likewise establishes the operative boundaries of an experiment and defines the limits for interpreting successes and failures. Finally, it discourages small bands of specialized investigators becoming what Bacon called the "Idols of the Tribe" who, for the most part, talk only to one another (see Chapter 1).

NULL HYPOTHESIS

As noted previously, for statistical purposes, hypotheses are generally stated in the null form. For example, our hypothesis might be stated: "there is *no significant relationship* between children's ages and the production of consonants in certain word positions" or "children of different ages *do not differ significantly* in their use of final position sounds." Having stated a proposition in the null form, we then apply statistical tests to determine if the null hypothesis can be rejected. By rejecting the null hypothesis, we conclude that whatever relationships or differences are observed among the measured variables of the study are indeed significant (owing to systematic influences instead of chance).

Many students who are unfamiliar with the use of the null hypothesis in statistical inference testing initially complain that such a proposition seems cumbersome, if not illogical. To them, it might sometimes appear that a fallacious proposition has been stated by an investigator merely to prove it wrong—simply setting up a "straw man" argument just to defeat it. In essence, this is indeed the principle underlying null hypothesis testing. Whereas our second research hypothesis stated above implies that two or more sampled age groups (e.g., three-, four-, and five-year-old children) represent *different* populations in their use of final position sounds, the null hypothesis says that they all must be considered representative of the *same* population until proved otherwise. In fact, there is a kind of inversion of logic surrounding null hypothesis testing because the usual purpose of research is not to determine that some difference in, for example, the mean scores between two groups is the result of chance. Instead, the goal of research usually is to prove the alternative proposition (research hypothesis) that the observed differences can be validly attributed to systematic influences within the experiment rather than to random fluctuations.

Statistical Logic of Null Hypotheses

The general logic underlying a null hypothesis (H_0) comes from evaluating its probable truth against the research hypothesis (H_1). This is made possible through statistical significance testing, which permits generalization from a sample of cases to the target population from which such cases were drawn. In statistical terms, a "target population" is a population to which a researcher wishes to generalize the results. The procedures employed in testing hypotheses in a prototypic experimental study are shown in Figure 4-2.

To simplify matters, assume that we wish to investigate the influence of phonological training in kindergarten on students' reading ability in the first grade. In setting up such an experiment, the first step would be to randomly *select* a sample of subjects from a population and randomly *assign* them to two groups designated as X and Y. Group X (the treatment

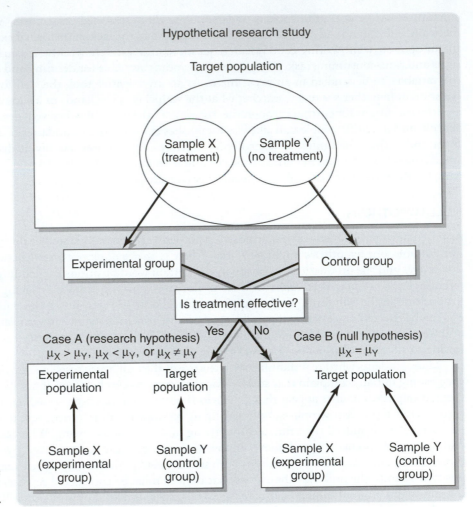

FIGURE 4-2

Relating the research hypothesis and the null hypothesis to the experimental results

group) will receive training, while group Y (the control group) will receive no training. Two situations or treatment outcomes are possible as the result of statistical testing of the differences between mean scores: either the null hypothesis or its logical alternative, the research hypothesis, will be supported. Our null hypothesis, as a *statement of equality*, might be stated as: there is no difference in the reading ability of those first graders who receive phonological training in kindergarten and those who do not, or symbolically,

$$\mu_X = \mu_Y \text{ (mean X equals mean Y)}.$$

The logical alternative to that prediction would be expressed as the research hypothesis, which is a statement of statistical difference:

$$\mu_X \neq \mu_Y \text{ (mean X does not equal mean Y)}$$

The first step in the decision-making process of a research study is to test the null hypothesis. Because the null hypothesis is the hypothesis of *no statistical difference*, if it is rejected, the alternative research hypothesis is supported. Thus, referring again to Figure 4-2, if phonological training has not been found effective, then Case B best represents the outcome wherein X is no different from Y. Alternatively, if Case A prevails (the treatment was effective), then the research hypothesis may be supported on the basis of finding a significant difference.

Keeping in mind that a research hypothesis is a prediction derived from a theory, there are cases in which a researcher might want to explicitly predict the *direction* of an expected difference. Using our previous example, the research hypothesis in Situation A could have been expressed as: $\mu_X > \mu_Y$ indicating that the mean of the treatment group is predicted to be greater than for the control group. In such a case, the implied null would read: $\mu_X \leq \mu_Y$ indicating that the mean of the treatment group is expected to be less than or equal to the control group.

In actual practice, null hypotheses are typically not stated explicitly in journal articles and related research reports unless predicting the direction of the differences. However, learning to formulate clear and concise hypotheses as a means of clarifying the purposes of an investigation is a valuable aid to inexperienced researchers such as students. Perhaps for this reason, the formal statement of null hypotheses is frequently required in theses, dissertations, and related academic projects designed to teach students how to conceptualize and investigate research problems.

Whether the null hypothesis is formally stated or simply implied, it must be formulated in a manner that allows for its rejection given certain probability estimates that are based on the results of statistical testing. As will be noted in Chapter 12, associated with null hypotheses are probability estimates for making certain types of statistical inference errors: either a **type I (alpha)** or **type II (beta) error** is possible. A type I error involves *rejecting a null hypothesis when it is true*. In such a case, one might conclude, for example, that Treatment A is significantly better than Treatment B when it is not. A type I error results in a **false positive conclusion.** On the other hand, one might instead make a type II error by *failing to reject a false null hypothesis*. In this case, it might be erroneously concluded that a particular treatment is no more effective than another. A type II error results in a **false negative conclusion.**

As noted in Chapter 12, researchers generally select an acceptable risk for error in the form of a **significance level** prior to an experiment. In the behavioral sciences, the conventional level of probability set by the researcher as the basis for rejecting the null hypothesis is either $p < .05$ or $p < .01$. Thus, for a finding to be *significant* (the basis for rejecting the null), the odds for making an inferential error must be quite small. However, the tolerance for making an error is greater when the significance level is set at 5% (one time in 20) than at 1% (one time in 100).

A rejected null hypothesis indicates that the research results are significant, leading to the acceptance of the research hypothesis. However, the failure to find a statistically significant result does not necessarily prove the null hypothesis to be true. All that can be said is that the accumulated data are as yet insufficient, casting doubt on the validity of the null hypothesis. Thus, the meaning of the term *nonsignificant* should be interpreted as "not yet proved" or "inconclusive." The failure to find significance can result because of many reasons, including a poorly designed study, experimenters' mistakes, instrument failure or insensitivity, sampling errors, insufficient subjects, and so on. In such cases, the best one can do is to live with the null hypothesis until it is otherwise proved invalid.

Conceptual Basis of Null Hypotheses

Science is concerned with discovering and documenting the "true nature" of objects and events in the real world and their lawful determination. In order to accomplish this, scientists have developed a philosophy that is aimed at divesting themselves from certain human limitations (e.g., prejudicial attitudes, personal preferences or beliefs, moralistic attitudes, emotions) that might otherwise bias the outcome of their work. Shaughnessy and Zechmeister (1994) have summarized well the attitude of most scientists:

> More than anything else, scientists are skeptical. Not only do they want to "see it before believing it," but they are likely to want to see it again . . . people make mistakes. (p. 19)

The skepticism of scientists is reflected in their use of the null hypothesis that contends, in effect, that nothing exists until proved to exist based on certain statistically defined levels of confidence. Some investigators have drawn analogies between null hypothesis testing and the legal system as it exists in the United States (Browner, Newman, Cummings, & Hulley, 1988). A major assumption in a court of law is that the accused is innocent until proved guilty. A prosecuting attorney must marshal evidence to prove that the accused is indeed "guilty beyond a reasonable doubt" prior to rejecting the null hypothesis of "not guilty." However, in deciding a case, it is possible for a jury to make one of two errors: an innocent defendant may be wrongly convicted (type I error) or a guilty defendant may not be convicted (type II error). These two errors are related. By increasing the likelihood of a guilty conviction, more innocent people will suffer the consequences (more type I errors). On the other hand, should the legal system render more lenient judgments, there is a greater likelihood that the guilty will go free (more type II errors).

According to the laws of the United States, it is better to allow a guilty person to go free than to falsely convict an innocent person. In statistical testing, the relative seriousness of one type of error over the other is a subject for debate. Purely on statistical grounds, it could be argued that the research error of missing the presence of a significant treatment effect is less serious than concluding incorrectly that one is present. The logic behind this preference might be based on the possibility of finding a truly significant treatment effect in future studies that are perhaps better designed.

Certainly, from a clinical perspective, there are potential negative consequences associated with both kinds of errors. On the one hand, a false positive identification, involving an incorrect diagnosis and/or unnecessary treatment, might also result in unwarranted anxiety, expense, or stigmatization. On the other hand, a false negative identification, associated with the failure to diagnose and provide appropriate treatment for a disorder or disease, could likewise result in deleterious consequences. Of course, the best policy is to make every reasonable effort to reduce the potential for both type I and type II errors whenever possible. This can best be done through carefully designed experiments and the use of appropriate sampling procedures including an adequate number of subjects.

Case for Personal Probabilities in Hypothesis Testing

Despite the best intentions of researchers to suspend their personal beliefs in favor of adopting objective attitudes in selecting and defining research problems, seldom does one begin an experiment without at least some tentative preconceived ideas about the possible outcomes. Prior information about a problem is often available to a researcher from many sources including theoretical knowledge, familiarity with the sample, documentation in the research literature, and subjective opinions of one's own or of other colleagues. Given this understanding, it is a fallacy to believe that a state of "mindlessness" is attainable or even desirable in the conduct of research. According to Hays (1963):

> The scientist does not operate in a vacuum . . . the experimenter has some initial ideas about how credible each of the hypotheses is . . . there are prior beliefs . . . that make some of the possibilities for a true situation a better bet than others for the experimenter. (pp. 347–348)

The foregoing remarks by Hays are in accord with the philosophy and methods of an alternative approach to null hypothesis testing based on directly determining the degree to which a prior belief fits with the actual facts of a subsequent observation. The **Bayesian method,** as it has come to be known, has existed longer than inferential statistics and null hypothesis testing, yet its applications and relevance to many research problems remain controversial.

First described by an English clergyman by the name of Thomas Bayes in 1763, the Bayesian method provides a mathematical basis for expressing one's beliefs in the language of probability prior to collecting data. Such a statement, called the **prior probability,** is akin to the research hypothesis discussed previously with the additional requirement of including a numerical or quantitative estimate or "bet" reflecting the *degree of belief* about a predicted result. The next step is to derive a **data probability** based on the sample of *data actually collected*. The data probability can be regarded as the conditional credibility of a particular view pending the calculation of a **posterior probability.** The latter probability, reflecting the updated credibility of an original opinion or viewpoint, is derived from a mathematical combination of the prior and data probabilities.

Advocates of null hypothesis testing have sometimes criticized if not denounced Bayesian methods. Such critics contend that subjective probabilities for a particular event may vary widely among different individuals. The rejoinder to this concern is that no statistical method, including null hypothesis testing, is free of the influence of prior opinion. Evidence of this fact can be found in the prior views of researchers that influence their choices in selecting and defining problems for study, in decisions about sampling procedures and the number of subjects to study, and in determining a particular significance level (e.g., .05 or .01). See Chapters 11 and 12 for a more detailed discussion of applications of Bayesian methods in deriving statistical probabilities.

Case Against Hypothesis Testing

Hypothesis testing is based on the tenets of inferential statistics as first expounded by Ronald Fisher and developed further by Neyman and Pearson in the early 1900s. Despite widespread acceptance of its philosophy of methods, the approach has often been criticized. Carver (1983) noted that inferential statistical testing has gained popularity because the users of such methods have advanced the illusion that a scientific decision can be made only if based on the results of a statistical calculation. More specifically, the convention has been to say that a result can be considered scientifically meaningful only if it leads to the rejection of a null hypothesis at what often appears to be one of two arbitrarily decided significance levels (i.e., .05 or .01 level).

There are at least two problems in viewing these probability values as the defining goals for scientific research. First, it is important to recognize that a scientifically important and statistically significant result is not one and the same. Virtually any study can yield a significant result at one of the conventional significance levels if it is replicated numerous times or if enough subjects are used. This can occur even though the actual difference in the size of the mean scores between two variables is minuscule. As noted by Young (1994), "the most serious limitation of statistical tests is thought to be the sample size problem. Generally, any difference between group means, no matter how small, may be statistically significant if based on a sufficiently large sample of cases" (p. 523).

For example, suppose a researcher administers an audiometric test to 5000 children, half of whom come from a low economic strata and the other half from a high economic strata. The question of interest is whether or not the hearing level of the two groups will differ significantly. Suppose further that a mean difference of 2 dB is found, leading to a rejection of the null hypothesis at a significance level of $p = .05$. Because of the very large size of the sample, this result may turn out to be statistically significant but lack practical value so far as having meaningful clinical implications.

The second point to bear in mind in evaluating the scientific importance of data is expressed in the following admonishment by Melton (1962), who said, "To insist upon the .05 level or .01 level is to talk about the science of business, not the business of science" (p. 137). Obviously, there must be some basis available for judging the scientific importance of data, but some scientists would argue against discounting a finding as trivial simply because it falls below some preordained probability value. In this respect, Morrison and Henkel (1970b) have argued that, instead of arbitrarily pronouncing a probability value that falls short of the .05 mark as "no difference," the finding should be reported relying on "the application of imagination, common sense, [and] informed judgment" (p. 311).

Several researchers have argued that hypothesis testing, whatever its nature or statistical methods, is an often misguided and counterproductive approach to developing a true science of behavior. For example, Sidman (1960) cautioned not "to fall into the error of insisting that all experimentation must derive from the testing of hypotheses. Such experimental activities can result in the piling up of trivia upon trivia" (p. 4). Sidman further advised the student to remember that what is most important in any experiment is a question that leads to "good data" that owes allegiance to no particular hypothesis or theory.

According to Bakan (1966) it is often the case that by the time a researcher, intent on proving a particular theory, finally gets to the stage of hypothesis testing, most of the important work has already been done. In a similar vein, Mishler (1983) offered a counterview to the common notion of exemplary scientific research as an enterprise involving "the elimination of plausible rival hypotheses to the preferred explicit hypothesis in any particular study" (p. 10). Instead, he proposed that the goal of behavioral science ought to be simply specifying the conditions under which lawful relationships of the form $Y = f(X)$ can be found and demonstrated.

Perspectives of Behaviorism

There is a school of behavioral science that holds that the determination of causal relations among variables, of the type described by Mishler, can best proceed when the main goal is to improve *observation, prediction* and *control* of behavior rather than to uncover or explain through hypothesis testing the factors that underlie its occurrence. The doctrine of this school has come to be known as **behaviorism,** and its methods are termed the **experimental analysis of behavior** or **applied behavioral analysis.** The defining feature of this approach is the emphasis it places on measuring the *effects* of manipulating aspects of the *observable behavior* of individuals.

The philosophical perspectives of behaviorism are rooted in a long effort among American psychologists to develop a science of learning beginning with William James (1890) who wrote at length "on the great law of habit." John Watson (1924) concluded that the *conditioned response* was the "fundamental unit of habit," and E. L. Thorndike (1938) later posited the "law of effect" to explain the influence of reward and punishment on behavior. The name of B. F. Skinner is most associated with the chief experimental method of behaviorism— **operant (instrumental) conditioning.** Although Skinner was influenced to some degree by Pavlovian principles of classical conditioning, his ideas incorporated to a much greater degree principles of trial and error learning and response reinforcement as mechanisms for shaping behavior. The so-called operant approach emphasized that behavior is best explained through the use of *controlled conditions* that demonstrate its *controlling variables*.

Hypothesis testing, inferential statistics, and the use of control subjects were all eschewed in favor of single-subject or small-N designs for controlling and monitoring the experimental situation. Skinner (1956) briefly summarized the essential steps of the operant paradigm as follows: "establish the behavior in which you are interested, submit the organism to a particular treatment, and look again at the behavior." As will be noted in Chapter 8, these three phases are commonly referred to as *baseline, conditioning,* and *withdrawal.*

The philosophical premises and experimental methods of behaviorism, particularly as reflected in operant conditioning, have been a subject of continuing controversy. The *Journal of Experimental Analysis of Behavior* was established in 1958 largely because of the refusal of other journals to accept small-N research studies for publication. As interest in the new field of *behavior modification* expanded, new journals and books began to appear that played an important role in developing applications that were therapeutically and educationally focused on a variety of human problems. *The Journal of Applied Behavioral Analysis,* first published in 1967, was devoted to human research in behavior modification and behavior therapy. New experimental methodologies and designs emphasizing small-N or single-subject research came into being and flourished throughout the 1970s (Krasner, 1971; Baer, 1975; Kazdin, 1978). The influence of these new developments also greatly impacted the field of communication sciences and disorders.

In support of the research strategies underlying the experimental analysis of behavior, Eysenck (1983) argued that its methods are likely to prove clinically more relevant and beneficial in the long run than therapies predicated on "nebulous hypotheses" or "unfounded theories." Some researchers have countered by arguing against the generalizability of the data of small-N or N-of-1 designs.

As we shall see in later chapters, obtaining generality of findings is a common problem in all studies regardless of the sample size. In the case of null hypothesis testing, we never can be absolutely sure that two sampled groups, to be compared on some variable, actually represent the *same* population. Because the variability of individual subject characteristics is unknown, the best we can do is to use the known variability in the sampled groups to *estimate* the unknown variability in the "assumed common population" (Carver, 1983). We must keep in mind that inferential statistics and null hypothesis testing are predicated on the use of average scores that reflect "typical," "usual," "normal," or "most representative" performance measures for comparing groups of subjects—not individual subjects themselves. More specifically, while it might be said that the group as a whole responded in a certain way to a particular treatment, the performance of individual subjects is typically not taken into account. In order to generalize the effect of a particular treatment from one individual to another, **systematic replication** of a research study would be required (i.e., a similar participant(s) would need to be evaluated, ideally by different researchers in different test settings).

SUMMARY

The primary purpose of a literature review is to relate the findings of previous research to a problem one might wish to investigate. Reading the research of others on a topic related to your own interest is the best means of learning how to write about your problem in a way that can be understood by others. In this chapter, we discussed the characteristics of a well-written literature review using examples from a published research article. The importance of a well-written literature review is that it makes clear the purpose of a study and establishes the basis for formulating research questions and/or hypotheses. The applications of research questions and hypotheses were discussed and examples given. How null hypotheses are used in research and their statistical logic was discussed. Alternative approaches to null hypothesis testing were also reviewed.

KEY TERMS

statistical equality
type I (alpha) error
type II (beta) error
false positive conclusion
false negative conclusion
significance level
Bayesian method
prior probability

data probability
posterior probability
behaviorism
experimental analysis of behavior
applied behavioral analysis
operant (instrumental) conditioning
systematic replication

SELF-LEARNING REVIEW

1. Once you have selected a problem, the next step is to define its parameters either in the form of a _____ _____ or a _____.
2. Having stated a hypothesis in the _____ form, we then apply a statistical test to determine if it can be _____.
3. Mathematically speaking, shortened expressions of the null hypothesis and its alternative, the research hypothesis, are _____ and _____, respectively.
4. If the mean of the treatment group (μ_X) was predicted to be greater than for the control group (μ_Y), the research hypothesis would have been expressed as _____. Alternatively, given the opposite prediction, it would have been read as _____.
5. Whether the null hypothesis is stated formally or simply implied, it must be formulated as to allow for its _____ given the results of _____ _____.
6. Concluding that Treatment A is better than Treatment B when it is not is an example of a _____ error. Concluding that Treatment A is no better than Treatment B when it is results in a _____ error.
7. A _____ error results in a _____ _____ conclusion while a _____ error results in a _____ _____ conclusion.
8. Other names for type I and type II errors are _____ and _____ errors, respectively.
9. When a finding reaches significance, the null hypothesis can be _____, typically at either p _____ or p _____ significance level.
10. The significance level that one selects should be decided _____ an experiment.
11. The meaning of the term "nonsignificant" should be interpreted as _____ _____ _____ or _____.
12. The skepticism of scientists is reflected in their use of the _____ _____.
13. A type I error leads to a _____ _____ conclusion. In a court of law, this is tantamount to _____ an _____ defendant.
14. Legally, a type II error associated with making a _____ _____ conclusion would result in a failure to _____ the _____.

15. A mathematical basis for expressing one's beliefs in the language of probability prior to data collection is called the _____ _____.
16. The above named method requires the establishment of three kinds of _____. These are: (1) _____, (2) _____, and (3) _____ probabilities.
17. Unlike inferential statistics, Bayesian methods incorporate within the analysis information from _____ samples.
18. Bayesian statisticians would argue against discounting a finding simply because it falls below a preordained _____ value.
19. A major strength of the Bayesian method is that it permits the comparison of _____ with _____ distributions of data over time.
20. A _____ shift involves a new way of "looking at the world."
21. According to Sidman, what is most important in any experiment is a question that leads in the end to good _____ owing allegiance to no particular _____ or _____.
22. Inferential statistics are predicated on comparing the performance of _____ of subjects—not _____ subjects.
23. One way to generalize the results of small-N research is by _____ _____.

QUESTIONS AND EXERCISES FOR CLASSROOM DISCUSSION

1. Go to the library and read the literature reviews of three journal articles of your choosing, but one in each of the areas of speech, language, and hearing. Having done so, note in writing whether or not the literature review made clear:
   - The history of the research problem in what appears to be a thorough and well organized review of past and current literature
   - The theoretical and practical importance of the research problem
   - Deficiencies in current knowledge about one or more aspects of the research problem
   - The purpose and direction of the present research by identifying the specific problem to be addressed
2. Distinguish between research questions and research hypotheses. Provide an example as to when one is more appropriately used than the other.
3. What criteria must a research hypothesis satisfy?
4. What is the statistical logic that underlies testing a null hypothesis and what is the result of rejecting it?
5. Why is the null hypothesis a statement of "statistical equality"? How is this stated in symbolic form?
6. Identify two types of errors that might result from rejecting or retaining the null hypothesis. Compare these errors to possible outcomes in a legal trial in terms of a "false positive" or "false negative" identification.
7. Discuss the meaning and interpretation of "significant" versus "nonsignificant."
8. How does the Bayesian method compare to the traditional null hypothesis testing approach to research?
9. Summarize the case that some researchers make against null hypothesis testing.
10. What is the perspective of behaviorism?
11. Formulate a problem that is of interest to you both in terms of a research question and a research hypothesis.

Sampling Theory and Methods

CHAPTER 5

CHAPTER OUTLINE

LEARNING OBJECTIVES

After reading this chapter, you should be able to identify, describe, or define:

- Fundamentals of sampling theory
- The importance of sampling

- Two types of populations
- Various types of random sampling methods
- Strengths and limitations of each type of random sampling method
- Various types of nonrandom sampling methods
- Strengths and limitations of each type of nonrandom sampling method
- Relationship between selection bias and sampling error
- Statistical theory in selecting a sample
- Statistical guidelines for determining sample size

CHOOSING A SAMPLE OF SUBJECTS

In most aspects of daily living, we form opinions and make decisions based on a sample of experience (limited information). The human brain is almost constantly engaged in some kind of sampling activity that leads us to anticipate certain outcomes. Wine tasters don't have to sip from every cask to pass judgment on a particular vintage. The same is true about the decisions all people make in judging the character of new acquaintances, in their choices pertaining to what food or clothes to buy, or whether or not to carry an umbrella on a cloudy day. By comparing our present observations with those of the past, we develop generalizations about the future.

Some Preliminary Concepts and Definitions

Researchers and statisticians use the term **population** to describe an all-inclusive data set about which they wish to draw a conclusion or causal inference. Typically, the term encompasses a large collection of animate or inanimate **elements** (people, objects, events, organizations, etc.) that share common attributes. In the field of communication sciences and disorders, a population might include all certified members of ASHA, all patients with whom they work, all patient files, all treatment facilities, and so on.

A population will include at least one common characteristic, but more can be defined as desired. For example, all certified members of ASHA would include all those holding the Certificate of Clinical Competence in the specialty speech-language pathology or the specialty of audiology. However, another population could be defined as only those who hold dual certification in both specialties. Should we decide to count all members belonging to one or the other of these populations, the resulting number would be referred to as a **parameter.** A parameter is a number or measured characteristic derived from the entire population.

A **sample** is a subset of a population ideally drawn in such a way that each member of the population has an equal chance of being selected. Thus drawn, such a sample is said to be **representative** of the larger population. In the example above, a sample could be drawn from the entire pool of certified members of ASHA or from the smaller population of members who hold both certifications. A **statistic** is a number derived from counting or measuring sample observations that have been drawn from a population of numbers.

Statistical methods allow researchers to make inferences about the characteristics of a population on the basis of information obtained from the sample. If the population consists of a finite number of observations, and provided that it is both possible and practical to count or measure each member of the data set, then variance for a particular population attribute also can be measured.

Conceivably, one might wish to determine the mean age for the entire population and then calculate the variance of each member from such an average measure (see Chapter 11).

Although such a task might be accomplished, to do so would be a tedious and highly laborious undertaking, particularly for an organization with more than a hundred thousand members.

A more feasible approach to this goal would be to draw a random sample to use as an estimate of the mean and variance of the **target population.** A target population can be defined as the population about which the investigator wishes to generalize. In so doing, the investigator must expect a certain degree of **sampling error,** which is the difference between the measures collected for a randomly selected sample and the population it is believed to represent. More specifically, sampling error can be defined as the expected amount of variance owing to *chance* alone rather than to *systematic* influences. The methods and statistical problems associated with sampling procedures are discussed more fully in Chapter 12.

Importance of Sampling to Research

One of the most important aspects of carrying out a research study is the selection of an appropriate sample of subjects. The main purpose of the majority of investigations conducted in the field of communication sciences and disorders is to generalize the findings obtained from the study of a relatively small group of subjects (sample) to a larger group of similar individuals (population) that the sample was chosen to represent.

For a smaller segment to represent the aggregate properties and characteristics of the whole, it must possess the same or highly similar "attributes." The ability of a sample to represent a population of interest is important because studying the latter is often difficult if not impossible. The target population might be so large as to preclude collecting data on each and every element (unit within a population) or there may be economic or time constraints that make doing so impractical. As a viable option, one can elect to study a sample presumed to represent the population. For example, in a study to examine the role of speech perception training in the correction of phonological errors, Rvachew (1994) randomly assigned preschoolers with phonological impairment (misarticulated /s/) to one of three groups involving various clinical treatments. In summarizing the results of her investigation, she concluded that ". . . this study demonstrates that interpersonal speech perception training can facilitate sound production learning for some children who are phonologically impaired." Rvachew's belief in the generalizability of her findings from a limited number of children to a larger population of similar children was reflected in her concluding statement,

> Although further research is required, some suggestions for clinical application of this approach can be made on the basis of the currently available information . . . Speech perception training should *probably* [ital. added] be provided concurrently with speech production training. (p. 355)

Rvachew's conclusion is indicative of having inductively inferred certain results to a *population* of children based on a *sample* of children who were believed to be representative of the population as a whole. The use of the word "probably" in Rvachew's concluding statement implies that consideration was given to the statistical probability of being wrong—one can not be sure that *all* children with such a pattern of phonological errors will respond to the treatment(s) found effective even though a significant number are predicted to respond favorably.

Random Assignment versus Random Selection

Rvachew's experiment is representative of a **random assignment** design in which an effort is made to form comparable groups prior to treatment. Random assignment is to be distinguished from **random selection** procedures. The goal of random assignment is simply to establish equivalent groups by balancing subject characteristics on the basis of the available subject pool. On the other hand, random selection involves drawing observations from a population defined as all members of any well-defined class of people, events, or objects in such a way that each observation has an equal chance of being represented (Kerlinger, 1973).

Types of Populations

In many investigations, there are actually two types of populations that an experimenter might wish to represent. First, there is an *infinite* number of observations that could conceivably be made in reference to certain populations of persons, objects, or events under specified conditions. Hypothetically, such a population is without limit, consisting of all possible observations of interest. For example, in the experiment discussed previously, an infinite population of preschoolers with /s/ misarticulations would consist of all similar children who could conceivably be subjected to the same treatment conditions. By definition, such a population must be conceptualized in *ideal* rather than *actual* terms because the probability that all possible members of a population could ever be studied is negligible. Furthermore, even if it were possible to accomplish, few investigators would undertake such an enormous task.

A second type of population can be defined in *finite* terms based on the number of individuals, objects, or events that are known to actually exist at a given time. It is the subset of an infinite population that is accessible for study. For example, such a population might consist of all preschool children with a particular type of phonological disorder living in a certain town or school district from which a smaller sample of children might be taken.

RANDOM SAMPLING METHODS

Random sampling methods are designed to eliminate or reduce systematic bias in the selection of subjects that otherwise might limit the generality of research findings (see Figure 5-1). Nonrepresentative samples can limit the ability of an investigator to form inferences that are internally and externally valid.

An **internally valid inference** is one in which the characteristic being studied in a particular sample can be generalized because it accurately represents the phenomenon of interest—say that the feature of specific language impairment (SLI) under investigation is indeed characteristic of this problem and not of a more global language disability. An **externally valid inference** is one that can be generalized from the sample to the finite population and, hopefully, to the infinite population as well. Conclusions about the validity of the latter inference are somewhat more subjective than the former. This is because, by definition, the complete set of people in the world presumed to illustrate a specified characteristic(s) is more geographically and temporally remote from the site of the investigation. As the distance between people increases geographically, you can be less and less sure they share the same demographic characteristics.

Several alternative methods are available for drawing a random sample so that it is representative of a given population. Four of these methods are discussed here.

Simple Random Sampling

There are two basic assumptions underlying a sampling approach called **simple random sampling** or, less commonly, *unrestricted random sampling*. First, each member of a population must have an equal chance of being selected. Second, one's chance for inclusion must not be diminished as the consequence of other individuals having been selected. Given these conditions, the probability of each element of a population being selected for study can be easily

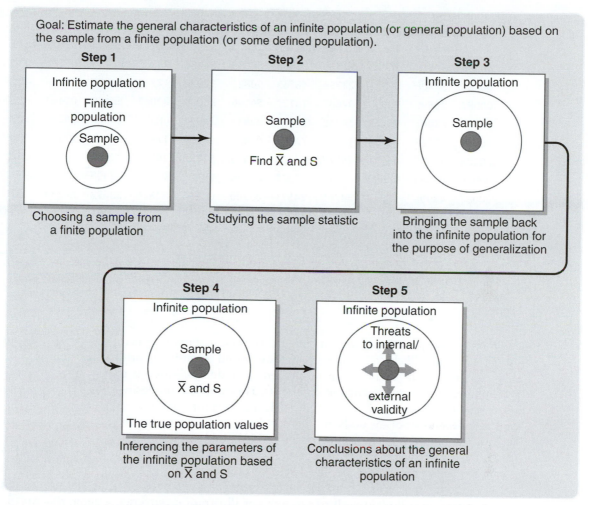

FIGURE 5-1   Steps in estimating a population parameter from a sample statistic. (Symbols $\bar{X}$ and S represent the mean and standard deviation, respectively.)

calculated. For example, given the wish of an investigator to obtain a sample of 300 people to survey from a population of 15,000, then the probability for selection of the sample is 300/15,000 or .02. This same probability would hold true for every person in the population.

One well known way for obtaining such a sample is the "hat technique," in which the names of all members of a population are written on individual slips (or more conveniently coded by numbers) and then drawn one by one from the hat or some other container after being thoroughly mixed. Each name or number would be returned after every draw in order to maintain equal probabilities for being chosen throughout the selection process until a sample of the desired size has been obtained. Failure to do may unwittingly bias the selection process. Another potential problem with pulling names or numbers out of the hat written on slips of paper relates to the order in which they were first put in the hat. Unless thoroughly

TABLE 5-1   Subset of Random Numbers

				Row Number					
00080	59580	06478	75569	78800	88835	54486	23768	06156	04111	08408
00081	38508	07341	23793	48763	90822	97022	17719	04207	95954	49953
00082	30692	70668	94688	16127	56196	80091	82067	63400	05462	69200
00083	65443	95659	18238	27437	49632	24041	08337	65676	96299	90836
00084	27267	50264	13192	72294	07477	44606	17985	48911	97341	30358
00085	91307	06991	19072	24210	36699	53728	28825	35793	28976	66252
00086	68434	94688	84473	13622	62126	98408	12843	82590	09815	93146
00087	48908	15877	54745	24591	35700	04754	83824	52692	54130	55160
00088	06913	45197	42672	78601	11883	09528	63011	98901	14974	40344
00089	10455	16019	14210	33712	91342	37821	88325	80851	43667	70883

Reprinted from *Basic Behavioral Statistics*, by D. E. Hinkle, W. Wiersma, and S. G. Jurs, 1982, Table 12, p. 387. Boston: Houghton Mifflin Company. Used with permission.

mixed—a subjective judgment at best—the slips located in the uppermost layers (those put in last) are more likely to be picked than those found toward the bottom (those put in first).

A more valid and convenient method of random selection is to use a table of random numbers available in many statistical texts. The numbers composing such lists are computer generated using special equations so that the odds for each number's placement in the list are independent of the odds for the preceding and following number. An example subset of random numbers taken from a random number table is shown in Table 5-1.

Suppose you are interested in randomly selecting children for audiometric screening in an elementary school system. The first step would be to clearly define the specific population of interest. Do you wish to sample all grades or a particular grade level? What proportion of the population do you wish to sample? For illustration purposes, assume that you have decided to limit your population to Grades 1–3, for which you have a list containing 90 names. You wish to evaluate one-third, or 30, of these children. The second step would entail assigning consecutive numbers to each member of the population. The third and final step would entail the actual use of the table in order to obtain a random sample of 30 children. The actual steps in using a random number table are illustrated below.

1. Close your eyes and bring the point of a pencil down at a place on the page chosen arbitrarily (see Table 5-1). Assume further that your pencil points to the third set of numbers in row number 00084, namely, 50264.
2. Proceed to select numbers in either a horizontal direction (rows) or a vertical direction (columns) as long as the direction does not change. Imagine that you have decided to proceed down the column in which 50264 is found.
3. Proceed to move down the column attending to only the first two numbers listed for each of the five-number digit sets. Only the first two digits of the number sets will be needed to meet our selection requirements of 30 subjects to be selected from the 90 names that constitute our sampling frame. Duplicate numbers and any number set exceeding 90 will be ignored.

4. The first number found in the column that can be used for selection purposes, to repeat, is 50264. However, as noted above, only the first two digits of this number is required for selecting a name for participation, namely, the 50th name on the list.
5. Repeat step four until you have randomly selected 30 names on the list. The first 10 randomly selected numbers used for this purpose are shown below:

Subject #:	Subject #:
50	75
06	23
15	18
45	13
16	19

Remember that the number of digits used depends on the number of subjects to be selected from a particular **sampling frame,** defined as a full listing of all subjects in a targeted population one wishes to sample. In the case of our example, the sampling frame consisted of 90 students from which the actual sample of 30 students was drawn. Had we wished to randomly select one hundred or more subjects from the sampling frame, we would have elected to use three-digit rather two-digit numbers while proceeding in the same manner as described.

Despite its moniker, "simple random sampling," to call this strategy *simple* can be highly misleading. This is because obtaining such samples from lists comprising relatively large populations can be difficult if not impossible. As Babbie (1990) observed, it is rarely the case that every element has a chance of being selected. This is due to the fact that lists compiled specifically for sampling purposes are seldom complete. Thus, an important caveat to remember is that a list of elements comprising a population can be viewed as *representative* of its members only so far as the list is complete. If incomplete, an effort should be made to locate and sample the unlisted members to the greatest extent possible. Having achieved this goal, still further difficulty may be encountered in assuring that the probability for selecting each listed element is equal. Accomplishing this task for a large population can be burdensome. Still another possible disadvantage is that this strategy cannot be used when an investigator wishes to sample more than one variable at a time. Because of the limitations described above, simple random sampling is not often employed for purposes of research.

Systematic Sampling

Another type of sampling method that may be viewed as an extension of simple random sampling is called **systematic sampling.** This strategy is a parsimonious way of drawing a sample from a large population when a membership list is available. For example, in a study designed to survey the attitudes of ASHA members toward some professional issue, every tenth name appearing in the membership directory could be selected.

In using this technique, investigators need to be wary of the potential danger of using a sampling interval that varies in some preordained fashion. If the ASHA directory was arranged so that every tenth name listed was a male, the survey might yield a very distorted view of the issue under study.

One means of reducing the possibility of some bias introducing an unwanted influence in sampling is to use a randomization procedure for deciding where in the list to begin the selection process. For example, if there are 30 names on the first page of the directory, use a random number table as described previously to select the name of the first person to be surveyed. Thereafter, use a **sampling interval** (the standard distance between the elements in a list) as a basis for inclusion in the sample. A mathematical means for this determination is by the following calculation:

- $K^{th} = N/n$, where K^{th} is the size of the sampling interval we wish to determine
- N is the size of the population
- n is the desired size of the sample

Suppose our desire is to study 100 (n) people selected from a population of 5000 (N), then $K^{th} = 5000/100 = 50$. Thus, you would randomly enter the list as noted above and select a number between 1 and 5000. Next, after a random start, you would select every 50th name on the list to include in your sample. However, it is important to recognize that the sequence of elements in a list may be affected by **periodicity.** This can occur if the elements in the list are arranged in a cyclical manner or particular pattern that might bias the outcome. Given the example above, such bias would operate if every 50th name on the ASHA list happened to be male, or Hispanic, or a new member, or whatever.

As noted, systematic sampling is usually a more convenient means of obtaining a sample of subjects for study when the population parameter is large. Consequently, it is commonly used in survey research. For studies in which the population to be sampled is relatively small, as in the majority of clinical studies, systematic sampling "offers no logistic advantage over simple random sampling, and in clinical research it is rarely a better choice" (Hulley et al., 1988, p. 24). Moreover, it should be remembered that the only random aspect of systematic sampling is the random start entailing the initial selection of an element on a list. Once selected, the remainder of the selection process is predetermined by a standard sampling interval.

Stratified Sampling

Still another form of sampling is called **stratified sampling.** This technique involves dividing a population into subgroups called *strata* in order to assure that certain segments of the population are adequately represented in a sample. By achieving this goal, stratified sampling can ensure a greater degree of representativeness than either simple random sampling or systematic sampling.

Suppose that in surveying ASHA membership attitudes regarding some issue, we wanted to assure adequate representation according to the factor of gender. For purposes of illustration, let us further assume that we learn that the professional membership is approximately 80% female and 20% male. Given this knowledge, we decide that we want our sample to represent this same gender proportion. One way to accomplish such a sampling distribution is to divide the population into two groups and then randomly select four females for every male using a random numbers table. This particular strategy is designed to proportionately represent elements of a population as these elements are found in the world or to create what has been called a "miniature of the population" (Kish, 1965). The same stratified random sampling procedure could be used to assure adequate representation of age, race, employment setting, and specialty area, among other factors. When the number of such stratified variables is large, it is often necessary to increase the size of the sample substantially to satisfy the minimum number of subjects that an investigator might wish to have in each category.

In cases where each variable sampled is to be independently examined, different sampling strategies may be employed. For example, simple random sampling might be employed for one or more category of variables and stratified sampling for other categories. When the sampling distribution involves a continuous variable (e.g., age) as opposed to a dichotomous variable (e.g., gender), the specific cutoff point for designating particular strata may be difficult to determine. For a discussion of the problems associated with the stratification of continuous variables, see Cochran (1977) and Jaeger (1984).

Cluster Sampling

In order to expedite the efficiency of data collection, **cluster sampling** may also be used in some combination with any of the sampling techniques mentioned above. Cluster sampling typically involves a multistage procedure in which smaller samples are selected from larger units or clusters. Referring once again to our attitudinal study of the ASHA membership, we might decide to conduct an area sampling survey in clusters of people based on geographical location. For example, using simple random selection procedures discussed earlier, we might initially select a predetermined number of states. Based on the states randomly selected (clusters), we would then randomly select from the appropriate geographical listings in an ASHA directory the desired number of names necessary for purposes of the survey. As noted previously, this could be done in combination with other sampling techniques. Although the use of clusters can reduce the time, effort, and expense involved in sampling, the risk for bias or sampling error can be relatively high, particularly when a small number of clusters are used. Thus, to optimize representativeness in sampling, the researcher should strive to form clusters that are as heterogeneous as possible.

A method for assuring that each element within a cluster has an equal chance for selection, regardless of cluster size, is called **probability proportionate to size (PPS) sampling.** According to Babbie (1990), the advantages of this method is that it provides for the sampling of more clusters, ensures that the elements contained within large clusters are represented, and equalizes the chance of selection of each element in the population. The probability for selecting a given element in PPS design may be calculated by the following formulae:

$$\frac{\text{Element}}{\text{probability}} = \frac{\text{Number of clusters}}{\text{selected}} \times \frac{\text{Cluster size}}{\text{Population size}} \times \frac{\text{Elements selected per cluster}}{\text{Cluster size}}$$

Thus, in our study of ASHA membership attitudes, let's assume that 20 states (clusters) are randomly selected for study with 100 elements (people) to be randomly drawn from each. Of these states, those with more people are likely to have more ASHA members than those with fewer people. How can we equate the probability for selection given the above formulae? For purposes of illustration, let us compare the results for California with Wyoming, assuming that these states were two of the twenty clusters randomly selected. Now we know that the *number of clusters selected* = 20, and *elements selected per cluster* = 100. As shown in Table 5-2, in California *cluster size* = 8683, and *population size* = 104,273. Thus, *element probability* is calculated as follows:

$$20 \times \frac{8683}{104273} \times \frac{100}{8683} = .01918 \text{ or } 1.918\%$$

Similarly, *element probability* for Wyoming is determined as follows:

$$20 \times \frac{225}{104273} \times \frac{100}{225} = .01918 \text{ or } 1.918\%$$

As shown above, regardless of the cluster size, element probability for California is equal to that for Wyoming. This calculation demonstrates that each of the elements in the population, regardless of the number within a particular cluster, have an equal probability for selection.

TABLE 5-2   Number of ASHA Members from California and Wyoming

ASHA Members (as of August, 2003)	
California	8683
Wyoming	225
Total population	104273

Cluster sampling is a convenient means of obtaining information, particularly from large-scale surveys of geographically diverse populations in which lists of the elements of the population are unavailable. However, a potential disadvantage is that this strategy is subject to a greater degree of sampling error than is simple random sampling or systematic sampling. This is because clusters of elements are by their very nature relatively homogeneous (i.e., people who live closer together are more similar in their demographic characteristics and cultural values than those living far apart). Therefore, in using this particular sampling strategy, investigators should sample as many clusters as possible in an effort to avoid underrepresenting various groups.

NONRANDOM SAMPLING METHODS

The sampling methods discussed thus far have involved random sampling procedures designed to distribute extraneous influences in a chance fashion that might otherwise produce differences between groups or treatments unrelated to the independent variable. Several other types of sampling techniques may be used in research studies, but their scientific application is more limited.

Consecutive Sampling

This technique involves selecting all individuals who agree to participate, provided they meet pre-established criteria, until the number of subjects desired has been recruited. For example, an author of this text once conducted a study of the verbal memory of adult dyslexics who were recruited by means of several techniques including appeals through newspaper and radio advertising. In order to qualify as subjects, several criteria had to be satisfied with respect to age, IQ level, educational achievement, history of remediation, mental and physical status, and scores on standardized tests of reading ability, among other factors.

Consecutive sampling can be highly useful when the available subject pool is limited or when using selection criteria so stringent as to reduce the number of subjects to a point that threatens the generality of findings. Although consecutive sampling methods are typically stronger than other nonprobability methods in controlling sampling bias, such confounding influence cannot be ruled out. **Response rate,** the proportion of subjects willing to participate of those selected, may also influence the validity of inferences. For instance, subjects who agree to participate may have different motivations or life circumstances than those who do not. Such bias can result in a nonrepresentative sample.

Convenience Sampling

Convenience sampling, sometimes called *"on-the-street"* or *opportunistic sampling,* is another technique commonly used by the media to poll attitudes or opinions about current events. Often, the general public may be invited to write or telephone to express their opinion about a particular issue. Obviously, such survey data is potentially fraught with bias because of the restricted pool of respondents who may *just happen* to be available at a given time.

Purposive Sampling

A third type of nonrandom sampling is variously called *purposive, judgment,* or *quota sampling.* Here, a smaller group of "key" individuals are targeted to focus or represent the attitudes, interests, or attributes of a larger group. In such a case, the researcher deliberately selects certain respondents based on knowledge of their characteristics. For example, one might make judgments about the suitability of recognized authorities in a particular field to summarize current clinical or research trends. This type of sampling is also used in the study of relatively infrequent phenomena such as rare genetic diseases or disorders as existing in individuals judged to be representative of the problem.

An advantage of purposive sampling is that a sample of subjects can be created that appears to have the major characteristics that an investigator wishes to study. Moreover, a quota of such people may be established so as to mirror or replicate the proportion of such characteristics found in the targeted population. For example, it might be predetermined that a certain percentage will have to be of a particular race, gender, age, socioeconomic status, and the like. Once the key characteristics are identified, sampling can proceed without having a population list.

A disadvantage of purposive sampling is that it is prone to the kind of biases that can result in an unrepresentative sample. We always must keep in mind that "appearances can be deceiving." Handpicking individuals because they *look* appropriate may be flawed by an investigator's personal prejudices or misperceptions in judgment. For example, certain subjects might be chosen because they seem to be especially motivated to participate or merely because of their greater accessibility. Furthermore, in the case of quota sampling, merely assuring that African-Americans or some other race represents a predetermined percentage of a sample will not assure adequate representation of their attitude, level of income, educational achievement, or any other population characteristic. As with other types of nonrandom sampling procedures, the generality of purposive samples may suffer if they fail to adequately represent the population as intended.

Snowball Sampling

Snowballing is a useful technique for recruiting a sample of subjects when an investigator has limited contact with a targeted population. In such cases, one or more identified participants can be asked to identify others in the population as prospective candidates for study. Through the use of such personal networks, the sample can be made to "snowball" or increase in size. For example, a client who stutters and happens to belong to a support group or knows other people who stutter might be asked to "spread the word." An obvious disadvantage of this strategy is that the network(s) sampled may not be representative of the larger population, thereby limiting the generalizability of findings.

Matched Samples

Another type of nonprobability sampling procedure used to establish equivalent groups in an experiment is called **matching.** Matching is a control procedure designed to restrict the degree to which subjects in different groups are allowed to differ by pairing them according to particular characteristics. Matching is frequently used in cases in which randomization is not possible or in experiments where the number of available subjects is so few that random selection and assignment cannot be trusted to achieve equivalent groups representative of the population.

Quasi-experimental designs commonly match subjects on key characteristics that are likely to exert some unintended systematic influence on the dependent variable over and above that intended by the independent variable under investigation (see Chapter 8). For example, in clinical studies designed to improve various aspects of language ability, subjects assigned to different groups are often matched on the basis of verbal intelligence factors in an effort to balance such potential mitigating influences. Such variables as age, gender, socioeconomic status, physical and emotional status, type and severity of disorder, and so on are among those frequently used in matching subjects to reduce potential between-group bias. To do so may be especially important when a researcher knows in advance that such pre-existing extraneous factors may impact the dependent variable. Indeed, this is essential for detecting a statistically significant difference between an experimental and control group that can be specifically attributed to the influence of treatment as opposed to some extraneous factor. For further information about how the data from experiments involving matched subjects is statistically analyzed see Chapter 12.

Blocking

Although matching techniques are often used in place of randomization, one procedure does not necessarily exclude the use of the other. Indeed, the strength of a design can be augmented by a combination of these methods. Liebert and Liebert (1995) described matched random assignment procedures, sometimes called **blocking,** as involving three steps:

1. Rank order the subjects on the variable for which control is desired.
2. Segregate the subjects into matched pairs (blocks) so that each pair member has approximately the same score on the variable to be matched.
3. Randomly assign pair members to the conditions of the experiment.

Blocking can also serve as an effective way to control for extraneous variables involving differences in subject characteristics by including them in the research design. For example, suppose the researcher wishes to know how gender might influence the outcome of a study involving a particular language development program designed to facilitate vocabulary development. In such a case, gender could be included as a second independent variable with two *levels* of analysis—male and female. After dividing the subjects into two groups based on gender, they would then be randomly assigned to the treatment conditions of the experiment as described above. This method, which allows for an analysis of particular subject attributes on a dependent variable, is called a **randomized block design** (see Chapter 8). In addition to a single attribute, various combinations of attributes (e.g., gender, age, intelligence, socioeconomic status, etc.) can be blocked, analyzed, and interpreted using this approach.

When matching procedures are used, they should be carried out on an *a priori* basis (i.e., before the actual treatments are administered). In cases in which the independent variable cannot be manipulated because the phenomenon of interest has already occurred, efforts to match individuals *ex post facto* (after the fact) can lead to serious errors in interpreting research findings. Conceivably, this could invalidate a case study of some communication disorder in which the investigator is looking to establish the relation between a certain predictor variable and currently manifested symptoms. Suppose we wish to examine the factor of age in relation to recovery of language in aphasia resulting from head trauma. After carefully matching subjects on the basis of the loci and severity of brain damage as determined from preexisting records, we conclude on the basis of current test results that the degree of language recovery is greater for children and adolescents than for middle aged and older adults. Such findings are explained on the basis of differences in brain plasticity—the ability of new brain regions to acquire functional abilities previously subsumed by others. However, such a conclusion is unwarranted because of the possible confounding influence of a third variable that is impossible to isolate on the basis of hindsight. Between-group differences in motivation, intelligence, type and extent of therapy, availability of family support systems, and pattern of recovery over time are but a few of the extraneous factors that might have influenced the outcome. Trying to second guess (ex post facto) which of these or other factors might have played a role in recovery, and thereby matching subjects accordingly in an effort to control potential confounding influences, is usually a waste of effort.

SELECTION BIAS AND SAMPLING ERROR

Various errors associated with the selection of subjects may undermine the validity of research investigation because of their biasing influences. With respect to selecting subjects, a **selection bias** may be defined as any variable that confounds the ability of chosen sample to represent the population parameter from which the sample was drawn. Selection biases result in systematic errors that cause the scores in a sampling distribution to lean more in one direction than another. Such errors are due to human or man-made influences that are known or unknown and are observed to occur in a lawful or predictable manner rather than in a random fashion (Kerlinger, 1986). Examples of such errors include those that stem from the unreliability of human observations. As we noted previously, there is a danger that the personal biases of an investigator, whether conscious or unconscious, may adversely influence sampling decisions. Other sources of error may result from inaccuracies in measurements or in the recording and coding of data that may result in a misclassification of subjects. While all such errors due to selection bias may adversely influence the sampling process, they are to be distinguished from what are commonly called errors in sampling. The latter type of error is best viewed as the degree to which a sample variable differs from the same variable as found in the population, due to random or chance factors alone. One should remember that such deviations are normally expected and are not due to mistakes on the part of the investigator.

Even if all sources of selection bias could be eliminated or effectively controlled, the characteristics of any one sample will not match exactly those found in the population. Perfect replication of a population parameter is highly improbable or impossible to achieve. For example, consider the population mean score for IQ, which is 100 on such tests as the Wechsler or the Standard Binet based on testing thousands of people. Now assume that you randomly select 20 samples for IQ testing, each consisting of 50 adults. Calculating the sample means for individual IQ scores within each of the 20 distributions, you find that the majority of them cluster around the population mean of 100, but some sample means may be considerable above or below the population mean. This distribution of means is called the **sampling distribution of the mean(s)** (see Chapter 12).

As a matter of practice, researchers do not generally draw numerous samples to estimate how a sample statistic varies from the population parameter. To engage in such a time-consuming and laborious task would defeat the purpose of sampling. Instead, probability theory can be used to determine how well a single mean is able to statistically estimate its population parameter. Determining the size of a sampling error (also called the *standard error of the mean*) is an important aspect of many statistical calculations used for determining the significance of research finding (see Chapter 12). Given our example of intelligence, it is sufficient to say that all of the sample mean scores would have had to have been exactly 100 for no sampling error to have occurred.

Minimizing Selection Bias and Sampling Errors

Ultimately, researchers hope to minimize errors in selecting subjects for a study to the greatest degree possible. Errors resulting from selection biases can best be dealt with by controlling confounding variables of the type previously described. Human capriciousness involving the attitudes, perceptions, and expectations of researchers or clinicians can be controlled to a large extent by using and adhering to well defined **inclusion criteria** that specify the age, gender, clinical characteristics, and the like of subjects. Likewise, thought should be given to **exclusion criteria** that will effectively eliminate unwanted individuals with the type of characteristics (e.g., certain psychological or physical impairments) that might bias a sample. When various tests or measurements are used to determine inclusion or exclusion criteria, make sure they are appropriate for the task and that the results are accurate and recorded correctly.

Also, be aware that the motives, values, and attitudes of persons who volunteer to participate in a study may differ substantially from those who do not. Based on this understanding, the reasons why people choose to participate may need to be evaluated.

In survey studies, it is often the case that the lower the rate of return of answered questionnaires, the greater the probability for biased results (see Chapter 9). This is because the respondents may have defining characteristics such as age, sex, occupation, education, and so forth that are not only different from nonresponders but also concentrated to a greater degree and of a type that might have a stronger impact in a smaller than in a larger sample.

One type of selection bias that is especially serious, perhaps due to naivety yet bordering on a breach of research ethics, is to examine the sample results of a study in progress, accepting those results that conform to a particular hypothesis while discarding those which do not. By discarding unfavorable results while continuing to draw a new sample, an investigator could bias the findings in any manner desired. Such a practice is tantamount to a fisherman, partial to a certain size or type of fish, throwing a less appealing catch back into the sea while continuing to bait the hook. This is not to imply that an investigator should refrain from examining a sample result that might have resulted from some form of measurement error and taking steps to eliminate the source of such errors as indicated. However, such corrections in sampling or in other methods of a study are best corrected before a study begins—not after the fact. Perhaps the most effective means of doing so is by running a pilot study (see Chapter 3). As noted previously, such a study can be viewed as a "practice run" or "miniexperiment" conducted to identify and correct possible methodological errors in advance of performing an actual investigation. While pilot studies are often an appropriate and useful means of improving the precision of the methods of an investigation, they should not be confused with flagrant and unacceptable forms of "fishing expeditions" as described above.

As we have attempted to make clear, confounding variables of various kinds can unduly bias the process of selecting an appropriate sample and/or assigning the individuals within such a sample to the treatment conditions of an experiment. When used effectively, randomization can guarantee that each element in a population has an opportunity for selection or assignment equal to all other elements. For this reason, probability sampling methods are likely to have greater fidelity in representing an observed phenomenon than nonprobability sampling strategies that are prone to selection biases of the kind discussed.

Despite the obvious advantages of probability sampling in achieving a representative sample and negating the influence of extraneous variables, there are some limitations in the assumptions underlying the use of such methods. For one thing, the assumption that the *process* of randomization (method used) has actually achieved its *intended result* (attainment

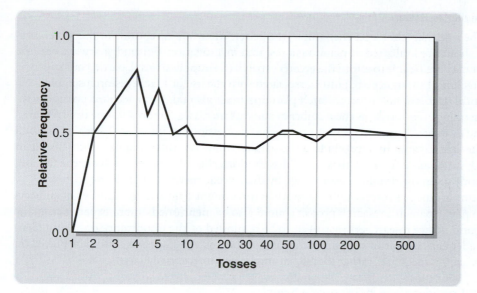

FIGURE 5-2

Given any number of coin tosses, the relative frequency of heads may differ from one-half but will approach this value in the long-run

Reprinted with permission from A Review of Biostatistics: A Program for Self-instruction *(4th ed), by P.E. Leaverton, 1991, Boston: Little Brown and Company.*

of randomness) is always open to question. As previously noted, the best we can do is to calculate the probability for such a result given the size of the sample.

When Bigger Is Better

According to Pedhazur and Schmelkin (1991), "Issues concerning sample size are germane to both random selection and random assignment" (p. 336). A sufficient number of observations must be incorporated within a sample to give randomization "a chance to work." If the sample size is too small, it may not be representative of a population.

Generally, it can be said that the larger the sample used in an investigation, the more accurate will be the estimate of the standard error (the smaller such an error is likely to be). This understanding is based on the so-called **Bernoulli theorem,** formulated by James Bernoulli in the eighteenth century. According to this theorem, the relative frequency of an observed event will approximate its probable frequency of future occurrence if observed over an indefinitely long series of trials. Stated differently, the more you observe a particular event, the more accurately you can judge the frequency of its future occurrence. This is why professional card-counting blackjack players may observe the game for a long time before joining the action.

To understand the Bernoulli theorem in more concrete terms, imagine that you are asked to determine the probability of a tossed coin turning up heads. In theory, provided that the coin is fair (unbiased), the probability of its turning up heads is 50%. Furthermore, the mathematical likelihood of the coin turning up heads will get closer and closer to 50% as the number of tosses increases. Thus, 5 tosses will typically yield results that conform to the expected outcome more often than 1 toss, 10 tosses more often than 5, and so forth (see Figure 5-2). Nevertheless, it is important to understand that such outcomes can be predicted with only relative degrees of confidence. Although improbable, it is still possible that 100 tosses may yield a more equal distribution of heads and tails than, let us say, 500 or more tosses of the same coin. Yet, to reiterate what we said previously, an estimate of a population parameter obtained from a sample statistic will be more accurate when the sample is large than when small. This presumes, of course, that the sample was drawn appropriately.

When Smaller Is Better

Despite the rule that "the larger the sample, the better," there are exceptions to this generalization that should be evaluated in planning a research investigation. For budgetary reasons, the researcher may not be able to afford the greater expense (for supplies, travel, participant stipends, costs for technical assistance, etc.) often associated with the use of a large research sample.

Practical decision making in research planning must also take into account possible temporal constraints. Obviously, as the number of subjects increases, so too does the time required to test and evaluate them in relation to the research questions of interest. Other responsibilities of the investigator may preclude an extensive time commitment. As we discussed in Chapter 3, students completing theses and dissertations should carefully evaluate the feasibility of a study given the deadlines established by their departments and graduate schools.

The importance of forethought as to where one might find a large number of subjects willing to participate in a research project should also be mentioned. In our experience, many students and novice researchers may need to be reminded of the importance of having identified an adequate sample of subjects before a study begins. An emphasis should be placed on finding what is "adequate" rather than what might be unnecessarily large.

Statistical Considerations in Selecting a Sample

Still, the question remains—what constitutes an adequate sample? How large or small should it be? The answer to this problem is influenced by a number of complex issues, some of which relate to *probability theory* and others to the purpose and design of the research study. With respect to the presumed advantage of a large sample over a small sample, McCready (1996) framed the question rhetorically: "After all, isn't bigger better?" He goes on to answer: "Not always!" The crucial question is not, "How big is the sample" but rather, "How are the elements of the sample selected?" (p. 107). In other words, more important than the size of the sample is the degree to which its quality and characteristics approximate those of the population.

Suppose you have a barrel full of apples, some of them red and others shades of yellow and green. If you hope to select a defined sample of red apples while blindfolded, the probability of your doing so will be greater when the proportion of red apples to the other colors is large than when small. The more **homogeneous** (alike) the apples in the barrel (population), the smaller the sample size needed to adequately represent the characteristic of interest. Conversely, the more **heterogeneous** (diverse) the apples in the barrel might be, the larger the sample required for adequate representation of the population. Thus, in choosing the size of a sample, a researcher must decide on the degree of *precision* desired in estimating a population parameter from a sample statistic. Of course, an informed decision can best be made based on knowledge of the variability within the population. The degree of this variability is commonly expressed statistically as the **standard deviation** and is calculated by determining the square root of the variance of all the scores in a distribution from their mean score (see Chapter 11). Nevertheless, as we noted earlier, information pertaining to the true population parameter is usually unavailable. In such cases, the sample standard deviation can be used to estimate the population standard deviation when calculating the standard error.

The standard error is incorporated into several different formulas for estimating the sample size needed to detect a significant finding, thereby avoiding statistical errors associated with hypothesis testing. As we discuss in Chapter 12, when sample size is excessively large, there is a danger in a test detecting a statistically significant result due to chance alone or to an otherwise quite trivial result lacking practical value (type I error). On the other hand, in cases where the sample size is very small, the power of a statistical test may be too slight to detect a significant effect when present (type II error).

In Appendix A-3, we provide a detailed discussion of a statistical method called **power analysis** for estimating both the size of a sample needed for a research study and the probability for committing a type II error. Power analysis allows for a consideration of the so-called **effect size** which, according to Cohen (1988), is the measure of "the degree to which the phenomenon is present in the population . . . or the degree to which the null hypothesis is false" (pp. 9–10). Meanwhile, you need only remember that when the expected differences between two or more groups in response to some treatment is large, relatively small samples may be adequate to reveal that such differences are statistically significant. On the other hand, in cases where only small between-group differences are predicted, large samples are more likely needed to uncover statistical significance.

Sampling and the Generalization of Findings

The main goal of sampling is to accurately represent a particular quality or characteristic as it exists in the population to the greatest extent possible. This is done with the hope of generalizing one's findings about the sample to the population. To the extent this is possible, the results can be assumed to be externally valid. Gay (1995) has proposed the following guidelines in deciding the size of a sample based on the type of study-design employed:

1. When the study is essentially descriptive in nature, as in a survey study, 10–20 percent of the population should be sampled, depending on the population size.
2. In the case of a correlational study seeking to establish associative relations between variables, the sample should include a minimum of 30 subjects.
3. Studies that entail a search for causal relationships by comparing groups on some treatment effect should include 30 subjects per group. It is noteworthy that the sampling distribution for group means approximates that of a normal curve for sample sizes of 30 or more subjects even when the population parameter is skewed (see Chapter 12).
4. In experimental studies that are well designed to exclude or control confounding variables, 15 subjects per group might constitute an adequate sample. In such cases, we recommend that the researcher demonstrate that the group variances are relatively equal. (See Chapter 12 for a discussion of the importance of establishing *homogeneity of variance*.)

In addition to using these statistical guidelines for determining sample size, you might also wish to use existing literature as a guide. McCready (1996) has recommended that relevant research projects completed in the past three years or so be reviewed for such guidance. He further advised beginning researchers to use the mean sample size of these studies as a pragmatic basis for establishing the size of one's own sample.

SUMMARY

In this chapter, we discussed some of the major theoretical principles and processes that underlie the selection of a subset of a population for inclusion in a research study. We noted that ideally such a sample should be drawn in a manner as to allow for it to truly represent the targeted population. In an effort to achieve this goal, various sampling methods are available for use. The best of these for eliminating or reducing bias and strengthening the validity of our inferences include various random (probability) sampling methods. We discussed some of the strengths and limitations of simple random sampling, systematic sampling, stratified sampling, and cluster sampling.

When a researcher is unable to determine the probability for inclusion of the elements of a population in the study sample, nonrandom sampling methods are used. Although the use of such methods may be necessary, they do not permit inferences about how representative the sample is of the population from which it was drawn. Another limitation of such methods is that their use precludes calculating estimates of the sampling error and, therefore, may violate some of the statistical assumptions pertaining to the analysis of sample data. Despite such limitations, nonrandom sampling procedures are used in many research investigations when random samples are unavailable or impossible to obtain. Nonrandom methods discussed in this chapter included consecutive sampling, convenience sampling, purposive sampling, snowballing, matched samples, and blocking.

Finally, we discussed several sources of selection bias and sampling errors associated with the selection of study samples and their statistical implications. In this context, issues germane to making decisions about sample size and how such decisions can impact the generalizability of the results obtained from a sample were likewise reviewed.

KEY TERMS

population
elements
parameter
sample
representative
statistic
target population
sampling error
random assignment
random selection
internally valid inference
externally valid inference
simple random sampling
sampling frame
systematic sampling
sampling interval
periodicity
stratified sampling
cluster sampling

probability proportionate to size (PPS) sampling
response rate
convenience sampling
snowballing
matching
blocking
randomized block design
selection bias
sampling distribution of the mean(s)
inclusion criteria
exclusion criteria
Bernoulli theorem
homogeneous
heterogeneous
standard deviation
power analysis
effect size

SELF-LEARNING REVIEW

1. Researchers and statisticians use the term _____ to describe an all-inclusive data set about which they wish to draw a conclusion or _____ _____. The term encompasses a large collection of animate or inanimate _____ that share common attributes.

2. A(n) _____ is a number or measured characteristic derived from the entire population. A(n) _____ is a number derived from counting or measuring sample observations that have been drawn from a population of numbers.

3. A(n) _____ _____ can be defined as the population to which the investigator wishes to generalize. In doing so, the investigator must expect a certain degree of _____ _____. More specifically, it can be defined as the expected amount of variance owing to _____ chance.

4. The goal of _____ _____ is to establish equivalent groups by balancing subject characteristics on the basis of the available subject pool.

5. An infinite population must be conceptualized in _____ rather than _____ terms because the probability that all possible members of a population could ever be studied is negligible.

6. A(n) _____ _____ _____ is one in which the characteristic being studied in a particular sample can be generalized because it accurately represents the phenomenon of interest. On the other hand, a(n) _____ _____ _____ is one that can be generalized from the sample to the finite and infinite populations.

7. There are two basic assumptions underlying a sampling approach called simple random sampling: (1) each number of the population must have a(n) _____ _____ of being selected, and (2) one's chance for inclusion must not be reduced because of others having been _____. Given the wish of an investigator to obtain a sample of 500 people to survey from a population of 20,000, then the probability for selection of the sample is _____.

8. The use of a random number table depends on the number of subjects to be selected from a _____ _____, defined as a full listing of all subjects in a(n) _____ population that one wishes to sample.

9. _____ sampling is a parsimonious way of drawing a sample from a large population when a membership is available.

10. The standard distance between the elements in a list is called a(n) _____ _____. A mathematical means for this determination is by the following calculation: Given N is the population size and n is the sample size, the size of the standard distance to be determined, denoted by K^{th}, is calculated as $K^{th} = $ _____; Suppose, we wish to study 200 people selected from a population of 4000, then $K^{th} = $ _____. Thus, you would randomly enter the list, selecting a number between _____ and _____. After that _____ start, you would select every _____ member of the list to include in your sample.

11. _____ can occur if the elements in the list are arranged in a cyclical manner or particular pattern that might bias the outcome.

12. _____ sampling techniques involve dividing a population into subgroups called _____ in order to assure that certain segments of the population are adequately represented in a sample.

13. _____ sampling involves a multistage procedure in which smaller samples are selected from larger units.

14. A method for assuring that each element within a cluster has an equal chance for selection, regardless of cluster size is called _____ _____ _____ _____ sampling, or simple _____ sampling. The probability for selecting a given element in this design may be calculated by the formula as follows: Element probability = _____ × _____ × _____.

15. Given that the number of clusters selected = 15, cluster size = 7000, elements selected per cluster = 200, and population size = 100,000, element probability is equal to _____.

16. A potential disadvantage of cluster sampling is that it is subject to a greater degree of _____ _____ than is simple random sampling or systematic sampling. This is because clusters of elements are _____.

17. _____ sampling technique involves selecting all individuals who agree to participate, provided they meet pre-established criteria, until the number of subjects desired have been recruited. This technique can be highly useful when the available subject pool is _____ or when using selection criteria so _____ as to _____ the number of subjects to a point that threatens the _____ of findings.

18. _____ _____, the proportion of subjects willing to participate to those selected, may influence the _____ of inferences.

19. _____ sampling is the technique commonly used by the media to poll attitudes or opinions about current events.

20. An advantage of _____ sampling is that a sample of subjects can be created that appears to have the major characteristics that an investigator wishes to study. A disadvantage of this sampling technique is that it is prone to the kind of biases that can result in a(n) _____ sample.

21. _____ is a useful technique for recruiting a sample of subjects when an investigator has limited contact with a targeted population.

22. A control procedure designed to restrict the degree to which the subjects in different groups are allowed to differ is called _____.

23. Blocking is a procedure that involves: (1) _____ _____ the subjects, (2) segregating the subjects into _____ _____, and (3) _____ assigning pair members to the conditions of the experiment.

24. Blocking can serve to control for extraneous variables involving _____ in subject characteristics by including them in the research design.

25. Suppose an investigator wishes to know how gender might influence the outcome of a study involving a particular type of fluency disorder. In such a case, gender is included as a(n) _____ variable with two _____ of analysis. After dividing the subjects into two gender groups, they would be _____ assigned to treatment conditions. This method, which allows for an analysis of particular subject attributes of a dependent variable, is called _____ _____ design.

26. When matching procedures are used, they should be carried out on a(n) _____ basis (i.e., before the actual treatment is administered).

27. In cases in which the independent variable cannot be manipulated because the phenomenon of interest has already occurred, efforts to march individuals _____ _____ _____ (after the fact) can lead to serious errors in interpreting research findings.

28. _____ _____ _____ are best viewed as the degree to which a sample variable differs from the same variable as found in the population due to random or _____ factors alone.

29. Human capriciousness involving the attributes of researchers can be controlled to a large extent by using and adhering to well-defined _____ _____ that specify certain characteristics of subjects. Likewise, thought should be given to _____ _____ that will effectively eliminate unwanted individuals with the type of characteristics that might _____ a sample.

30. A(n) _____ _____ can be viewed as a "practice run" or "miniexperiment" conducted to identify and correct possible _____ errors in advance of performing an actual investigation.

31. According to the _____ theorem, the relative frequency of an observed event will approximate its probable frequency of future occurrence if observed over a(n) _____ long series of trials.

32. The more _____ the population is, the _____ the sample size needed to adequately represent the characteristic of interest. The more _____ the population is, the _____ the sample required for adequate representation of the population.

33. In choosing the size of a sample, a researcher must decide on the degree of _____ desired in estimating a population parameter from a(n) _____ _____.

34. Power analysis allows for a consideration of the _____ _____, that is, the measure of the degree to which the phenomenon is present in the population.

35. In deciding the size of a sample based on the type of study and design used, Gay (1995) had suggested: (1) when the study is descriptive, as in a survey study, _____ to _____ percent of the population should be sampled, depending on the population size; (2) in the case of a correlational study, the sample should include a minimum of _____ subjects; (3) studies that entail a search for causal relationships by comparing groups on some treatment effect should include _____ subjects per group; and (4) in experimental studies that are well designed to exclude or control confounding variables, _____ subjects per group constitutes an adequate sample.

QUESTIONS AND EXERCISES FOR CLASSROOM DISCUSSION

1. Distinguish between a population and a sample using an example in the field of communication sciences and disorders.

2. What is the statistical meaning of the term *sampling error?*

3. Distinguish between random selection and random assignment and provide an example of each.

4. Provide an example of an infinite and a finite population. In practice, what is the importance of understanding the difference between them?

5. What are the two types of validity pertaining to the generalization of research findings from a study sample to a population, and which of the two is more limited because of geographic and temporal factors?

6. List four types of random sampling methods. Provide a brief description and example of each.

7. Why are random sampling methods more powerful than nonrandom sampling methods?

8. Distinguish between the terms *selection bias* and *sampling error*. How can these errors be minimized?

9. Discuss the ethical implications of examining the sample results of a study in progress.

10. What is the importance of the Bernoulli theorem to sampling?

11. With respect to sample size, what are the implications of using one that may be too large versus one that may be too small? Discuss two types of statistical errors associated with such choices.

12. Of what relevance is the standard error to calculating sample size?

13. What are four general guidelines that can be used in deciding the size of a sample?

14. Given the example of the attitudinal study of ASHA membership cited previously, assume that 25 states (clusters) are randomly selected with 150 elements (people) to be randomly drawn from each cluster. Using the ASHA Web site (www.asha.org) to locate the distribution of ASHA constituents by state and certificate status, calculate and compare the results of *element probability* for New York and Oregon.

15. Suppose we wish to study the vocabulary development of 30 preschool children selected from a population of 180 such children. Find the sampling interval (K^{th}).

Controlling, Measuring, and Recording Variables

LEARNING OBJECTIVES

After reading this chapter, you should be able to identify, describe, or define:

- Types of variances in a research study
- Methods of controlling errors in a research study
- The utility of measurements
- Concepts of measurement reliability and validity
- Relationship between measurement reliability and validity
- Four common scales of measurement
- Methods of recording behavioral/physiological responses
- Types of response measures

CONTROLLING VARIABLES

In addition to thinking carefully about how to obtain an appropriate sample of subjects, an investigator must also decide how best to regulate or control the variables in a research study so as to arrive at valid and reliable conclusions. We previously defined a variable as any factor capable of assuming different values. Stated somewhat differently, a variable may be generally defined as any attribute of people, objects, or events that is subject to variation.

From the perspective of designing research, a variable is anything having *observable characteristics* that can be described, predicted, or caused to change. Examples of such variables include: age, height, weight, gender, intelligence, anger, aggression, motivation, speech, language, hearing, or even today's weather. As we have repeatedly emphasized, for such constructs to be scientifically useful, they must be operationally defined.

Systematic Variance

In earlier chapters, we noted that studies limited to describing or predicting the attributes of variables are classified as nonexperimental research because no effort is made to explain causal relationships. On the other hand, experimental research seeks to determine how one variable may be "controlled" as to cause a change in another. As discussed in Chapter 2, the variable considered to cause variation in some other variable is called the *independent variable* because it is independent of any influence by the phenomenon under investigation. The *dependent variable* is generally viewed as the measured variation in behavior caused by the independent variable.

Known causes of variation in an experiment are termed **systematic variance (between-group variance).** Variance of this kind is usually reflected in systematic differences between the scores of two groups resulting from the *assignment* or *active manipulation* of independent variables by the experimenter. In the typical experiment, the variance between at least two groups is examined.

If we wish to examine the relative effect of varying amounts of a particular independent variable on the dependent variable, one means of doing so is by assigning individuals possessing different levels of the independent variable to two or more groups. For example, suppose that we wish to investigate systematic variations in stuttering severity in relation to different levels of anxiety. One way to accomplish this would be to divide subjects into two groups consisting of "low anxious" and "high anxious" individuals based on their scores obtained on an anxiety questionnaire such as the Speech Situation Checklist (Brutten, 1975).

Between group variance on measures of stuttering severity, such as those found on the Stuttering Severity Instrument (Riley, 1986) could then be examined. A frequent difficulty surrounding the interpretation of between-group differences based on assignment can result from the so-called **directionality problem.** This problem is associated with the inability of an investigator to determine which of two variables causes a change in the other. With respect to the hypothetical study just discussed, we would be unable to determine whether or not any observed between-group differences in stuttering severity resulted from or was a cause of between-group differences in anxiety. Such problems in determining the causal relations between two variables are discussed further in Chapter 7.

In order to avoid or diminish such "cart before the horse" dilemmas in making causal inferences, many investigators tend to favor a design strategy that allows for the active manipulation of independent variables if possible. Designs that involve the active and systematic manipulation of one or more independent variables are called **controlled experimental studies.** Such experiments allow for a more direct determination of causal relations than do methods that are based solely on the between-group assignment of independent variables according to preexisting subject characteristics. For instance, several studies have explored the relationship between anxiety and stuttering by varying (manipulating) the difficulty of reading tasks or speaking situations while recording changes in autonomic arousal. In the majority of these experiments, no consistent relationship between changes in such anxiety measures as palmar sweating, galvanic skin response, heart rate, or pulse volume and the frequency of stuttering behavior was found (Bloodstein, 1987).

Some independent variables, such as those involving relatively stable physical or psychological characteristics, are not subject to active experimental manipulation. Examples of such **organismic variables** might include age, gender, height, weight, auditory and visual acuity, motor skills, intelligence, memory, and health status. By and large, such intrinsic subject characteristics would be impossible or unethical to alter in human investigations; their influence on dependent variables can be better controlled or investigated through group assignment.

Error Variance

Effective problem solving involves not only the determination of systematic relations among variables but the degree to which random fluctuations in measured observations occur as a result of unidentified and uncontrolled circumstances. In the opening pages to *Moby Dick,* Herman Melville set out to explore the often-hidden and disorderly forces in nature by stating, "The classification of the constituents of chaos, nothing less here is essayed."

Whether and to what extent randomness actually exists in the universe is a continuing debate among scientists. As noted earlier, a primary tenet of science is that the relations among objects and events are causally determined by lawful and orderly processes that are subject to discovery. Given this mind set, the idea that some element of chaos is to be found within the workings of all biological and physical systems is difficult to accept. Nonetheless, researchers are aware that relatively small unsystematic changes in variables, owing to random fluctuations of unknown factors, commonly exist in experiments. Influences that cannot be held constant from subject to subject and that do not systematically favor any one particular treatment over another are *random sources of error.*

One way to think about error variance is that it is the amount of variation that still remains after all known sources of systematic variance have been eliminated (Kerlinger, 1973). Conceptually, tests of the significance of difference between groups, such as the *F* test,

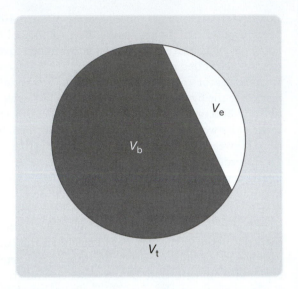

FIGURE 6-1

Total variance constituted of sources of variation between groups, owing to (1) systematic influences (V_b) and (2) unknown causes of uncontrolled influences (V_e). As V_e increases, the between-group variance attributable to systematic influences (shaded area) decreases.

can be defined as the ratio of systematic variance (denoted by V_b) to error variance (denoted by V_e) (see Chapter 12). Symbolically, this ratio can be written as:

$$F = \frac{V_b}{V_e}$$

The larger the denominator (error variance or V_e) in relation to the numerator (systematic variance or V_b), the less likely it would have been that the independent variable produced a true between-group difference (or a true treatment effect). The relationship of systematic variance to error variance is depicted in Figure 6-1.

Sources of systematic variance tend to produce a directional effect in a set of scores—either a measurable increase or decrease in their values. Conversely, sources of error variance can cause scores to fluctuate in a willy-nilly fashion. As noted previously, such residual variance is typically ascribed to random or chance factors.

One possible source of error variance that we previously discussed is *errors in sampling*. As the result of chance alone, the sample result may be higher or lower than for the population as a whole. One should remember that such deviations are normally expected and are not due to experimenters' mistakes.

A second source of uncontrolled variation of the dependent variable can arise from **errors of measurement.** Suppose you wish to compare the voice initiation times of stuttering participants as compared to normal speakers. A means of doing so might entail using a stopwatch to measure the two groups' response latencies in vocalizing the schwa vowel in response to a defined visual or auditory cue that signals the onset of vocalization. In such a study, an important question to raise is to what degree efforts to measure response latency accurately reflect subject performance. Are there any inconsistencies related to errors within the experimenter in starting and stopping the watch? Other errors in measurement might result from instability in the measuring devices themselves.

A third class of error variance can result from **fluctuations in testing conditions.** Imagine that different experimenters are collecting data on different subjects who stutter as noted previously. Variations in scoring *between* experimenters as well as *within* experimenters could account for chance errors of measurement. Other sources of variation in the test conditions such as distracting noises, unwanted interruptions, changes in temperature or lighting, or alterations in the appearance of the test environment are additional examples of uncontrolled variations that might unduly influence the outcome of an experiment. In Chapter 12, statistical procedures will be described that allow us to evaluate the relative influence of systematic variance versus error variance in accounting for the results of an experiment. This evaluation is of great importance for two reasons:

- Significant differences observed between the measured values of two or more groups or treatment conditions can result as the consequence of random sources of error.
- The converse is also possible: the failure to find significant differences can likewise result from random sources of error.

Sources of Variance

Two major sources of variance must be calculated in any experiment. As noted previously, the first of these are the effects of systematic influences that contribute to *between-group variance*. The second source involves **within-group variance,** consisting primarily of error variance plus variations owing to differences within individual subjects that constitute the group. According to strict definition, error variance is a random phenomenon that is beyond the control of the experimenter. However, secondary influences involving individual differences among subjects within a group can be controlled to some degree. Because the main goal of any experiment is to demonstrate that the assignment or manipulation of an independent variable influences the dependent variable, it is desirable that the subjects within a group be as closely alike as possible. The importance of this principle can be readily understood in relation to the assessment of the efficacy of our diagnostic or treatment procedures. Given significant within-group differences that might result from individual variations in cognitive level, degree of motivation, severity of the problem, and the like, how could valid answers to these or other significant questions ever be obtained? The difficulty in doing so is the reason that secondary sources of variance must be reduced as much as possible. Because it is often difficult to separate sources of error variance from variance resulting from secondary influences, they are considered jointly in statistical calculations.

Maximizing Experimental Systematic Variance

The systematic influence of the independent variable can best be maximized by assuring that the treatment effect is sufficient to produce the intended result. In considering an independent variable for use in an experiment, some factors to evaluate are:

- The amount or strength of the stimulus variable to be administered
- The number of trials or sessions involved
- The duration of treatment
- The degree to which treatment influences can be operationally specified and linked to changes in the dependent variable

Ultimately, an investigator must answer questions, based on the best information available, pertaining to what type of independent variable to use in an investigation, how much of it to administer, and for what period of time. If the choice of independent variable is inappropriate for the question or hypothesis under investigation, the study will lack internal validity. If the magnitude of the independent variable is too small or applied for too short of a time period to exert an effect on the dependent variable, then a type II error may result (failure to find a significant effect when present).

Provided that preexisting studies or clinical experiences suggest that a particular level of an independent variable is effective, such studies might be used as a basis for selecting a particular stimulation value for use in an investigation. In the absence of such guidelines, a pilot study might be useful as a means of exploring different levels of the independent variable and which among these might be appropriate for an investigation (see Chapter 3). Once manipulation of a particular level of the independent variable has been shown to be sufficient to produce changes in the dependent variable, such a level may be selected for use. However, its influence on the dependent variable should first be demonstrated. Experimental variations or refinements in an independent variable, to determine the range of its effectiveness in producing desirable changes in behavior, typically are explored in more advanced stages of research. To use a medical analogy, a drug must first be found to be effective at *some dosage level* before answering questions as to *which dosage level* is most effective.

Minimizing Random and Systematic Errors

Earlier, we discussed the concept of error variance resulting from haphazard fluctuations in scores. Such variance is associated with **random errors** owing to unknown factors. Systematic variance, on the other hand, includes sources of variance resulting from **systematic errors** that consistently *cause* the scores in a distribution to lean in one direction or another. Both types of errors culminate in the wrong result but, whereas random errors are due to chance alone, systematic errors are the result of a certain bias that may or may not be known to the experimenter. While no research study is immune to the influence of certain types of errors, the ultimate goal is to maximize the internal and external validity of its findings to the greatest extent possible (see Chapter 7).

Random Errors

Control of random errors can be partially achieved through the **method of constancy.** Factors that can undermine constancy in an experiment include:

- Inconsistency in measurements
- Inconsistency in subject responses during the repeated performance of the same task
- Inconsistency in the conditions of testing

To illustrate efforts to control errors arising from inconsistency in measurement, imagine that you wish to investigate the duration of stuttering moments during oral reading. Prior to such a study, observers could be trained in the use of a stopwatch to improve their *intraobserver reliability* (consistency within self) and *interobserver reliability* (consistency with others) in starting and stopping the watch in accordance with task demands. Without such training, observers might start and stop the watch at different times even though subject responses remain the same. Also, clear agreement must be established among observers as to the units of behavior to be measured and exactly how measurements are to be made. In measuring instances of stuttering, it is important to know whether *whole word* or *part word* disfluencies are to be counted; perhaps some combination of these features will be evaluated in conjunction with such *accessory behaviors* as facial tics, dysrhythmic phonation, interjections, and so forth. Will measurements be made under a standard set of recording conditions involving direct observation or will a tape recorder or audio-video tape be used? Of course, the calibration and precision of all measuring devices (stopwatch, electronic timer, etc.) should be determined before the experiment.

Efforts must also be made to reduce individual subject variability resulting from uncontrolled influences. At the outset of an experiment, some amount of variation in subject responses can always be expected due to a myriad of factors such as innate learning ability, attention, emotional state, motivation, fatigue, and so on. Nevertheless, consistency in performance can often be improved by training trials designed to familiarize and give subjects prior practice with a similar task to that required in the actual experiment. For example, if we wish to investigate stuttering severity in relation to some variable like *voice initiation time,* all subjects could be given training prior to studying potential group differences to improve "readiness to respond." Such preliminary training may also be used in conjunction with a pretest or to establish a baseline of responding that can be compared to subsequent behavior changes observed in response to treatment.

Another source of random error can result from failing to hold constant the conditions of testing in an experiment. Uncontrolled variations can arise from numerous sources such as distracting noise, breakdowns in equipment, marked changes in temperature, physical rearrangements in the testing environment, or the researcher failing to treat all subjects participating in a particular condition in the same manner. The latter problem is less likely to occur if the researcher gains practice in administering the experimental procedures prior to an experiment. For this reason, as noted in Chapter 3, a pilot investigation can be useful in planning and rehearsing exactly how the independent variables are to be administered, how measures of the dependent variables are to be recorded, and how subjects can best be instructed on the tasks they are asked to perform. A written protocol or outline that specifies all experimental procedures and the sequence for carrying out each step can greatly expedite precision of control over the variables of a study. The main worth of pilot investigations is that they aid in solving many problems that might otherwise be unanticipated in the course of an actual experiment.

Systematic Errors

As noted previously, uncontrolled systematic errors can bias the findings of an experiment so that it is impossible to separate the intentional effects of the independent variable from inadvertent influences. One means of controlling the potential biasing influence of one experimental treatment or condition preceding another is by a **method of counterbalancing** their presentation. Suppose you wish to investigate the influence of some tranquilizing drug like haloperidol (treatment X) against a placebo (treatment Y) on the severity of stuttering behavior wherein each participant receives both treatments. A problem of **within-subject designs** of this kind involves **order effects**—that is, interactions arising from one treatment variable preceding another. If treatment X precedes Y, there is the possibility of a drug residue being carried over to influence performance during the placebo condition. On the other hand, should treatment Y precede treatment X, certain pretesting factors such as practice may combine with the effects of the drug to augment its apparent influence on performance. To counterbalance such interactions, the researcher can reverse the order of treatments from one subject to the next. Thus, the first subject would be given treatment X followed by treatment Y; the second subject would then receive treatment Y followed by treatment X; and thereafter treatments would alternate in this manner for each new subject as shown:

Subject # 1: Pretest . . . Drug (X) . . . Posttest 1 . . . Placebo (Y) . . . Posttest 2
2: Pretest . . . Placebo (Y) . . . Posttest 1 . . . Drug (X) . . . Posttest 2 etc.

As can be seen, subject 1 received the drug before receiving the placebo. The second subject received the placebo before the drug. Subsequent subjects 3 and 4 would receive the same order of treatment as subjects 1 and 2, respectively. This same counterbalancing sequence would continue until all participants in the experiment had been treated. Provided that subjects who received the drug treatment showed greater improvement than those who received the placebo treatment, we could be relatively confident that the drug had a therapeutic effect.

The use of counterbalancing in conjunction with other types of research designs is discussed further in Chapter 8.

Another control procedure for dealing with systematic sources of error is the **method of elimination.** Obviously, the very best way to rule out the influence of extraneous variables, that might otherwise confound accurately interpreting the influence of the independent variable on the dependent variable, is to remove them from the experiment. One common means that audiologists use for this purpose is a soundproof room. Extraneous noise sources can be virtually eliminated by the acoustic insulation in the walls of such chambers. Other laboratory settings may be designed to eliminate visual or other forms of distracting stimulation.

When extraneous variables cannot be eliminated from the test environment, then the researcher generally attempts to maintain the **constancy of conditions** so far as possible. Thus, hearing might be evaluated in the quietest test environment available. Subjects might be tested in the same room and perhaps at the same time of day.

As we have noted, confounding factors pertaining to differences in subject characteristics can best be controlled through random assignment or matching techniques aimed at producing homogeneous samples. Obviously, if your goal is to examine a particular element of language processing in children with a *specific* type of learning disability, you would want to exclude those children with *gross* cognitive impairment. Nevertheless, despite the researcher's wish to achieve group equivalence, there are some experiments in which naturally occurring categories of variables such as intelligence, age, race, gender, and the like cannot be eliminated. In some studies (particularly if participants are expected to benefit), it may be unethical to exclude people who might possess one or another of these traits merely for the sake of experimental constancy. In other cases, groups might have been formed with little attention as to how these or other factors might influence the dependent variable under investigation. Perhaps the experimenter had hoped that randomization or matching would equally distribute extraneous variables among the control and experimental group(s).

Sometimes, the influence of secondary influences or unwanted variables in an experiment can best be dealt with through **statistical control methods.** One such method is the **analysis of covariance (ANCOVA),** designed to remove the influence of extraneous variables when they can be identified. This is accomplished by treating secondary variables that are predicted to have such an influence as **covariates** to be measured and then, through the use of combined correlation methods and analysis of variance procedures, removing their influence as uncontrolled sources of variation. In essence, the analysis of covariance is a mathematical correction procedure for controlling extraneous variables statistically.

A study conducted by Erler and Garstecki (2002), who examined the degree of stigma that women in three age groups attached to hearing loss and hearing aid use provides an example of how ANCOVA can be employed to control for a potentially confounding covariate. The three groups of women were asked to complete statements designed to assess their perceptions related to hearing loss and hearing aid use. Although all participants in the study were determined to have hearing within normal limits based on age-related norms, the ANCOVA was used to control for the effect of hearing variations across the three groups (the unwanted covariate). This was done so that a true age-related difference in the perceptions of the three groups of women could be detected, if present, uncomplicated by the covariate of their own hearing ability. The manner in which this was accomplished is portrayed graphically in Figure 6-2. The results of the study indicated that younger women perceive greater stigma related to hearing loss than older women, among other findings. See Chapter 12 for additional information about the statistical theory and methods underlying ANCOVA.

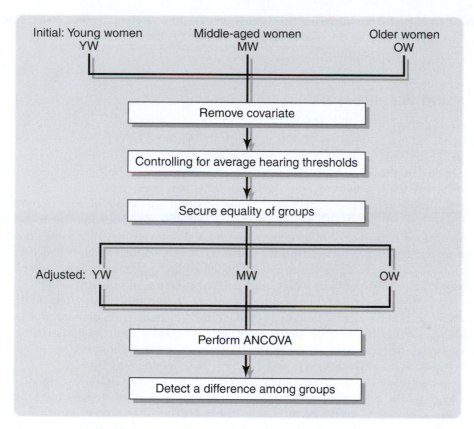

FIGURE 6-2   Use of ANCOVA to control for a potentially confounding covariate involving variations of hearing of three age groups of women

Still another technique that has statistical control implications, more so for random errors than systematic errors, is simply to increase sample size, thereby augmenting the likelihood of finding a significant result if present. Problems related to the process of selecting a sample of subjects for study were discussed in an earlier chapter. We noted that decisions pertaining to the selection of an appropriate sample size for detecting a significant association or difference between variables are complex (see also Chapter 12). Nevertheless, as a general rule, remember that as sample size increases, the likelihood decreases that certain chance factors or selection biases will threaten the validity of inductive inferences.

Finally, an important control procedure designed to reduce or eliminate the potential influence of **experimenter bias** should be mentioned. Imagine that a particular researcher has a vested interest in proving the effectiveness of some clinical program over another. To improve the potential for drawing objective conclusions, perhaps three graduate students are appointed to judge treatment outcomes. Yet, if the judges are aware of which subjects receive the favored treatment versus those who receive the alternative approach, they may be prone to see more improvement in the former cases than in the latter. Using independent judges who are unaware (*blind*) of the anticipated outcome and to which treatment a particular subject was assigned can control these biasing influences. An even greater degree of control can be achieved in a **double-blind investigation.** For example, in the hypothetical study of the effect of haloperidol on stuttering mentioned previously, *both* the judges and the subjects would be kept blind as to the type of treatments (drug or placebo) being used as well as to the results that might be anticipated.

SPECIFYING MEASUREMENTS

Clinical scientists, no matter their professional background, hope to make good decisions based on a rational evaluation of reliable and valid evidence. In this process, we strive to increase the odds of being correct while decreasing the odds of being incorrect. To this extent, we could be described as "odds makers" who assess, interpret and apply information in such a way as to forecast probable outcomes. While some fields of research place less emphasis than others on the use of numeric values to quantify observations of people, objects, or events, the majority of research investigations do incorporate some form of measurement toward this end. An obvious advantage of measurement, as opposed to merely relying on one's own subjective impressions and verbal descriptions, is that it helps to reduce ambiguity in defining the phenomenon of interest. The assignment of numbers to such phenomena is not a haphazard process but occurs in accordance with certain rules or conventions (Stevens, 1968).

It is sometimes said that human beings are simply too complex to comprehend through measurement. However, this is a fatuous argument because researchers do not seek to understand human beings as a *whole* but instead to study their various *attributes*. By assigning numbers to such attributes and applying various measurement techniques, we can obtain relatively precise information.

A major concern in any experimental study is the manner of measurement of the dependent variable. Such measurements are a means for numerically representing the characteristics of objects or events of interest to the researcher. The type of information one wishes to record largely determines the measurement procedures selected.

In selecting a particular measurement for an experiment, four important factors that should be considered pertain to its (1) utility, (2) reliability, (3) validity, and (4) scaling power.

Measurement Utility

The first and perhaps most important question to ask in assessing the overall usefulness of a measurement is whether or not it is *appropriate* given the aims of the study. If the desire of a researcher is to investigate the role of memory in language comprehension, it is important to specify further which *kind* of memory and language comprehension processes one actually wants to examine. Is the type of memory operation of interest related to short-term phonological memory or to long-term semantic memory? What aspect of language will be evaluated in reference to memory proficiency—oral or written comprehension? And what specific tasks and performance measurements are most appropriate given the particular investigative goals? For these questions to be answered, the aims of the study must be stated as clearly as possible and in operational terms that define the parameters of the independent and dependent variables. Only then can suitable measurements be selected.

The utility of measurements can also be evaluated in reference to the sensitivity and specificity of test results. A **sensitive test** is one that rarely fails to identify a disorder or disease. In mathematical terms, such a test can be defined as the proportion of people who test positive on a screening test to those people with a disorder or disease.

In a study by Jerger and his colleagues (1993), the utility of acoustic reflex measurements in predicting hearing threshold levels was examined in 1043 ears. The overall sensitivity of reflex testing was found, in the words of the authors, to be "amazingly good." Of the 453 ears that showed some level of audiometric hearing loss, 372 ears were correctly predicted to have abnormal audiograms. This result, corresponding to the sensitivity of the acoustic reflex screening test, was calculated as 372/453 = 82.12%. As in the case of this example, a sensitive test is one that "casts a wide net," rarely missing people who have a disorder or disease.

Test sensitivity must also be evaluated in relation to test specificity. A **specific test** is one that seldom erroneously identifies a person as having a disorder or disease when they do not. Mathematically, this translates into the ratio of people who test negative on a screening test to those people without the disorder or disease. Referring again to the study just mentioned, of 590 ears that showed normal audiometric test results, 349 ears were correctly predicted to have normal hearing. This result, corresponding to the specificity of the acoustic reflex screening test, was calculated as 349/590 = 59.15%. Thus, apparently, this test has greater diagnostic sensitivity than specificity.

Generally speaking, a "good test" is one that is both sensitive and specific. Nevertheless, the practical reality is that leveraging a test in one direction correspondingly diminishes its utility in the other. With increased sensitivity, more false-positive identifications are likely as opposed to a highly specific test in which false negative identifications prevail. In addition to test sensitivity and test specificity, other indices of the accuracy of a test relate to its predictive value (see Chapter 9).

Closely related to the concepts of test sensitivity and specificity are **ceiling effects** and **floor effects.** Ceiling effects result when scores on a test pile up at the high end of a distribution because the test is too easy or the dependent variable is too sensitive to the treatment employed. Conversely, a floor effect occurs when the majority of scores fall near the lower limit of a distribution, indicating that the test may be too difficult or perhaps the dependent variable is insensitive to the experimental treatment. Both ceiling and floor effects are undesirable sources of variation that can obscure the influence of the independent variable on the dependent variable.

Reliability of Measurement

The *reliability* of measurement pertains to the constancy of a test instrument, whether mechanical or human, in rendering consistently similar or identical values on repeated applications or observations. The lack of such consistency is reflected in *variability* of measurement.

According to the definition of reliability reviewed in the *Standards for Educational and Psychological Testing,* prepared by a joint commission of the American Educational Research Association, American Psychological Association, and National Council on Measurement in Education, "Reliability refers to the degree that test scores are free from errors of measurement" (1985). In a mathematical sense, this definition casts the concept of reliability as a problem requiring the determination of just how far such errors might have caused the **observed test score** to vary from the **true test score.**

Keeping in mind that a true test score is a hypothetical or idealized score that might be expected under perfectly controlled conditions, while the observed test score is the actual score obtained, then the difference between the two can be said to constitute **measurement error.**

There are actually two components of measurement error that can be associated with an observed score. The first of these, **systematic error,** results when the same error is made consistently throughout the entire process of measurement—for example, you make the same numerical mistake repeatedly or apply the wrong measuring instrument over and over again. Although such errors are likely to seriously undermine the validity of your test, they have little impact on the issue of measurement reliability. By definition, such errors are in fact "reliable" because of their consistency. However, the second error component associated with observed scores, called an **unsystematic error,** can seriously impair the reliability of observed test scores. The size of such errors, resulting from random fluctuations in observed test scores due to factors unknown to the investigator or beyond his or her control, can be small or large. Variations within subjects (attention span, motivation, testing skills, the test environment, the manner in which the test is administered, or sheer luck in guessing the correct answer) are sources of error that might compromise measurement reliability. Because such errors can never be eliminated entirely, the best we can do is to take them into account in our calculations of measurement reliability. Such a calculation can be represented as:

$$\text{Reliability of observed score} = \frac{\text{True score}}{\text{True score} + \text{Error score}}$$

As the error score portion of this equation decreases, the portion reflecting the reliability of the observed score gets larger. Conversely, as the size of the error score increases, the reliability of the observed score decreases. Ideally, with an error score of zero, such an equation would be equal to 1, although such perfection is highly unlikely if not impossible to achieve.

The reliability of a test is expressed mathematically as an *absolute* magnitude of a correlation coefficient, denoted by $|r|$, can range in value from 0.0 to 1.0. A correlation between .80 and .90, which is the benchmark for many tests used for educational, clinical, and research purposes, would be considered a very strong correlation. Correlations extending below this range would be viewed as becoming progressively weaker in reflecting the association between variables. See Chapter 11 for a further discussion of correlation coefficients including their *relative* values.

Types of Reliability

As a theory of error arising from the study of the relations among test variables, it is inappropriate to speak of "the reliability of *the* test measure" as though only one source of error might exist (Pedhazur & Schmelkin, 1991). In fact, there are several approaches used for estimating the reliability of a test score as appropriate for the particular source of error of concern (see Table 6-1).

Test-Retest Reliability

Test-retest reliability is concerned with how consistent or stable a test measure is over time. Giving an individual or group of individuals a test and then administering the same test at some subsequent point assesses this. Provided that the scores obtained on the second test occasion are in close agreement (highly correlate) with those obtained on the first test, high test-retest reliability can be established. In other words, we can conclude that the test is measuring a relatively stable trait as opposed to one that might otherwise fluctuate significantly as the result of error variance.

Although high test-retest reliability can be used as an indicator that a particular test is capable of yielding stable test results, finding that test scores change significantly from one occasion to the next does not necessarily indicate that the *test* is unreliable. Indeed, it is well known among both clinicians and researchers, that the so-called **practice effect,** associated with increased knowledge or familiarity with test items, can operate to boost test scores with repeated testing. Thus, it is possible for scores to show a reliable *change in direction* from one test period to another (see Figure 6-3). One possible means of avoiding or reducing the practice effect is to extend the time period between the test and retest. Commonly, one month or more is allowed to pass between test periods to counter the influence of memory.

When low test-retest reliability is found, the result usually reflects instability in either (1) the trait being measured, (2) the test instrument or manner of its administration, or

TABLE 6-1   Types of Reliability

Type	Definition	Process of Establishment	Statistical Method(s)
Test-Retest	The consistency or stability of a measurement	Administering the same test on two different occasions to the same individuals and examining the correlation between their test-retest scores	Pearson Product Moment Correlation denoted by r or the Spearman Rank Order Correlation denoted by ρ
Alternate Forms	The extent to which two forms of the same test yield relatively equivalent test results	Administering two different forms of the same test to the same individuals and examining the correlation between scores on the two test forms	Pearson Product Moment Correlation denoted by r or the Spearman Rank Order Correlation denoted by ρ
Internal Consistency	The degree of relatedness among the items on a particular test	Splitting a test into two or more parts and determining the correlation between the scores	Spearman–Brown Prophecy formula, Cronbach's alpha, or Kuder–Richardson's formula 20
Observer	*Intraobserver* reliability is related to the stability of judgment within a person while *interobserver* reliability is related to the accuracy of judgment between persons	Having the same person score the same test on two occasions and examining the degree of intra-observer agreement. Having two different persons score the same test and examining the inter-observer agreement	Percentage of agreement of kappa statistic

(3) some combination of these factors. Logically, it makes sense to assess the test-retest reliability of a measuring instrument when it has been developed to assess a particular trait in people that is relatively fixed or unchanging. Examples of such traits would include intelligence or personality that is presumed to be relatively stable over time. On the other hand, the assumption of such stability with respect to various clinical disorders is highly questionable. Indeed, many forms of communication disorders may show marked variations in the frequency and intensity of various signs or symptoms, given a host of factors. Furthermore, depending on the efficacy of treatment and the course of the underlying pathology, the severity of such disorders might be expected to change over time. In such cases, applying the criterion of test-retest reliability to a measuring instrument would hardly seem fair or appropriate.

Alternate-Forms Reliability

This type of reliability, also known as *parallel* or *equivalent forms reliability,* is concerned with measuring the consistency of a test based on its content. In essence, establishing alternate-forms reliability is accomplished by showing that two forms of the same test containing equivalent yet different test items yield highly similar results. Although the specific items on the two forms of the test may differ, the same rules are used in developing each. In both cases, the items are designed to measure an identical construct and are determined to be relatively equivalent in their level of difficulty.

An example of a commonly used test for which alternate-forms reliability has been established is the Peabody Picture Vocabulary Test (PPVT-III). This was accomplished by

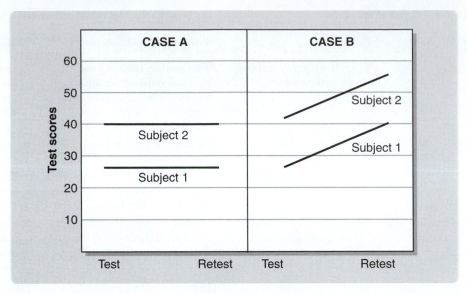

FIGURE 6-3 Test-retest scores for two subjects in two situations. In situation A, the two subjects obtained the same scores on retest as obtained on their initial tests. In situation B, the same two subjects obtained scores on retest that differed from their initial test scores. However, in both situations, the difference between the two subjects' test and retest scores were reliable when compared to one another. Therefore, test-retest reliability for both situations are identical.

administering two forms of the test (forms IIIA and IIIB), separated by a short period of time, to all persons in the standardization sample. As shown in Table 6-2, *coefficients of equivalence* between the two test forms were calculated for various age groups, yielding coefficients ranging from .89 to .99 computed from raw score data (median = .95) and from .88 to .96 (median = .94) computed from standard scores. (See Chapter 12 for a discussion of how standard scores are calculated.) In both cases, these coefficients were judged as showing a high correspondence between results yielded by the two test forms.

From both a clinical and research perspective, tests that have established alternate-forms reliability can have great utility, particularly when there is a need to evaluate the same subject characteristic over a relatively short period of time. By establishing that two forms of the same test yield highly equivalent scores, concerns pertaining to the potential biasing influence of giving the same test twice (practice effect) can be obviated or reduced. Moreover, the availability of alternate forms of the same test can sometimes eliminate the need for a control group by allowing each subject to serve as his or her own control (within-subject design). Provided the correlation between the two test forms is found to be sufficiently high, using an appropriate statistical measure, alternate-forms reliability can be demonstrated. Unfortunately, in the field of communication sciences and disorders, the number of tests that have established such reliability is quite small.

Internal Consistency Reliability
Another reliability method specifically designed to determine the internal consistency of the items within a test is the **split-half reliability estimate.** The procedure entails splitting the items on a test in half with the odd numbered items constituting one half of the test and the even numbered comprising the other half. Alternatively, the whole test may be split down

TABLE 6-2   Alternate-Forms Reliability Coefficients and Standard Errors of Measurement for Raw Scores and Standard Scores, by Age

Age Group	N	Reliability Coefficients	
		For Raw Scores	**For Standard Score Equivalents**
2-6–2-11	100	.89	.88
3-0–3-5	100	.90	.90
3-6–3-11	100	.93	.93
4-0-4-5	100	.94	.94
4-6-4-11	100	.95	.95
5-0-5-5	100	.93	.93
5-6–5-11	100	.93	.93
6-0-6-5	100	.94	.94
6-6–6-11	100	.92	.91
7	100	.95	.95
8	100	.93	.93
9	100	.94	.93
10	100	.95	.95
11	100	.96	.96
12	100	.95	.93
13	100	.95	.95
14	100	.96	.95
15–16	150	.96	.95
17–18	150	.96	.94
19–24	150	.94	.92
25–30	125	.95	.94
31–40	125	.97	.94
41–50	125	.99	.95
51–60	100	.96	.91
61–90+	100	.97	.89
Median		.95	.94

the middle, deriving an equal number of items from the upper and lower halves. Whatever the method used in splitting a test into two parts, the ultimate goal is to determine the correlation between the two halves. However, the problem with treating the scores in such a direct statistical fashion is that the two tests derived from the original each contain only half the number of items. In an effort to adjust for this problem, the **Spearman-Brown Prophecy formula** (named after the two statisticians who developed it) is often used to estimate the reliability coefficient for the entire test. The formula used for this purpose is:

$$\text{Reliability of test} = \frac{2 \times \text{reliability of } \frac{1}{2} \text{ test}}{1 + \text{reliability of } \frac{1}{2} \text{ test}}$$

Assuming that the correlation between the two halves of a test instrument was .68, by applying the Spearman-Brown formula, then:

$$\text{Reliability of test} = \frac{2(.68)}{1 + .68} = \frac{1.36}{1.68} = .81$$

Despite the increased gain in the size of the coefficient resulting from the application of the Spearman-Brown formula, such an adjustment does not resolve all the problems associated with the use of split-half reliability estimates. There are many rules that might be applied in splitting a test into an equal number of items, and who can say with certainty that one method is better than another? Suppose a diagnostic test is constructed in such a way that the "easy items" are even-numbered and the "difficult items" are odd numbered. The biasing influence of such an arbitrary rule is obvious. The presumption that one can simply split the items of a test in accordance with some predetermined method and thereby achieve test item equivalence is ill-founded. Furthermore, pretending to estimate the reliability of a whole test by splitting its items in half, and then attempting to make up for the resultant loss in statistical accuracy by means of the Spearman-Brown formula or some other method, is a weak substitute for alternate-forms reliability estimations. The latter methods, which examine what are presumed to be equivalent forms of the same instrument, are statistically more accurate because they include within the analysis twice the number of items analyzed by split-half reliability procedures. Unfortunately, because of the time and costs involved in developing and evaluating the reliability of alternative forms of the same test, split-half reliability estimation may be used instead.

Still other methods for evaluating the internal consistency of a test, so far as the ability of its items to examine the same construct, are based on the methods of **Kuder and Richardson's formula 20** (1937) and **Cronbach's alpha** (1951). Kuder and Richardson's formula is used with dichotomous test items while the so-called Cronbach's alpha is more appropriate for continuous data. The advantage of these methods over the split-half approach is that both procedures are based on calculating the averages of all possible combinations of inter-item correlations. The higher the resulting correlations, the greater will be the internal consistency of the items.

Observer Reliability

Professionals in clinical fields often are interested in assessing their reliability in administering diagnostic tests or treatment programs. Two types of *observer reliability* (also known as rater or scorer reliability) are typically of interest in any clinical study or research investigation. The first of these, termed **intraobserver reliability,** is the degree of internal consistency of an individual observer with her or himself in administering the proscribed tests or experimental procedures and in measuring and assessing the results. Fluctations within the observer, such as those resulting from extraneous distracters or changes in one's mental or physical state, can impair intraobserver reliability.

While intraobserver reliability is related to the *stability* of judgment, another form of reliability that is of equal or greater importance to assess in most clinical studies or experiments is concerned with the *accuracy* of judgment. This is termed **interobserver reliability** and is often expressed as a percentage reflecting the proportion of agreements to disagreements between two or more observers. Suppose that two clinicians independently evaluate the speech of 30 randomly selected children born with a cleft palate one year after pharyngeal flap surgery. The clinicians decide to rate each child according to his or her degree of perceived nasal resonance. Assume that the ratings are assigned to one of four categories based on a numerical scale where 0 = normal resonance, 1 = mild hypernasality, 2 = moderate hypernasality, 3 = severe hypernasality. Hypothetically, the distribution of ratings for the two clinicians could have looked something like the following:

Case #	1	2	3	4	5	6	7	8	9	10	11	12	13	14	15	16	17	18	19	20
Rater A	1	0	1	3	2	2	1	1	3	1	1	1	0	0	1	2	1	1	0	1
Rater B	2	0	1	2	2	1	1	1	2	1	1	2	0	0	1	2	0	1	0	1

One simple means of calculating interobserver reliability given the above data is to count the frequency of agreements between the two clinicians and divide this value by the total number of observations, or:

$$\frac{\text{Agreements}}{\text{Agreements} + \text{Disagreements}} = \frac{14}{20} = 70\% \text{ agreement}$$

A problem with this method is that when the number of observed cases decreases, the probability of observers agreeing by chance alone increases. To overcome this problem, techniques have been developed that calculate the probability for such a chance error and then subtract this probability in calculating interobserver reliability.

One relatively simple and useful method for measuring agreement between two observers in making judgments about behaviors that are assigned to one category or another is based on the so-called **kappa formula** (Cohen, 1988). The method has relevance to many clinical situations in which clinicians might wish to measure their agreement in diagnosing a particular disorder based on judgments of the *presence* or *absence* of abnormality. Such dichotomous results can be expressed as either "normal" or "abnormal" outcomes in leading to a diagnosis.

Imagine that two clinicians independently evaluate 100 children suspected of stuttering and render judgments about the normality or abnormality of disfluent speech using the same diagnostic criteria. Hypothetical data based on their observations can be cast in the form of a 2 × 2 contingency table (Table 6-3). Based on the results shown, we can proceed to illustrate the calculation of kappa (k), defined as the agreement beyond chance divided by the amount of agreement *possible* beyond chance, such that

$$k = \frac{0 - c}{1 - c}$$

where o = the observed agreement, and c = the chance agreement. The actual steps involved in calculating kappa (k) are outlined below.

Step 1: Calculate the observed agreement (o):

o = [(# of "normality agreements") + (# of "abnormality agreements")]/the grand total
= (60 + 18) /100
= 78/100 (.78) or 78% = (o)

Step 2: Calculate the chance agreement (c):

a. Calculate how many observations the clinicians may agree are abnormal by chance, determined by multiplying the number each clinician found abnormal and then dividing by the grand total of 100 observations: (30 × 28)/100 = 8.4.

b. Calculate how many observations the two may agree are normal by chance, as determined by multiplying the number each found normal and dividing by the grand totals of 100 observations: (70 × 72)/100 = 50.4.

TABLE 6-3   Observed Agreement on Judging Disfluent Children as "Normal" or "Abnormal"

| | Clinician B | | |
Clinician A	Abnormal	Normal	Subtotal
Abnormal	18	12	30
Normal	10	60	70
Subtotal	28	72	100

   c. Add the two numbers found in the first two steps and divide by 100 to obtain the proportion of chance agreement: $(8.4 + 50.4)/100 = 0.588$ or $58.8\% = c$.

Step 3: Calculate kappa (k)

   a. Given that the observed agreement (o) is 78%, or 0.78, the agreement beyond chance ($o - c$) is $0.78 - 0.588 = 0.192$, representing the numerator of k.
   b. The potential agreement beyond chance is 100% minus the chance agreement of 58.8%, or $1 - .588 = .412$, the denominator of k. Thus, in our example, $k = 0.192/0.412 = 0.47$ or 47%.

For a two-category system (or 2 by 2 categories) of the type described above, chance would dictate that the observers would agree .25 or 25% ($1 \div 4$ categories) of the time. Thus, based on the results of our hypothetical example in which a kappa of 47% was found, we can conclude that the extent of agreement between our two clinicians well exceeded chance expectations by approximately 22% ($47\% - 25\%$).

The kappa formula represents a convenient and straightforward method for calculating the degree of reliability based on probability theory. Other more complex statistical procedures such as tests of correlation are available for determining the accuracy and stability of observations; some of these will be discussed in Chapter 11. Meanwhile, remember that with respect to measurement considerations in research, the concept of reliability relates to the need for assessing errors resulting from inaccurate or unstable recording devices, including our own eyes and ears as they too may be used for such purposes.

Validity of Measurement

As a concept, validity of measurement applies to issues involving both the accuracy and reliability of a test instrument. For a measurement to be valid, it must accurately reflect the nature of the underlying variable that it is intended to represent. To be reliable, it must do so consistently with repetition over a span of time.

Relationship of Validity to Reliability

Establishing the reliability of a test is a necessary condition for establishing its validity—nothing can be true unless it is trustworthy. However, reliability alone is insufficient to establish validity. A case in point is a poorly calibrated audiometer that *reliably* produces *invalid* results in the measurement of hearing acuity. While validity pertains to the *accuracy* of a test result, reliability only pertains to its *replication*.

The relationship between reliability and validity is illustrated in Figure 6-4. Using a bull's-eye target as an analogy, we can see that validity is based on how "true" one's aim is in

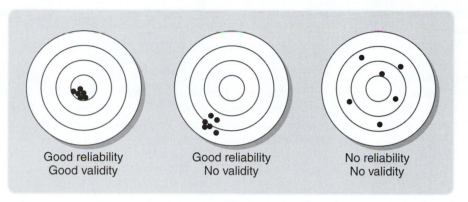

FIGURE 6-4   Using a bull's-eye target as an analogy to describe the relationship between reliability and validity

hitting the center of the target. On the other hand, reliability can be assessed solely on the basis of how closely the hits cluster to one another independent of their proximity to the bull's-eye. In other words, validity can exist only to the degree that scores reliably cluster near the center of the target. On the other hand, reliability can exist independent of accuracy so long as the scores are not widely dispersed.

Generalizing from our bull's-eye analogy, we can say that the reliability of measurement is primarily concerned with determining certain types of errors associated with the interpretation of test scores.

Definition of Validity

The term *validity* is roughly synonymous with the word *truth*. If you look up the meaning of the noun *truth* in the *Oxford American Dictionary* (1980), you will find a kind of circular reasoning: "truth is the quality of being true; something that is true." Because of the tautology associated with such a definition, your next step might be to look up the adjective *true* (truer, tru-est) that describes a condition of being in agreement with *accepted* facts, principle, or standards. According to this definition, an important element of validity (being true) resides within the eye of the beholder. Certainly, in establishing truth, your own perceptions and the degree of their congruence with those of other people should be taken into account. But so-called **face validity,** based merely on the surface appearance of things (the earth's surface appears flat), can be quite wrong.

Suppose you develop a test protocol for measuring the severity of stuttering while reading a standard passage. You decide to calculate the number of words stuttered by two speakers and find that Speaker A stuttered many more times than Speaker B. On the face of it, it may appear that Speaker A's problem is more severe than Speaker B's. Such a conclusion might have merit as long as you and perhaps other clinicians are content with such a narrow definition based on a single behavioral criterion—namely, frequency of stuttering during oral reading. Yet, such a restricted view of stuttering does not permit consideration of other parameters of stuttering severity. What, for example, might more frequent stuttering, exhibited by a particular speaker during an oral reading task, predict about his or her level of anxiety during social encounters or overall confidence as a communicator? Is Speaker A more avoidant of certain speaking situations than Speaker B, or vice versa? What might the frequency of stuttering, per se, predict about educational or vocational achievement?

The point is that simply because a test "appears" to accurately measure limited aspects of a phenomenon doesn't make it a valid test. Because of the limitations surrounding the meaning of so-called face validity, in its *Standards for Educational and Psychological Testing* (1999), the joint committee of the American Educational Research Association, American Psychological Association, and the National Council on Measurement in Education excluded the construct as a basis for drawing inferences. Keep in mind that "on the face of it" interpretations of test results, based on simple logic or so-called common sense are often fraught with error.

Over the past 50 or more years, much controversy has surrounded the meaning of validity as a scientific construct. Although a review of these controversies is beyond the scope of this chapter, the interested reader might wish to consult relevant commentaries (Cureton, 1951; Cronbach, 1971; Messick, 1988; Kaplan and Saccuzzo, 1997). Essentially, some of the difficulties surrounding the definition stem from the fact that the meaning of *test validity* differs from concepts of validity related to research design (see Chapter 7). According to the American Psychological Association's *Standards for Educational and Psychological Testing* (1999), test validity ". . . refers to the appropriateness, meaningfulness, and usefulness of the specific inferences that can be made from test scores. Test validation is the process of accumulating evidence to support such inferences." More briefly, validity can be thought of as the extent to which a test instrument or experimental method achieves the purpose(s) of the research.

Types of Validity

Despite its position that test validity is best seen as a "unitary concept," the joint committee referred to above has suggested a tripartite classification scheme for conceptualizing various aspects of validity with the caveat that these "types" are not to be viewed as mutually exclusive or exhaustive categories. Furthermore, it was recommended that each type should be taken into account for purposes of test validation. These types of test validity include the following: (1) content validity, (2) criterion validity, and (3) construct validity (see Table 6-4).

Content Validity

Content validity refers to how well a test adequately represents the various content domains the test was designed to assess. Suppose you want to develop a general test of receptive and expressive language abilities that will span the range of language functions including morphology, syntax, and semantics. To the extent that your subtests adequately represent each of these areas, your test might be said to have "content validity." Content validity is sometimes called **sampling validity,** referring to the ability of a test "to provide an adequate, or representative, *sample* of all *content,* or elements, or instances of the phenomenon being measured" (Monette et al., 1998, p. 108). Content validity is best established by efforts to conceptualize the entire content domain prior to developing a test and by a careful analysis of the final content, making sure that all relevant domains are included. Although the establishment of content validity presumably depends on a more comprehensive analysis of the concepts underlying a test than does face validity, these types are related in that both are determined on the basis of subjective opinion. Should the majority of your professional colleagues decide that your so-called *general* or *wide-range* test of language abilities inadequately represents the full gamut of language domains, perhaps because it failed to include content for the assessment of pragmatics or some nonverbal area of language functioning, the test might be judged as lacking content validity. Therefore, any developer of a new test is well

TABLE 6-4   **Types of Validity**

Type	Definition	Process of Establishment
Content	The extent to which a particular test or measurement is judged to be representative of the behavior or skills it is designed to assess.	Seek out expert opinion and advice to see if the test items assess what you want them to.
Criterion	There are two subtypes of criterion validity. Predictive validity relates to the ability of a given test to predict an outcome that is consistent with the theoretical construct that underlies the test. Concurrent validity is concerned with how well a test estimates present performance.	In predictive validity, a researcher establishes a criterion and correlates scores on the test with scores on the criterion in the future. In concurrent validity, a researcher established a criterion and correlates scores on the test with scores on the criterion in the present.
Construct	The degree to which a particular test or measuring instrument actually measures the theoretical construct under investigation.	It pertains to establishing the meanings of the test results in relation to the theoretical constructs upon which the test is based. In other words, a researcher asks "to what degree does this test truly test the particular thing of interest?"

advised to seek out expert opinion and advice before making final decisions as to the content domains that the test should cover.

While the weakness of content validity lies in its lack of objective or quantifiable evidence, its subjective qualities involving good logic, intuitive skills, and perseverance are vitally important not only in the initial stages of developing a test instrument but also in revising test items on a continuing basis (Kaplan & Saccuzzo, 1997). Remember that the content of a test is good (valid) only so long as the test items adequately represent the concepts underlying the test as a whole. As concepts change, so too must the test items in which they are reflected. Thus, if the goal is to construct a test of vocabulary recognition, including a stimulus item such as a picture of a typewriter might be inappropriate in this computer age.

Criterion Validity

Criterion validity refers to how well a test can predict a particular outcome. Such an outcome might be educational achievement, job success, psychosocial adjustment, physical health, or any other criterion one might wish to predict. The major focus of criterion-related validation is on the ability of a test to successfully predict a phenomenon rather than explaining its occurrence.

Test developers often seek to establish two subtypes of criterion validity. The first of these, **predictive validity,** relates to the ability of a given test to predict an outcome that is consistent with the theoretical construct that underlies the test. For example, if a test presumes to assess one's competence in oral language, then these same skills should be reflected in speech production. To use another example, many programs of graduate study require that students take the Graduate Record Examination (GRE). This test is given because its content domains are considered to predict something about success or failure in graduate school. What might actually constitute the criteria for success is a matter for debate . In the case of the predictive value of GRE scores, the chosen criterion for success is typically based on academic rather than clinical performance. This is because predictions about academic performance reflects the theoretical constructs underlying GRE scores, whereas clinical performance includes many other skills, as in certain various psychosocial domains, that are not reflected in such scores.

As Wallace (1965) succinctly noted, because of the difficulties associated with defining and qualifying some performance criteria, researchers and policy makers often elect to use "criteria that are predictable rather than appropriate" (p. 411). In a similar vein, Kaplan and Saccuzzo (1997) stated: "criterion validity studies mean nothing at all unless the criterion is valid . . . the criterion should relate specifically to the use of the test" (p. 139).

Another subtype of criterion validity is called **concurrent validity.** In order to establish concurrent validity, the results from a new test must agree with those of existing tests that are presumed to be valid. Suppose you decide to develop a test to diagnose the presence of a sensorineural hearing loss. For the test to have concurrent validity, the results obtained should be highly associated with the results of other tests known to be valid indicators of sensorineural hearing loss. The audiometric profile that a person obtains on one test, although perhaps not identical, should be highly similar to results of the other test. Logically, this would be expected provided that the two tests are measuring the same phenomenon—sensorineural as opposed to some other form of hearing loss.

Of the criterion-related measures, predictive validity is typically more difficult to establish than concurrent validity. As the name implies, predictive validity is concerned with forecasting some future performance variable or test result. Temporal constraints, particularly for data that cannot be collected for a long period of time, often militate against the establishment of predictive validity. Such constraints operate to a lesser degree for the comparison of test scores that can be collected *concurrently* or in closer proximity to one another. Unlike indicators of content-related validity, the measures of critierion-related validity typically lend themselves to objective analysis or quantification.

Construct Validity

Constructs can best be thought of as internal representations of the world that people use in the process of reasoning and explaining various phenomenon. Construct validity is a metamorphic type of validity that embraces all other types. It pertains to establishing the meaning of test results in relation to the theoretical constructs upon which the test is based. Essentially, when we question a test's construct validity, we ask "to what degree does this test *truly* test the particular thing of interest?"

Construct validation is especially important in the early stages of developing a new test when the meaning of the test results is still unclear. The process entails the use of two types of evidence. The first of these types is called **convergence evidence.** If you wish to develop a test for verbal intelligence, the results from the various measures used to assess this construct (e.g., vocabulary development, reading comprehension, memory for words and sentences, etc.) should be shown to be related (converge). Stated in statistical terms, we hope to find strong *intercorrelations* among the various test items, thereby providing evidence that they are all measuring a single construct, namely, verbal intelligence.

Keeping in mind that the process of construct validation continually searches for additional evidence to support the construct in question, we might decide to broaden our definition of verbal intelligence to include other measures of oral and written language, related perhaps to the use and understanding of complex syntax or abstract language such as analogies and metaphors. The greater the number of verbal measures that converge within the framework of a single test, the stronger (more meaningful) it becomes in representing a particular construct.

Another means to validate a test instrument is by marshalling **discriminant evidence.** As a part of construct validation, such evidence is used to establish the case that test items normally considered to be unrelated to the construct in question are, indeed, unrelated to it.

Thus, further validation of our verbal intelligence construct could be achieved by including test items that assess skills outside its domain. Such skills might include visual-motor integration, map reading, object assembly abilities, and so forth. To the degree that low correlations would be found among such nonverbal test items and the verbal test scores, we would have established some level of discriminant evidence in support of our construct.

While convergent evidence helps to prove that certain tests are measuring an aspect of the same construct, divergent evidence shows the opposite—namely, that the tests are measuring something other than the construct in question. Together, these forms of evidence function reciprocally to show that our test is measuring what it was designed to measure and not measuring things unintended. A statistical means of examining these aspects of validity simultaneously is by constructing a **multitrait-multimethod matrix.** First introduced by Campbell & Fiske (1959), the method is complex to use and often very time consuming, yet it can be highly valuable in establishing the validity of a test. For an excellent step-by-step illustration of the techniques used in constructing an MTMM, see Jabs (http://trochim.human.cornell.edu/jabs/mtmm).

Applying Reliability and Validity Measures to Psychometric Assessment

Now that we have discussed important aspects of validity and reliability as they relate to test construction, let us now examine how these measures relate to the assessment of an actual clinical test. Each of these indices is typically assessed in evaluating and selecting a test instrument for use whether for diagnostic or research purposes.

The psychometric assessment of the reliability and validity measures discussed previously is exemplified by the Childhood Autism Rating Scale (CARS) developed by Eric Schopler and his colleagues (1988). The main purpose of this scale is to distinguish children with the autistic syndrome from children with other developmental disorders.

In standardizing this scale, three aspects of test reliability were assessed. The first of these, *interobserver reliability,* was assessed by correlating individual item scores obtained from two trained independent observers. The overall interobserver reliability was calculated to be .71 based on an average correlation coefficient for 15 individual CARS items. In order to assess *test-retest reliability,* scores on the first administration of the test were compared with those obtained from a second administration approximately one year later. The resulting correlation of .88 indicated that the CARS yielded temporally stable measurement. The *internal consistency of reliability* of the CARS was also assessed to determine the degree to which the 15 scale items were related to one another as opposed to representing different facets of behavior. The resulting correlation of .94 provided justification for combining scale item scores into a single score.

Three aspects of validity that are important in assessing the accuracy of measurement procedures were also assessed. As noted previously, *predictive validity* concerns the success of a measurement in accurately estimating a particular outcome. Such validity is based on the extent to which test results are correlated with performance measures. Although such validity was not assessed in the case of the CARS, it might have been by evaluating how successful it actually was in predicting educational achievement, language development, emotional adjustment, or other significant factors. As we have discussed, predictive validity is often difficult or unfeasible to establish because prospective studies of subjects may be needed requiring data analysis over a lengthy time span.

When predictive validity is not established, the next best alternative is to establish *concurrent validity*. Such validity is established by collecting test measurements along with other criterion data almost simultaneously to determine their degree of agreement. Referring once again to the CARS, concurrent validity was established by comparing total scores to clinical ratings of the degree of abnormality made during the same diagnostic sessions. The resulting correlation was .84, indicating high validity with respect to the criterion clinical ratings.

Perhaps the most desired yet difficult to establish form of measurement validity is termed *content validity*. Such validity must be based largely on subjective opinion as to whether or not a test actually measures what it has been designed to test. Using the CARS once again to illustrate this concept, the scale ought to reflect the underlying attributes of autistic syndromes in a true and comprehensive manner. Commenting on this matter, Prizant (1992) noted that a strength of the CARS is that its content was derived from behavioral characteristics of autistic children over the last four decades. He further noted that a content weakness is found in its failure to sufficiently emphasize measurement of reciprocal social relations, communication, and imaginative activity. Such criteria are weighted heavily in current diagnoses of autistic syndromes. Prizant's review of the CARS appears in the *Buros Mental Measurement Yearbook,* a standard and highly useful reference for gaining reliability and validity information relating to published tests and measurements in current use.

Measurement Scales

Measurement involves the assignment of numerical values to observations made directly by an investigator or indirectly by a test instrument or recording device. Underlying the theory of measurement are certain assumptions pertaining to the suitability and power of different numerical scales for representing the data of an investigation. These assumptions form the basis for a set of rules that specify the admissible operations for the mathematical manipulation and statistical analysis of data that can be (1) named or categorized only, (2) ordered or ranked, (3) arranged along a numerical line, possessing equal intervals and an arbitrary zero point, or (4) treated as a ratio, possessing all the previous features in addition to a nonarbitrary zero point. Each of these classes of data along with their respective measurement scales are discussed further in Chapter 11.

RECORDING MEASUREMENTS

Researchers in the field of communication sciences and disorders are primarily interested in the speech, language, and hearing abilities of human subjects and the means of their measurement. A major avenue of recording data with respect to these and related phenomena entails the observational use of the sensory apparatus of the observer—that is, his or her own eyes and ears. Such observations often require binary judgments about the *presence or absence* of certain characteristics that are important in categorizing various types of disorders and related attributes of the subjects' physical or psychological makeup (e.g., age, gender, cognitive functioning, etc.).

In many studies, simple checklists are sufficient for satisfying the purpose of coding the targeted behavior, perhaps supplemented by the use of tape recorders, audio-video recordings, or hand-held computers. In more complex investigations, where a number of behavioral or physiological responses may be of interest, electrical or mechanical devices can often facilitate the precision and accuracy of recorded observations.

An example of a useful method for recording overt verbal or nonverbal behaviors as they occur in social interactions was developed by Robert Bales, who designed a 12-category system for classifying different types of goal-oriented and social-emotional interactions among

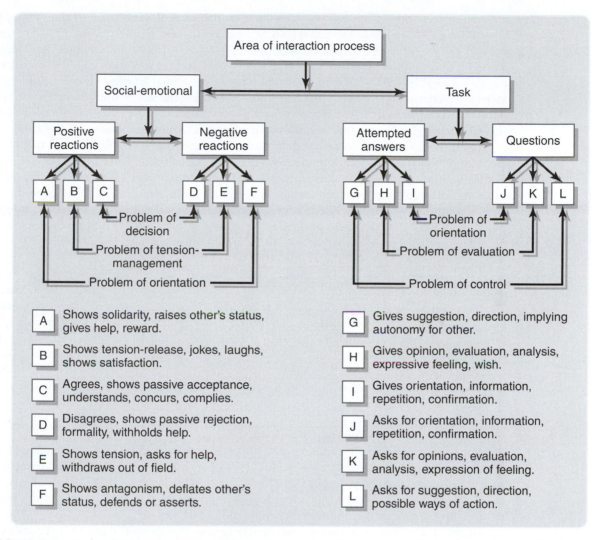

FIGURE 6-5   A schematic representation of Bales' category system for assessing and recording goal-oriented and socioemotional interactions

(adapted from Interaction Process Analysis, *by R. Bales. 1950, p. 9. Chicago: University of Chicago Press.)*

individuals in small group settings (Monette, Sullivan, & DeJong, 1998). To expedite the goals of such studies, Bales developed a recording device that consisted of a driving mechanism and a movable tape that rolled across the top surface of the casing at a constant speed. Space was provided for an observer to tabulate interactions according to the 12 categories within which a unit of behavior was judged to fall (see Figure 6-5).

Assessment procedures of the type developed by Bales would also appear to have relevance for researchers interested in developing taxonomies for observing and recording aspects of verbal and nonverbal communicative behavior. One example of an approach used to assess young children's social interactions has been developed by Brown et al. (1996). Called the *System for Observation of Children's Social Interactions* (SOCSI), the authors note that the recording system can be used to ". . . generate information about social goals occurring in interactions, behavioral strategies that children use when addressing those goals, and the success of children in achieving their goals" (p. 29). Table 6-5 lists several types of behavioral strategies used in children's social interactions, the manner in which they are coded using the SOCSI, and research literature upon which they are based. As can be seen, a range of behavioral strategies can be recorded with this system, ranging from simple gestural communication to more complex verbal requests.

Computerized event recorders and software systems are now available that are capable of recording frequencies or durations of several categories of behavior. Observations pertaining to the qualities of various social interactions can be recorded at regular intervals in response to a series of simple keyboard commands. Brown et al. (1996) describe a number of contemporary computer technology systems for recording behavioral data. One of these systems, called the *Multi-Option Observation System for Experimental Studies* (MOOSES) is adaptable for collecting and analyzing a wide array of behavioral data as involved in children's play and social interactions (Tapp, Wehby, & Ellis, 1995).

Videotape technology provides another avenue for recording observational data. One such system called the *Professional Tape Control, Coding, and Analysis System* (PROCODER) includes hardware and software adaptations that allow for "frame-accurate" coding of behavioral events (Tapp and Walden, 1993). An example of a commercially available software program that can be used for the systematic analysis of any kind of videorecorded behavior of interest is INTER-ACT (2004), available from Mangold Software and Consulting (http://www.mangold.de/). One or several behavioral codes can be assigned to any event that happens at a particular time (*event sampling*) or during a predefined time interval (*time sampling*). The program includes basic statistics for the calculation of frequencies, sequences, durations, and the like of observed behavior. Software is also available for identifying patterns inside the observational data, such as the order, duration, or relative position of behavioral events.

For a description of still another general purpose software package that can be adapted to a wide range of observational data see Noldus (1991). For various physiological measurements, such as heart rate, electromyography (EMG), or electroencephalography (EEG), *biotelemetry techniques* now make possible the remote recording of responses from sensors and electrodes with the resulting signals fed to computers or analog-to-digital converters.

In the discussion to follow, we will briefly review four general types or categories of response measures to include the following: (1) frequency, (2) latency, (3) duration, and (4) amplitude/intensity.

Response Frequency

The most common unit of measurement in the behavioral sciences is **response frequency,** referring to the total number of response units observed to occur. Perhaps the popularity of this measure is due to its relative simplicity of use and broad range of research and clinical applications. Frequency measures are especially useful in describing the characteristics of dichotomous observations having only two categories (nominal data) or that can only be ranked according to which observation occurred more often than another (ordinal data). In the field of communication sciences and disorders, we are typically interested in measuring the number of correct versus incorrect responses with respect to various types of speech, language, or hearing behavior. We might also wish to use the frequency of certain errors to rank a disorder according to severity level (e.g., mild, moderate, or severe).

TABLE 6-5   System for Observation of Children's Social Interactions (SOCSI)

15 Behavioral Strategies	
1. Affilatives/affection (AF)	Makes prosocial physical contact with peer (e.g., hugs, kisses, hold hands) (K&R, HG&C, T, S, B, O)
2. Calling (CA)	Verbally addressing a peer by name or role with no other message included (e.g., "Bobby!"). This may also be a single word exclamatory statement ("Hey!"). When this behavior is paired with another message in the statement, the order message should be coded. (K&R)
3. Comments (CO)	Directing a declarative statement to peer about peer's or self activity, behavior, or other condition. (C&P-B, H, K&R, P&K)
4. Complimentary statement (CS)	Conveying a prosocial verbal message to a peer (e.g., "You are nice," "I like you") (B, O, S, T)
5. Gestural communication (GC)	Directing a gesture to a peer to convey a message (OMO&B)
6. Need statements (NS)	Stating to a peer that the speaker wants or needs an object or needs help with an activity
7. Object aggression (AGO)	Taking an object away from a peer, or destroying an object of another peer (K&R, O, S&T, T)
8. Personal aggression (AGP)	Hitting, pushing, pinching a peer (HG&C, K&R, O, S&T, T)
9. Physical assistance (PA)	Through a nonverbal, physical action, the child helps a peer with an activity, task, or other action (O, T)
10. Play noises (PN)	Directing noises to a peer that are associated with the play theme in which the speaker or peer is/are engaged (K&R)
11. Questions (Q)	Directing an interrogative statement to a peer ("Will you help me?") (G&P-B, P&K)
12. Requests/command (RQ)	Imperative statement to a peer to perform or not to perform an action ("Stop that!") (G&P, B, P&K)
13. Role assignment (RA)	Directing a peer or self to perform or not to perform an action ("You be the dad!") (K&R, O, S, T)
14. Share/trade (ST)	Gives an object to a peer (O, S, T)
15. Suggestions (SG)	Proposes an activity for a peer in a conditional manner (e.g., "You could . . . ") (K&R)
Outcomes of Interactions	
1. Successful (+)	Child accomplishes the apparent function of the interaction (K&R)
2. Unsuccessful (−)	Child does not accomplish the apparent function of the interaction (K&R)

Investigators Using Behavioral Codes Included in SOCSI

D = Dore (1979)	OMO&B = Odom, McEvoy, Ostrosky, & Bishop (1987)
G&P-B = Guralnick & Paul Brown (1980)	P&G = Putallaz & Gotman (1981)
HG&C = Hartup, Glazer, & Charlesworth (1967)	P&K = Prutting & Kirschner (1987)
HW = Howes (1988)	R&K = Rubin & Krasnor (1987)
K&R = Krasnor & Rubin (1983)	S = Strain (1983)
B = Brown, Ragland, & Fox (1988)	S&T = Strain & Timm (1974)
O = Odom, Hoyson, Jamieson, & Strain (1985)	T = Tremblay, Strain, Hendrickson, & Shores (1981)

Reprinted from "Observational Assessment of Young Children's Social Behavior With Peers, by W. H. Brown, S. L. Odom, and A. Holcombe, 1996, *Early Childhood Research Quarterly, 11*, p. 30, with permission from Elsevier.

To have meaning, the frequency of an observed event must be specified in terms of some time frame. Thus, we often describe the rate of responding as the total number of occurrences per unit of time (minutes, hours, days, etc.) A simple formula for converting response frequency to response rate is calculated as follows:

$$\text{Response rate} = \frac{\text{Response frequency}}{\text{Time}}$$

For example, a clinician might wish to record the number of misarticulated phonemes during a 30-minute clinical session. Assuming that 18 such errors occurred during this period, response rate would be calculated as 18/30 = 0.6 per minute.

In discussing the history of time series research, McGuigan (1993) cited B. F. Skinner, who said that, with respect to progress in the behavioral sciences, his development of rate of responding measures was the most important of his own contributions. Single-subject research paradigms often display the results of an experiment in the form of a cumulative graph (see Chapter 8). Such a graph shows the total frequency of responses whereby changes in the dependent variable are attributed to systematic changes in the independent variable.

Frequency measures also have utility in studies of auditory physiology such as investigations of the characteristic frequency of discharge (Cfs) of cochlear neurons in response to acoustic stimuli. Figure 6-6 is neurogram representing the Cfs of 50 individual neurons in response to brief clicks. Recordings of neurons having Cfs in the lower-frequency range (cochlear apex) are located toward the front of the neurogram, whereas those with higher frequency Cfs (cochlear base) are located toward the rear.

Response Latency

Measurements of **response latency** are also used in recording physiological or behavioral observations in accordance with some predetermined unit of time. Such measures are

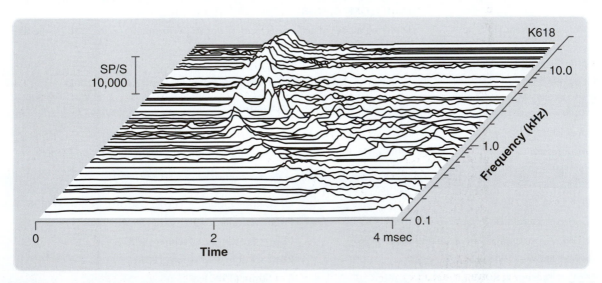

FIGURE 6-6   Neurogram display of spike activity for 50 individual neurons in a single animal. The stimulus was a brief click presented at a peak SPL of 100 dB

From "Stimulus Representation in the Discharge Pattern of Auditory Neurons," by N.Y.S. Kiang. In: D.B. Tower, ed. The Nervous System, *vol. 3 of* Human Communication and Its Disorders, *New York: Raven Press.*

recorded according to how long it takes for a specified response to occur following some specified event. In the neurogram shown in Figure 6-6, Cfs with the shortest latencies in response to clicks are located toward the rear of the neurogram, whereas those with the longest latencies are found toward the front.

Another relevant example of a useful latency measurement in the field of audiology involves the assessment of brainstem auditory evoked responses (BAERs), also called brainstem auditory evoked potentials (BAEPs), or auditory brainstem responses (ABRs). BAER is a non-invasive diagnostic test useful for evaluating the functional integrity of the auditory system from the ear through the brainstem. Auditory potentials are recorded from an array of electrodes placed on the scalp evoked by auditory stimulation typically consisting of click sounds presented rapidly to the ears. The evoked potentials, consisting of 1000 to 2000 responses, are averaged by a computer and displayed as a series of five waveforms (see Figure 6-7). These waves are believed to have relatively distinct anatomical loci as to where they are generated along the auditory pathway: Wave I is thought to represent neural activity emanating from the distal portion of the cochlea, Wave III arises from the superior olive, while Wave V is believed to reflect neural activation of the upper portions of the brainstem near the inferior colliculus. As can be seen in Figure 6-7, these waves can be plotted in such a way as to reflect the temporal progression of auditory neural activation from one generator site to the next.

The absence of waves or increased latencies along their time-base can indicate the presence of brain stem tumors, hearing loss, or neurological diseases such as multiple sclerosis. Figure 6-8 compares normal and pathologic BAER records from patients with surgically confirmed acoustic tumors.

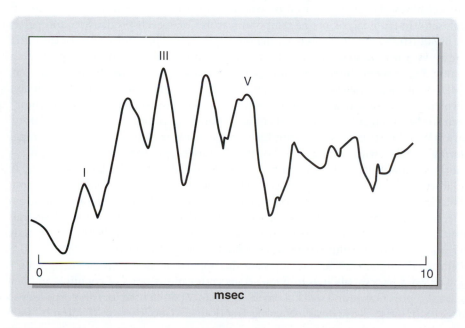

FIGURE 6-7   Illustration of auditory evoked potential. Latency measures are taken on the horizontal axis.

(adapted from Short-Latency Auditory Evoked Potentials, *by T.J. Glattke, 1983, p. 82, figure 7-3. Baltimore, MD: University Park Press.)*

FIGURE 6-8

ABR recorded from patients with surgically confirmed acoustic tumors. The top waveform in each panel is from a normal ear. The lower waveform in (A) shows the prolonged I–V interval from a patient with an acoustic neuroma. The lower waveform in (B) shows an absence of waves beyond Wave II from a patient with meningioma in the cerebello-pointine angle.

(adapted from Short latency auditory evoked Potentials *by American Speech–Language–Hearing Association. (1987). Rockville, MD: Audiologic Evaluation Working Group on Auditory Evoked Potential Measurements.)*

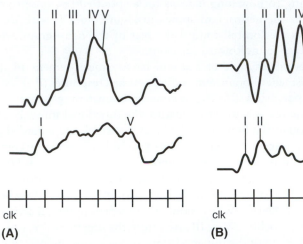
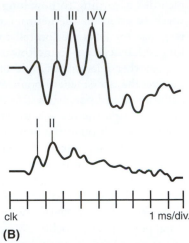

(A)   **(B)**

Latency measures likewise have many applications in acoustic studies of speech. For example, in studies of the acoustic cues that may be used in making perceptual distinctions among speech sounds, measures of voice onset time (VOT) have been employed often in conjunction with sound spectrography. According to Kent and Read (1999) VOT denotes the ". . . interval between the articulatory release of the stop and the onset of vocal fold vibration" (p. 108). VOT values can range from negative to positive depending on whether the consonantal feature of the stop is voiced or voiceless, respectively. Sound spectrograms can be highly useful in the analysis of the temporal features of speech production and perception. Figure 6-9 illustrates the VOT intervals, denoted by a vertical bar and arrow, for the initial consonant in *dad* for four speakers. The first spectrogram (A) is for a normal speaker, and the remaining 3 spectrograms (B–D) are for speakers with apraxia of speech. As can be seen, VOT intervals for the neurologically impaired speakers have negative values, indicating increments in prevoicing durations in stop productions. In the examples shown, the latency (time lapse) between the beginning of the laryngeal event (initiation of phonation) and articulatory event (plosive release burst) is relatively long for neurologically impaired speakers as compared to the normal speaker, with speaker (D) showing the longest prevoicing duration. This suggests that in the normal speaker there was a close coordination between the laryngeal event and the articulatory event, so VOT is close to zero. However, in the apraxic speakers, such coordination is lacking or less precise. Spectrograhic records such as these can help to make possible an objective examination of a variety of speech disorders. In addition to VOT, several other reaction time measures of response latency have been employed in studies of laryngeal dynamics in the study of speech fluency disorders (Adams, Freeman, & Conture, 1984).

Behavioral response latency measures are also applied in clinical studies designed to assess naming or word retrieval abilities in populations with various types of cognitive and language disorders. A representative and well known test instrument often used for this purpose by speech-language pathologists is the Boston Naming Test (Kaplan, Goodglass, & Weintraub, 1983).

Response Duration

Measures of **response duration** also have utility in both behavioral and physiological studies. A common measure of stuttering severity involves recording the duration of stuttering moments as assessed, for example, on the Riley Stuttering Severity Instrument for Children

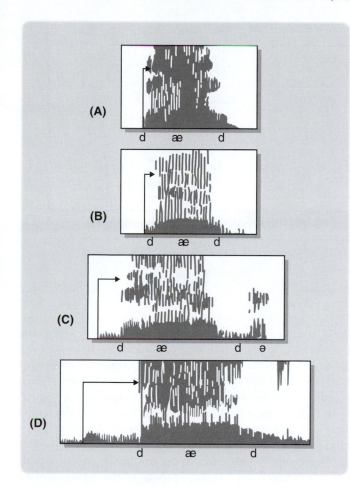

FIGURE 6-9

Spectrograms of the word *dad* produced by (A) a person with normal speech, and (B–D) persons with apraxia of speech. The interval marked by the arrow is the prevoicing duration of the interval |d| in |dad|. This represents the response latency time lapse between alaryngeal event (prevoicing duration) and an articulatory event (plosive release burst).

Reprinted with permission from The Acoustic of Speech, *by R. Kent and C. Read, 1992, San Diego: Singular Publishing Group.*

and Adults (1994). A simple stopwatch may be used for this purpose, or more sophisticated instrumentation such as sound spectography could be employed in the analysis of the separate elements of stuttering as shown in Figure 6-10. **Total response duration** can also be expressed as a proportion (percentage) of time spent in emitting a particular behavior during a defined period. For example, we might wish to calculate the proportion of speaking time marked by stuttering behavior during a 60-minute session. If the total response duration, based on measuring all stuttering moments was found to be 10 minutes, then the proportion of time spent stuttering would be calculated as 10/60 = .17 or 17%. Because some stuttering moments are likely to be longer than others, we might likewise wish to calculate their *mean duration*. This would involve a simple matter of dividing the total response duration time for stuttering by the number of stuttering moments noted to occur.

Response Amplitude-Intensity

The final measure that we wish to mention is based on physical or behavioral recordings of the **amplitude** or **intensity** of a response. Using a sound level meter with the decibel (dB) as a standard unit of sound measurement, we might set about to investigate the average intensity level of conversational speech (about 60 dB) as compared to shouting (about 75 dB) or very quiet speech (approximately 35–40 dB) as measured 3 feet from the sound source

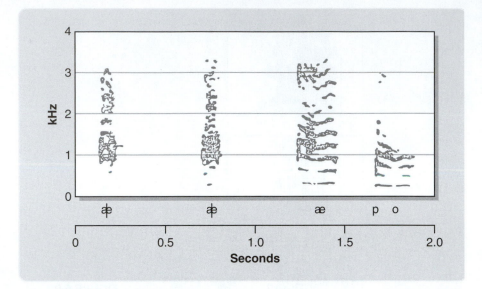

FIGURE 6-10

Sound spectrography of separate elements of stuttering

Reprinted with permission from Elements of Stuttering, *by C. Stromsta, 1986, Kalamazoo, MI: Atsmort Publishing, p. 74.*

(Fry, 1979). We might compare these values to inanimate sound sources such as a jet plane (130 dB at a distance of 120 feet) or the ticking of a watch next to the ear (20 dB).

Alternatively, we might decide to measure the amplitude-intensity function of the ear itself in response to sound. An illustrative application of the response of the auditory system to a sound wave is based on recordings of the acoustic reflex, the magnitude of which increases with the intensity of the stimulus. Figure 6-11 shows the acoustic reflex for a normal ear and an ear with eighth nerve disorder. Note that the maximum amplitude reflex of the abnormal ear is substantially reduced when compared to the normal ear.

A more general meaning of amplitude-intensity pertains to the amount or level of a quality as it is perceived or judged to exist by an observer. We might speak of the intensity of an anxiety reaction in a speaker and apply various rating scales such as low anxiety, moderate anxiety, or high anxiety based on our observation of a prescribed set of behaviors.

In considering all of the response measures discussed above, remember that no one of these is better than another but is selected as appropriate for recording the specific characteristics of the particular dependent variable under study. Furthermore, no matter how precise they might be, empirical measurements cannot replace the perspicacious judgments of the human observer who is ultimately responsible for analyzing and interpreting the recorded data in a reliable and valid manner.

SUMMARY

This chapter has focused on three research processes that can influence the reliability and validity of a study. We began by discussing the importance of controlling variables in order to determine the influence of the independent variable on the dependent variable. This can best be achieved through controlled experimental studies that allow for the active manipulation of one or more independent variables. In the process of such manipulation, the researcher seeks to maximize experimental systematic variance while minimizing random and systematic errors. We noted that random errors can be controlled to some degree through the method of constancy, which attempts to reduce inconsistencies in measurements, subject responses, and the conditions of testing. Systematic sources of error that can bias an experiment were also

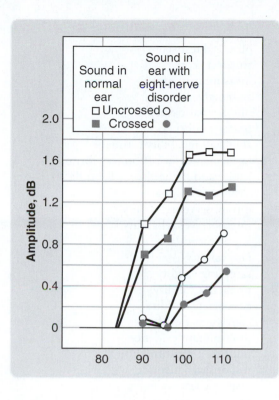

FIGURE 6-11

Amplitude-intensity function for acoustic reflex amplitude in a patient with an acoustic tumor

---

Reprinted with permission from Clinical Audiology: The Jerger Perspective, *B.R. Alford and S. Jerger, eds, 1993, p. 357, San Diego: Singular Publishing Group.*

discussed along with several methods for reducing them including counterbalancing, elimination of extraneous variables, statistical control, and blinding techniques.

A second research process reviewed in this chapter pertains to the selection and specification of measurements appropriate for the dependent variable(s) of an experiment. We noted that the first question a researcher should ask about a measurement concerns its utility. Is the measurement sensitive enough to identify a disorder or disease when present yet specific enough so as to seldom err in such identification? To what degree is the measurement free of the influence of ceiling effects (test is too easy) and floor effects (test is too hard)?

In deciding to use a particular measurement, the researcher also must evaluate its reliability and validity. Problems in the measurement of reliability stem largely from errors in determining how far an observed score varies from a true score. The means of calculating systematic errors (consistent errors) in relation to unsystematic errors (random errors) was discussed. Several types of reliability (test-retest, alternate-forms, internal consistency, and observer reliability) were reviewed, as well as approaches for assessing each type.

Whereas the concept of reliability essentially pertains to the consistency of a measurement, validity pertains to its accuracy. Types of validity (content, criterion, and construct validity) and approaches to their measurement were likewise considered in this chapter. We noted that the nature of the data in an experiment (whether it is nominal, ordinal, interval, or ratio) will determine the type of statistic used in its analysis.

The third and final research process we discussed concerned various approaches to recording measurements by the use of simple checklists and coding schemes or by means of computerized event recorders and their associated software programs. Four common measurements of behavioral/physiological responses were identified and described (frequency, latency, duration, and amplitude/intensity).

KEY TERMS

systematic variance
between-group variance
directionality problem
controlled experimental studies
organismic variables
errors of measurement
fluctuations in testing conditions
within-group variance
random errors
systematic errors
method of constancy
method of counterbalancing
within-subject designs
order effects
method of elimination
constancy of conditions
statistical control methods
analysis of covariance (ANCOVA)
covariates
experimenter bias
double-blind investigation
sensitive test
specific test
ceiling effects
floor effects

observed test score
true test score
measurement error
systematic error
unsystematic error
practice effect
split-half reliability estimate
Spearman-Brown Prophecy formula
Kuder and Richardson's formula 20
Cronbach's alpha
intraobserver reliability
interobserver reliability
kappa formula
face validity
sampling validity
predictive validity
concurrent validity
convergence evidence
discriminant evidence
multitrait-multimethod matrix
response frequency
response latency
response duration
total response duration
amplitude (intensity)

SELF-LEARNING REVIEW

1. The variable considered to cause variation in some other variable is called the _____ variable because it is independent of any influence by the _____ under investigation. The _____ variable is generally the measured variation in behavior caused by the _____ variable.

2. Known causes of variation in an experiment are termed _____ _____ or _____-_____ _____.

3. A frequent difficulty surrounding the interpretation of between-group difference based on assignment can result from the _____ problem.

4. Designs that involve the active and systematic manipulation of one or more independent variables are called _____ _____ _____.

5. Some independent variables, such as those involving relatively stable physical or psychological characteristic, are not subject to active experimental manipulation. They are called _____ variables.

6. Conceptually, tests of significance of difference between groups, such as the F test, can be defined as the ratio of _____ _____ to _____ _____. Symbolically, we write $F =$ _____.

7. Uncontrolled variation of the dependent variable can arise from _____ of measurement and _____ in the conditions of testing.

8. _____-_____ variance consists of error variance plus variations owing to differences within individual subjects that constitute the group.

9. Systematic variance includes sources of variance resulting from _____ _____ that consistently causes the scores in a distribution to lean in one direction or another.

10. Control of random errors can be partially achieved through the method of _____. Factors that can undermine this method in an experiment include: (1) inconsistency in _____, (2) inconsistency in _____ _____ during the repeated performance of the same task, and (3) inconsistency in the conditions of _____.

11. _____ reliability refers to the consistency of judgments within the same observer, based on measurements made at different points in time. _____ reliability refers to the consistency of judgments between two or more observers based on measurements made at the same point in time.

12. One means of controlling the potential biasing influence of one experimental treatment or condition preceding another is through the method of _____.

13. _____ _____ are interactions arising from one treatment variable preceding another.

14. The very best way to rule out the influences of extraneous variables is to _____ them from the experiment. Such a control procedure is called the method of _____.

15. When extraneous variables cannot be eliminated from the test environment, then the researcher generally attempts to maintain the _____ of _____ as far as possible.

16. Confounding factors pertaining to differences in subject characteristics can best be controlled through random assignment or matching techniques aimed at producing _____ samples.

17. _____ of _____ is designed to remove the influence of extraneous variables when they can be identified.

18. A(n) _____-_____ _____ is designed to reduce or eliminate the potential influence of experimenter bias.

19. In mathematical terms, a(n) _____ test can be defined as the proportion of people who test positive on a screening test to people with a disorder or a disease. A(n) _____ test translates into the ratio of people who test negative on a screening test to people without the disorder or disease.

20. _____ _____ result when scores on a test pile up at the high end of a distribution because the test is too easy or the dependent variable is too _____ to the treatment employed. Conversely, a(n) _____ _____ occurs when the majority of scores fall near the lower limit of a distribution, indicating that the test may be too difficult or the dependent variable is _____ to the experimental treatment.

21. There are two components of measurement error that can be associated with an observed score, namely a(n) _____ error and a(n) _____ error. Because such errors can never be eliminated entirely, the best we can do is to take them into account in the calculation of measurement reliability. The formula is given by: Reliability of Observed Score = _____.

22. _____ reliability is concerned with how consistent or stable a test measure is over time. _____-_____ reliability is concerned with measuring the consistency of the test results from two equivalent test forms.

23. One reliability method specifically designed to determine the internal consistency of the items within a test is called the _____-_____ _____ _____. The Spearman-Brown Prophecy formula is often used to estimate the internal consistency reliability coefficient for the entire test. Assuming that the correlation between the two halves of a test instrument is .75, by applying the Spearman-Brown formula, then the reliability of the test is _____.

24. In evaluating the internal consistency of a test, Kuder and Richardson's formula is used with _____ test items whereas the Cronbach's alpha is more appropriate for _____ data. The advantage of these methods over the split-half approach is that both procedures are based on calculating the _____ of all possible combinations of _____ _____.

25. While intraobserver reliability is related to the _____ of judgment, interobserver reliability is concerned with the _____ of judgment.

26. The formula for calculating interobserver reliability is _____.

27. The calculation of kappa (k) is calculated as _____.

28. _____ validity refers to how well a test adequately represents the various content domains that the test was designed to assess. It is sometimes called _____ _____.

29. _____ validity refers to how well a test can predict a particular outcome. There are two subtypes of such validity. The first of these, _____ validity, relates to the ability of a given test to predict an outcome that is consistent with the _____ _____ that underlies the test. Another subtype, _____ validity, refers to the results from a new test agreeing with those of existing tests that are presumed to be _____.

30. _____ validity is a metamorphic type of validity and pertains to establishing the meaning of test results in relation to the theoretical constructs upon which the test is based.

31. The process of developing a new test, especially when the meaning of the test result is unclear, entails the use of two types of evidence. They are _____ evidence and _____ evidence.

32. Frequency measures are especially useful in describing the characteristics of _____ observations or _____ data.

33. Measurements of _____ _____ are used in recording physiological or behavioral observations in accord with some predetermined unit of time.

34. _____ _____ _____ can be expressed as a proportion of time spent in emitting a particular behavior during a defined period.

35. A more general meaning of _____-_____ pertains to the amount or level of a quality as it is perceived or judged to exist by an observer.

QUESTIONS AND EXERCISES FOR CLASSROOM DISCUSSION

1. What is the experimental meaning of "systematic variance"? Provide two examples, one relevant to the *assignment* of the independent variable and another relevant to its *active manipulation*.

2. Distinguish between systematic variance and error variance.

3. What is a "controlled experimental study"? Why is such a study generally inappropriate for the study of organismic variables?

4. Discuss the "directionality problem" and provide at least two examples pertinent to research in communication sciences and disorders.

5. Given the formula: $F = V_b/V_e$, discuss the meaning of this ratio in interpreting the influence of the independent variable on the dependent variable. How does it relate to the calculation of between-group and within-group variance?

6. Discuss three sources of errors of measurement and provide an example of each as it might operate in a hypothetical experiment.

7. In considering how systematic variance might be maximized, what are some factors to consider?

8. By strict definition, random errors are due to chance alone. Yet, these errors can be partially controlled. Discuss the factors that can undermine *constancy* in an experiment and what can be done to improve it.

9. Define systematic errors and describe the means of their control.

10. Identify and describe four important factors to consider in selecting a particular measurement for use in an experiment.

11. Distinguish between a *sensitive* and a *specific* test and note the importance of each to the definition of a "good test."

12. What is the difference between a *ceiling* and a *floor* effect, and what are the implications of each for test construction?

13. How does the reliability of a test differ from its validity?

14. Identify and discuss four types of measurement reliability and provide an example of each.

15. Identify and discuss three types of measurement validity and provide an example of each.

16. Distinguish between the four scales of measurement.

17. Identify and discuss four common measures of behavioral/physiological responses.

Causal Inferences and Threats to Their Validity

CHAPTER 7

CHAPTER OUTLINE

LEARNING OBJECTIVES

After reading this chapter, you should be able to identify, describe, or define:

- The concept of causality
- How causal relationships differ from correlational relationships
- The statistical meaning of a coefficient of correlation
- How the "directionality" and "third variable" problems can complicate causal determination
- Three criteria for causal determination
- Four types of research validity and threats to their establishment

DETERMINING CAUSALITY

The use of controls as described in the previous chapter is an essential feature of any research methodology that seeks to explain the cause or causes of a particular observation. Before discussing the types of experimental designs employed for this purpose, let's first consider some scientific principles that underlie the quest to identify the causes of phenomena or "why things happen."

Philosophers have debated the nature of causality for centuries. Some, like David Hume and Immanuel Kant, have questioned whether cause-effect relationships between variables truly exist in the universe or instead represent the tendencies of the human mind to mistakenly attribute one event to another based merely on their co-occurrence. Most modern day scientists embrace an earlier view espoused by Aristotle that some observations in nature are not merely correlated in time and space but are dependently related so that a change in one object or event produces a change in another object or event. As we discussed in Chapter 1, the ultimate goal of science is to determine cause-effect relationships by systematically manipulating an independent variable (the cause) and observing the influence of this manipulation on the dependent variable (the effect) under controlled conditions.

One of the first steps in establishing a causal relationship between two or more observations is through what is referred to as the **method of association.** Using various correlational techniques (see Chapter 11), the correspondence between two or more sets of data can be determined. More specifically, by arranging pairs of observations according to the relative magnitude of one or the other factor, it is possible to determine the degree to which the factors covary or the degree to which a change in X factor is *correlated* with a change in Y factor. In statistical terms, the relations between X and Y can be expressed as a **coefficient of correlation** denoted by the letter r ranging from -1 to $+1$. Such a coefficient indicates the strength of a relationship between X and Y. Furthermore, the $+$ or $-$ sign indicates the direction of the relationship between X and Y. A plus sign means a positive relationship to the degree that the X and Y variables move in the same direction; thus if one variable increases so too will the other. On the other hand, a minus sign indicates a negative relationship in the sense that the two variables move in an opposite direction; as one goes up the other goes down.

As noted above, the numerical value r is expressed as a decimal value that ranges from -1 to $+1$. A coefficient of correlation of $r = -1$ describes a perfect, one-to-one negative relationship such that as each X score increases, each Y score will corresponding *decrease* by the same amount. By the same token, $r = +1$ describes a perfect, one-to-one positive

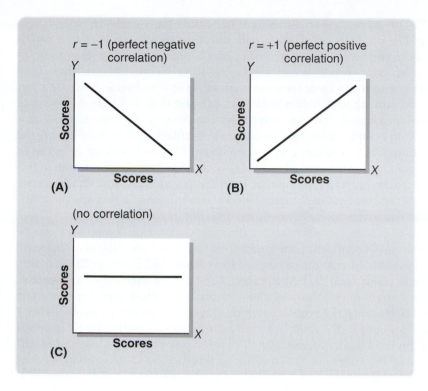

FIGURE 7-1

Examples of three different correlations: (A) perfect negative correlation, (B) perfect positive correlation, and (C) no correlation

relationship such that as each *X* score increases, each *Y* score will correspondingly *increase* by the same amount. Should *r* = 0, the two variables will be totally unrelated to one another (see Figure 7-1).

Although a correlation may suggest the existence of some type of relationship between two or more data sets, it is impossible to conclude on this basis alone that factor *X* influences or changes factor *Y*. This is because such a relationship may represent what researchers call a **spurious association** (one that is false) as opposed to reflecting a true causal influence. As mentioned in Chapter 3, one problem that can result in a spurious association involves the *directionality problem* that plagues much of correlational research. Recall that the directionality problem results when equally plausible (rival) explanations can be offered to explain the cause of the outcome of an investigation. For example, we might ask if competence in reading is *caused* by one's oral language ability or vice versa. The difficulty in discerning which of two variables is the *cause* and which is the *effect* is known in the common vernacular as the "chicken or the egg" dilemma. A second dilemma in interpreting the meaning of correlations can result from a spurious association involving the **third variable problem.** This problem occurs when an investigator concludes that there is a causal linkage between two variables when the true cause(s) is quite distinct from the variables under investigation. Thus, a child might illustrate deficits on tests of both reading ability and oral language ability because of such other variables as poor motivation, inattention, depression, anxiety, or some combination of these factors.

The possibility that the cause for a particular outcome might be the result of a set of interrelated factors, as opposed to a single factor, always must be borne in mind. According to Russell (1948), "... a 'thing' or a piece of matter is not to be regarded as a single persistent substantial entity, but as a string of events having a certain kind of causal connection with each other" (p. 475). This point is especially relevant in considering disorders of speech, language, and hearing. The products of human communication are the result of vast neural linkages among sensory-end organs and motor-end plates coordinated by higher order association areas within the brain. Theories regarding the linguistic rules that govern a myriad of interactions occurring within this complex system are as yet incomplete. Indeed, the sheer number of associations among its variables may be so complex that no single theory could ever account for all of their causal relations. Nevertheless, the history of science suggests that the challenge of solving complex problems more often stimulates rather than lessens the interest and motivation of researchers as they seek to determine how one event gives rise or brings about definite changes in the next. Meanwhile, we should proceed with caution in formulating causal inferences, keeping in mind that both the directionality and third variable problems are examples of how rival hypotheses lend credence to what is perhaps the most-often cited dictum of research practice: "Correlation does not imply causation."

By what means, then, can causality be determined? Unless rival hypotheses can be excluded with some degree of confidence, the internal validity of a study must be questioned. According to the logic expounded in the writings of John Stuart Mill (1806–1873), causality can be inferred, all else being equal, by two methods. The first, the **method of agreement,** states: *if X occurs then Y occurs.* In other words, when the presumed cause is present the effect should be present also. However, the problem with this logic as a proof of causality is that Y might occur in the absence of X. Thus, the observed relationship might be entirely spurious in nature. Aware of this limitation, Mill formulated a second proof called the **method of difference,** which states: *if not X then not Y.* According to this premise, Y occurs *only* when X occurs—Y fails to occur in the absence of X. This does not exclude other possible causes of Y. However, when such other influences are absent or under control (all things being equal), X is inferred as *sufficient* to cause Y.

Most scientists agree that still a third condition, called **temporal precedence,** must be met to determine causality. To conclude that X is sufficient to cause Y, X should *precede* the occurrence of Y. This is the same as saying that the "cause" must precede the "effect." Together, these three premises form the touchstone for most modern research hypothesis-testing procedures in which at least two effects are typically examined—the first when preceded by the presumed cause (experimental group) and the other when the presumed cause is absent (control group), or

$$X \longrightarrow Y \text{ (Presence of independent variable—experimental group)}$$
Compared to
$$\text{No } X \longrightarrow \text{No } Y \text{ (Absence of independent variable—control group)}$$

VALIDITY OF RESEARCH DESIGNS

Although causal inferences are always subject to some uncertainty, their validity can best be assured through the use of previously discussed controls to exclude as many rival explanations for the obtained results as possible. In Chapter 6, we discussed the meaning of the term *validity* in reference to interpreting various tests and measurements. Other meanings of the term pertain to the overall validity of a research investigation. Four types of validity relate to the accuracy of the conclusions or inferences made on the basis of scientific research, namely, (1) internal validity, (2) external validity, (3) statistical validity, and (4) construct (theoretical) validity (Campbell & Stanley, 1966; Cook & Campbell, 1979). Before discussing the relative merit of various research designs employed by researchers to test their research hypotheses, we will discuss each type of validity and the threats to each type.

Internal Validity

Internal validity refers to the extent that causal inferences are justified based on observed changes in a dependent variable in response to systematic variations in an independent variable. As we have noted, in order for a conclusion to be drawn with confidence, other plausible causes involving extraneous variables must be eliminated or controlled. Failure to do so could result in a **confounding effect** as a result of two variables being allowed to vary simultaneously. For example, if you wish to evaluate the comparative effectiveness of two therapy programs for treating aphasia, you could avoid the potential confounding effect of age on performance by matching subjects on this variable prior to their group assignment.

In estimating the internal validity of a research study, Cook and Campbell (1979) emphasized the importance of: "a deductive process in which the investigator has to systematically think through how each of the internal validity threats may have influenced the data . . . the researcher has to be his or her own best critic, trenchantly examining all of the threats he or she can imagine" (pp. 55–56). We agree with this position but would add that thought should also be given to potential sources of invalidity in the planning phase of a research study. Whereas the need for careful reflection in evaluating data is undeniable, it is more important to consider how threats to internal validity can be eliminated or controlled in planning and designing an experiment from the outset. As in the case of caring for one's own health, weak or ill-conceived research plans are better treated prospectively than lamented posthumously.

Threats to Internal Validity

The purpose of most experimental studies is to establish conditions that allow an investigator to conclude with confidence that an observed *effect* is the consequence of a particular *cause*. In other words, an investigator wishes to establish the internal validity of his or her research. To establish internal validity, various research designs are selected to maximize the intended systematic influence of the independent variable on the dependent variable while controlling or eliminating extraneous influences that might otherwise invalidate conclusions.

Several threats to internal validity can be identified according to two broad classes of statistical comparisons that were briefly discussed in Chapter 6. The first of these is called a **within-subjects design** (repeated-measures design). Such a design involves a comparison within the same subjects under circumstances in which they were exposed to two or more treatment conditions. Suppose you wish to investigate the influence of verbal reward on some aspect of children's pragmatic language skills such as appropriate turn-taking during conversations. You decide to measure such skills prior to introducing the treatment condition and after the treatment condition has been in effect for some period of time. A "within-subjects comparison" can be completed by examining each participant's "before and after" performance records. An obvious advantage of this design is that there is no need for matching subjects on extraneous variables since each subject serves as his or her own control.

Instead of opting for a within-subjects design, you could have decided to investigate the same problem using a **between-subjects design.** Such a design involves the comparison of groups that have been treated differently on some independent variable. Typically, subjects are randomly assigned to one of two or more treatment conditions or are carefully matched prior to their assignment. In the case of our example, the performance of one group of subjects exposed to verbal praise could have been compared to a second group who was not exposed. The statistical comparison of scores *between* groups exposed to different treatment conditions constitutes a between-subjects comparison.

We will now discuss several threats to internal validity associated with each of these designs.

Within-Subject Sources of Internal Invalidity

History Effect

Two types of subject variation due to historical influences, or history effects, may alter the validity of a study. The first of these, called **proactive history,** relates to *preexisting differences* due to learned or inherent abilities that subjects might bring to an investigation. Differences related to gender, personality, intelligence, motivation, learning experiences, and the like are potential sources of such variation that might invalidate a study.

> **Example:**
>
> An entering class of graduate students is tested on matters pertaining to their knowledge of communication disorders and related issues of a professional nature. The faculty are surprised that the class as a whole seems less knowledgeable than students entering the previous year. Should the faculty be apprehensive about the academic capability of the new class? Not without checking the educational backgrounds of the students as compared to the year before. It just might turn out that a relatively large number of the new students had undergraduate majors in fields other than communication disorders as compared to the class of the previous year.

Because of the great variability that can preexist in subject characteristics, researchers must give careful thought as to how it can be controlled. When the size of the sample (n) is sufficiently large, say a sample size of greater than 30 ($n > 30$) subjects in each group, proactive history effects can best be controlled through randomization. For smaller samples of 30 or fewer subjects ($n \leq 30$), strategies designed to eliminate or hold subject characteristics constant might be more effectively employed.

Another type of historical influence, termed **retroactive history,** relates to change-producing environmental events, tangential to the purposes of an experiment, that intervene between two observations or measurements (e.g., between a pretest and posttest).

> **Example:**
>
> We wish to determine the effect of completing a research and statistical methods course on graduate students' attitudes about the importance of such content to their future day-to-day work as clinicians. Attitudes are pretested at the beginning of the course and posttested upon completion. In the interim, the coordinator of graduate studies circulates a memorandum with study tips for students preparing for comprehensive examinations, many of whom are presently enrolled in our course. The memorandum states, among other things, that the "ability to critically evaluate research literature will be emphasized and necessary in order to satisfy the academic standards of the program."

Of the factors that can potentially invalidate a research study, the historical influences related to changing events in people's lives involving daily living circumstances (physical and mental status, social and economic conditions, etc.) are perhaps the most difficult to control. Because the likelihood of such changes often increases with the passage of time, the interval between a pretest and posttest should be as brief as possible given the aims of a study.

Maturation Effect

Maturational effects are internal biological or psychological changes within subjects that may occur over a span of time resulting in performance variations unrelated to the treatment of interest.

Example:

At the beginning of the school year, you decide to evaluate the efficacy of an articulation training program for a group of first-grade students who have yet to acquire correct production of the /s/ phoneme. You pretest the children in September before commencing treatment and provide therapy until June of the following year, when you posttest their performance. Happily, for most, a significant reduction in the severity of frontal lisping has occurred. Perhaps coincidentally, because of the full eruption of their central incisors, the dental appearance of many of these children has likewise greatly improved! Such maturational changes in dentition might account, in whole or in part, for the observed improvement in articulation.

As in the case of retroactive history, maturational influences are more likely to confound internal validity the longer the period between the pretest and the posttest. In addition, to the extent that they reflect endogenous progression in mental or physical ability resulting from developmental changes, maturational effects are likely to grow stronger with the passage of time. Obviously, maturational effects cannot be eliminated. However, their potentially biasing influence can be equated through the use of a control group.

Sleeper Effect

This source of invalidity is a change in a dependent variable due to a treatment effect that is not immediately observable but tends to become increasingly observable over a span of time.

Example:

The therapeutic benefits of antibiotics in treating ear infections may not immediately improve hearing acuity, but gradually, over several days or weeks, hearing may be observed to improve as the result of a reduction in inflammation and swelling, in fluid in the ear, and so on. Thus, it would be invalid to conclude that a particular antibiotic is not effective simply because no instantaneous improvement in hearing is observed.

Testing Effect

Previous testing on performance measures can have a facilitative influence, called the **testing effect,** accruing as the result of familiarity, practice, or learning with repeated exposure to the same or similar test.

Example:

There is evidence that people tend to score better on IQ measures merely as the result of repeated testing (Anastasi, 1988). Some measures of verbal ability, such as the Peabody Picture Vocabulary Test, attempt to offset the potential for such a *practice effect* by developing two standardized forms of this particular instrument. Of course, there also is the familiar refrain of students proclaiming to their instructors after taking the first test of the semester, "Now that I know what to expect, I'll do better the second time around."

While the use of an alternative form of the same test can help diminish the confounding influence of the practice effect, it is not likely to eliminate the effect entirely. As we shall see later in the next chapter, some experimental designs eliminate a pretest or account for its potential effects by including a non-pretested control group as a part of the design.

Order and Carryover Effects

When the effects of two or more treatments are being compared within the same group of subjects, the sequence in which the treatments are presented might confound interpreting the results.

Example:

Suppose you wish to determine which of two therapies, A or B, is the more effective of the two. You decide to administer therapy A first, followed by therapy B. The subjects' performance during therapy B might improve solely as a result of practice or decline solely as a result of fatigue independent of a treatment effect (**order effect**). Moreover, whatever positive or negative effects that resulted from having received therapy A first might carryover to therapy B so that the latter response measures reflect the residual influence of therapy A singly or the combined effects of both treatments (**carryover effect**). More simply stated, therapy B could appear more or less effective than it would have if administered alone.

A procedure mentioned in Chapter 6, called *counterbalancing,* is frequently employed to control for order and carryover effects. Such effects can be controlled by distributing them equally across treatment conditions. Thus, subject 1 might be given treatment A followed by treatment B, while subject 2 would receive treatment B followed by treatment A. In the case of only two treatment conditions, the treatment sequence would be altered so that half of the subjects would end up receiving treatment A first followed by treatment B and the other half would receive treatment B first followed by treatment A. Obviously, interaction effects pose a threat to internal validity only when more than one treatment effect is under investigation. For additional information about methods for counterbalancing, see Chapter 8.

Instrumentation Effect

Changes can occur in the accuracy or precision of measuring devices or human observations. This produces an **instrumentation effect** that undercuts validity.

Example:

The calibration of an audiometer is altered or an electrical short in the wiring of a headphone produces intermittent static noise during an experiment. The audiologist conducting the experiment develops an ear infection accompanied by tinnitis (ringing sensations) that is likely to interfere with his or her own accuracy in judging and recording subject responses during speech discrimination testing.

Sources of invalidity arising from errors in mechanical or electrical measuring devices can best be eliminated by proper calibration and equipment maintenance throughout the course of a study. In cases where the recording instrument is a human observer, training such observers until they obtain a predetermined criterion of accuracy in making reliable judgments should occur in advance of the investigation. To discover later that such observers are neither accurate nor reliable obviously will invalidate the results. Ultimately, errors resulting from instrumentation, regardless of the source, must be attributable to what the experimenter did or failed to do. Such errors are not the result of flaws in the design of a study per se.

Statistical Regression

In the nineteenth century, Francis Galton observed from hereditary studies of nature that the characteristics of phenomena not only evolve but end up clustering in such a way as to be more similar than dissimilar. Statistically, this is reflected in the tendency for extreme scores in a data set, on repeated testing, to move toward the average score of the distribution, or **statistical regression.**

Example:

A researcher wishes to examine voice onset times in two groups of stuttering children that differ in severity. Subjects whose severity scores are atypical of their average level of disfluency may be inappropriately delegated to one group or the other. Greater regression is likely for subjects whose scores are the most extreme. Given a large number of such subjects, resulting comparisons between the two groups would be inappropriate because the groups tend to be more alike than initially believed.

Because the natural tendency of most phenomena is to statistically regress toward an average observation, the effect is difficult if not impossible to eliminate in most research studies. One means of controlling for this tendency is in the statistical analysis of the data. By subdividing control and experimental groups on the basis of their performance scores into, let's say, "high" and "low" achievers, statistical comparisons may lead one to find significant differences between them when none were found by comparing the groups as a whole.

Between-Subject Sources of Internal Invalidity

Selection Bias

Selection is a process of assigning subjects to different groups or conditions of an experiment (see Chapter 5). The goal in most experiments is to equate subject characteristics through random assignment or through such nonrandom means as matching subjects on characteristics that might otherwise confound the interpretation of findings. However, preexisting factors may preclude or interfere with the establishment of equivalent groups so that it cannot be assumed that the operative influences or treatments in an experiment differ systematically only with respect to the independent variable. In other words, a **selection bias** might operate.

> **Example:**
>
> You wish to determine the effectiveness of a parent-counseling program in facilitating the language acquisition of preschool children judged to be mildly delayed on standardized language tests. You ask for volunteers and divide children into two groups based on their parents' participation in counseling or the lack thereof. Some months later, posttesting reveals that the children whose parents participated in the counseling program made significant gains in language development whereas the children of the nonparticipating parents did not. Can you conclude that parent counseling was effective in achieving the intended goals? You cannot.

One major problem relates to the volunteer status of the parent participants who may have been more highly motivated to provide direct assistance to their children despite the counseling program. Furthermore, the children of the parent volunteers may have come from cultural or socioeconomic backgrounds in which greater emphasis is placed on developing the very same type of verbal skills measured by the testing procedures.

Differential Attrition

Although sometimes referred to as *experimental mortality,* we prefer to call this extraneous variable **differential attrition** because subjects may terminate their participation in an experiment for reasons other than that implied by the more ominous term. Hopefully, when the loss of subjects occurs, as often happens, especially in the course of lengthy experiments, it will be for reasons related to ordinary living circumstances (e.g., job changes, family or school demands, moving from the area, temporary illness, etc.). Whatever the reason, the differential loss of subjects from comparison groups can seriously impair an experiment.

> **Example:**
>
> Suppose you wish to study the speed and accuracy of sentence comprehension in two groups of subjects, one group during a quiet condition and the other under a condition of ambient noise. You know or suspect that a subject's performance may be related differentially to such

extraneous factors as age, intelligence, motivation, attention, and so forth. As a means of controlling these extraneous variables, you may attempt to distribute their effects equivalently in the two groups through random assignment or try to control for such influences through careful matching of groups on all-important variables so that they differ only with respect to the independent variable. Despite your best efforts to achieve control, subjects drop out from one group in significant numbers, invalidating the assumption of group equivalency. The resulting imbalance is reflected not only in a disproportionate number of subjects constituting the comparison groups, but in the loss of control over important variables that are likely to differentially impact group performance.

The validity of a research study can be seriously jeopardized by the loss of subjects, particularly when the attrition rate is large. This is because the assumption of having achieved group equivalence through the randomization or matching of subject characteristics (e.g., gender, race, age, education, motivation, health status, etc.) may no longer hold true. While the loss of subjects sometimes can be dealt with through statistical adjustments, researchers hope to avoid the necessity of doing so. The larger the number of subjects recruited to participate and the lengthier the time period required to complete a study, the greater this threat is likely to be.

Compensatory Rivalry

Unwanted competition between the groups of an experiment—**compensatory rivalry**—can inadvertently emerge to confound the interpretation of a treatment effect.

> **Example:**
>
> Suppose we divide the mothers who volunteered for the parent-counseling program discussed above into two subgroups. We are interested in evaluating the extent to which a packet of specially designed therapy materials might augment the goals of counseling. One of the parent subgroups (experimental subjects) is given this packet during their counseling sessions and instructed as to how such materials can be used at home to foster language development in their children. The second subgroup of parents (control subjects) comes to the clinic for counseling related to the problems of their children just like the first subgroup, but does not receive any materials for supplemental use at home. Suppose that conversations among a mix of these parents during clinic visits lead some to learn about the existence of the homework packet given to other parents but not to themselves. Consequently, such parents may choose to work extra hard with their own children at home, be more sensitive to their children's needs, or alter their style of parent–child interaction in other ways in an effort to compensate for a perceived deficiency in facilitating their children's language development. Compensatory rivalry of this kind is sometimes called the "John Henry effect" after the legendary steel driver who, upon learning of the invention of a new machine, competed to outperform it and died of overexertion in the process.

The best means of dealing with compensatory rivalry is to avoid exposing control and experimental subjects to one another throughout the period of a research study. If this cannot be avoided, subjects should be asked to refrain from discussing the nature of their involvement with other participants.

Resentful Demoralization

A confounding factor associated with an outcome just opposite to that of compensatory rivalry can occur when some subjects in an experiment perceive that other subjects, as compared to themselves, are receiving a more favorable treatment.

Example:

Referring once again to the parent-counseling experiment described above, knowledge by some parents that other parents had been singled out for special treatment may cause resentment, anger, and decreased motivation. In this event, the net effect might lead them to be less effective in addressing the language problems of their children. Thus, although exerting opposite influences, both **resentful demoralization** and compensatory rivalry can confound the interpretation of a treatment effect that might otherwise be demonstrated.

As in the case of compensatory rivalry, avoiding circumstances that allow experimental and control subjects to discuss the nature of their research participation can best prevent resentful demoralization.

Experimenter Bias (Rosenthal Effect)

Whereas well-designed experiments are effective at eliminating most, if not all, threats to their internal validity, some pitfalls are sometimes difficult, if not impossible, to avoid no matter how well the study is planned. Such threats are often due to inherent biases within the investigator rather than to structural faults in the research design.

Rosenthal and Jacobson (1968) have documented several sources of such bias. **Experimenter bias** often exists in the form of expectations about what the results of an investigation *ought to be* that can lead an investigator, perhaps unknowingly, to treat subjects differently in certain respects or to favor a particular outcome.

Example:

An early awareness of the power of such "self-fulfilling prophesies" is contained in the story of Clever Hans, the horse who was believed to be able to understand words, spell, and perform arithmetic in response to his trainer's instructions. What first were considered remarkable abilities were later discovered to represent conditioned responses to subtle movements and related cues unintentionally provided by the trainer.

The practical implication of this story is represented in the problems resulting from labeling school children as "cognitively impaired," "learning disabled," "conduct disordered," and so on. Research has demonstrated quite clearly that such labels can mold teachers' expectations in ways that influence their evaluation of student performance (Rosenthal & Jacobson, 1968).

As the name implies, experimenter bias is directly attributable to the experimenter and not to a flaw in research design. In Chapter 6, we discussed the means of controlling such bias by blinding procedures that prevent an experimenter's expectations from influencing the outcome. We noted that one of these procedures, called *double-blinding*, can prevent subjects' expectations, as well as those of the experimenter, from biasing the results of a study. It is also known that such awareness may limit the generality of finding to other subjects, settings, or treatment circumstances. Such limitations pertain to the external validity of research data—the next topic of our discussion.

External Validity

External validity pertains to the degree to which the results from a specific sample are generalizable to one or more populations, settings, treatment variables, or measurement variables (Campbell & Stanley, 1966). Establishing external validity is predicated on the existence of internal validity. Obviously, when there is reason to doubt the accuracy of experimental results, questions pertaining to their generalization are moot. However, in most investigations, the researcher is faced with balancing the often conflicting or competitive demands for establishing both external and internal validity. Efforts to achieve relevancy can result in the loss of experimental control over important variables. On the other hand, gains in experimental control can reduce the meaning of the results as they might otherwise apply to the outside world. In addressing the problem of external validity, we are asking about the usefulness of our findings to the world beyond the narrow domain of our own investigation. As noted above, it is possible for data to be internally valid but lack external validity. For example, we know that it is often possible to achieve marked reductions in stuttering behavior within the clinic or laboratory but also difficult to generalize these same results to other speaking conditions. The same could be said for many other types of cases and treatment programs in the field of communication disorders. A common argument for the use of inclusion models of therapy intervention, as commonly practiced in many school systems, is that such programs are purported to foster improved functioning in more "real life situations" than can be provided in relatively "artificial settings" as the therapy room. Yet, a study's prospects of replication are of major concern in matters pertaining to its external validity. If a study cannot be replicated, it has little or no scientific value regardless of the internal validity of its results.

Threats to External Validity

When one asks about the external validity of a particular study, the question pertains to the limits of how far the results can be extended beyond the confines of a particular study to other persons, settings, or circumstances. Just as the factors that jeopardize internal validity must be weighed, threats to the generality of research findings require careful evaluation. Citing philosopher David Hume (1711–1776), Campbell and Stanley (1966) noted there is in fact no logical basis for ever making generalizations beyond the limits of a particular study in absolute terms. This is because the precise characteristics of subjects, conditions, or circumstances surrounding the time and place of an original experiment can never be fully duplicated. The best a researcher can do is to make the best guesses possible about what pitfalls might undermine the generality of the results of an experiment. Several factors can restrict or invalidate the generalizability of research finding.

Subject Bias

Subject bias refers to the fact that the mere awareness by subjects that they are being observed or evaluated can influence their performance. Relevant to an understanding of subject bias is the **Hawthorne effect,** named after a production plant of the Western Electric Company where the effect was first observed in a study of factors influencing worker productivity. It was found that any change in the lighting condition, whether an increase or decrease in illumination, seemed to improve worker performance. Such improvements appeared to be related to the workers' awareness that they were being "singled out" for observation rather than to the particular manipulation employed by the experimenter (change in level of illumination). Although the reasons for the effect are no doubt complex, it is believed that the action of an independent variable can alter the behavior of subjects based on how they perceive the experimenter might expect or hope they will behave (Franke & Kaul, 1978). In such cases, subjects' presumptions about the intended effect of an independent variable may turn out to be quite different from the effect intended by the experimenter.

The lesson to be learned from the Hawthorne effect is that subjects should not be viewed as *passive* objects in an experiment but as participants who are potentially *reactive* to factors in addition to the treatment (independent variable). The attributes of the people studied (age, gender, education, attitude, motivation, anxiety, experience, etc.) may interact with treatment(s) as to limit generalizations. As noted previously, there is evidence that the preconceptions of subjects as to how they should behave in a study can influence the outcome. Orne (1959), who did some of the earliest work in this area, identified what has come to be known as the **good subject effect**—descriptive of subjects who try hard to perform in accordance with what they believe are the expectations of the experimenter. Thus, some subjects participating in hypnosis research, might act out and even exaggerate certain trance-like characteristics of a hypnotized person because of certain preconceptions about what the experimenter might want them to do. Alternatively, some researchers (Silverman, 1977; Jourard, 1968) have identified the **negativistic** or **perverse subject effect**—subjects who may be hostile toward a particular research project and attempt to undermine what they perceive its goals to be by their dishonest or uncooperative behavior.

All of the forms of subject bias noted above are difficult to control. Whenever possible, yet within the codes of ethical research practice, the amount of information given to subjects about the treatment they receive and the reasons for it should be as limited as possible.

Pretest Sensitization

The threats to external validity discussed thus far result from certain biasing influences involving subjects' attitudes, expectations, or perceptions about their role in a particular experiment. **Pretest sensitization,** another biasing factor similar to those just reviewed, also can interact with experimental treatments, leading to invalid generalizations. For example, suppose you wish to investigate the vocational acceptability of adults born with a cleft lip and palate. You administer an attitudinal test to potential employers followed by an informational film about various aspects of the birth defect (its causes, physical and psychological consequences, treatment, etc.). Subsequently, you administer the attitudinal test again. Even though a change in attitudes is evident on the posttest, you are unable to conclude that the film caused it. Items on the pretest may have sensitized the subjects to the influence of the film, causing a positive or negative modification in attitudes that might not have occurred in the absence of the pretest. On the other hand, merely giving the pretest might have altered attitudes in the absence of the film. Whatever the final results, the confounding influence of pretesting cannot be ruled out.

Still other sources of external invalidity can result from certain restrictions resulting from errors inherent in an experimenter's assumptions about the appropriateness of the sampling, measurement, or treatment procedures used in an experiment. A brief description of each of these restrictions is provided next.

Sample Restrictions

Sample restrictions, that might adversely affect the external validity of an experiment, relate to the representativeness of the subjects used (see Chapter 5). More specifically, a question that must be raised pertains to the degree that a sample of subjects truly reflects the behaviors, physical and mental attributes, socioeconomic status, motivation, level of skill, and the like as the target population to whom we wish to extrapolate our findings. If a sample of subjects is not representative of the population, there is no justification for inductively inferring the meaning of an experiment beyond the immediate results. A reasonable safeguard is to clearly identify the specific population characteristics of the population for which generalization is desired *prior to* an experiment. Having done so, the next step is to implement sampling procedures estimated to yield a subject pool as much like the population of interest as possible. Nevertheless, we must also keep in mind the difference between our ability to generalize *to* a population as opposed to *across* a population (Cook & Campbell, 1979). While it may be possible to apply our conclusions to a population as a whole, there may be subgroups within the population to which the results do not apply. For example, a particular therapy approach shown to be effective in treating dysphagia may lack utility for certain disorders or diseases despite the fact that subpopulations of individuals having such disorders or diseases were included in the study sample. Statistically speaking, the "average" score for a sample characteristic may not adequately represent the same tendency found in any one segment of the population frame.

Measurement Restrictions

Measurement restrictions are those in which the measure selected to represent a dependent variable is not truly representative of the phenomenon that the experimenter wants to assess. Imagine an experimental study of people who stutter designed to explore the level of anxiety associated with speaking in the presence of photographs of certain individuals. The investigator selects galvanic skin response or palmar sweating as the measure of anxiety to be recorded at predetermined times during the experiment. The question is whether or not the degree of physiologic (autonomic) arousal is the variable that was actually of interest to the investigator. After the experiment, a problem arises should he or she decide to the contrary. For example, it might be decided that the more intriguing issue pertains to the nature of the threats posed by the photographs *as consciously perceived* by the speaker. In this case, cognitive measures of apprehension or rating scales of avoidance about speaking engendered by the photographs might have proved more useful in examining the "real" question of interest. Before initiating an experiment, it is important to determine the degree to which a selected measure is appropriate for its intended use and thus capable of producing relevant (generalizable) results.

Treatment Restrictions

Treatment restrictions that might involve, for example, the selection of an independent variable that is unsuitable for generalizing results, can also limit the external validity of an experiment. In our example above, it could be argued that the use of photographs to examine speech related anxiety is an *artificial research arrangement* having little or no relevance to actual speaking situations; that is, individuals typically speak to other people directly rather than having imaginary conversations in response to the photographs of such people. Based on this line of reasoning, the investigator might alter the experiment by substituting actual listeners in place of photographs in an effort to create testing conditions more like "real-life" speaking circumstances. While admitting that the generality of results could be improved by such an alteration, critics might still contend that any testing arrangement involving experimental research is artificial to the degree that it departs from natural occurring circumstances or ordinary experience. Although such a conclusion is technically correct, the internal validity of some research studies simply cannot be evaluated short of the controls and constancy imposed by the structure of a laboratory experiment. The investigator is generally faced with alternative choices that require perspicacious judgment in weighing threats to external validity against internal validity. As the risks to external validity increase because of the artificially of a treatment or setting, the influence of extraneous variables threatening internal validity often decrease. The reverse is also found.

Threats to Statistical Conclusion Validity

A third category of validity important to establish in a scientific study, statistical conclusion validity, pertains to the relative truth upon which its statistical conclusions are based. In most investigations, statistical methods are used for collecting, organizing, analyzing, and interpreting the results of a study in a mathematical form. A characteristic of such data that usually interests the researcher is its variability. More specifically, a major concern is the degree to which data are indicative of intended systematic influences as opposed to uncontrolled chance factors. Based on the available information, an educated guess in the form of a hypothesis is formulated as to the likely outcomes (statistical findings) of the experiment.

In the vernacular of statistics, hypotheses are generally formulated in the *null* form. A null hypothesis is one formulated for the specific goal of statistical significance testing, thereby permitting generalization from a sample of cases to the population from which such cases were drawn. Briefly defined, the word *null* means "no difference" and generally refers to a predicted finding of no significant differences between or within groups of subjects or treatment conditions (see Chapter 4).

Associated with null hypotheses are probability estimates for making certain types of statistical inference errors (sampling errors): *type I* or *type II errors*. Recall that a *type I error* involves rejecting a particular null hypothesis when it is true. For example, there is a chance of erroneously concluding that treatment A is significantly better than treatment B when it is not. On the other hand, one might make a *type II error* (retaining a null hypothesis when it is false) by erroneously concluding that a particular treatment is no more effective than another.

As discussed previously, the researcher typically selects an acceptable risk for error in the form of a significance level (i.e., alpha = .05 or alpha = .01, where the term "alpha" represents a type I error) prior to initiating an experiment. For a finding to be regarded as "significant" the odds for making an inferential error must be quite small—no greater than 5% of the time in the case of the first probability value noted above (.05). In the case of the second value (.01), an inferential error would be expected only 1% of the time.

Remember that statistical significance testing involves *estimating the odds* for a systematic influence controlled by the experimenter against the expected amount of deviation in the measures of interest owing to chance alone. As a part of null hypothesis testing, errors of inference can and do occur. The nature of such errors and their statistical relevance for formulating and testing null hypotheses is discussed more fully in Chapter 12.

Threats to Construct Validity

The final type of threat to research validity that we wish to discuss pertains to the notion of the truth of a construct or theory. In Chapter 6, we discussed the meaning of *construct validity* in relation to developing new tests and measurements. In addition, researchers use this term to describe the extent to which the results obtained from a new research investigation converge with those found in other investigations of the same phenomenon to support a particular theory.

For example, numerous researchers have attempted to study anxiety in individuals who stutter because of its presumed theoretical relevance in explaining characteristics of the behavior. The inconclusive nature of the research findings about the role of anxiety in stuttering may be the result of employing widely differing methods that measure unrelated things. Physiological measures of autonomic arousal, like galvanic skin response or palmar sweating, may tap into aspects of anxiety that are quite distinct from other indicators based on anxiety questionnaires, subjects' expectancies of stuttering, ratings of word or situational avoidance, or certain behavioral observations. Because of discrepancies among the results of several pertinent experiments, the role of anxiety and its theoretical importance in reference to various aspects of stuttering behavior can be said to lack construct validity. Construct validity can only be established based on evidence accumulated from several studies performed by different researchers employing the same operational definitions or criterion measures of anxiety. Because of the diversity of the methods and measurements employed by researchers to investigate a particular problem, construct validity is often hard to establish.

Statistical methods have been developed that allow for the analysis and summary of the results of independent experiments. In the future, such a sophisticated group of statistical procedures, called *meta-analysis,* will no doubt play a critical role in helping to validate the theoretical constructs that serve as a basis for explaining and managing problems in numerous professional fields, including communication disorders (see Chapter 12).

SUMMARY

An underlying assumption of modern day science is that causal relationships exist among variables. Much of scientific work is aimed at discovering such relationships. In the process of such discovery, it is necessary to distinguish between relationships that are merely correlational in nature versus those that are causally determined. Three means for this determination were discussed in this chapter including the method of agreement, the method of difference, and temporal precedence.

As we shall see in the next chapter, the search for causality occurs within the framework of experiments in which an independent variable is systematically manipulated to determine the influence of such manipulation on a dependent variable. In the process of doing so, the influences of extraneous variables that can invalidate an experiment are controlled as completely as possible. Four types of threats to validity that are typically of concern in research studies were reviewed including:

- Internal validity: the extent to which causal inferences are justified based on observed changes in a dependent variable in response to systematic variations in an independent variable.
- External validity: the extent to which the results from a specific study sample of cases are generalizable to one or more populations, settings, treatment variables, or measurement variables.
- Statistical conclusion validity: the relative truth of the statistical findings from a study.
- Construct validity: the relative truth of the theory used to explain the statistical findings.

KEY TERMS

method of association
coefficient of correlation
spurious association
third variable problem
method of agreement
method of difference
temporal precedence
internal validity
confounding effect
within-subjects design
between-subjects design
proactive history
retroactive history
maturation effect
sleeper effect
testing effect
order effect

carryover effect
instrumentation effect
statistical regression
selection bias
differential attrition
compensatory rivalry
resentful demoralization
experimenter bias (Rosenthal effect)
external validity
subject bias (Hawthorne effect)
good subject effect
negativistic (perverse) subject effect
pretest sensitization
sample restrictions
measurement restrictions
treatment restrictions

SELF-LEARNING REVIEW

1. One of the first steps in establishing a causal relationship between two or more observations is through the method of _____, or the _____ method.

2. In statistical terms, the relations between X and Y can be expressed as a _____ _____ denoted by the letter $+r$ or $-r$.

3. Statistically, the numerical value r is expressed as a decimal value that ranges from _____ to _____.

4. A perfect one-to-one negative relationship between X and Y can be expressed as $r =$ ____. If $r =$ _____, the two variables will be totally unrelated to one another.

5. Although a correlation may suggest the existence of some type of relationship between two or more data sets, it is impossible to conclude on this basis alone that factor X influences factor Y due to the possibility of a _____ _____ as opposed to reflecting a true causal influence.

6. The difficulty in discerning which of two variables is the cause and which is the _____ is the so-called _____ problem that plagues much of correlational research.

7. The third variable problem is another dilemma in interpreting the meaning of a _____.

8. According to John Stuart Mill, causality can be inferred, all else being equal, by two methods. The first method, called the method of _____, stated: if _____ occurs, then _____ occurs. The second method is called the method of _____, which states: if not _____, then _____ _____.

9. Most scientists agree that still a third condition must be met to determine causality, called _____ _____. To conclude that X is _____ to cause Y, _____ should precede the occurrence of _____.

10. _____ validity refers to the extent that causal inferences are justified based on observed changes in a dependent variable in response to systematic _____ in an independent variable.

11. Failure to eliminate plausible causes involving extraneous variables could result in a(n) _____ _____ as a result of two variables being allowed to vary simultaneously.

12. Several threats to internal validity can be identified according to two broad classes of statistical comparisons. A(n) _____-_____ design involves a comparison within the same subjects under circumstances in which they were exposed to two or more conditions. On the other hand, a(n) _____-_____ design involves the comparison of groups that have been treated differently on some independent variable.

13. Two types of subject variation due to historical influences may alter the validity of a study. _____ _____ relates to preexisting differences due to learned or inherent abilities that subjects might bring to an investigation. _____ _____ relates to change-producing environmental events, tangential to the purposes of an experiment, that intervene between two observations or measurements.

14. _____ refers to internal biological or psychological changes within subjects that may occur over a span of time resulting in performance variations unrelated to the treatment of interest.

15. _____ _____ refer to a change in a dependent variable due to a treatment effect that is not immediately observable but tends to become increasingly observable over a span of time.

16. _____ _____ refer to the tendency for an initial measurement in a research study to influence a subsequent measurement.

17. A procedure called _____ is frequently employed to control for order effects and _____ effects. Such effects can be controlled by distributing them _____ over all treatment conditions.

18. Changes in _____ refer to changes in the accuracy or precision of measuring devices or human observations.

19. Sources of invalidity arising from errors in mechanical or electrical measuring devices can best be eliminated by proper _____ of equipment and equipment _____ throughout the course of a study.

20. _____ _____ is the tendency for individuals or groups selected on the basis of initial extreme scores on a measurement instrument to behave less atypically the second and subsequent times on that same instrument.

21. Between-subject sources of internal invalidity include _____ _____, _____ _____, _____ _____, and _____ _____.

22. _____ _____ exists when preexisting factors may preclude or interfere with the establishment of equivalent groups for comparison.

23. _____ _____ occurs if subjects terminate their participation in an experiment for reasons other than that implied by the more ominous term_____.

24. _____ _____ refers to unwanted competition between the groups of an experiment that can inadvertently emerge to confound the interpretation of a treatment effect.

25. _____ _____ is a confounding factor associated with an outcome that can occur when some subjects in an experiment perceive that other subjects, compared to themselves, are receiving a more favorable treatment.

26. _____ effects often exists in the form of expectations about what the results of an investigation ought to be that can lead a researcher to treat subjects differently in certain respects or to favor a particular outcome. Such an effect is also called the _____ effect.

27. _____ validity pertains to the degree to which the results from a specific study sample of cases are generalizable to one or more populations, settings, treatment variables, or measurement variables. _____ bias refers to the fact that the mere awareness by subjects that they are being observed or evaluated can influence their performance. Relevant to an understanding of this is the _____ effect, named after a production plant of the Western Electric Company.

28. A description of subjects who try hard to perform in accordance with what they believe are the expectations of the experimenter is called the _____ subject effect.

29. Subjects who are hostile toward a particular research project and attempt to undermine what they perceive its goals to be are examples of the _____ subject effect.

30. Threats to external validity include _____ sensitization, _____ restrictions, _____ restrictions, and _____ restrictions.

31. _____ _____ is the tendency for an initial measurement in a research study to influence a subsequent measurement.

32. _____ restrictions might adversely affect the external validity of an experiment related to the representativeness of the subjects used.

33. _____ restrictions are those in which the measure selected to represent a dependent variable is not truly representative of the phenomenon that the experimenter wants to assess.

34. The selection of an independent variable that is unsuitable for generalizing results can also limit the external validity of an experiment. Such a threat is called a _____ restriction.

35. The word _____ means "no difference" and generally refers to a predicted finding of no significant differences _____ or _____ groups of subjects or _____ conditions.

36. Type _____ error involves rejecting a particular _____ hypothesis when it is true. Type _____ error involves retaining a _____ hypothesis when it is false.

37. _____ _____ is perhaps the most abstract and difficult type of validity to establish.

QUESTIONS AND EXERCISES FOR CLASSROOM DISCUSSION

1. What is the "method of association" and its statistical relevance?
2. What does a coefficient of correlation denote?
3. Describe the idea underlying the concept of causality.
4. Distinguish between the "directionality" and "third variable" problems and give an example of each.
5. Describe three methods for determining causality.
6. Identify two major sources of internal invalidity and list the kinds of threats to a study that can operate in each category.
7. Identify the threats to external validity discussed in this chapter and provide relevant examples of each type.
8. In a general way, describe what statistical testing involves.
9. Describe the potential statistical errors associated with statistical testing.
10. What is necessary to establish construct validity?

Experimental Designs

CHAPTER 8

CHAPTER OUTLINE

LEARNING OBJECTIVES

After reading this chapter, you should be able to identify, describe, or define:

- Different ways to classify research designs
- Three broad types of experiments and the relative power of each
- The basis for distinguishing true experiments from quasi-experiments
- The Campbell and Stanley system for symbolizing experiments
- A classic example of a true experiment and the method of data analysis
- Why the Solomon four-group design has greater strength than traditional two-group designs
- Why some experiments are called ANOVAR designs
- The meaning of the term "factorial design"
- Main effects versus interaction effects
- The shared goal of randomized control trials (RCTs)
- Three advantages of random assignment
- Completely randomized versus randomized block designs
- Repeated measures (within-subjects) versus parallel group (between-subjects) comparisons
- How to control for order and carryover effects in a repeated measures design
- Mixed experimental design
- Three types of quasi-experiments including their strengths and weaknesses
- Three types of preexperiments and the limitations of each
- Primary aims of single-subject research
- Advantages of single-subject designs
- Comparison of the A-B-A-B design over other withdrawal designs
- Reversal design versus alternating treatment design
- Main steps in using a multiple baseline design
- How a changing criterion design is similar to a multiple baseline design
- The means of determining treatment efficacy in single-subject research

WAYS TO CLASSIFY RESEARCH DESIGNS

The term *research design,* when used in its broadest sense, pertains to most of the details of how a study is to be conducted. Such details generally involve specification of the characteristics of the subjects to be studied and their manner of selection and assignment to groups, the means of controlling experimental and extraneous variables, the specific measurements to be taken, and the methods used for recording data. In this chapter, we focus on a more restrictive meaning of the term "research design," perhaps best conceived as the specific "blueprint" employed by an investigator to answer questions or test research hypotheses. As the plans or schemes that researchers use in meeting the aims of various types of investigations, some designs are tightly organized and highly detailed; others are loosely sketched.

Sorting out the multitudinous terms and taxonomies used to classify various research designs is a formidable task even for seasoned researchers. Designs are commonly classified according to:

- *The number of subjects employed*—whether groups are studied extensively to examine between-subject variations or individuals are evaluated intensively for within-subject variations.

- *The purpose or aim of a study*—whether to merely describe or seek associative or causative relations.
- *The place of occurrence*—whether in a laboratory, clinic, or field (natural) setting.
- *The dimension of time*—whether phenomena are studied prospectively (longitudinally) as they continue to unfold or retrospectively after they occur.
- *The degree to which quantitative versus qualitative observations and judgment are emphasized*—whether numerical values or more subjective interpretations serve as the primary basis for data analysis.
- *The type of statistical approach applied in analyzing data*—whether for comparing the influence of a single independent variable against a control group or the influence of two or more independent variables against a control group.
- *The degree to which the variables under investigation are experimentally controlled*—whether cause-and-effect relationships among them can be determined as opposed to merely describing their particular attributes, associative relations, or predicting their future occurrence.

Of these various approaches to categorizing research, we prefer the latter classification scheme with its emphasis on experimental control. As we have emphasized throughout this book, the ultimate goal of science is the determination of causality—how and to what degree the controlled manipulation of an independent variable causes a change in a dependent variable. For conclusions to be drawn from such observations about which one can have confidence, the influence of confounding factors must be ruled out or effectively controlled.

CHOOSING A RESEARCH DESIGN: EXPERIMENTAL METHODS

The threats to research validity discussed in Chapter 7 can individually or in some combination weaken or entirely undermine the credibility of a research study. Some research designs are better at eliminating or controlling such threats than others. The best of these are experimental designs. As defined by Pedhazur and Schmelkin (1991):

> An experiment is a study in which at least one variable is manipulated and units—e.g., people, households, groups, schools, factories, etc.—are randomly assigned to the different levels or categories of the manipulated variable(s). (p. 252)

As summarized in Table 8-1, *true experiments* are the strongest of the research designs because they include (1) random assignment of participants, (2) deliberate and active manipulation of independent variables, and (3) use of control groups as a basis for evaluating the influence of an independent variable. *Quasi-experiments* are like true experiments with the important exception that subjects are not randomly assigned to groups. In discussing what many believe to be the widespread use of quasi-experimental designs, Pedhazur and Schmelkin (1991) quoted Campbell (1984a), who noted that "experiments move to quasi-experiments, and on into queasy experiments, all too easily" (p. 33). Such "queasy" experiments, called *preexperimental* designs, sometimes referred to as "pseudoexperimental designs," are by far the weakest of all in controlling for pitfalls that can invalidate an experiment. Such designs, particularly one-group studies, should only be undertaken when nothing better can be done and the essential goal is to explore or describe new phenomena rather than to explain their causes.

In the discussion to follow, we review some of the commonly employed experimental designs from each of these categories along with their strengths and weaknesses. In addition to the name of a particular design, we have used the well known notation system of Campbell and Stanley (1963), wherein the symbols R = randomization, X = treatment by the independent variable, and O = observation.

TABLE 8-1   Ways to Classify Various Types of Research

Type of Research	Characteristic	Relevant Examples in Communication Sciences and Disorders
Quantitative	The collection of numerical measures of behavior under controlled conditions that can be subjected to statistical analysis	Examining acoustic characteristics of crying behavior in preterm and full-term infants
Qualitative	Strategies that emphasize nonnumerical data collection methods such as observations, interviews, etc.	Vocational choices of adults with cleft palate
True Experimental	Research methods that investigate a true cause and effect relationship, i.e., random assignment of subjects to at least two groups, use of a control group, and active manipulation of an independent variable	The effect of speaking rate on fluency of normal speaking children as compared to children who stutter
Quasi-experimental	Research methods that investigate a causal relation ship whenever true experimentation is impractical or impossible to perform. The study satisfies all of the requirements of a true experiment without random assignment.	Differences of language comprehension between normal attending children and children with attention deficit
Nonexperimental	Research in which causal relations cannot be established. Many of them involve qualitative approaches. The study in which no attempt is made to achieve randomization nor manipulation of a variable.	Relationship between premorbid intelligence and recovery of language skill in persons with expressive aphasia
Clinical	A particular research design that involves collecting data in the context of the clinical setting.	Survey of the degree of clients' satisfaction with therapy outcomes

True Experimental Designs

As we noted above, in addition to randomly assigning subjects to the conditions of a research investigation, so-called true experimental designs entail the active manipulation of one or more independent variable by the experimenter. Through such manipulation, the potential effect on a dependent variable can be established provided that a *statistically significant* effect is found.

Pretest-Posttest Control Group Design: $RO_1\ X\ O_2$
$$RO_3\quad O_4$$

A classic example of a true experimental design is the **pretest-posttest control group design.** Here two groups of subjects are randomly selected from a population and then randomly assigned to either an experimental condition, in which they will receive treatment (X), or to a control condition in which no treatment will be given. Pretests and posttests are given to the experimental group (O_1 and O_2, respectively) and to the control group (O_3 and O_4, respectively). This allows for the difference between the pretest and posttest in the experimental condition to be compared to the difference between the pretest and posttest in the control condition for each subject (see Table 8-2). The calculation of these so-called **difference scores** or **gain scores** can proceed as follows:

1. Subtract the pretest score from the posttest score for each subject to determine the degree of change.

TABLE 8-2   Method for Calculating Difference (Gain) Scores

Subject	Pretest	Posttest	Difference Scores
1	X_1	Y_1	$Y_1 - X_1$
2	X_2	Y_2	$Y_2 - X_2$
3	X_3	Y_3	$Y_3 - X_3$
.	.	.	.
.	.	.	.
.	.	.	.
n	X_n	Y_n	$Y_n - X_n$

$$\text{Mean of the difference scores} = \frac{\left(Y_1 - X_1\right) + \left(Y_2 - X_2\right) + \cdots + \left(Y_n - X_n\right)}{n}$$

2. For each group, sum these difference scores and divide by the number of subjects in each group to determine the means of the difference scores.
3. Calculate the significance of the difference between these means (see Chapter 12).

Because the design under discussion involves the comparison of only two groups, it is likely that a statistical analysis involving a *t-test* would be carried out to determine if the independent variable had a significant effect. Such a statistical analysis typically entails the evaluation of a null hypothesis that states: "no population difference exists," which is the same as saying in statistical terms: ($H_0: \mu_1 = \mu_2$). Provided these differences are large enough, the null hypothesis will be rejected in favor of a significant finding (see Chapter 12). Consequently, the observed between-group differences can be causally attributed to the influence of treatment.

The statistical assumption underlying this two-group design is that the difference between the pretest and posttest scores in the experimental group should be larger for the treated subjects (those who received the independent variable) than for the control subjects (those who did not receive it). To determine the probability that such a difference in the dependent variable reflects a *systematic influence* as opposed to a mere *random fluctuation,* a ratio representing the amount of between-group variation (B_v) to the amount of within-group variation (W_v) can be calculated as: B_v/W_v. The dividend in this equation, reflecting the measured difference in the dependent variable between the groups, can be attributed to the systematic influence of the independent variable. The divisor, reflecting the amount of fluctuation of the dependent variable due to uncontrolled extraneous variables, is the difference between the scores within the groups. The larger B_v is in relation to W_v, the greater the probability that the independent variable exerted a systematic influence on the dependent variable. Stated differently, the probability that the observed variation resulted from chance factors would be less likely. Thus, a value of 1.25 would be less likely to be associated with a significant effect than, say, 2.80. Researchers need not actually calculate the probability for the occurrence of a certain B_v/W_v ratio since this information is already available in *t tables.* Once a *t*-test has been completed, the significance of the resulting value can be readily determined by consulting such tables (see Appendix A-1).

In some cases the use of a control group, from whom a potentially beneficial treatment is withheld, cannot be justified on ethical grounds. Furthermore, a researcher might be interested in comparing one form of intervention to a second form of intervention in order to determine which of these is most effective. In such a case, the design of the study would be represented as follows:

$$RO_1 \, X_A \, O_2$$
$$RO_3 \, X_B \, O_4$$

As can be seen, participants are randomly allocated to receive one of two forms of intervention, namely, either X_A or X_B. Both groups are given a pretest and are then posttested after receiving one or the other form of treatment.

Campbell and Stanley (1963) pointed out that researchers often incorrectly analyze the data from pretest-posttest designs of the kind discussed by performing two t-tests, one that compares the difference between the pretest measures for each group and another for the difference in their posttest measures. The "logic" behind doing so is that if the difference between the groups' pretest scores is not statistically significant while the difference between their posttest scores is significant, a causal effect can be tied to the independent variable. However, such a conclusion involves an indirect, rather than a direct, analysis of the influence of the independent variable that is essentially unjustified, thereby threatening statistical conclusion validity.

In addition to the procedure involving the analysis of difference scores between the pretest and posttest as we described above, Campbell and Stanley (1963) suggested that an even better method is to use an analysis of covariance (ANCOVA) to analyze between-group differences while treating the pretest scores as covariates. We briefly mentioned the use of this method for controlling extraneous variables in Chapter 6. For additional information about how to conduct an ANCOVA, see Chapter 12.

A major strength of the randomized pretest-posttest design is that it increases the probability that the subjects assigned to groups are relatively equal on all variables with the exception of the independent variable. As a consequence, the majority of threats to internal validity can be eliminated or minimized, with the caveat that the study must be properly conducted. The primary threat to external validity is pretest sensitization (see Chapter 7).

Posttest Only Control Group Design: $R \, X \, O_1$
$$R \quad O_2$$

An even more basic version of a true experiment is the **posttest only control group design.** The rationale for this design is based on the assumption underlying random assignment procedures intended to minimize extraneous preexisting differences between groups. If such procedures are truly effective in accomplishing this goal, then pretesting subjects could seem redundant and unnecessary (Cambell & Stanley, 1963). Furthermore, posttest only designs are advantageous when pretesting is impossible to accomplish or when the effect of such testing might unduly sensitize subjects to the experimental treatment or bias posttest scores as the result of repeated measurements.

Despite the legitimacy of the posttest only design for many experimental situations, it is not widely used, perhaps because of the prevailing belief in the value of a pretest as a "fail-safe mechanism" to guard against the possible failure of randomization to establish group equivalency. Indeed, the argument that this design cannot always guarantee that random assignment has effectively controlled selection bias is quite legitimate. Nevertheless, it can also be said that the probability of balancing, through random assignment, subject characteristics between the groups of an experiment is relatively great when large samples are used—say, when $n > 30$.

The statistical analysis of this research design can proceed in a straightforward manner simply by comparing the posttest scores for each group. The significance of difference between the posttest scores can be accomplished by the use of a *t*-test as discussed above. Alternatively, or in addition to a *t*-test of between-group differences, an ANCOVA can be performed on the posttest scores of the groups with certain potentially confounding variables serving as covariates.

Solomon Four-Group Design: $R\ O_1\ X\ O_2$

$$R\ O_3\ \ \ O_4$$
$$R\ \ \ \ X\ O_5$$
$$R\ \ \ \ \ \ O_6$$

A popular experimental design that incorporates aspects of both the previously discussed pretest-posttest and posttest-only control group designs is the **Solomon four-group design.** Notice that the first two groups constitute a pretest-posttest control group design, while the last two groups are identical to a posttest-only control group design. The strength of this design lies in its ability to control for certain interactions between a pretest and an independent variable that combine to affect a dependent variable in a way that neither might have done when operating alone.

To use a concrete example of such an unwanted interaction, imagine that you wish to investigate the attitudes of classroom teachers toward providing direct assistance to children with speech or language disorders by reinforcing the goals and procedures of a therapy program designed by a speech-language pathologist. Suppose further that you develop a questionnaire to uncover positive and negative attitudes toward such involvement; it is completed by a targeted sample of first-grade teachers in a school system. Subsequently, these same teachers will be assigned to either an experimental group or a control group. Teachers assigned to the experimental group will participate in a workshop to learn about various speech and language disorders and how communication deficits can impede educational achievement. Teachers assigned to the control group will not participate in the workshop. Thereafter, both groups are posttested, and the results indicate that teachers who completed the workshop now show a significant reduction in negative attitudes and a reciprocal increase in positive attitudes. No such changes are found in the control group.

Although you may be inclined to conclude from the results that the workshop had a favorable effect in altering attitudes, such a conclusion may not be valid because of a possible interaction between the pretest and the experimental treatment. More specifically, in the course of completing the workshop, the experimental group may eventually surmise that the purpose of the experiment is to alter their attitudes in a particular manner, leading them to respond accordingly on the posttest. Thus, their posttest performance actually reflects the insights gained from the *combined influence* of pretesting and exposure to treatment.

The Solomon design can be viewed as a special case of a **factorial design** that can be defined as any design in which more than one treatment factor is investigated. Technically speaking, our example falls short of this definition since only one treatment factor was used, namely, the workshop administered to half of the teachers. However, in the case of the Solomon design, it is also possible to evaluate whether or not the pretest acted as a *factor* to sensitize subjects since it is given to only half of them. By casting the results from the design in the form of a two-by-two contingency table (see Table 8-3), the statistical permutations can be better visualized. Such a table helps to make clear that two categories of effects can be analyzed using the Solomon design. The first of these are the so-called **main effects** for (a) the pretest versus its absence and (b) treatment versus its absence. Using this design, it is also possible to analyze the results to determine whether or not a statistically significant **interaction effect** occurred. Comparing the posttest results of the two experimental groups and

TABLE 8-3   Two-by-two contingency table illustrating how the Solomon four group design can be used for analyzing two categories of effects in which one group has been pretested and the other group has not been pretested

		Treatment	
		Yes (Experimental)	No (Control)
Pretest	Yes	O_2	O_4
	No	O_5	O_6

making the same comparisons for the two control groups accomplishes the latter goal. The experimental and control groups are arranged in pairs with one pair pretested and the other pair not pretested. If the posttest results of the two experimental groups are comparable, you can be relatively confident that the interaction effects of pretesting and treatment were negligible. Statistically, these data can be best evaluated by employing an ANCOVA using the pretest scores for each group as a covariate (see Chapters 6 and 12).

Despite the obvious strengths of the Solomon design in accounting for the influence of pretest sensitization on a dependent variable, it is infrequently used. This is no doubt due to the relatively large number of participants required for random assignment to four separate conditions, as well as the time consumed in executing the various components of this design.

Multigroup and Factorial Designs

With the exception of the Solomon design, which, as noted above, is a modification of a pretest-posttest experiment tailored to assess pretest sensitization, the designs discussed thus far have employed only two randomized groups. Designs that require the comparison of three or more such groups are sometimes called **ANOVAR designs** because they involve the use of statistical techniques called an **analysis of variance (ANOVA).** Using such multigroup designs, it is possible to investigate the influence of one or more independent variables on a dependent variable. Such designs would be appropriate for comparing the relative efficacy of three or more different therapy approaches. Further, the question posed might concern whether or not the effectiveness of a single treatment approach varied as a function of the number of therapy sessions per week (e.g., one, two, three). A multigroup design that employs only a single independent variable is typically evaluated by a *one-way* analysis of variance; if two independent variables are to be evaluated, a *two-way* analysis of variance is employed, and so on.

Designs that employ more than one independent variable are called, to repeat, *factorial designs*. Factorial designs can be used to examine not only *different* treatment effects resulting from alternative independent variables but also such treatment effects at different levels of the *same* independent variable. This allows not only for the study of two or more independent variables acting separately (main effects) but the possible interaction effects between them. More specifically, within the framework of this design, different *treatment factors* and *level effects* can be studied simultaneously. Given the example provided above, we might choose to study the interaction of three treatment factors (therapy approaches A, B, or C) administered at three levels (once, twice, or three times a week) on a clinical outcome. The treatment factor and the levels of their administration constitute two main effects. We can also identify a possible interaction effect resulting from a combination of two or more of the

TABLE 8-4   General Structure of Three-by-Three Factorial Design

	Treatments		
	A	**B**	**C**
1	A_1	B_1	C_1
2	A_2	B_2	C_3
3	A_3	B_2	B_3

For example, A_1 represents a subject who received treatment A and 1 session, A_2 represents a subject who received treatment A and 2 sessions, and so forth.

main effects. Thus, our example can be described as a 3×3 factorial design (see Table 8-4). Such a design allows us to address the following questions:

1. Are the treatments equally effective (main effect 1)?
2. Are there differences in the outcome due to the frequency of sessions (main effect 2)?
3. Are there combinations of the main effects that influence the outcome (interaction effect)?

Theoretically, there is no limit to the number and levels of independent variables that can be employed in an experiment. However, for most clinical questions, the complexity of the experiment is unlikely to exceed a 3×3 design. By studying the influence of multiple independent variables within the framework of a single experiment, both the *efficiency* and *effectiveness* of the research process is facilitated. Greater efficiency is accomplished by saving time and money. Greater effectiveness is possible because the interaction between two or more variables can be simultaneously evaluated. However, the complexity of statistical analysis will grow exponentially with increments in the number of interactions to be investigated. Because of the complexity of the statistical calculations required, computer assistance can greatly ease the burden of what might otherwise prove to be an onerous and time-consuming task (see Chapter 12).

Randomized Controlled Trials

All of the designs discussed thus far entail randomization. Such experiments are commonly referred to as **randomized controlled trials (RCTs).** Although numerous terms are used to describe and classify RCTs, the shared goal of all such experiments is to allow for a valid interpretation of the influence of the independent variable by controlling for confounding variables.

Altman et al. (2001) summarized three major advantages of random assignment:

- First, it eliminates selection bias in the assignment of subjects to treatment groups. Without such safeguards, the conscious or unconscious prejudices of experimenters might favor the assignment of certain participants to one group or another.
- Second, random assignment can facilitate blinding of both the investigators and the subjects with respect to the treatment received.
- Third, random assignment allows the use of probability statistics to determine the likelihood that the differences found between treatments groups are the consequence of experimental manipulations as opposed to chance variations.

Two types of randomization methods are often used for purposes of allocating subjects to experimental and control groups. The first of these, called a **completely randomized design,** places no restrictions on how participants are allocated to the study groups as long as they meet the inclusion criteria. Thus, assuming that we wish to compare the efficacy of two experimental therapy programs for a particular type of communication disorder (Treatments A and B), we might ask for volunteers from several treatment centers Hypothetically, let's suppose that 30 individuals from a pool of 50 volunteers met the inclusion criteria related to such factors as physical and mental status, severity of symptoms, age, socioeconomic level, and so forth. Half of this number would then be randomly allocated to Treatment Group A and the other half to Treatment Group B.

A second method for allocating subjects to the groups of an experiment is called a **randomized block design.** It is useful when we suspect that some factor(s) other than the treatment under investigation might influence the outcome of an experiment. The first step in using this design requires that all participants be stratified into *blocks* on the basis of one or more potentially confounding variables—say, age, cognitive ability, severity of disorder or disease, or something. Such variables are often viewed as a "nuisance" to the degree that they can exert an unwanted or *secondary treatment effect* on the results of an experiment, leading to errors in interpreting the *primary treatment effect* of interest. Having stratified (divided) the participants into homogenous blocks based on a potentially confounding variable, the second step would be to randomly assign them to different groups or treatment conditions.

To borrow from our previous example, suppose we wish to evaluate the influence of Treatment A against Treatment B within the framework of a randomized block design while taking into account the severity of a particular disorder—a suspected confounding variable. More specifically, perhaps the severity of the participants' disorder might cause them to be more or less sensitive to the influence of a particular treatment. To control for the possibility of such a secondary influence, we decide to block our subjects into homogeneous subgroups constituted of mild, moderate, and severe participants based on the results of clinical testing. Subsequently, the participants are randomly assigned to each of these blocks. A comparison of the randomized block design with a simple random design is illustrated in Figure 8-1.

The statistical assumption underlying the randomized block design is that by controlling for within-subject variability through the use of homogeneous subgroups, between-group differences owing to the intended treatment effect can be validly assessed. This assumption is appropriate only so far as the blocking procedures results in subgroups that are more homogeneous on a confounding factor than the sample as a whole. If the subgroups happen to be highly variable on important confounding factors that the researcher failed to identify, blocking will be of little or no benefit. For this reason, researchers need to think carefully about the types of confounding variables that might operate before undertaking an experiment, so that experimental errors can be prevented to the greatest extent possible.

When well designed and executed, perhaps the chief value of RCTs is their potential for eliminating selection bias and other confounding variables (Altman et al., 2001). Recognizing that many experiments employ inadequate methodologies for achieving this purpose, a group of scientists and journal editors developed a set of standards for reporting clinical trials called the Consolidated Statement for Reporting Randomized Trials (CONSORT). The revised version of the CONSORT statement contains a checklist of items designed to improve the internal and external validity of trials (Altman et al., 2001). An associated Web site can be found at: http://www.consort-statement.org.

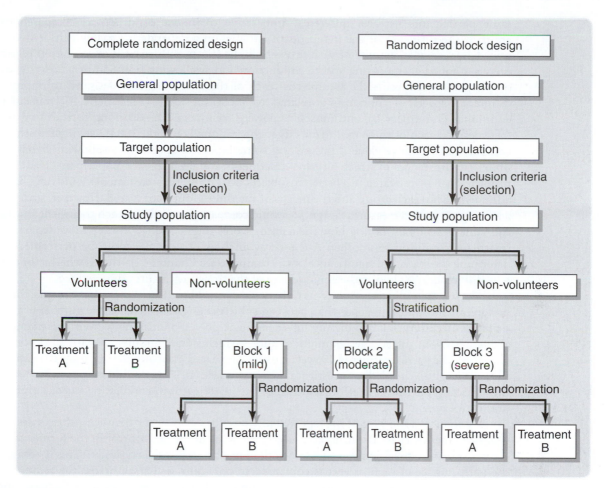

FIGURE 8-1   Comparison of a complete randomized design with a randomized block design. As opposed to a complete randomized design, participants are stratified into three blocks prior to their random assignments to either Treatment A or Treatment B.

Repeated Measures (Within-Subjects) Designs

Whatever method of randomization employed, the majority of RCTs use a **parallel group design**—another term for experiments that entail between-group comparisons of the type discussed above. As we have noted, such experiments generally employ at least two randomly assigned independent groups of participants, each of whom receive only one of the treatments (independent variables) under investigation. Earlier in this chapter, we briefly discussed an alternative to such between-group comparisons that entails taking repeated measurements on the *same* participants as they receive *different* treatments. A more detailed account of this design is provided here.

The defining aspect of a **repeated measures design** is that each participant is exposed to all the treatments administered in an experiment according to a randomly assigned sequence, and the effects of these treatments are compared within each individual. A repeated measures design is also called a *within-subjects design* because each participant serves as his or her own control as a basis for evaluating different treatment effects. Given that the same participants perform differently under one treatment condition as compared to another, the influence of the independent variable on a dependent variable can be determined. For example, suppose we wish to ascertain the effects of three types of strength-training exercises aimed at improving speech production and swallowing function in patients with dysphagia. More specifically, assume that each of these treatments is designed to improve different aspects of functioning related to muscular force (Treatment A), muscular endurance (Treatment B), and muscular power (Treatment C). Assuming further that we have defined each of these treatment targets operationally (Clark, 2003), we might wish to compare their relative value in improving some aspect of speech or swallowing behavior under circumstances in which all three treatments are given to each participant. Had this problem been investigated in a between-subjects design, only one treatment would have been administered to each group and the means of the three groups compared. However, since we are using a repeated measures design, we would compare the results of each treatment within the same individuals, noting how their mean scores might change as they move from one treatment condition to another. A three-way analysis of variance could be performed to determine the statistical significance of the findings (see Chapter 12)—that is whether or not true differences resulted as the consequence of the three treatments administered.

Because each subject serves as his or her own control in repeated measures designs, these designs are more advantageous than between-subjects designs in so far as the number of participants necessary for conducting an experiment goes. For instance, given the example above, a between-subjects design might require the inclusion of 60 subjects, with 20 allocated to each of the three treatments. However, using a repeated measures design, only 20 of these subjects might be needed to investigate the same question. This would also prove economical regarding the time and effort required of the investigator in conducting various aspects of the experiment.

A statistical advantage of the repeated measures design over the between-subjects design is also frequently cited. Because each subject serves as his or her control in the former case, greater statistical precision can be attained than in a between-subjects design. This is because the performance of each subject is compared to only him- or herself across the treatment conditions. On the other hand, in a between-subjects design, the error variance factor might be substantially larger as the consequence of individual differences among the groups. Stated differently, the size of error variance ought to be reduced to a greater degree when the same individuals are compared to themselves than when compared to different individuals.

Two major problems, called *order effects* (practice effects) and *carryover effects,* are often associated with the use of a repeated-measures design. As we noted in Chapter 7, the first of these problems, order effects, result from the repeated exposure of participants in an experiment to the same order of treatments over and over again (e.g., Treatment A followed by Treatment B, Treatment B followed by Treatment C, etc.). Exposure to such an order of treatments administered to each participant sometimes can result in performance changes that are not attributable to the treatments alone. It is possible that performance changes among treatments might simply result because of increased familiarity with the task or learning how to perform it more efficiently. In other words, performance gains observed in later treatment conditions might be due, at least in part, to skills practiced and acquired in earlier treatment conditions. Changes in performance as the result of practice do not always reflect positive gains. It is also possible for a decline in performance to occur because of boredom or fatigue.

Order effects are to be distinguished from a second source of bias commonly associated with repeated measures designs resulting from carryover effects. While order effects relate to *general changes* in performance that occur independently of the particular sequence of the

TABLE 8-5   Relative Efficacy of Two Treatments for Reducing Stuttering Using a Repeated Measures Design

	Results of a Repeated Measures Design		
	First Period	**Second Period**	**Difference**
Mean frequency stuttering	A → 25	B → 10	15
Mean frequency stuttering	B → 18	A → 12	6
where A = counseling, B = speech therapy			

Note: Half of the subjects were initially assigned to counseling. The reduction in stuttering was substantially greater when counseling preceded speech therapy, indicating the presence of a significant carryover effect before receiving the speech therapy. The remaining half of the participants were first assigned to receive speech therapy before receiving the counseling. Reduction in stuttering occurred from the first period to the second in this group as well, but to a lesser extent.

treatment given, carryover effects result from *specific changes* caused by one or more earlier treatments interacting with later treatments (Keppel et al., 1992).

To further clarify how carryover effects can bias the outcome of a study, consider an example in which we might wish to compare the relative efficacy of two treatments aimed at reducing stuttering using a repeated measures design. Half of our subjects are randomly assigned to a counseling program aimed at ameliorating speaking apprehension and avoidance (Intervention A), during the first period to be followed during the second period by speech therapy designed to enhance fluency skills (Intervention B). The remaining half of the participants is randomly assigned to receive Intervention B first before crossing over to Intervention A.

Hypothetical results for such an experiment are displayed in Table 8-5, in which the reduction in the mean percentage of stuttering is shown subsequent to each treatment period. As can be seen, a reduction in stuttering occurred from the first period to the second period irrespective of the treatment sequence. However, the reduction in stuttering was substantially larger when counseling preceded speech therapy than when this sequence was reversed. Such a finding would indicate the presence of a significant carryover effect. More specifically, the findings would suggest that a significant interaction occurred between the two treatment factors, that is the effect of the treatment factors acting together was greater than each factor acting independently of the other.

In addition to counterbalancing treatment conditions, another means to control for carryover effects is to use a so-called **washout period.** This is a time interval interposed between successive treatments to allow for the dissipation of treatment effects. Obviously, the length of this time interval will vary as a function of the type and magnitude of the treatments given. Generally, to avoid carryover effects, the washout period should be long enough to allow for a particular treatment effect to dissipate before introducing another. Finally, to use a repeated measures design, the dependent variable under investigation should be relatively stable through time to avoid **period effects.** If the disease or disorder is regressing, progressing, or fluctuating up and down, it will be impossible to conclude that the level of the dependent variable was relatively the same during the time period preceding each treatment intervention. Given such circumstances, a fair comparison of different treatment effects would not be possible. All of the requirements cited above can place major constraints on the clinical utility of repeated measures designs.

TABLE 8-6   All Possible Treatment Combinations for a Three-Treatment Repeated Measures Design

Treatment 1	Treatment 2	Treatment 3
A_1	A_6	A_{11}
A_2	A_7	A_{12}
A_3	A_8	A_{13}
A_4	A_9	A_{14}
A_5	A_{10}	A_{15}

The table illustrates that 15 subjects were randomly assigned, 5 each to three treatments. Research Question: Are there any significant differences between the three treatments?

As we noted above, the biasing influence of both order effects and carryover effects can often be minimized by *counterbalancing* the treatment conditions such that each participant is exposed to each treatment an equal number of times and the sequence of such treatments varies for different participants. In the simplest case, involving the comparison of two treatments, participants either receive Treatment A first followed by Treatment B or vice versa. Moving from one such treatment to another is termed **crossover.** To qualify as an RCT, the order in which participants receive the treatments in such trials must be randomized. The time during which each intervention is administered is called the **treatment period.** In the simplest case of two treatments (A and B), approximately half of the subjects would receive Treatment A during the first period, then crossover to Treatment B during the second period.

For the counterbalancing treatments to be complete, all possible orders of the treatment periods must be represented. Table 8-6 illustrates all such possible combinations for a three-treatment repeated measures design. A major limitation in constructing a complete counterbalanced design as shown is that the complexity of such a design increases progressively as the number of the treatments increases. For instance, in the case of four treatments, 24 sequences of treatment are required. When five treatments are to be investigated, 120 sequences are required; six treatments require 720 sequences to accomplish a complete counterbalanced design.

To reduce the number of treatment sequences required for a complete counterbalanced design, investigators often use a **Latin square design,** in which only selected treatment sequences are used for purposes of counterbalancing. A Latin square design can be defined as a matrix consisting of equal numbers of rows and columns that contain a subset of all possible treatment sequences in a multiple treatment experiment. Although a Latin square design can be useful in partially counterbalancing treatment effects, a limitation of the design illustrated in Figure 8-2(A) is the cyclical pattern of the treatments. As can be seen, Treatment B always follows Treatment A, Treatment C always follows Treatment B, and so on. Thus, order effects are not completely eliminated in the case of this particular Latin square. An improvement in this design is illustrated in Figure 8-2(B). This design is called a **balanced Latin square** because all treatments precede and follow each other only once, thereby minimizing order effects to a greater extent.

Treatments

Subjects	1	2	3	4
1	A	B	C	D
2	B	C	D	A
3	C	D	A	B
4	D	A	B	C

(A)

Treatments

Subjects	1	2	3	4
1	C	D	B	A
2	D	A	C	B
3	A	B	D	C
4	B	C	A	D

(B)

FIGURE 8-2

(A) Example of the Latin square design, illustrating the cyclical pattern of treatments (e.g., Treatment B always follows Treatment A, Treatment C always follows Treatment B, etc.). (B) Example of a balanced Latin square design in which all treatments precede and follow each other only once

Mixed Experimental Design

Thus far, we have discussed a variety of experimental designs in which (a) participants are randomly assigned to two or more groups where each of them is exposed to one treatment only (between-subjects design), or (b) two or more treatments are administered to the same participants (within-subjects design). Some designs are said to be "mixed" to the degree that a mixture of these designs is employed. Referring to our hypothetical study of stuttering discussed above, we might wish to compare the two forms of treatment (counseling versus speech therapy) in the context of a within-subjects design as discussed previously. Suppose further that we wish to evaluate each therapy approach against two levels of stuttering severity. For the latter purpose, we divide our subjects into two distinct groups of participants based on their diagnosis, those with mild stuttering and those with severe stuttering. A schematic representation of this design is shown in Table 8-7. Sometimes called a **split-plot design,** this design evolved from agricultural investigations of the effect of different fertilizers (treatments) applied within each of several plots of land (Shavelson, 1988). In the case of our hypothetical study, the two main plots are analogous to the within-subjects and the between-subjects portions of the experiment. Each of these plots can be subdivided so that the within-subjects portion is constituted of the treatments administered to each subject, while the between-subjects portion reflects the severity levels. By randomly assigning the subjects to a particular treatment sequence, this would qualify as a true experiment.

TABLE 8-7 An example of a mixed (split plot design) for the evaluation of within-subject and between-subject effects

Severity (Between-Subjects)	Subject	Order (respectively)	Treatment (Within-Subjects) Counseling (C)			Speech Therapy (S)		
			Pre	Post	Diff (D)	Pre	Post	Diff (D)
	1	(C, S)	X_1	Y_1	$Y_1 - X_1 (DM_1)$	X_1	Y_1	$Y_1 - X_1 (DM_1)$
Mild (M)	2	(S, C)	X_2	Y_2	$Y_2 - X_2 (DM_2)$	X_2	Y_2	$Y_2 - X_2 (DM_2)$
	3	(C, S)	X_3	Y_3	$Y_3 - X_3 (DM_3)$	X_3	Y_3	$Y_3 - X_3 (DM_3)$
	.	.						
	.	.						
	.	.						
	1	(C, S)	A_1	B_1	$B_1 - A_1 (DSV_1)$	A_1	B_1	$B_1 - A_1 (DSV_1)$
Severe (SV)	2	(S, C)	A_2	B_2	$B_2 - A_2 (DSV_2)$	A_2	B_2	$B_2 - A_2 (DSV_2)$
	3	(C, S)	A_3	B_3	$B_3 - A_3 (DSV_3)$	A_3	B_3	$B_3 - A_3 (DSV_3)$
	.	.						
	.	.						
	.	.						
Between-Subject Difference					$DSV - DM$			$DSV - DM$

Reprinted with permission from "Schematic representation of a mixed design: Pretest-posttest control group design," by Richard J. Shavelson, 1998, Statistical Reasoning for the Behavioral Sciences, (2nd ed.), Needham Heights, MA: Allyn and Bacon, p.466.

Quasi-Experimental Designs

Quasi-experiments are those that satisfy all of the requirements of a true experiment *with the exception of random assignment.* The general ethic is to use the very best method possible aiming at "true experiments," "But where randomization is not possible . . . we must do the best we can with what is available to us" (Campbell, 1969, p. 411).

As noted in Chapter 6, matching is often used to equate the participants of an experiment on potentially confounding influences when randomization of such influences across the groups of an experiment is impossible to achieve. The determination of just what factors should be considered in matching groups will vary among experiments. Generally, an experimenter will consider the potential biasing influences of age, gender, socioeconomic status, cognitive ability, physical and mental status, and the like, as such factors might bear on a particular attribute of speech, language, or hearing targeted for study.

Although quasi-experimental designs are generally considered to be less powerful than true experiments in meeting the assumption of *group equivalence,* quasi-experiments are rated second best, particularly in cases in which (1) only preformed groups or specific individual cases are available for study, and/or (2) ethical issues may preclude withholding treatment from certain individuals. For example, this might be the most appropriate design in a clinical situation in which you wish to evaluate the effect of a specific treatment for a group of cases already admitted to therapy as compared to the absence of such treatment for other cases on a waiting list. Often, the assemblage of such comparison groups is the natural consequence of scheduling factors beyond the control or interests of the experimenter. In other words, lacking randomization, such a design allows for "when and to whom" certain measurements are made but not "when and to whom" treatment is given (Campbell & Stanley, 1966).

Nonequivalent Comparison Group Design: O_1 X O_2
$$O_3 \quad O_4$$

A design typical of the type discussed above is known as a **nonequivalent comparison group design.** It entails the use of at least two nonrandom comparison groups who are pretested with respect to some dependent variable. The experimental group is then treated according to the independent variable, while the control group goes untreated. Subsequently, a posttest is again administered to both groups, and their performance scores are compared. If statistical testing indicates that the performance of the experimental group is significantly better than that of the comparison group, some level of confidence can be placed in the efficacy of the treatment in question. In the case of nonequivalent groups, a *t-test for two independent groups (unpaired t-test)* could be used for this purpose (see Chapter 12).

Although this design is commonly used when randomization is not possible, it must be borne in mind that initial equivalence in the groups under study cannot be assumed. Therefore, whatever confidence we are able to have that an observed change in the dependent variable represents a true treatment effect is tied to elimination of sampling errors. In other words, we wish to assure that our experimental and control groups are equivalent on all variables with the exception of how they are treated on the independent variable. To the extent this is not achieved, the validity of the study design will suffer.

Other threats to this design that must be considered include history, maturation, and pretest sensitization (see Chapter 7). In an effort to control for these possible confounding variables, a time-series design can be used.

Single Time-Series Design: O_1 O_2 O_3 O_4 X O_5 O_6 O_7 O_8

Other types of quasi-experimental studies include **single time-series designs** in which repeated measures of a dependent variable are made prior to and subsequent to the administration of an independent variable. More specifically, this design involves periodic measurements over a time span in order to establish either an *average* performance value (in the case of groups) or a *baseline* (in the case of individual subjects) prior to introducing an experimental treatment. Subsequently, a series of ongoing measurements are taken to determine whether or not a change in the dependent variable has occurred.

An advantage of this design over the nonequivalent comparison group design is due to the use of several pretests and posttests for evaluating treatment effects as opposed to judging such effects by the use of a single pretest and posttest. Some treatment effects, such as *sleeper effects,* might not be immediately apparent but tend to become evident over a period of time (see Chapter 7). This is particularly true for disorders in which the severity of the problem varies from one time period to the next, such as stuttering. By repeated observation of the behavior over a span of time, more valid conclusions might be drawn as to the true efficacy of a treatment effect.

Although an advantage of this design over the nonequivalent comparison group design lies in its ability to collect numerous pretest and posttest measures to use in the evaluation of a treatment effect, this same ability might also threaten the validity of findings. More specifically, administering several pretests and posttests possibly could result in a greater degree of test sensitization than giving a single pretest and posttest. Still another design weakness results from the lack of a control group against which to compare a treatment effect.

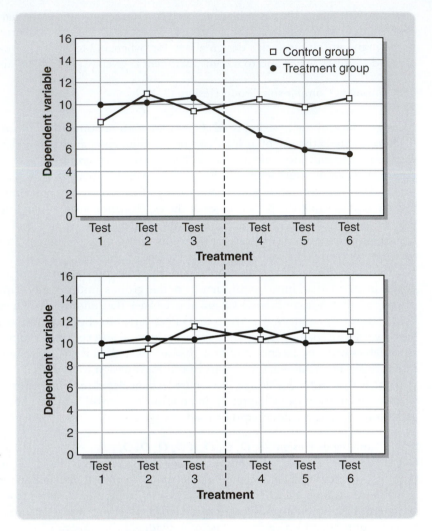

FIGURE 8-3

Two possible outcomes of a multiple time-series design. *Top*, results suggest that treatment had an effect on the dependent variable; *bottom*, results supply no evidence that treatment affected the dependent variable.

Reprinted with permission from Research Methods and Statistics for Psychology, *by W.A. Schweigert, 1994, Pacific Grove, CA: Brooks/Cole Publishing Company (Part of the Thomson Corporation), p. 308.*

Multiple-Time-Series Design: $O_1\ O_2\ O_3\ O_4\ X\ O_5\ O_6\ O_7\ O_8$

$O_1\ O_2\ O_3\ O_4\quad O_5\ O_6\ O_7\ O_8$

As opposed to a single time-series design, a multiple group design can be used to control extraneous variables that might bias the interpretation of a treatment effect. The basic concept of what is called a **multiple time-series design** for group experiments is graphically portrayed in Figure 8-3. In addition to accounting for sleeper effects, the inclusion of a control group allows for a better determination of a true treatment effect resulting from the independent variable as opposed to a spurious effect resulting from some simultaneously occurring extraneous variable.

Both the single and multiple time-series designs require a large number of observations to statistically estimate a change in behavior over time. When only a few data points are available, the alternative solution is to increase the number of time periods used in pretesting and posttesting the behavior of interest. Another descriptive approach to evaluating treatment effects is simply by means of visual inspection of graphs.

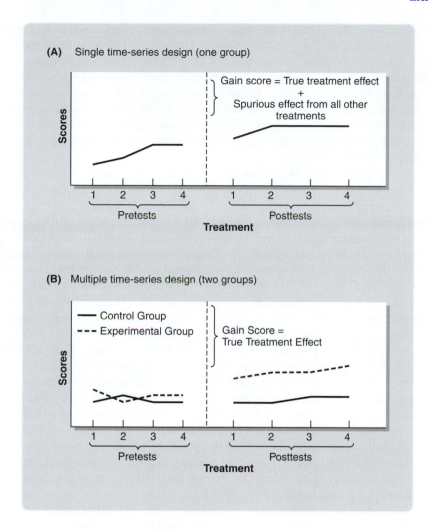

FIGURE 8-4

Comparison of (A) a single time-series design (one group) with (B) a multiple time-series design (two groups). A weakness of design (A) is that it is subject to spurious effect from all other treatments, that is, potentially confounding variables that may bias the true treatment effect. By the inclusion of a control group, design (B) can better account for minimizing a spurious effect

Figure 8-4 provides a graphic comparison of (A) a single group time-series design and (B) multiple time-series designs. These designs incorporate the dimension of time by administering multiple pretests and posttests with respect to a treatment. By incorporating the dimension of time, a multiple time-series design is simply an expansion of the nonequivalent comparison group design.

Single-Subject Designs

Some quasi-experimental studies entail the use of what are variously called **single-subject designs,** single-case designs, small-N designs, $N = 1$ designs, idiographic (intensive, long-term, individually focused) designs, and the like. The central focus of such research is the use of systematic methods for applying various treatment interventions and documenting their effects repeatedly in single individuals over a period of time. For this reason, such studies also can be broadly viewed as a special category of the repeated-measures and time-series designs discussed earlier.

As we noted in Chapter 2, the origin of single-subject research owes much to the scientific philosophies and methods for the experimental analysis of behavior developed by B. F. Skinner and many other early advocates of what has come to be broadly known as the "operant conditioning approach." Despite the use of such methods for half a century or more, some researchers continue to confuse single-subject designs with "one-shot case studies." The latter methods have little scientific merit for reasons we will discuss later in this chapter. On the other hand, single-subject designs have been increasingly seen by researchers and clinicians in many behavioral, educational, and medical fields as a valid means of contributing toward scientific knowledge.

Indeed, there are practical reasons why single-subject designs sometimes might prove more advantageous than group research methods. First, the availability of a large numbers of individuals for the study of certain problems can be limited. This is often true for a field such as communication sciences and disorders where the number of people available who might fit into a well defined category of dysphagia, aphasia, cerebral palsy, autism, cleft lip and palate, and so forth might be quite small. The large physical and functional variations among the subjects falling into such categories can often confound the search for systematic treatment effects.

A second advantage of single-subject over group designs is that the methods employed are more adaptable to many clinical research problems in which the main interest is in assessing the effect of therapy on individual patients over an extended period of time. Such specificity of focus allows for predicting whether or not an individual participant might or might not benefit from a particular intervention. Taking into account the needs and abilities of specific individuals, while continuously measuring the influence of treatment, can increase what is called *intrasubject control,* thereby ruling out many sources of internal invalidity. In single-subject research, aggregating performance measures into averages across heterogeneous individuals is avoided because of the possibility of obscuring or concealing variations in treatment effects in such individuals. Instead, an emphasis is placed on collecting a large amount of data from a single subject or a limited number of such subjects. Group studies, on the other hand, by focusing on the overall or average performance of large numbers of people, on each of whom a small amount of data is collected, have major limitations when it comes to making their findings apply to therapeutic situations within individuals. In the process of attempting to assure generality of group data to the targeted population, investigators typically employ sampling procedures designed to include *all* relevant population characteristics in the sample. In so doing, the relevance of such data to specific subjects may be substantially diminished (Herson & Barlow, 1976). Statistically, this is comparable to observing that many individual scores in a distribution may depart substantially from an average score used to represent such a distribution as a whole.

Still a third advantage of single-subject designs is that they are well adapted for satisfying the goals of quality-assurance established by public and private health care providers (Medicaid, Medicare, profit and nonprofit insurance companies, etc.). Questions pertaining to both the short-term and long-term benefits of various treatment interventions can be answered because of the ability of such designs to profile treatment results for individual clients. As Robey et al. (1999) aptly noted, the movement toward the adoption of forms of experimentation and evidence will lead to ". . . greater acceptance by (a) the public, (b) those influential in the creation of public policy, and (c) public and private reimbursers of therapy services that treatments of communication disorders are demonstrably effective as evaluated through stringent scientific criteria" (p. 445).

The major goals of single-subject research are to:

1. gain precise control over the experimental conditions of an investigation by eliminating extraneous variables
2. establish a stable level of responding (baseline) before administering a treatment condition (independent variable)
3. record the treated behavior of interest (dependent variable) within a given time period
4. perform a visual and/or statistical analysis of the data to determine the treatment outcome

Several representative paradigms for single-subject research are reviewed next.

A-B Design

The most basic of the time-series designs involving individuals is the **A-B design.** In this paradigm, observations of single individuals are made over a period of time to establish a baseline of retest data during period "A." No treatment is administered during this period. Subsequently, during period "B," a treatment is introduced and changes in the dependent variable from the baseline period are noted. Generally, there is no universally applied criterion for determining the length of the baseline period or the treatment period that follows. With respect to the baseline period, the stability of the dependent variable is the deciding factor in determining when to apply the independent variable. The definition of *response stability* should be decided prior to the experiment according to the degree of response variability that the experimenter has judged to be acceptable. For example, an experimenter might decide that response variability should not exceed 5% of all responses made over some number of sessions during the baseline period. Once such a performance standard is met, a treatment condition could be introduced and continued across some number of consecutive sessions until a *response plateau* is reached, that is, no further improvement in performance is evident.

Suppose we might wish to study the effect of a verbal cueing procedure on the naming ability of patients with Broca's aphasia. Using an A-B design, one could establish a baseline during pretreatment phase A; treatment then could be introduced during phase B in an effort to increase the number of correct responses (see Figure 8-5). If the number of correct

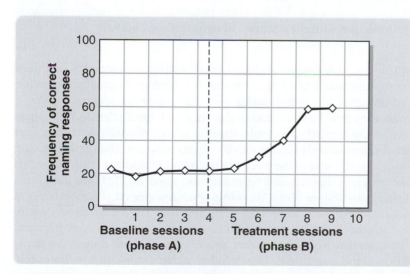

FIGURE 8-5

Illustration of A-B design demonstrating an increment in correct naming responses from the baseline period (phase A) to the treatment period (phase B). Alternative explanations for the treatment effect might include the practice effect, placebo effect, or other changes within the participant or experimental environment.

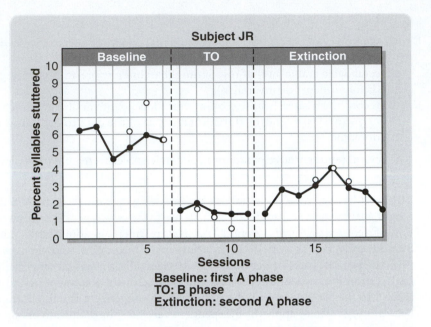

FIGURE 8-6

%SS scores for Subject JR. Filled circles are the investigator's data, and open circles are the independent clinician's data.

Reprinted with permission from "Control of Children's Stuttering with Response-Contingent Time-Out. Behavioral, Perceptual, and Acoustic Data," by M. Onslow and A. Packman, 1997, Journal of Speech, Language, and Hearing Research, *40, p. 125.*

responses observed during phase B is greater than in phase A, you might be tempted to attribute such a response change to the effect of the treatment. However, the validity of such a conclusion could be challenged. Perhaps the observed change in the behavior would have occurred in the absence of the treatment administered. Alternative explanations to a true treatment effect might include the practice effect, the placebo effect, or other changes within the participant or experimental environment known or unknown to the experimenter. Because of such problems, the A-B design is generally considered to be the weakest of the single-subject designs for determining causality. However, its explanatory power can be substantially enhanced by replicating one or more of its phases during additional time periods while continuing to observe changes in behavior. Some possibilities for observing *replication effects* are discussed in connection with the next two designs reviewed below.

A-B-A Design

A marked improvement in the basic design can be achieved by adding a second A in a third phase of the experiment in which the dependent variable is measured again after treatment has been withdrawn. The advantage of this **A-B-A design** over the simpler A-B approach is that it affords greater experimental control. By withdrawing the treatment during the second A phase and observing the effect on the dependent variable, the researcher can conclude with greater confidence that the independent variable was responsible for the observed change in behavior.

An example of this design is found in the work of Onslow and Packman (1997) in which a behavior modification program that entailed time-out from speaking (TO) was used in an effort to control stuttering (see Figure 8-6). Following a baseline period (first A phase) in which percent syllables stuttered (%SS) were relatively stable, the TO condition was introduced (B phase). TO, which required a brief pause in speaking contingent on every perceptible stuttering event, was applied while the subject spoke a monologue during 3-minute sessions. Visual inspection of the graphic data clearly indicate that a substantial reduction in the rate of stuttering occurred contingent on TO that began with the first treatment session and continued throughout treatment. During extinction (second A phase), note that %SS

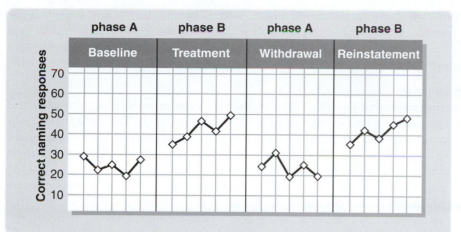

FIGURE 8-7
Representative A-B-A-B design. The addition of a fourth phase enhances the internal validity of the treatment effect, demonstrated in phase 2, by restoring the desirable behavior following the withdrawal of treatment (phase 3).

initially increased during the first couple of sessions when the TO contingency was withdrawn and then declined again in subsequent sessions. However, as the authors point out, the overall degree of stuttering was still lower than during the baseline period.

A-B-A-B Design

Still a further elaboration of the A-B design is the **A-B-A-B design,** which is one of the most frequently employed designs in behavioral or "operant" research. By adding a second B phase, the last two phases of the design are a replica of the first two phases. Thus, A-B-A-B studies are sometimes called **replication designs.** A common form of this design involves withdrawal of treatment during the third phase so that phase one represents *baseline,* phase two represents *treatment,* and phase three represents *withdrawal (extinction)* as in the A-B-A design. However, the A-B-A-B design adds a fourth phase in order to determine what happens to the dependent variable when the treatment is *reinstated* (see Figure 8-7). In effect, the A-B-A-B sequence involves the study of the treatment effect as it both *precedes* and *follows* a baseline condition. Clinically, the fourth phase of such a design is highly desirable since it avoids the negative consequences of the A-B-A experiment that leaves the participant/client at the end of the study as they were in the beginning—namely, in a state comparable to their original baseline level of responding.

Numerous variations of the A-B-A-B are available to address other kinds of research problems. For example, should you wish to compare the effectiveness of two different treatments (B and C) the design might be extended (A-B-A-A-C-A).

Still another application of the design might entail the inclusion of a "placebo" condition against which to compare a particular treatment effect as in an A-B-C-B design. This might be important since neither the A-B nor the A-B-A-B design is able to rule out entirely the possibility that *anything* (even a sugar pill) might have caused a performance change. To deal with this problem, instead of instating a withdrawal condition and returning to baseline during the third phase of the experiment, a treatment considered to be ineffectual (C) could be substituted. Should the response measure return to the baseline level during phase C, while showing a change as predicted during the final B phase, you could be relatively confident that the treatment of interest exerted the intended influence on the dependent variable.

In addition to ending with the subject in a treatment intervention, the major advantage of the A-B-A-B design over the A-B-A design is that it allows for demonstrating the influence of the independent variable on two occasions. Based on this fact, it has been said to provide ". . . the most powerful demonstration of causality available to the applied researcher" (Tawney & Gast, 1984, p. 202). A possible ethical concern for some clinicians might relate to withholding treatment when a second baseline condition is used. If the treatment appears to be working, one might ask "Why remove it?" The answer is to gain more confidence in its potential efficacy by demonstrating its positive influence during a second treatment period.

Alternating Treatment Design

In an **alternating treatment design,** sometimes called a "between-series design," the effect of two alternating treatments are studied, first A then B. Instead of using a baseline as traditionally defined, two or more treatments (A, B, etc.) are simply presented randomly or counterbalanced with respect to their order of presentation. The ability to discern treatment differences early in a study and to respond accordingly should be appealing to clinicians.

An example of an alternating treatment design in which the relative efficacy of two language treatment methods was compared can be found in an investigation by Weismer and associates (Weismer, Murray-Branch, & Miller, 1993). Two teaching methods, modeling versus modeling *plus* evoked production techniques, were taught in a semirandom order during group and individual instruction. Although not a required component of an alternating treatment design, the authors chose to use a baseline phase before individual (but not group) instruction. This was done ". . . to further document the lack of target vocabulary in a child's repertoire before teaching" (p. 1040). As shown in Figure 8-8, more correct productions

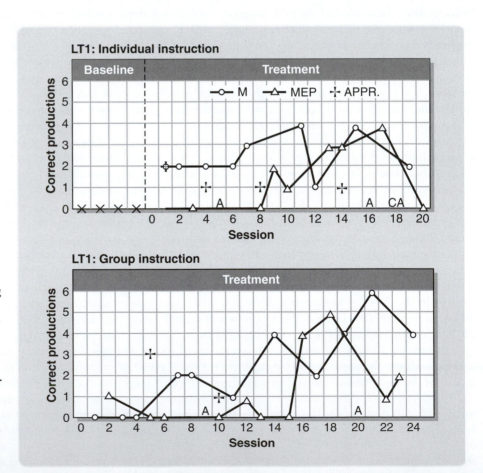

FIGURE 8-8

Frequency data for subject LT1 on the production probes following individual instruction (top panel) and group instruction (bottom panel). M = modeling treatment; MEP = modeling plus evoked production treatment; APPR = approximation; A = subject absence; CA = clinician absence.

Reprinted with permission from "Comparison of Two Methods for Promoting Productive Vocabulary in Late Talkers," by S. E. Weismer, J. Murray-Branch, and J. F. Miller, 1993, Journal of Speech and Hearing Research, 36, *p. 1043.*

generally occurred in response to modeling alone than for the combined treatment approach. This was true under individual as well as group instruction, although overlap in the curves for the two treatments is evident for both types of instruction.

A clinical advantage of this design is that some type of treatment is always being used in contrast to withdrawal designs that return to baseline following treatment. Thus, treatment effectiveness can be assessed by comparing differences between alternative treatments for a comparable series of data points. Another advantage of the design is that different effects of the interventions can be more rapidly determined than in other designs. More specifically, decisions to modify or terminate a study can be made more quickly if the interventions of interest appear to be ineffective.

All studies that involve within-subject comparisons entailing the comparison of two or more treatments, whether large *n* or small *n* in nature, face threats to their internal validity stemming from what are called **multitreatment interference effects.** This is a general term that describes the influence of one treatment on another in cases in which the same subject is exposed to each of them. More specifically, it is possible for preceding treatments to make successive treatments more or less effective. As we noted earlier in this chapter, this may be due to the *order* in which treatments are given or to that influence of a specific treatment that *carries over* to another.

In addition to allowing for the comparison of the effectiveness of two or more interventions, with or without the inclusion of a baseline condition, the strength of alternating treatment designs is that both order and carryover effects can be minimized by the use of randomization or counterbalancing techniques that allow for the rapid alternation of treatments. Without such controls, the validity of the findings obtained from an alternating treatment design would be questionable due to multiple-treatment interactions. Still another possible limitation of alternating treatment designs pertains to their practical applications. Seldom do clinicians switch rapidly from one therapy to the next in administering treatments to clients.

Reversal Design

The **reversal design** is similar to the withdrawal designs discussed previously, with one important exception. During phase 3, instead of withdrawing treatment, a second form of intervention can be applied and the effect of the two treatments then compared. For example, two incompatible behaviors such as fluency and disfluency in a stuttering individual might be selected for treatment (see Figure 8-9). After establishing a baseline in phase 1, the first contingency could be applied (e.g., reward of fluency/punishment of disfluency). Subsequently, in phase 3, these contingencies might be reversed (reward of disfluency/ punishment of fluency). Phase 4 of the reversal design typically entails reinstatement of the same treatment contingency as administered in phase 2 in order to terminate the experiment by once again producing the desired treatment effect. In the case of our hypothetical experiment, this would involve rewarding fluency and punishing disfluency. Although a strength of the reversal design is its power in illustrating the efficacy of a clinical intervention, a weakness is the possibility of being unable to reverse some negative consequence associated with the effort to demonstrate experimental control over the targeted behavior (Gelfand & Hartmann, 1984). Thus, for practical and ethical reasons, caution should be exercised in the use of this particular design.

Multiple-Baseline Design

In cases where it is undesirable to leave the research participant in the original baseline state or to augment some behavior incompatible to the intended treatment outcome merely to demonstrate the ability to reverse such a negative effect, a **multiple-baseline design** might be used instead. Commonly used variations of this design are applicable to the study of

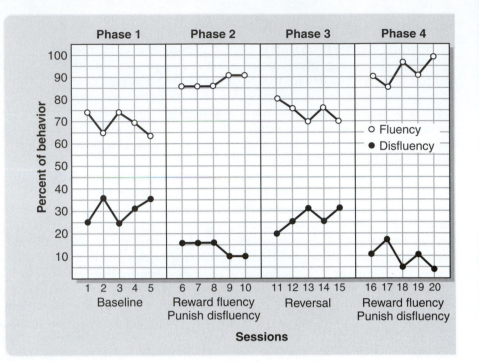

FIGURE 8-9

Reversal design for treating stuttering and hypothetical results. The contingencies of phase 2 (reward of fluency/punishment of disfluency) were reversed in phase 3 (reward of disfluency/punishment of fluency). In phase 4, the phase 2 contingencies were reinstated.

efforts to modify different behaviors across two or more situations or the same behavior across two or more situations.

A simplified graphic representation of the basic paradigm for a multiple-baseline design is shown in Figure 8-10. As illustrated, a stable baseline is established on two or more behaviors in the series. After a predetermined number of sessions, the treatment is next applied to the second behavior in the series while the first behavior also continues to receive treatment. In this manner, sequential applications of treatment continue across all behaviors to be assessed. Similarly, treatment efficacy can also be evaluated across two or more situations, settings, or time periods by the sequential application of the intervention to different baselines. As Kazdin (1982) pointed out, multiple-baseline designs are essentially "mini A-B experiments" involving successive comparisons between treatment and no-treatment conditions. More specifically, he noted: "Each time the intervention is introduced, a test is made between the level of performance during the intervention and the projected level of the previous baseline" (p. 128). In this way, each baseline serves as a control condition against which the influence of subsequent interventions can be evaluated.

Typically, these designs involve "keeping data on two or more behaviors that are to be modified sequentially with the same treatment procedure" (Gelfand & Hartmann, 1984, p. 69). The main steps in the use of any multiple-baseline design are as follows:

1. Establish reliable and stable baselines on all behaviors selected for modification.
2. Randomly select a behavior (or subject or setting) for treatment while simultaneously observing an untreated behavior (or subject or setting).
3. Randomly select another untreated baseline and introduce the experimental treatment.
4. Continue until all baselines have been treated.
5. Demonstrate treatment effectiveness by showing systematic modifications in performance across more than one baseline.

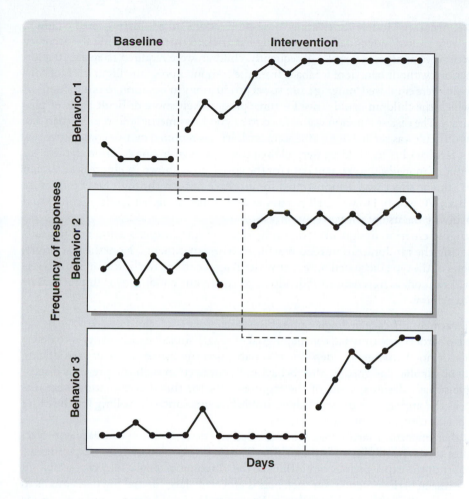

FIGURE 8-10

Hypothetical data for a multiple-baseline design across behaviors in which the intervention was introduced to three behaviors at different points in time

Reprinted with permission from Single Case Research Designs: Methods for Clinical and Applied Settings, *by A. E. Kazdin, 1982, New York: Oxford University Press, p. 127.*

A major advantage of multiple-baseline designs is that they do not necessitate withdrawal of treatment in order to demonstrate treatment efficacy. Thus, they are well suited to a variety of clinical applications, particularly when the clinical researcher is interested in monitoring several target measures concurrently. A potential disadvantage associated with their use arises when different baselines are not independent, so that the effects arising from treating the first behavioral target or situation/setting spread across to influence performance in other experimental conditions. Other problems might arise from the inability to achieve stable baselines prior to intervention and the large amount of time that may be needed to collect data.

Changing Criterion Design

Like the multiple-baseline design discussed previously, the **changing criterion design** uses each phase of an experimental treatment to evaluate subsequent phases of treatment. However, in the latter design, a step-wise criterion rate of responding is determined for each phase of treatment, which subsequently serves as a baseline for the next phase in the series.

An example application of a single-subject multiple-baseline design that incorporated a changing criterion is found in a study by Pratt and her associates (Pratt, Heintzelman, & Deming, 1993). Specifically, these researchers investigated the efficacy of the IBM Speech

Viewer's Vowel Accuracy Module for treating vowel productions in hearing impaired children. The children were treated individually by providing feedback to them concerning the accuracy of 10 productions of a targeted vowel. Subsequently, children were required to make 10 additional productions without benefit of feedback from the computer program. Eight levels of contextual difficulty were employed, ranging from vowel productions in isolation to productions in phrases, in which the children could strive for three progressively more difficult levels of production accuracy. The easiest criterion was defined as a "goodness metric" of no more than 3.0, and the most difficult was set at 1.4. An 80% accuracy level was required on two consecutive sessions without feedback before children were allowed to progress from one criterion to the next.

An example of individual treatment data for the vowel /u/ is shown in Figure 8.11. As can be seen, a treatment effect was demonstrated for all three criteria through Level 6 (picture labeling with a CVC word). However, all criteria were not met at higher levels of contextual difficulty involving the use of the vowel in phrases.

The changing criterion design, like other single-subject quasi-experimental designs, falls short of meeting the randomization requirement of true experiments. Nonetheless, single-subject designs of the type discussed have many useful applications to clinical or applied settings in which random assignment of individuals to treatment conditions is impractical or impossible to achieve.

Evaluating Treatment Efficacy in Single-Subject Research

As in the case of group experiments, the major goal of single-subject experiments is to determine whether or not a change in a dependent variable was the consequence of introducing an independent variable designed to alter behavior. In connection with the previous discussion of single-subject designs, some of the requirements for this determination were discussed, such as the importance of establishing stable baselines and controlling for the order of treatments and treatment interaction effects.

Still another important factor that can confound the determination of treatment effectiveness relates to the possibility of experimenter bias. As in the case of group experiments, bias on the part of the experimenter can influence the outcome in single-subject research. In single-subject research, the potential for such bias is especially large in making decisions as to when treatment is to be applied and withdrawn. For example, should the experimenter decide to initiate treatment prior to the establishment of a stable baseline, the treatment result might be unreliable. The same could be said about decisions pertaining to the withdrawal of treatment based on the assumption that the response of interest has reached a plateau; that is, no further changes in performance are expected. To deal with the possibility of bias influencing such decision making, the length of the baseline, treatment, and withdrawal periods should be specified in advance of beginning the experiment.

To help guard against researchers' "seeing" what they might expect or hope to see, additional observers can be used in data collection who are otherwise naïve as to the purpose of the experiment. Such observers are often graduate or undergraduate students who are trained to a high level of proficiency in accurately identifying and recording the targeted behavior. A number of observational recording methods are available as appropriate for the dependent variable selected for study and the aims of the research. Some of the more common of these procedures are summarized in Table 8-8.

Visual (graphical) analysis.   The most commonly employed method for determining the efficacy of treatment in single-subject research is **visual (graphical) analysis.** Tawney and Gast (1984) have provided general guidelines for inspecting and interpreting line-graphed single-subject research data:

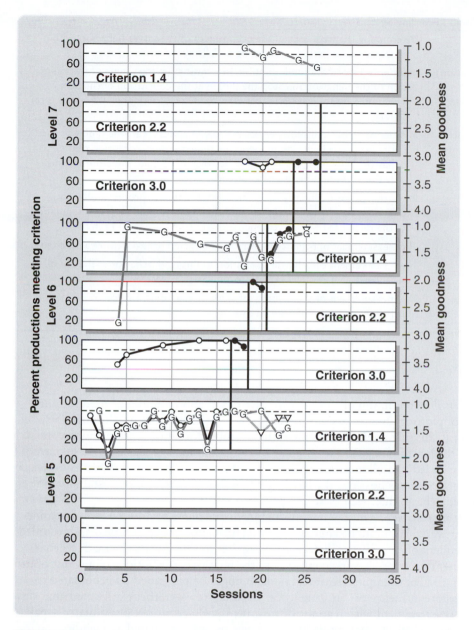

FIGURE 8-11

Individual treatment data for Subject 1 for vowel /u/. The open circles represent pretreatment data points, the filled circles treatment data points, and the inverted open triangles represent posttreatment data points; all are referred to the left-hand axis. The letter G represents the average goodness of the productions and is referred to the right-hand axis. The 80% level of performance is marked by a dashed line. Four of the five judges indicated an overall treatment effect.

Reprinted with permission from "The Efficacy of Using the IBM Speech Viewer Vowel Accuracy Module to Treat Young Children With Hearing Impairment," by S. R. Pratt, A. T. Heintzelman, and S. E. Deming, 1993, Journal of Speech and Hearing Research, *36, p. 1067.*

TABLE 8-8   Direct Observational Recording System

Event recording:	Determining the frequency of the occurrences of the target behaviors within an observation period by counting or tallying it.
Duration recording (total duration):	In order to record the total duration, one must start the timing at the initiation of the behavior and stop the timing at the conclusion of the behavior. The timing device is *not* reset between behaviors, therefore yielding the total duration.
Duration recording (duration per occurrence):	In order to record duration per occurrence, one must start the timing at the initiation of the behavior and stop the timing at the conclusion of the behavior. The timing device *is* reset between behaviors, therefore yielding only the duration per each occurrence.
Latency recording:	In order to measure latency, one must start the timing promptly after the directions for the task are given, and the timing should stop upon initiation of the response behavior. Latency should be measured for each trial.
Interval recording:	The measurement of behavior in relation to targeted behavior *during* a set interval.
Time sample recording:	The measurement of behavior in relation to targeted behavior at the *end* of a set interval.
Placheck recording:	The measurement of the quantity of subjects exhibiting a targeted behavior at the *end* of a set interval.

Adapted from Tawney and Gast, 1984

1. *Phase length.* A minimum of three consecutive observations should be used for purposes of plotting data points during each phase of the experiment, although, by necessity, this rule might be modified when withholding intervention could jeopardize the health of a participant. Some investigators such as Sharpley (1986) have recommended a baseline length of between 5–10 sessions to avoid problems in visual inference. So far as possible, the baseline phase should continue until stability in the targeted behavior has been established.

2. *Change one variable at a time.* When moving from one phase to another, only one independent variable should be altered so that its influence can be observed and recorded independent of any other influence. An exception to this rule can be made when a "treatment package" is being compared to the relative contributions of any one of its procedures. For example, Treatment A *and* B might be combined and compared to the separate influence of Treatment A *or* B alone. However, the relative contributions of any one treatment within an intact treatment package cannot be evaluated separately from another—such a treatment package must be evaluated as a whole.

3. *Level.* Refers to the magnitude of the data points on a graph. Typically, measures of the dependent variable (frequency, duration, percentage, etc.) are referenced to the vertical or *y* axis, called the *ordinate,* while time measures (sessions, days, weeks, etc.) are shown on the *x* axis, called the *abscissa.* Two aspects to examine include the *level stability* and *level change* of data.

The range of the data point values determines level stability *within* a particular phase of the experiment regardless of whether it is a baseline phase or treatment phase. As a general guide, Tawney and Gast (1984) note that ". . . if 80%–90% of the data points of a condition fall within a 15% range of the mean level of all data point values of a condition, applied researchers will consider the data stable" (p. 161). In Figure 8-12(A), two different

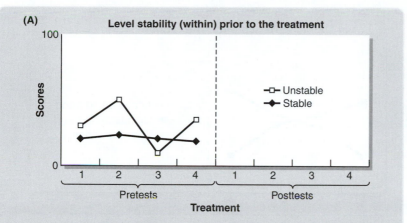

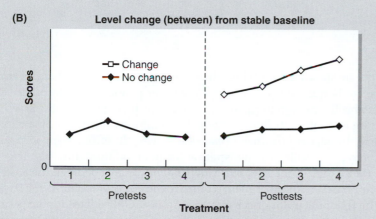

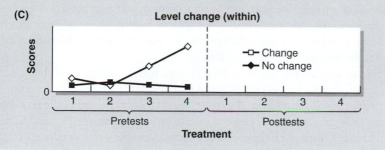

FIGURE 8-12

In (A), two different series of data points are shown for a baseline phase. One series of data points is stable from one measured time period to the next, while the other lacks stability.

In (B), two different changes in the level of the scores following the establishment of a stable baseline are illustated. One series of data points shows very little change from the baseline to the treatment phase, while the other shows considerable change.

In (C), two different changes in the level of a score within a baseline phase are illustrated. One series of data points shows little difference between the first and last data point, while the other shows a substantial increment from the first to the last data point.

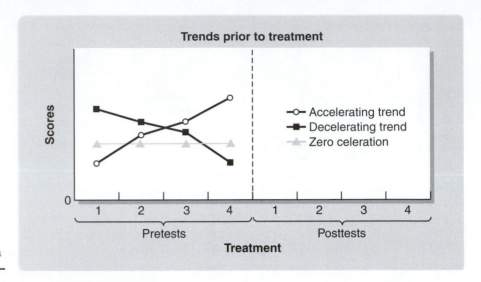

FIGURE 8-13

Three different trend characteristics that can be found in single-subject data

series of data points are shown for a baseline phase. As can be seen, one of these series of data points appears to be quite stable across measured time periods while the other illustrates considerable fluctuation from one measured time period to the next. Level stability is important to establish before changing the conditions of the experiment as from the baseline to the adjacent treatment phase. Otherwise, the effectiveness of a particular treatment may be difficult to demonstrate at the point of intervention.

To determine the change in the level of the dependent variable between the baseline and treatment phases of an experiment, compare the last data point of the baseline phase with the first data point of the treatment phase. Only adjacent phases can serve as valid comparisons of data points. Generally, the *sooner* a change in response level is observed following the introduction of treatment and the *greater* its magnitude in relation to baseline, the more confidence we can have in the treatment effect. Figure 8-12(B) illustrates two different changes in the level of the dependent variable following the establishment of a stable baseline.

It is also possible to identify the degree of level change within a particular phase. A simple way to accomplish this is to (1) identify the first and last data points of a phase, (2) subtract the smaller of the values from the larger, and (3) observe whether the change in level is in a positive or negative direction based on the treatment objectives. Figure 8-12(C) illustrates two different changes in the level of a dependent variable within a particular phase with little difference between the first and last data point in one case and a substantial increment from the first to the last data point in the other case.

4. *Trend*. This term refers to the *slope* of the data points on a graph. Such a slope can illustrate one of three characteristics with respect to the direction of data points across time (sessions, days, weeks, etc.) displayed on the abscissa (horizontal or *x* axis) of a graph (see Figure 8-13). The data points can be said to be *accelerating* (increasing with respect to their ordinate values), *decelerating* (decreasing with respect to their ordinate values), or show *zero celeration* (data points are level with abscissa). Figure 8-13 illustrates these three trend characteristics found in single-subject data.

The trend of the data points in a single-subject experiment can be difficult to interpret. Generally, if the slope of the data points in the baseline phase, as compared to their slope in the adjacent treatment phase, move in opposite directions (one moves in a positive direction and the other moves in a negative direction), a treatment effect is thereby demonstrated. However, should the slopes of the data points in adjacent phases move in the same direction (both move in either a positive or negative direction), it is difficult to detect a treatment effect under such circumstances. This is because such a change simply may be due to an extraneous variable such as maturation, history, and the like. Furthermore, should the data points illustrate a large degree of fluctuation during the baseline phase, the number of trials during this phase should be increased until either (1) a stable response rate is demonstrated or (2) the trend of the direction of behavior of interest is opposite to that of the intended treatment effect.

It is also possible to estimate the slope of the trend. To accomplish this analysis, the most commonly used visual approach is to draw a straight line that most closely approximates the majority of the data points in a series. Such a line is called a **celeration line.** The instructions for drawing such a line for a hypothetical series of data points are shown in Figure 8-14.

Despite the common use of visual inspection as a tool for the analysis of single-subject data, several studies provide evidence to suggest that such methods are often unreliable (Crosbie, 1993). Even among experienced judges, a lack of high inter-observer agreement can be found when the degree of variability in the data is great. Such low reliability might also result from lack of consistency in interpreting changes in the trends of data or in the use of decision rules for visual analysis (Wolery & Harris, 1982). Applying standardized methods to the analysis of graphic data obtained from single subject experiments, as opposed to merely "eyeballing" the results, should improve the reliability of an experimenter's observations and the inferences from them.

Statistical analysis.   In place of or in combination with visual inspection methods, a variety of statistical analyses can be performed on single-subject research data. Descriptive statistics can include the use of means, ranges and standard deviations to summarize and compare performance values within and between phases (see Chapter 11). For purposes of drawing statistical inferences about the significance of the difference between data values, a variety of parametric and nonparametric statistics can be employed (see Chapter 12).

Much controversy has surrounded the analysis of single-subject data. As we discussed above, the primary means of data reduction is based on visual inspection. According to Parsonson and Baer (1986), visual analysis is a dynamic process that allows for the examination of patterns of performance over time. They commented that such methods are better suited for determining "clinical significance" as opposed to "statistical significance."

Despite the widespread use of graphic presentations and visual inspection approaches to the analysis of single-subject data, Kazdin (1978) commented that a limitation of visual inspection techniques is their tendency to encourage subjectivity and inconsistency in the evaluation of treatment effects. In view of the poor interrater reliability that has been documented for single-subject research data (Johnson & Ottenbacher, 1991; Ottenbacher, 1992), this criticism seems warranted. Despite this limitation, Parsonson and Baer (1986) noted that a possible advantage of visual analysis is that it is relatively insensitive to weak treatment effects. To the extent that only strong treatment effects are likely to be observed and reported, the probability of a type I error (concluding the existence of a treatment effect when there is none) might be expected to be reduced when evaluated only through visual analysis (Parsonson & Baer, 1986). At the same time, according to Ottenbacher (1992), small

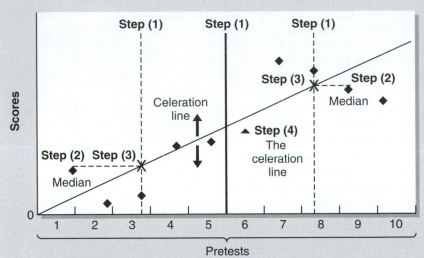

FIGURE 8-14

How to draw a celeration line

X represents the intersection point between the median data point and the dashed vertical line.

Step 1. Count the total number of data points in the baseline phase (pretest 1 to pretest 10) and divide this number so that half fall on one side of a solid vertical line and the remaining half fall on the other side. As can be seen, the solid line falls directly in the center of the graph. Next, draw a second dashed vertical line on each side of the solid vertical line that again divides the data points in half.

Step 2. Identify the median score for the data distribution on each side of the solid vertical line. The median is the middle value of the data points with respect to their magnitude.

Step 3. Draw a dashed horizontal line through the median data point on each side of the solid vertical line so it intersects the dashed vertical lines.

Step 4. Draw a straight solid line by connecting the two points of intersection (denoted by X) passing through the solid vertical line. This final step completes the construction of the celeration line. In this case, we can visually determine that the trend of the data points is accelerating. However, based on such a visual analysis alone, we cannot determine the *rate of change*—how fast the dependent variable changes over time. This determination can only be made by the use of statistical methods that are beyond the scope of the present chapter.

yet consistent and statistically significant effects might go undetected when employing only visual analysis, resulting in a type II error (concluding the absence of a treatment effect when there is one).

While Bloom and Fischer (1982) argued that visual inspection of data can serve as a useful starting point, they went on to state that other statistical methods of data analysis should be employed as well. As noted above, several types of parametric and nonparametric statistical tests have been applied to the analysis of single-subject data, many of which are discussed in Chapter 12. A straightforward approach to statistical analysis might entail the use of a paired *t*-test to compare mean scores across phases of an experiment. For example, in an AB design, the significance of the difference between the mean scores obtained from observations during phase A and phase B could be determined though the use of such a test. Alternatively, analysis of variance techniques in the form of an *F* test might be employed to examine statistical differences among mean scores across *multiple phases* of an experiment as in an A-B-A design, or A-B-A-B design. According to Sharpe and Koperwas (2003), such tests would be appropriate only if the so-called **autocorrelation** among data points has been found to be negative. Autocorrelation is a problem involving serial dependency in a temporally ordered sequence of data points so that preceding data points are likely to predict subsequent data points in time-series experiments. In other words, the temporally ordered scores obtained on successive trials tend to be highly related (correlated with) one another. As Todman and Dugard (2001) point out, such "positive autocorrelation will result in many more significant findings than justified" (p. 7). To avoid the likelihood of such type I errors, they noted that the "onus" should be on the researcher to rule out autocorrelation before using such classical parametric statistics as described above.

Still another statistical method that is commonly used in the analysis of single-subject data is termed *time-series analysis*. This statistical method involves the analysis of a sequence of measurements taken on a response that tends to vary over time. In single-subject research, time-series analysis can be employed to detect changes in one or more recorded behaviors from one phase of treatment to the next. More specifically, the main goals of time-series analysis are to (1) forecast future values of particular responses based on a series of observations made in the past or in prior phases of the experiment, and (2) evaluate any substantial changes in the *level* or *trend* in adjacent phases of treatment. From a statistical standpoint, the most distinguishing feature of time-series analysis, as opposed to other statistical methods as discussed above, is that the observations are not assumed to vary independently. Therefore, time-series analysis is a valid and effective means of detecting a treatment effect when autocorrelation exists among several observations or data points within a particular treatment phase. Despite this advantage, it is sometimes difficult to implement a time-series analysis that is suitable for the characteristics of a particular series of data points. In such a case, Cook and Campbell (1979) noted that the particular time-series that an investigator hopes to implement may have to be discarded and new models tried out in an effort to increase accuracy of forecasting. To determine the "best fit," 50 or more observations may be required for a time-series analysis. The method for calculating a time-series analysis in a single-subject research design is illustrated in Appendix A-2.

Generality of findings.   A limitation of single-subject research frequently mentioned in textbooks and journal articles pertains to the generality of findings. It is often said that, just as the findings of group experiments cannot be generalized to specific individuals, neither can the findings from single subjects be generalized to a population. Perhaps the best way to establish the generality of research findings from single-subject experiments is through replication. Wolery & Ezell (1993) identified several factors that can influence replication success:

- Descriptions of subject characteristics and the experimental procedures employed in the original study being precise and complete
- The degree to which the new study actually duplicated the procedures of the original study
- The similarity and description of the relevant setting variables

- All potential sources of variability associated with conducting an experiment being identified and controlled to the greatest extent possible

In addition to demonstrating the reliability of a study's findings, replication can demonstrate the generality of a treatment effect under different conditions and with different people (Kratochwill and Levin, 1978). To the degree this actually occurs, the treatment effect is said to be *robust*.

Preexperimental Designs

Preexperimental designs involve studies that fail to meet at least two of the criteria of a true experiment. As forerunners of stronger experimental designs, the present day value of such studies is limited because of their almost total lack of control of numerous extraneous variables that can invalidate an experiment.

One-Group Posttest Design: $X\ O$

Among the preexperimental designs, the weakest of all is the **one-group posttest design,** which has practically no scientific value for drawing causal inferences. This approach, also known as the *one-shot case study,* involves studying the presumed effect of an independent variable in a single group of subjects by administering a posttest after some intervention(s). Although used extensively in various clinical studies, there are serious pitfalls to this approach. Suppose you are treating a number of cases whose clinical progress is below your level of expectation. You decide to increase the number of clinical contacts from one to two therapy sessions per week. After a certain time period, you measure the achievement of these cases and observe improvements as consistent with your therapy goals. Can you conclude that increasing the amount of therapy (level of the independent variable) was an effective strategy? Unfortunately, in the absence of the use of a pretest and a control group, there is no valid basis for drawing this conclusion.

One-Group Pretest-Posttest Design: $O_1\ X\ O_2$

One major hindrance to determining causal relations in a one-shot case study is the lack of a pretest so that conclusions must take the form of retrospective suppositions about what the results might otherwise have been in the absence of the independent variable. Most clinicians are knowledgeable about the importance of pretesting; most, therefore, would have wisely included this step in our hypothetical study. Had this occurred, the design would be called a **one-group pretest-posttest design.** Is this design, by virtue of including a pretest, markedly improved over the one-shot case study? Again, we must say no. There are still many extraneous variables that can seriously confound the interpretation of findings. Indeed, by the inclusion of a pretest, this design introduces another potential problem not present in the posttest only design, namely, that of pretest sensitization with the possibility of accompanying interaction effects that are impossible to evaluate because of the absence of an appropriate comparison group. Posttest scores may simply reflect the influence of practice or learning how to be a better "test taker" the second time around. In order to avoid this complication, one might decide to omit the pretest and use a control group.

Static-Group Comparison Design: $X\ O_1$
$$O_2$$

Opting for the control group approach, perhaps our clinicians would select a design called **static-group comparison** wherein two preformed groups would be selected, one group receiving additional therapy sessions and the other not. However, this goes back to the problem of lacking two important criteria for inferring causal relations. What is now missing is *both* random assignment *and* the use of a pretest as a control mechanism. Should we decide to add both factors to our study design, we have once again established the requirement for performing a true experiment!

Because appropriate statistical comparisons cannot be performed on the results of preexperimental studies, such investigations are essentially limited to describing outcomes. Perhaps such studies might be more appropriately described as **pseudoexperiments** that sometimes convey the misleading impression of belonging to more rigorous and powerful kinds of experimental methodologies that are better equipped for observing lawful relationships and drawing plausible explanations with greater confidence.

SUMMARY

We began this chapter by noting that different types of experimental designs are available for testing hypotheses given various research interests. As discussed, the most powerful of these are true experiments which entail the randomized allocation of subjects to two or more comparison groups. In at least one of these groups, an independent variable is actively manipulated to determine its influence on a dependent variable. Generally, whether or not such a treatment effect occurred is decided by comparing the results for a treatment group to a control or placebo group. Several types of two-group and multigroup designs involving betweengroup and within-group comparisons that are appropriate for such purposes were reviewed along with their strengths and weaknesses. Despite their obvious advantages over other forms of experiments, true experiments are not as frequently employed because of the sizable number of subjects required to meet their statistical assumptions and because of possible ethical issues arising from randomly assigning participants to nontreatment or placebo conditions.

Quasi-experiments fall short of being true experiments because of the lack of randomization. Instead, matching procedures are typically used in an effort to equate participants on potentially confounding variables prior to their group assignment. However, possible errors in identifying significant confounding variables and assuring that those identified are equally distributed, as these might influence the dependent variable, weaken the power of this design. Despite this fact, quasi-experiments are often the best means available for investigating a problem and are the most commonly used research design in the behavioral sciences, including communication sciences and disorders.

A special category of quasi-experiments is a single-subject experiment. Several types of these experiments were reviewed along with their strengths and limitations. These experiments are commonly used in the field of communication sciences and disorders because of their clinical appeal. Compared to group studies, often it is possible to achieve a greater degree of experimental rigor in single-subject experiments because a subject serves as his or her own control in evaluating a treatment effect, thereby eliminating many threats to internal validity. With respect to external validity, the ability to generalize the findings from a single subject to a larger number of individuals as they exist in a population is problematic. The best way to augment the generality of research findings from single-subjects experiments is through replication. Several factors that can influence replication success were discussed.

The weakest of the experimental designs are preexperiments, sometimes called pseudoexperiments because they give the impression of constituting credible scientific studies but are characterized by numerous sources of invalidity. We reviewed several of these methods primarily to call attention to their "fools gold" appeal.

KEY TERMS

pretest-posttest control group design	nonequivalent comparison group design
difference scores (gain scores)	single time-series designs
posttest only control group design	multiple time-series design
Solomon four-group design	single-subject designs
factorial designs	A-B design
main effect	A-B-A design
interaction effect	A-B-A-B design
ANOVAR design	replication design
analysis of variance (ANOVA)	alternating treatment design
randomized controlled trial (RCT)	multitreatment interference effects
completely randomized design	reversal design
randomized block design	multiple-baseline design
parallel group design	changing criterion design
repeated measures design	visual (graphical) analysis
washout period	celeration line
period effects	autocorrelation
crossover	preexperimental design
treatment period	one-group posttest design
Latin square design	one-group pretest-posttest design
balanced Latin square design	static-group comparison
split-plot design	pseudoexperiments

SELF-LEARNING REVIEW

1. Control of variables in an experimental study is achieved by _____ of independent variables, _____ or inclusion of extraneous variables, and _____ control of extraneous variables.

2. _____ experiments are the strongest of the research designs because they include _____ _____ of units, deliberate and active manipulation of _____ _____, and a basis for evaluating the influence of a(n) _____ _____.

3. _____-_____ are like true experiments with the important exception of the absence of _____ _____.

4. _____ designs are by far the weakest of all in controlling for pitfalls that can invalidate an experiment. They are also called _____ experimental designs.

5. Because _____-_____ _____ group design involves the comparison of two groups, it is likely that a statistical analysis involving a(n) _____ test would be carried out to determine if the independent variable had a significant effect. Such a statistical analysis typically entails the evaluation of a(n) _____ _____ that states that no population mean difference exists, and is symbolically written as _____. In this design, the difference between two scores is termed _____ scores.

6. The statistical assumption underlying the two-group design is that the difference between the pretest and posttest scores in the experimental group should be larger for the _____ subjects than for the _____ subjects. To determine the probability that such a difference in the dependent variable reflects a(n) _____ _____ as opposed

to a mere _____ _____, a ratio representing the amount of _____-_____ variation can be calculated, and is symbolically written as _____.

7. In addition to the procedure involving the analysis of difference scores between the pretest and posttest, Campbell and Stanley (1963) suggested that an even better method than a *t*-test is to use a(n) _____ _____ _____ to analyze between-group differences while treating the pretest scores as _____.

8. A major strength of the randomized pretest-posttest design is that it increases the _____ that the subjects assigned to groups are relatively _____ on all variables with the exception of the _____ _____.

9. The rationale for posttest only control group design is based on the assumption underlying _____ _____ procedures intended to minimize _____ _____ differences between groups. Furthermore, this design is advantageous when _____ is impossible to accomplish or when the effect of such testing might unduly _____ subjects to the experimental treatment or bias posttest scores as the result of _____ _____.

10. The strength of the _____ _____-_____ design lies in its ability to control for certain _____ between a pretest and an independent variable that combine to affect a dependent variable in a way that neither might have done when operating alone. This design can also be viewed as a special case of a(n) _____ _____ which can be defined as any design in which more than one treatment factor is investigated. This design also has two categories of effects that can be analyzed, namely _____ _____ for (a) the pretest versus its absence, (b) treatment versus its absence, and (c) an _____ _____.

11. One of the major limitations of the use of the Solomon design is that it requires a relatively _____ number of participants for random assignment to _____ separate groups as well as the _____ consumed in executing the various components of this design.

12. Designs that require the comparison of three or more groups are sometimes called _____ designs because they involve the use of a statistical technique called a(n) _____ _____ _____, or ANOVA.

13. The most complex of all the experimental designs are called _____ designs because they allow for administering more than one independent variable at a time to a subject. Within the framework of this design, different _____ factors for between-subject and _____ effects can be studied simultaneously.

14. Quasi-experiments are those that satisfy all of the requirements of a true experiment with the exception of _____ _____.

15. By studying the influence of multiple independent variables within the framework of a single experiment, both the _____ and _____ of the research process is facilitated. Greater _____ is accomplished by saving time and money, whereas greater _____ is possible because the interaction between two or more variables can be simultaneously evaluated.

16. The goal of _____ _____ trials is to allow for a valid interpretation of the influence of the independent variable by controlling for _____ variables.

17. According to Altman et al. (2001), three major advantages of random assignment are (1) it eliminates _____ bias in the assignment of subjects to treatment groups; (2) it can facilitate _____ of both the investigators and the subjects with respect to the _____ received; and (3) it allows the use of probability statistics to determine the

_____ that the differences found between treatment groups are the consequence of experimental manipulations as opposed to _____ variations.

18. A(n) _____ _____ design places no restrictions on how participants are allocated to the study groups as long as they meet the inclusion criteria.

19. A(n) _____ _____ design is useful when we suspect secondary treatment effect other than _____ treatment effect.

20. The statistical assumption underlying the randomized block design is that by controlling for ____-____ variability, through the use of _____ subgroups, between-group differences owing to the intended treatment effect can be validly assessed.

21. Whatever method of randomization might be employed, the majority of randomized controlled trials use a(n) _____ _____ design, another term for experiments that entail between-group comparisons.

22. A(n) _____ _____ design is one in which each participant is exposed to all the treatments administered in an experiment according to a randomly assigned sequence and the effects of these treatments are compared within each individual. This design is also called a(n) ____-____ design.

23. In a repeated measures design, greater _____ _____ can be attained than in a between-subject design because the performance of each subject is compared to only him- or herself across the treatment conditions.

24. In a repeated measures design, _____ _____ result from specific changes caused by one or more earlier treatments interacting with later treatments, whereas _____ _____ relate to general changes in performance that occur independently of the particular sequence of the treatment given.

25. One way to control for carryover effects is to use a(n) _____ period. This is a time interval interposed between successive treatments to allow for the dissipation of treatment effects.

26. In a repeated measure design, if a particular disorder is regressing, progressing, or fluctuating up and down, it will be impossible to conclude that it was relatively the same during the time period _____ each treatment intervention. Such effects are called _____ effects.

27. The biasing influence of both order effects and carryover effects can often be minimized by _____ the treatment conditions. When a design involves the comparison of two treatments, participants either receive treatment A first followed by treatment B, or vice versa. Moving from one such treatment to another is termed _____. To qualify as a randomized controlled trial, the order in which participants receive the treatments in such trials must be _____. The time during which each intervention is administered is called the _____ period.

28. For purposes of counterbalancing, investigators often use a(n) _____ _____ design that can be defined as a matrix consisting of equal numbers of rows and columns that contain a subset of all possible treatment sequences in a multiple treatment experiment.

29. A(n) ___-____ design evolved from agricultural investigations of the effect of different fertilizers applied within each of several plots of land.

30. The ____ comparison group design entails the use of at least two ____ groups, the members of which are ____ before administering treatment. The statistical analysis of this design requires a(n) _____ ___-____.

31. Designs in which repeated measures of a(n) _____ _____ are made prior and subsequent to administering an independent variable are called _____-_____ designs. More specifically, this design involves periodic measurements over a time span in order to establish either an average performance value or a(n) _____ prior to introducing an experimental treatment.

32. The strength of the time-series design is to control for _____ effects that might not be immediately apparent but tend to become more evident over a period of time. The limitation of the design is that the validity of findings might be threatened due to a greater degree of test _____.

33. A(n) _____ _____-_____ design for group experiments can not only control for sleeper effects but also the inclusion of a control group allows for a better determination of a true treatment effect resulting from the independent variable as opposed to a(n) _____ effect resulting from some simultaneously occurring extraneous variable.

34. The primary aims of a single-subject research are to (1) gain precise control over the _____ conditions of an experiment by eliminating extraneous variables, (2) establish a stable level of _____ before administering a treatment condition, (3) record the _____ _____ of interest within a given time period, (4) perform a(n) _____ and/or a(n) _____ analysis of the data to determine the treatment outcome.

35. The most basic time-series design involving individuals is called the ____-___ paradigm. An elaboration of this design in which the dependent variable is measured again after withdrawing treatment is the ___-__-__ design.

36. The A-B-A-B design can involve both _____ and _____ of treatment. This makes the design clinically more appealing than the A-B-A design.

37. A design used in evaluating alternative treatment approaches is the _____ _____ design. In such a design, _____ treatments are alternated _____. A limitation of the alternating design pertains to _____-_____ interactions. This is the effect that one treatment has on the effectiveness of one that follows it.

38. _____ _____ effects is a general term that describes the influence of one treatment upon another in cases in which the same subject is exposed to each of them.

39. A design in which alternative incompatible behaviors can be treated is called _____.

40. _____-_____ designs fail to meet at least two of the criteria of a(n) _____ _____. A major advantage of such designs is that they do not necessitate _____ of treatment in order to demonstrate treatment _____. A potential disadvantage associated with their use arises when different baselines are not _____, so that the effects arising from treating the first behavioral target spread across to influence performance in other experimental conditions.

41. Like the multiple-baseline designs, the _____ _____ design uses each phase of an experimental treatment to evaluate subsequent phases of treatment. However, in this design, a(n) _____-_____ criterion rate of responding is determined for each phase of treatment, which subsequently serves as a baseline for the next phase in the series.

42. The major goal of _____-_____ experiments is to determine whether or not a change in a dependent variable was the consequence of introducing an independent variable to change behavior.

43. Another important factor that can confound the determination of treatment effectiveness relates to the possibility of _____ bias.

44. The range of the data point values determines level stability _____ a particular phase of a single-subject experiment regardless of whether it is a(n) _____ phase or

_____ phase. As a general guide, if ___–____% of the data points of a condition fall within a(n) _____% range of the mean level of all data point values of a condition, applied researchers will consider the data stable.

45. Level stability is important to establish _____ changing the conditions of the experiment as from the baseline to the _____ treatment phase.

46. To determine the change in the level of the dependent variable between the baseline and treatment phases of an experiment, compare the _____ _____ point of the baseline phase with the _____ _____ point of the treatment phase. Only _____ phases can serve as valid comparisons of data points.

47. It is possible to identify the degree of level change within a particular phase. A simple way to accomplish this is to (1) identify the _____ and _____ data points of a phase, (2) subtract the _____ of the values from the _____, (3) observe whether the change in level is in a(n) _____ direction or _____ direction based on the treatment objectives.

48. _____ refers to the slope of the data points on a graph. It can be _____ (increasing with respect to their ordinate values), _____ (decreasing with respect to their ordinate values), or show _____ celeration (data points are level with abscissa).

49. In addition to demonstrating the reliability of a study's findings, _____ can demonstrate the generality of a treatment effect under different conditions and with different people. To the degree this actually occurs, the treatment effect is said to be _____.

50. Preexperimental designs fail to meet at least two of the criteria of a(n) _____ experiment. The weakest of these is the ___–____ _____ _____.

51. The ___–____ ____–___ design is similar to the one-shot case study except for the inclusion of a(n) _____. The limitation of this design pertains to _____ _____ with the possibility of accompanying _____ effects that are impossible to evaluate because of the absence of an appropriate comparison group.

52. A preexperimental design that omits both random assignment and the use of a pretest is called a ____–___ comparison.

QUESTIONS AND EXERCISES FOR CLASSROOM DISCUSSION

1. Discuss several ways to classify research designs.

2. Define the term _experiment_ and explain how this type of research differs from other research studies.

3. What are three characteristics of a true experiment and why are quasi-experiments and preexperiments considered to be less powerful in determining causality?

4. Why might a randomized posttest only control group design be considered as powerful as a randomized pretest-posttest control group design? Compare each of these designs to the Solomon four-group design and identify what advantages the latter has over the former.

5. What is the appropriate method for analyzing the results from a randomized pretest-posttest control group design with respect to the statistical comparisons?

6. Compare the steps involved in implementing a completely randomized design to those for a randomized block design using hypothetical research problems of your own choosing to represent each.

7. How does a repeated measures (within-subjects) design differ from a parallel groups (between-subjects) design? Formulate a research problem that might be investigated by applying *either* of these designs. Why would you choose one of these methods as opposed to the other?

8. What are two unwanted effects that can be especially troublesome in repeated measures designs? What steps can be taken to control for these problems?

9. What is a Latin square and what purpose does it serve?

10. Why is a mixed experimental design sometime called a "split-plot design"?

11. When would a quasi-experimental design be chosen as opposed to a true experiment?

12. Discuss three types of quasi-experimental designs and formulate a research problem to represent the use of each type.

13. List and briefly discuss the types of single-subject designs reviewed in this chapter. In your judgment, which of these has the greatest clinical appeal?

14. What are the major strengths and limitations of single-subject research as compared to group research?

15. Locate and critique two research articles pertaining to a communication disorder that employed different types of single-subject designs.

16. What is the primary basis for determining treatment efficacy in single-subject research?

17. Identify and discuss the two major means for visually evaluating single-subject data.

18. List and briefly describe the preexperimental designs discussed in this chapter and the shortcomings of each. Why would the use of such methods cause some researchers to feel queasy?

Nonexperimental Research Methods

CHAPTER 9

LEARNING OBJECTIVES

After reading this chapter, you should be able to identify, describe, or define:

- The basis for distinguishing nonexperimental from experimental designs
- Strengths and limitations of case studies and case series research
- Two types of cohort studies and their relative advantages and disadvantages
- The difference between cohort studies and case-control studies
- Incidence rate versus prevalence rate

■ The nature of causal-comparative (ex post facto) studies
■ The steps in developing a survey
■ Cross-sectional, longitudinal, and prevalence/incidence survey designs
■ How to construct a questionnaire
■ The Likert, Guttman, and Thurstone scales
■ Strategies for maximizing survey response rate
■ Measures of response rate and their calculation
■ Types of interviews and their relative advantages and disadvantages
■ The accuracy of a diagnostic test
■ Test sensitivity, test specificity, and predictive values and their calculation

In the previous chapter, we discussed a number of experimental research designs appropriate for investigating causal relationships among variables. Such studies entail an active and deliberate manipulation of one or more independent variables in order to assess the influence of such manipulation on one or more dependent variables under conditions controlled by the experimenter. Most scientific researchers are of the opinion that such methods are the only means for *directly* inferring causal relations among variables. However, there are several types of research questions that can only be answered through the use of nonexperimental methods. This would be the case in circumstances where an independent variable is not subject to manipulation or an effort to do so would breach ethical standards.

For example, suppose we are interested in studying the relationship of otitis media in children to some aspect of language acquisition. Obviously, no effort would be made to directly manipulate the independent variable (otitis media). Instead, to examine this problem in relation to a particular parameter of language development (dependent variable), an investigator might choose to divide a population of children into two groups based on their medical histories (those with and those without the disease) and proceed to compare them on the language factor of interest (dependent variable). If unable to perform an experiment, describing the characteristics of an observed behavior, correlating its occurrence with some other variable(s), or determining the probability for its future occurrence may be all that a researcher can presently do.

In addition to limitations imposed by variables that can't be manipulated, use of the experimental method may not be feasible due to constraints stemming from an inadequate number of subjects, limited material or financial resources, or insufficient time to conduct the project. In this chapter, a variety of nonexperimental research methods are reviewed, along with their strengths and limitations. Nonexperimental research is comprised of several types of studies in which the investigator observes and describes an outcome as it happens or has happened sometime in the past. Before science can proceed to a level of knowledge grounded in an understanding of causal relations, the major activities of science must first focus on observation, description, and empirical testing.

CASE STUDIES AND CASE SERIES

Perhaps the simplest and most familiar of these approaches is the **case study,** in which a single individual or a few individuals sharing similar characteristics are studied and the findings reported. This approach should not be confused with single-subject designs discussed in the previous chapter. Although case study observation may serve as a basis for *forming* a hypothesis about the nature or treatment of a particular disorder or disease, such cases are not often used to actually *test* a treatment hypothesis. Nevertheless, case studies can yield insight about the mechanisms underlying pathology and point the way toward treatment.

A variety of data-gathering techniques can be used in an effort to understand the problems pertaining to a particular case including observation and recording of behavior, interviews with the case and significant others, results from clinical and laboratory tests, results of previous educational and medical assessments, progress reports, and so on. Ultimately, the goal is to sift through such data to focus more narrowly on the issues that are currently of interest and that may be relevant to understanding future cases of a similar kind.

The field of aphasiology is replete with instances in which the case study approach has helped to elucidate the neural basis of various disorders of oral and written language. An example of such studies is well represented in a paper by Armstrong and MacDonald (2000), who described an effort to help a young aphasic man "overcome what had appeared to be intractable written language expression difficulties." After briefly reviewing the literature pertaining to the methods to be employed in their study and the study goals, the authors proceeded to provide "case information" including the relevant medical history, a description of language recovery following surgical removal of a hematoma, a review of previous therapy methods and outcomes, the assessments given prior to administering the treatments currently of interest, the postassessment results, and a discussion of language therapy that the authors emphasized could best be measured "in *this* [italics added] man with chronic aphasia." Recognizing the limits of their study, the authors were careful to restrict their conclusions to the case they reported.

The format of the case study reported by Armstrong and McDonald is typical of the approaches used to investigate many other types of communication disorders in which detailed observations and descriptions of clinical and laboratory findings for single patients often serve as a basis not only for diagnosis but for treatment planning as well. Although case reports can sometimes help to facilitate understanding of various clinical problems, they also are susceptible to bias on the part of the reporter. Furthermore, because of their narrow focus on a single or a few selected individuals, the generality of findings from such studies is limited. An investigator's reluctance to infer causal relations on the basis of case study findings is always warranted because such studies provide no basis for determining the future probability for an observation or event in another person(s) beyond the case(s) studied. Perhaps the chief value of case reports is that they can serve as a basis for systematically investigating the same or similar problems in a larger population.

Although there is no specific rule as to how many cases can be included in a case report, three or more cases are often described as a collective case study or, more commonly, as a **case series** (Jenicek, 1999). In Chapter 2 we noted how initially studying a few individuals with various patterns of orofacial malformations can lead to the identification of specific syndromes and their possible genetic basis such as the velocardiofacial syndrome. Starting with a limited number of what are sometimes called *index cases*, investigators began to study the frequency of various clinical manifestations in a larger number of such patients. Through the case series approach, we have learned that this syndrome is associated with a high prevalence of learning disabilities (99%), cleft palate (98%), pharyngeal hypotonia (90%), cardiac anomalies (82%), and retrognathia (80%), as well as many other physical and functional abnormalities (Goldberg et al., 1993).

Different types of case series studies are possible, depending on how the cases are assembled. Such studies can be based on cases:

1. Investigators have observed themselves
2. Seen by others in several clinical facilities
3. Derived from a systematic review of isolated cases presented in the literature

Also, case series studies can be classified according to the time domain in which they are performed. They can be a **cross-sectional study,** in which observations are made at a particular point in time, or they can be a **longitudinal study,** in which repeated observations are made over an extended period of time.

While studies involving a case series of selected individuals are likely to yield more valid and reliable information than focusing on a single case, the absence of a control or comparison group weakens the value of both of these approaches. Such studies cannot be used as proof of cause or proof of the efficacy of treatment (Jenicek, 1999).

COHORT AND CASE-CONTROL STUDIES

Two observational strategies that permit stronger inferences about possible cause and effect relations than do case study methods, yet still fall short of directly demonstrating causality, are called **cohort studies** and **case-control studies.** Such studies entail the comparison of two or more groups based on their differing exposures to particular **risk factors** *believed to be* related to the occurrence of certain disorders or diseases. Risk factors may be environmental, behavioral, social, or genetic in nature. Associated with both cohort and case-control studies are certain advantages and disadvantages that determine their value as research designs.

In a cohort study (also known as an incidence study, follow-up study, or longitudinal study), individuals having known characteristics are assembled for study and then observed for some period of time. Selection for participation in such a study may depend on the presence or absence of a risk factor(s) believed to influence a particular outcome. People may be divided into groups given the presence or absence of one or more risk factors and then followed to determine who among them are more or less likely to illustrate the particular outcome of interest. A famous example of a cohort study was undertaken in Framingham, Massachusetts, in 1949. A representative sample, consisting of more than 5000 men and women, were studied to determine risk factors related to developing heart disease. None of these people had coronary heart disease at the outset of the study. Subsequent examination of this cohort on a biannual basis revealed that the risk for developing such disease was greater among people who smoked and had high blood pressure and elevated serum cholesterol.

An example of a cohort study relevant to the field of communication sciences and disorders was conducted by Catts et al. (2002), who investigated predictors of reading outcomes in young children. The study participants included 604 children whose language, early literacy, and nonverbal cognitive abilities were assessed in kindergarten. Subsequently, the reading achievement of these children was assessed in the second grade. Participants were then divided into children with and without reading problems. Statistical analysis of the findings revealed that five variables (letter identification, sentence imitation, phonological awareness, rapid naming, and mother education) best predicted reading outcomes. More specifically, of *the risk factors studied,* weaknesses in these particular areas were those most likely to be associated with reading difficulty.

Both of the studies cited above are examples of **prospective (concurrent) cohort studies.** In such a study, the cohort is selected using *current information* about the people comprising it, who are then tracked forward in time to determine their *future status.* Despite the power of prospective cohort studies in determining the risk for a particular disorder or disease, such studies are often expensive and inefficient designs for accomplishing this purpose. This is particularly true when the occurrence of the disorder or disease is rare.

Sometimes, it is also possible to perform a **retrospective (historical) cohort study** based on *past records* where the outcome is already known. From such historical records, individuals are selected for the study of factors that might explain their *present status*. A study by Carter et al. (2003), who investigated the occurrence of speech and language impairments following severe malaria in Kenyan children, is representative of this latter approach. The study participants included 25 children previously exposed to malaria and 27 children that were not exposed. All were assessed for the occurrence of a wide range of speech and language impairments at least two years after children exposed to malaria were admitted to the hospital. The exposed children were found to have significantly lower scores than unexposed children on several of the language measures. The researchers concluded that such linguistic deficits might be "under-recognized" sequelae of the disease.

An advantage of a retrospective cohort study over a prospective cohort study is that the former can be completed faster and more economically because it is based on existing data. In the study of malaria noted above, the investigators were able to assemble the cohort of exposed and nonexposed subjects into two comparison groups because of the availability of past diagnostic records. These groups were examined subsequently to determine the present incidence of speech and language disorders in relation to the risk factor. A possible disadvantage of a retrospective cohort study, as compared to its prospective counterpart, is that the validity of its findings is dependent on the integrity of preexisting records. If such records are incomplete or inaccurate, the conclusions may not be valid (Knapp & Miller, 1992). Furthermore, of the two types of investigations, only prospective cohort studies yield a *direct estimate of risk* for a particular disorder or disease—that is, the probability that a healthy individual will develop the disease over a specified time period.

Another type of observational study, sometimes confused with cohort studies, is called a case-control study. The manner in which subjects are selected is the major factor that distinguishes between these two experiments (Schesselman & Stolley 1982). In cohort studies, subjects are selected who are, at least conceptually, free of a disorder or disease at the outset. These subjects are then tracked into the future to determine their disorder or disease rates based on the presence or absence of their exposure to a risk factor(s). On the other hand, in a case-control study subjects are selected at the outset based on whether they have or do not have a particular disorder or disease of interest. A search is then undertaken for risk factors in the past that might account for a particular outcome (why cases were affected and controls were not). Whereas cohort studies explore the relations between variables by proceeding in the direction of the *presumed cause* to the *presumed effect,* case-control studies reverse this paradigm by proceeding from the *presumed effect* to the *presumed cause*. Figure 9-1 provides a comparison of the cohort studies discussed with case-control studies in relation to the dimension of time.

A good example of a case-control study design is found in an investigation of familial aggregation in specific language impairment (SLI) conducted by Tallal and her colleagues (2001). Two groups of subjects were chosen for study after meeting operationally defined inclusion criteria. The proband group was constituted of 22 students receiving speech-language therapy; a comparable control group of 26 students was ascertained from the local schools. The proband group met both the family-inclusion criteria and the diagnostic criteria for SLI, while the control group met only the family-inclusion criteria. The study compared impairment rates in the mothers, fathers, sisters, and brothers of SLI probands to control families without SLI. Based on testing, the SLI probands were significantly more likely to have a positive family history of SLI (59.1%) than the control group (19.2%).

An advantage of case-control designs over the prospective cohort design is that the former are more practical for studying rare disorders or diseases. An investigator does not have to wait for such problems to emerge at some point in the future but can proceed to assemble

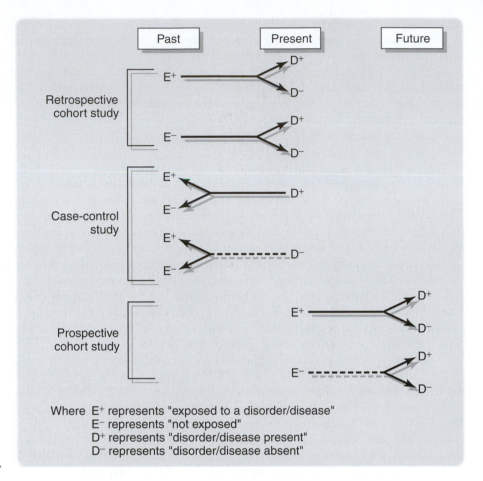

FIGURE 9-1

Comparison of retrospectivec cohort study, prospective cohort study, and case-control studies for determining a risk of a disorder or disease in relation to the dimension of time

observations for study based on cases that might be currently available. However, because cases are selected for study *after* the disorder or disease has occurred, case-control studies are more subject to bias than prospective cohort studies. At the outset of prospective cohort studies, we do not know who among the participants might develop the disorder or disease. During the course of the study, *all* of the participants are systematically examined for the emergence of the disorder or disease, and occurrence rates are related to the presence or absence of particular risk factors. By contrast, in case-control studies, cases are sampled in which a disorder or disease has been previously diagnosed—perhaps correctly, perhaps incorrectly. Only such cases and selected controls believed suitable for comparison are included in the study.

In mathematical terms, the conclusions drawn in cohort studies are based on the **incidence rate** (number of new cases) that emerge in a defined population during the course of the study, whereas case-control studies draw conclusions based on the **prevalence rate** (number of existing cases) in a defined sample at a particular point in time. Thus, the potential for both selection and sampling bias is substantially greater in case-control than in cohort studies. According to Cole (1979), it is possible to reduce such biasing influences by assuring that control subjects are as similar to case subjects as possible, with respect to their potential for exposure to a particular risk factor, during the time period for such risk.

CAUSAL-COMPARATIVE (EX POST FACTO) STUDIES

The majority of the disorders and diseases that investigators wish to study in the field of communication sciences and disorders preexist in a population. In other words, the dependent variable has already occurred, so its relationship to other variables can only be studied ex post facto (after the fact) of such an occurrence. Such studies are often called **causal-comparative studies.** As opposed to true experiments, where the level of explanation for the findings proceeds from cause to effect, in causal-comparative studies the researcher begins by defining the effect as it currently exists and then looks backward in an effort to explain the cause.

An article entitled "Auditory Temporal Processing Impairment: Neither Necessary nor Sufficient for Causing Language Impairment in Children" (Bishop et al., 1999) is representative of a causal-comparative investigation. The authors point out that the problem investigated is one that has "raged for many years over the role of auditory perceptual impairment in the genesis of developmental language disorders" (p. 1295). The study was undertaken to correct what the authors presumed to be weaknesses and poor agreement among previous investigations stemming from low validity and reliability in measurement and the heterogeneity of the population under study. The subjects included 14 twin pairs, aged 8–10 years, 11 of whom were assessed as having language impairment (LI), 11 control children matched on nonverbal ability and age, and 6 co-twins who did not meet criteria for LI or control status. The auditory processing abilities of the LI and control group samples were compared on a range of different auditory measures. The overall findings of the study indicated that were no significant differences between the LI and control groups on any auditory measure. This outcome was determined by the use of analysis of variance (ANOVA) statistical methods (see Chapter 12 for a detailed discussion). Although substantial individual variation in children's performance was found on auditory temporal processing tasks, such variation was largely attributed to the intellectual demands of the psychophysical procedures and to training effects. The authors concluded, "We found no evidence that auditory deficits are a necessary or sufficient cause of language impairment" (p. 1295). In discussing the findings, the authors go on to say "Nevertheless, it would be dangerous to conclude simply on the basis that children with auditory deficits have normal language, that auditory deficits play no role in LI" (p. 1308).

As noted previously, the study just discussed is representative of investigative methods that proceed from effect to cause—in this case, from an observation of an effect (LI) to an inference about the cause of the effect (auditory processing disorder). Strictly speaking, the interpretation of the results from such studies can violate a major scientific premise for determining causality called *temporal precedence* (the presumed cause must precede the effect). Suppose significant statistical findings had been found in the Bishop et al. study instead of nonsignificant findings. In such an event, the authors would have been in no better position to conclude that auditory processing disorders are a cause of LI because of the possibility of the "cart coming before the horse"—perhaps LI was a cause of poor auditory processing rather than the other way around. Moreover, depressed performance on both variables might have resulted from some unidentified third (confounding) variable such as problems in paying attention to task.

In addition to evaluating the size of between-group differences on some presumed dependent variable (e.g., auditory processing), causal-comparative studies often examine the *strength of association* between variables thought to contribute to such differences using various correlational statistics (see Chapter 11 for a detailed discussion). By using such methods in the Bishop study discussed above, the correlation between the composite measures of language ability were not found to be significant on certain measures of auditory processing, while other variables, such as age, nonverbal ability, and performance on an auditory repetition test were found to be significantly correlated with auditory processing.

Another commonly used statistical procedure in causal-comparative studies is called **multiple regression** (see Chapter 11 for a detailed discussion). Essentially, investigators employ such statistical methods when a single dependent variable (called the criterion variable) is believed to be influenced by multiple independent variables (predictor variables) instead of a single independent variable. The method allows for determining the relative power of the predictor variables as each contributes to the magnitude of the criterion variable under investigation. To determine which variables made a "separate independent contribution" to predicting outcomes on several auditory processing measures, multiple regression analyses were also conducted in the Bishop et al. study. For example, on one of these measures involving the determination of backward-masked thresholds, language composite scores were not found to be significant predictors of outcomes, while scores on the sentence repetition test were found to be significant predictors.

As with other observational studies we have reviewed, causal-comparative investigations draw conclusions primarily on the basis of associative relations found to exist among variables. As Cochran (1965) noted, the most that such conclusions can end with is an expressed opinion or judgment about causality as opposed to a statement of proof. Despite this caveat, the conclusions drawn from an earlier study of the associative relations among variables can be strengthened by *replication* of findings in subsequent studies. Conversely, diverse studies that fail to replicate the findings of earlier investigations weaken the credibility of such evidence.

In the field of communication sciences and disorders, as in many other behavioral and biological fields of study, multiple causes typically underlie the effects observed in both research and clinical practice. The search for single causes is generally too simplistic if not a futile undertaking. Certainly, this holds true outside the confines of carefully crafted experiments.

SURVEY RESEARCH

Survey research is one of the most commonly used nonexperimental research methods in the field of communication sciences and disorders. Broadly defined, surveys consist of various methods for collecting information about the characteristics and practices of individuals or the groups they form. Such information can be used for descriptive or predictive purposes (Goddard & Villanova, 1996).

Surveys are often designed to sample the feelings, beliefs, and opinions of people with respect to various problems encountered in their daily lives. Asking clients or significant others to judge the effectiveness of particular therapy methods or professionals to rate their degree of their job satisfaction on a particular scale exemplify *attitudinal approaches* to survey research. Other survey research methods are more empirical in orientation, focusing on *demographic characteristics* (age, gender, medical history, geographical location, etc.) that might relate to occurrences of particular disorders or disease or to the policies and programs that impact the health, education, or socioeconomic welfare of people.

Steps in Developing a Survey

To derive valid and reliable results from any survey study, each step of the process must be carefully thought out in advance. The success of each step will depend on how successfully the previous steps were accomplished (Goddard & Villanova, 1996). A flow plan of the major activities to be performed in survey research is illustrated in Figure 9-2. These steps are discussed more fully below using examples from relevant literature.

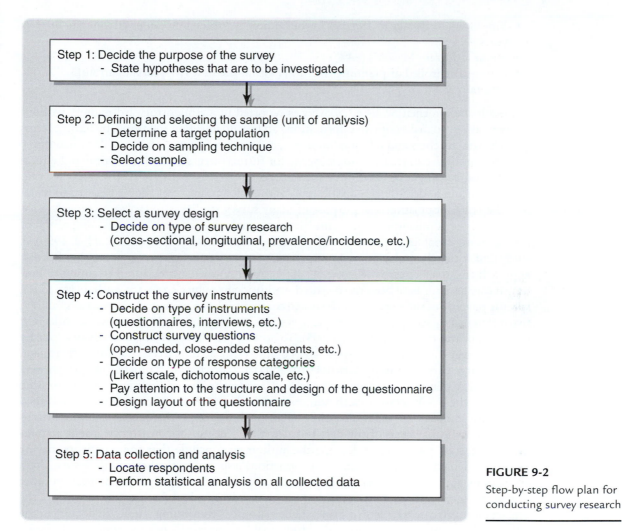

FIGURE 9-2

Step-by-step flow plan for conducting survey research

Step One: Decide the Purpose of the Survey

The purpose of the survey should be made clear with respect to its importance, and the hypotheses or questions to be investigated should be stated in specific terms. The purpose of some surveys is simply to describe particular characteristics or attributes according to their manner of distribution in a population without resorting to explanations as to why such a distribution exists. For example, a comprehensive employment survey was mailed to 4490 ASHA constituents in 2000. A 54% response rate was obtained on the Audiology Survey of certified, full-time employed audiologists. The survey sample was stratified (see Chapter 5) according to seven primary employment facilities: school, college/university, hospital, nonresidential health care facility, residential health care facility, industry, and agency/organization/research facility. The employment demographics of the respondents broke down as follows:

- Primary employment function—77% clinical service provider
- Secondary employment function—38% administrator

- Employed an average of 19 years in the audiology profession, ranging from 1 to 50 years
- Highest degree—Master's (84%)
- Currently enrolled or planning to enroll (within the next five years) in an AuD program—53%

Although the information listed above was reported in a straightforward manner without interpretation, such descriptive information can be valuable. For one thing, by having access to such data, teachers and administrators in graduate programs are better able to determine what to emphasize in training audiologists for future careers and what clinical and educational resources might be needed for such purposes.

In addition to describing a distribution of traits for a sample of people believed to represent the larger population, the purpose of many survey studies is to *explain* or to *make assertions* about the population based on **multivariate analysis**—the simultaneous comparison of two or more variables believed to differentially influence some outcome (Babbie, 1990). A study that entailed a multinational comparison of aphasia management practices typifies this approach to survey research (Katz et al., 2000). After reviewing literature pertaining to how health care systems have been restructured worldwide to reduce costs, the authors stated the specific purpose of their study, which was: to compare aphasia management practices "among five different English-speaking healthcare systems . . . to gain insight about what works best for patients and their clinicians" (p. 305). To accomplish this goal, the authors developed a 37-item survey that focused on several areas of interest related to access, diagnosis, treatment, and discharge patterns among patients with aphasia. Three hundred ninety-four surveys were distributed to clinicians working in Australia, Canada, the United Kingdom, the U.S. private sector, and the U.S. Veterans Health Administration. The 175 surveys completed and returned (44%) were compared across health care systems with respect to the questions under investigation. Statistical analysis of the data revealed a high degree of consistency among respondents on certain survey items, leading the authors to conclude that some patients may be "routinely denied treatment" because of restrictions imposed by the health care system. Such restrictions appeared to operate to a greater degree in the U.S. private sector than in other health care setting. Based on the results, the authors advocated professional monitoring of the impact of health care restructuring on patients, as well as continuing studies to document the efficacy of clinical practice. Neither the study goals of this survey nor the conclusions drawn from achieving them would have been possible to achieve in the absence of a clear understanding of the purpose of the investigation at the outset.

Step Two: Define and Select the Sample (Unit of Analysis)

Although survey techniques can be applied to anyone, the *ones* under study, called the **units of analysis,** require careful definition and selection (Babbie, 1990). As we noted in Chapter 5, the unit of analysis is typically a person, and such units are aggregated into samples as a whole that are more or less representative of a population of similar persons, depending on how the sample was drawn. In Chapter 5 we also reviewed the types of sampling techniques that can be used in selecting a sample of participants in any research study (surveys included) with respect to two broad categories of techniques called *probability random* and *non-probability nonrandom* sampling methods. The former category of methods is by far the more powerful of the two in achieving a *representative* sample for reasons we previously discussed.

In the same way that it is important to arrive at a clear statement of the purpose of a survey study before it is undertaken, so too must the units of analysis and their manner of selection be clearly identified at the outset. For example, in the Katz et al. study cited above, the units of analysis were identified as clinicians who were mostly women (89.7%), licensed as speech-language clinicians (81.1%), who worked full-time (85.0%) in settings with three or fewer clinicians (55.9%), all of whom had at least a bachelor's degree and had worked for at least one full year providing services to patients with aphasia (100%). The units of analysis were further subdivided according to each health care system investigated (Australia, Canada, UK, U.S.-private, U.S.-VA). Membership lists from the professional organizations within each of these health care systems were obtained. These lists were then used to construct a *sampling frame* constituted of all members of the populations from which the samples were drawn.

In considering the feasibility of a survey study, the adequacy of a sample must be considered both in terms of the **representativeness of the sample** and the *potential response rate.* How representative the sample is of the population is related to the *ecological validity* of a study. More specifically, the selection of participants should yield units of analysis that are appropriate for answering the questions asked. This is not to say that the constituents of the sample should be equal in all respects. However, they should share characteristics that are relevant to the problem under investigation. This is particularly important for statistical analyses predicated on probability theory that allows for the examination of sample differences from a population on one or more defined variables when *all else* is considered equal. If sample differences exist that are unknown, ill defined, or otherwise beyond the control of the investigator, the statistical validity of a study is likely to suffer.

In planning to select participants for a survey study, potential response rate also should be an area of concern. Generally speaking, the more interesting and personally or professionally relevant the survey is to the lives of potential respondents, the greater will be their cooperation. Although a theoretical assumption underlying statistical inferences based on survey data is that *all* units of a surveyed sample are included in the data analysis, in actual practice this rarely happens. Instead, considerably fewer than 100% of the people surveyed in a typical study complete and return their questionnaires. The lower the response rate, the more likely it is that sampling bias will occur. Although response rates vary greater across survey studies, Babbie (1990) has offered the following guidelines in evaluating rates of return:

- *Adequate response rate:* at least 50%
- *Good response rate:* at least 60%
- *Very good response rate:* at least 70%

These guidelines should be considered as "rules of thumb" instead of hard and fast statistical criteria. Furthermore, if your sample is inherently flawed so that it does not adequately represent the population of interest, a high response rate will be meaningless.

Step Three: Select a Survey Design

Once an investigator has determined the purpose of a survey and identified the sample for study, the next step is to select an appropriate research design. Three major categories of designs used in survey research are **cross-sectional designs,** longitudinal designs, and prevalence/incidence designs.

Cross-sectional survey designs. In cross-sectional surveys, the sample data is collected at a particular point (cross-section) in time for purposes of describing variables and their patterns of distribution. The Katz et al. (2000) study discussed previously is an example of such an approach in which various therapy practices were surveyed for a cross-section of clinicians working with aphasic patients in different health care settings. Still another example of such a study in the field of audiology was an effort to document hearing-aid fitting practices for children with multiple impairments (vision impairment, mental retardation, physical

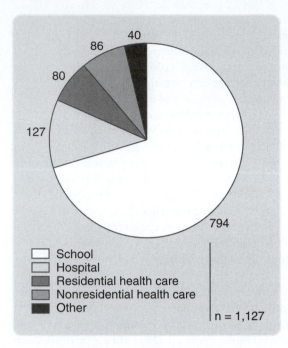

FIGURE 9-3

Distribution by primary employment facility of speech-language pathologists who are employed full time and who provide clinical service

Reprinted with permission from ASHA omnibus survey, by Survey and Information team (J. Janota et al.), ASHA, 2003.

impairment, autism spectrum disorder) (Tharpe et al., 2001). The survey instrument was comprised of several multiple-part questions designed to extract information from a cross-section of audiologists working throughout the United States who see children in their practice on a regular basis. The survey was sent to 6000 (approximately half) of the audiologists certified by ASHA. The authors noted that the response to the survey was "widely and evenly distributed" with the respondents appearing to adequately reflect the "profile" of the targeted audiologists since most had master's degrees, (84%), worked full time (79%), primarily performed clinical duties (95%), and so forth. Of this group, 27% were found qualified to complete the entire questionnaire, having met preestablished criteria of experience with pediatric hearing-aid fitting. The findings indicated that the fitting practices for children with various handicapping conditions did not appear to be different for children with hearing loss only. For various reasons that they discussed, the authors found several findings from this survey "alarming," leading them to recommend "additional training in the unique characteristics and amplification needs of children with handicapping conditions in addition to hearing loss" (p. 39).

Longitudinal survey designs.   Survey studies that collect information over an extended period of time are called longitudinal surveys. Two major subtypes of such studies are trend surveys, and cohort surveys, briefly reviewed below with relevant examples of each approach.

Trend survey studies: Such studies can be used to evaluate one or more attributes in a population by sampling such attributes over an extended time period. For example, each year or two the American Speech-Language-Hearing Association (ASHA) conducts an omnibus survey of its membership on various topics of professional interest. During 2003, a survey was sent to 7500 of ASHA's constituent members, using stratified sampling methods (see Chapter 5). Of this number, 4387 (58%) responded to the survey. Of these respondents, 1127 were identified as certified speech-language pathologists (SPL) who were working full time. One type of information obtained from the sample data related to the percentage distribution of this group according to employment setting (see Figure 9-3). The data was further evaluated to derive information pertaining to *case load* and *case characteristics* within such settings. For example, the average case load of SLPs working in school settings was approximately 50. Of these cases, close to half had articulation/phonological problems. Appropriate data of a similar kind is also obtained on a regular basis for ASHA members working in the field of audiology. By sampling such characteristics of our membership over a period of time and comparing one time period to the next, we can learn about "trends" affecting the profession.

Cohort survey studies: In contrast to studies of a trend in the general population, where *different* people are usually sampled from one time period to another, cohort surveys study the *same* people from one time period to the next. An example of such a survey was a cohort study conducted by Rosenfeld et al. (1997) that evaluated the changes in health-related quality of life for 186 children with otitis media. The "quality of life" issues, assessed on a survey instrument, pertained to six items including the degree of estimated physical suffering, hearing loss, speech impairment, emotional distress, activity limitations, and caregiver concerns. The survey was completed by each child's caregiver upon entry to the study and again at least 4 weeks later after the child had been clinically treated. Change scores on the survey instrument were found to be well correlated with the degree of clinical change as assessed by such measures as tympanometry, audiometric thresholds, and the like. Based on these findings, the authors concluded that the survey instrument is a valid and reliable measure of quality of life issues for children with otitis media.

Table 9-1 summarizes some of the advantages and disadvantages of cross-sectional as compared to longitudinal research studies, including surveys.

Prevalence/incidence survey designs.   Survey methods are often used by researchers and clinicians to gain information on the risks for certain disorders or diseases by estimating their rates of occurrence in the population. Earlier in this chapter, we briefly mentioned two common measures that are used for this purpose, called prevalence and incidence. Although these terms sometimes are confused in their usage, they have different meanings and applications for determining the frequency with which disorders and diseases occur.

Prevalence is a statistical measure descriptive of the proportion of the people in a population surveyed or examined that have a disorder or disease at a given point in time. Such

TABLE 9-1   Advantages and Disadvantages of Cross-Sectional as Compared to Longitudinal Research Studies, Including Surveys

	Cross-Sectional	**Longitudinal**
Advantages	Well suited for studies of existing attributes in different people	Well suited for studies of attributes in the same people
	Economical	Well suited for developmental studies of dynamic processes
	Can be completed quickly	
	Low attrition rate	
Disadvantages	Ill-suited for developmental studies of dynamic processes	Expensive
		Can take a long time to complete
		High attrition rate

TABLE 9-2   Method of Calculating Prevalence and Incidence Rate

	Prevalence	Incidence
Numerator	Number of existing cases of the disorder or disease	Number of new cases of the disorder or disease
Denominator	Total number of people at risk	Total number of people at risk
Time	Single point	Duration of the period
Method of measure	Cross-sectional study	Longitudinal study
Formula	$\dfrac{\text{Numerator}}{\text{Denominator}}$ per time period	

a "point in time" is analogous to a static snapshot or a single frame of a motion picture that could capture a combined image of such persons (Knapp & Miller, 1992). Cross-sectional surveys generally provide the kind of data from which such prevalence information can be obtained.

As shown in Table 9-2, prevalence can be calculated based on a fraction or proportion of people identified with a disorder or disease (numerator) to the total population (denominator). The numerator includes the number of diagnosed cases for a particular point in time. The denominator can be thought of as the number of persons *at risk in the population* for the disorder or disease of interest.

The term *population* can be defined in different ways depending on the purpose of a particular study. The definition of a population might include all persons living in a large geographical region or might be limited to only those found in a particular clinical facility. Suppose an audiologist wishes to determine the prevalence of suspected hearing loss based on the results of newborn infant screening. The records of a local hospital indicate that of the 100 infants tested during a six-month period, 5 were identified as having a hearing loss. Entering this information into the formula for prevalence in Table 9-2, we can determine the prevalence of suspected hearing loss to be $5/100 = .05$ or 5% for children screened in this facility.

In contrast to prevalence, which measures the number of *existing* cases identified at a given point of time, incidence refers to the number of *new* cases of a disorder or disease that emerge over a period of time in people initially observed to be free of the disorder or disease in question. Using a photographic analogy once again, whereas measures of prevalence yield static images of disease frequency, measures of incidence provide a more dynamic assessment, much like a movie reel that captures new images (cases) as they unfold during a specified time period. Incidence surveys are appropriate for longitudinal studies in which the same cohort of people are followed and assessed periodically.

Mathematically speaking, incidence can be expressed as a fraction or proportion wherein the numerator represents the number of new cases during a specified time period whereas the denominator is the number of people at risk during a specified time period.

Some survey research studies are designed to obtain both prevalence and incidence information. An example of this type of effort was an epidemiological study of stuttering across the entire life span (Craig et al., 2002). Stratified and random sampling methods (see Chapter 5) were used to obtain a sample of households in the state of New South Wales, Australia. During a telephone interview, respondents were asked if any person living in the household stuttered: If such a person was identified, that person was taped over the telephone for purposes of detection. Collaborative questions were also asked, such as "Has the stuttering persisted for more than three months?", "Has the stuttering caused fear and avoidance?", and "Has the person consulted a speech professional?"

Table 9-3 Breakdown by age of stuttering cases (SC), prior stuttering cases (PSC), prevalence, male-to-female stuttering ratios, and an estimate of the incidence or risk of stuttering

Age (yrs)	SC	PSC	Total N	# males	Prevalence (95% CI)		M:F ratios	Risk (95% CI)	
2–5	10	10	720	389	1.4%	(0.54–2.26)	2.3:1	2.8%	(1.6–4.0)
6–10	13	18	902	465	1.44%	(0.66–2.22)	3.3:1	3.4%	(2.2–4.6)
11–20	10	32	1,881	1006	0.53%	(0.20–9.86)	4:1	2.2%	(1.5–2.9)
21–50	42	71	5,405	2607	0.78%	(0.55–1.01)	2.2:1	2.1%	(1.7–2.5)
51+	12	45	3,207	1556	0.37%	(0.16–0.58)	1.4:1	1.8%	(1.3–2.3)
All ages	87	176	12,131	6023	0.72%	(0.57–0.87)	2.3:1	2.2%	(1.3–2.3)

Note: There are 16 missing cases in the 2–5 age breakdown as children less than 2 years old where not included in the analysis.

Adapted with permission from "Epidemiology of Stuttering in the Community Across the Entire Life Span" by A. Craig, K. Hancock, Y. Tran, M. Craig, and K. Peters, 2002, *Journal of Speech, Language, and Hearing Research, 45,* p. 1102. © American Speech-Language-Hearing Association.

The sample included 4689 families who were interviewed, consisting of 12,131 persons. Table 9-3 shows prevalence rates for all age categories. Prevalence was highest in the 2–5 (1.4%) age group and 6–10 (1.44%) age group, with an overall prevalence of .72%. The male–female sex ratio was 2.3:1. Table 9-3 also includes prior cases of stuttering (those believed to have stuttered in the past). Inclusion of this data allowed for the *estimation of the incidence* over the entire sample as 2.2%. The data in Table 9-3 also allow for the determination of recovery rates (remission of stuttering). Of the 263 persons identified with stuttering in the past (87 SC plus 176 PSC), the recovery rate over the entire life span was 176/263 or 67%. For additional information on methods for calculating prevalence/incidence rates based on the data of this study, see Appendix A-5.

Step Four: Construct the Survey Instruments

Careful attention should be given to the construction of the measuring instruments used in survey studies because the quality of these tools will significantly affect the reliability and validity of the results. Two common tools used for collecting survey data are questionnaires and interviews. Essentially, these instruments can be distinguished according to their manner of administration and method for recording data. A questionnaire is typically self-administered. The person surveyed reads instructions, responds to questions in a pencil-and-paper format, and then returns the questionnaire to a designated person. On the other hand, in an interview, an interviewer reads the instructions and questions to the respondent and records the answers. Some approaches to surveying combine these techniques. Each of these methods have certain advantages and disadvantages.

Because they are usually self-administered, questionnaires can be forwarded through the mail, allowing for a survey to be made of a large and geographically dispersed population. As compared to interviewing respondents face to face, questionnaires can be cost saving despite the ever increasing expense of mail services. An additional advantage of questionnaires over interviews is that respondents are allowed more time to think about their responses in the comfort of their own surroundings. Under circumstances of complete anonymity, their responses may be more forthcoming and valid, particularly in regard to sensitive or emotionally laden topics.

Unfortunately, flexibility as to when and under what conditions a questionnaire can be completed may turn out to be a disadvantage, particularly when the questionnaire is lengthy. There is evidence that respondents may not complete questionnaires that they consider time consuming—response rates and the quality of responses begin to decline significantly after

125 items (Dillman, 1978). Obviously, such a conclusion must include a consideration of respondents' level of motivation that may either diminish or augment the reliability and validity of their responses. Still another disadvantage of questionnaires is that the respondent may seek the opinion of others in responding to questions, therefore introducing the potential for sampling bias.

Several factors must be considered in developing the items and format for a questionnaire that will hopefully elicit reliable and valid answers from respondents. First, an investigator must develop questionnaire items appropriate for the aims of the study. If the primary goal of a survey is to assess the attitudes of potential employers toward hiring people with certain speech, language, or hearing handicaps, the researcher should refrain from probing other attitudes tangential to that specific purpose, such as whether employers would choose to socialize with such people or lobby politicians to pass legislation on their behalf.

The items on the questionnaire should be free of jargon, clearly and simply stated, and designed to sample information within the realm of respondents' abilities to provide such information. Obviously, an exception to this latter requirement would exist in cases where the main goal of the survey is to determine how much knowledge respondents might have about a particular problem. Three types of questions that must be avoided are **double-barreled questions, loaded questions,** and **leading questions:**

- *Double-barreled questions* contain two queries that are impossible to untangle with respect to the intended answer. For example, given a survey item that reads "Do you believe that men and women are compensated fairly in the field of communication sciences and disorders?" and a negative response to this query, you would not know which gender had been perceived as being discriminated against—women, men, or both. Questions that use the words "and" or "or" can lead to problems of this kind.
- *Loaded questions* contain emotionally charged language. Asking "Do you believe profit-driven health care companies are devoted to expanding services for people who suffer from communication disorders?" is an example of this kind of question.
- *Leading questions* tend to guide or channel a response in a particular direction, such as "I agree with ASHA's position that insurance providers should increase their reimbursement schedules for services provided to people with communication disorders." Check the box below:

strongly agree	agree	uncertain	disagree	strongly disagree
[ ]	[ ]	[ ]	[ ]	[ ]

Decisions as to whether to ask participants to respond to **open-ended questions,** or **closed-ended questions,** or to express agreement or disagreement with statements indicative of a particular attitude must be carefully evaluated. Open-ended questions ask respondents to answer questions in their own words. For example, should a researcher wish to sample public awareness of aphasia, open-ended questions such as "What causes aphasia?" or "What do you think might be done to help people with aphasia?" might be asked. Alternatively, closed-ended multiple-choice questions might be used in response to which participants might choose from a list of preselected answers. For example, such a question might read:

Is aphasia caused by?
a) Brain damage
   [ ] yes
   [ ] no
   [ ] not sure

b) Emotional problems
   [ ] yes
   [ ] no
   [ ] not sure
c) Impaired intelligence
   [ ] yes
   [ ] no
   [ ] not sure
d) etc.

Still another option would be to use both open-ended and closed-ended questions as did Simmons-Mackie et al. (2002) in their survey of the same problem (public awareness of aphasia), in which the authors collected data in face-to-face interviews with respondents.

Generally speaking, structured, closed-ended questions are the predominant type used on most self-administered surveys, although open-ended questions may be used as well. Problems with open-ended questions can include incomplete, inconsistent answers that can impair reliability in coding and interpreting responses. Despite such limitations, open-ended questions are the best choice when it is impossible to predict in advance all the possible answers that a respondent might give to a particular question. For example, if clinicians were asked to specify the reason for choosing a career in communication sciences and disorders, the reasons could be so many that open-ended questions might best be used to allow for a broad range of possible answers. Sometimes, this problem can be dealt with by including on a closed-ended questionnaire of preselected items a bracketed option designated as [ ] *other*. When using this option, the researcher should also include the words "please specify" to learn what the selection of the option might mean.

Decisions pertaining to the type of questions to ask in survey research can be complex given the diverse goals of different researchers. In cases where multiple answers are likely to exist to the same question and the number of such questions is large, open-ended questions would be the best type to administer, preferably in the context of a face-to-face interview or over the telephone. Under such conditions, the interviewer can probe more deeply to gain additional information or clarify the respondents' answers as warranted.

In addition to questions, statements that summarize particular attitudes are often included in surveys, and respondents are asked to express their degree of agreement or disagreement on a numerical scale such as a **Likert scale.** This scaling method is often used in conjunction with of a series of statements, each followed by a number of alternative responses such as "strongly agree," "agree," "neutral or undecided," "disagree," or "strongly disagree." A study that incorporated a Likert type scale was conducted by Rodriquez and Olswang (2003), who investigated the cross-cultural and intracultural diversity of mothers' beliefs and values regarding child rearing, education, and the causes of language impairment. One of the questionnaires completed by all mothers in this study was the *Parental Modernity Scale*. The scale is a 30-item questionnaire that asks parents to express their degree of agreement or disagreement on a scale ranging from 1 (strongly disagree) to 5 (strongly agree). The scale contains statements such as "It's all right for my child to disagree with me," reflecting the idea that children should be encouraged to express their own opinion. Other statements on the questionnaire reflect a more traditional, authoritarian view of child rearing practices (e.g., "The most important thing to teach children is absolute obedience to parents."). The findings of the study indicated that "Mexican-American mothers held more strongly traditional, authoritarian, and conforming educational and child rearing beliefs and values than Anglo-American mothers" (p. 452).

By using a Likert scale, it is possible to summate ratings of respondents in numerical terms according to their ordinal properties of measurements (see Chapters 6 and 11). Ordinal numbers are those ranked from highest to lowest according to an assigned numerical value. Scaling techniques of this kind allow a researcher to assess the *range of variation* in the strength of peoples' attitudes or the opinions they might hold in numerical terms.

Attention must also be paid to the *structure and design* of the questionnaire used in a survey. Almost all surveys will contain items relating to such demographic information as age, gender, ethnicity or race, education, and employment. As noted previously, such questions should be worded clearly and carefully and should seek no information beyond that which is necessary to satisfy the aims of the study. There is evidence that the order in which questions are presented can affect the outcome of the survey results, although there is also some disagreement about the best way to handle such problems (Sudman & Bradburn, 1982). Some researchers might ask respondents to first answer questions related to their demographic characteristics, saving what might be viewed as more sensitive items until the end of the questionnaire. A possible pitfall to beginning a questionnaire with such questions is that some respondents might judge some questions as boring and be less inclined to complete the entire questionnaire. On the other hand, other respondents might view certain kinds of demographic information as "sensitive," preferring to keep such matters confidential. Therefore, in deciding the order of questions to be asked, it is important for the researcher to consider the nature of the population to be surveyed in relation to the topic studied. As a rule of thumb, items that are likely to be interesting to the respondent and that are more salient to the purposes of the survey should come first in an effort to maximize the number of surveys completed and returned (response rate).

Another design strategy for maximizing response rate is by the use of **contingency questions** that allow respondents to skip from one question to the next as appropriate. Because respondents are more likely to answer questions that are relevant to themselves, contingency questions are formatted to guide respondents to relevant questions and away from irrelevant ones. Babbie (1990) has recommended that contingency questions be indented on the questionnaire, set off in boxes, and connected with the previous question by arrows leading from appropriate responses. Figure 9-4 illustrates such a format for the inclusion of contingency questions as might be relevant to the purposes of a particular survey.

The physical layout of the questionnaire is also important to consider. Questions should not be cramped together and should be easy to follow from one page to the next. Most surveys will include a separate cover sheet that provides written directions for completing the questionnaire. The clarity of such instructions is particularly important in mail questionnaires, when the researcher is not present to provide assistance. A cover letter should always accompany the questionnaire, written by the researcher and/or the sponsor of the research (professional organization, educational institution, hospital, etc.). To maximize the return rate, the letter should summarize all aspects of the survey in understandable terms, including:

1. The purpose of the research and its importance
2. Why the respondent was selected for participation and who else was selected
3. Who might benefit from the research
4. Payment terms or other incentives if included
5. Steps taken to safeguard privacy of respondents
6. Statement of deadline date for return and the importance of adhering to it
7. The fact that a stamped return envelope has been enclosed to cover the cost of mailing

Question 1. Are you licensed to practice in Massachusetts?

[   ] Yes (go to question 2)
[   ] No

  (a) In which state are you licensed to practice? _____

  (b) How many years have you been licensed to practice in your state? _____

    _____

  (c) Are you a member of American Speech-Language-Hearing Association?_____

Question 2. Do you hold a PhD in speech-language pathology?

[   ] Yes (go to question 3)
[   ] No

  (a) ----

  (b) ----

  etc.

FIGURE 9-4   Example of a format for the use of contingency questions in a survey

Step Five: Collect and Analyze Data

Once the steps described above have been taken, the researcher can move to the final step of survey research that entails collecting and analyzing data. In cases where the survey tool was a self-administered questionnaire mailed to a sample of potential respondents, the process of collecting the desired data is sometimes an arduous undertaking. Steps that can be taken in the initial mailing to maximize the response rate were described above. However, in actual practice, follow-up efforts are often needed. Chadwick, Bahr, and Albrect (1984) have offered several recommendations for maximizing response rate as follow-ups to the initial mailing. Approximately two weeks after the initial mailing, a postcard, consisting of a brief version of the initial cover letter should be sent. The postcard should list the researcher's phone number and should invite respondents to call the researcher if they have questions or have misplaced the questionnaire. A toll-free number should be provided if respondents reside outside the area code. When the response to the postcard reminder is presumed to have worn off (approximately two weeks later), an entire new packet should be sent including another copy of the cover letter for the survey along with a return envelope. The letter should acknowledge the earlier effort to solicit participation, restate the importance of the research, and once again express a strong appeal for participation. If still no response is forthcoming, some researchers might opt to send another postcard reminder and then may go so far as sending a third and final mailing of the complete survey and supportive materials. This final effort is undertaken when returns have seemed to stop or slowed to a trickle. The point of this is to say that doing survey research involving the collection of questionnaire data often requires persistence and hard work.

Calculating response rate.   Once the cut-off date established by the researcher for receiving returned questionnaires has passed, analysis of the data can begin. As a first step, response rate should be calculated. Actually, response rate is a broad term that encompasses a number of rate measures (Neuman, 2000). To aid understanding of these measures, assume that a researcher wishes to survey the degree of satisfaction with services provided by a particular clinic based on an available list of the names of 400 adults seen during a particular year.

- *Location rate* is calculated as the number of located respondents from the entire sample. Provided that the addresses for the entire sample were found in clinic files, the location rate would be 400 out of 400, or 100%. However, if only 350 of the addresses were found, the location rate would be 350/400 = 87.5%.
- *Contact rate* is the number of respondents contacted out of the number located. Thus, assuming that 350 addresses were located, if 250 of this number responded to the questionnaire, the contact rate would be 250 out of 350, or 71.4%. Contact may not have been made with 100 of the people located for a variety of reasons (they could have moved, been ill, out of town, etc.).
- *Completion rate* is the proportion of respondents who begin a survey and complete all items. Thus, of the 250 people who responded to the questionnaire, if 215 completed all items, the completion rate would be 215/250 = 86%.
- *Total response rate* is the number of respondents who completed the questionnaire out of all possible respondents. The total response rate in our example would be 215 people out of all possible respondents, 215/400 = 53.8%.

Various methods are used for the analysis of questionnaire data that go beyond merely reporting percentages of respondents' answers that fall into particular categories. Alphabetic and coding schemes are often employed for transforming respondents' answers on survey forms into variables that can be treated statistically. Some variables evaluated in surveys are *nominal* (categorical) in nature. In such cases, a number is used to code a particular attribute such as race: Black = 1, White = 2, Asian = 3, Hispanic = 4. The numbers assigned have no quantitative meaning. A letter or other symbol could have been used instead of numbers to designate the categories of interest. Other survey variables can have *ordinal* characteristics that allow them to be ranked as well as categorized. As mentioned above, the Likert scale, commonly used in survey research to quantify attitudes and opinions, has ordinal characteristics. Respondents are typically given a list of statements and asked to rank the degree to which their attitude or opinion agrees with a statement made, on some scale having a range of numerical values. We mentioned that the data values obtained from such scales are *summative*—an overall score can be calculated by adding up the points from each item, provided that the items are shown to have **internal consistency** (shown to be measuring the same attribute). A statistical technique called Cronbach's alpha can be used to assess the correlation among all items on a Likert scale (see Chapter 11).

Despite the popular use of Likert scales in survey research to assess the strength of attitudes and opinions, some researchers could argue on technical grounds that such scales are statistically limited. This is because they only allow for ordering evaluations of statements according to assigned numerical values. The relative size of the intervals between the assigned numbers is unknown and, therefore, cannot be assumed to be mathematically equivalent. In the absence of demonstrating such equivalence, whether or not statistics such as means and standard deviations should be used for the analysis of Likert scale data can be debated (Spector, 1992).

Another scaling method that has ordinal properties like the Likert scale but can be used in cumulative scaling of statements of increasing intensity is called a **Guttman scale.** The scale is said to be *cumulative* in character because if a response achieves a ranked score signifying agreement (or disagreement) with an item at a certain level of intensity, the response will signify agreement (or disagreement) with all other items ranked at lower levels of intensity. This pattern of responding will hold true provided that the respondent is internally consistent with him/herself. For example, a respondent could be asked to agree or disagree with each of the following statements:

Circle the letter of every statement that you agree with:
a. Vocal abuse can cause hoarseness.
b. Vocal abuse is an important cause of hoarseness.
c. Vocal abuse is a very important cause of hoarseness.
d. Vocal abuse is the most important cause of hoarseness.

As noted previously, the respondent's score on a Guttman scale is cumulative based on the total number of items for which agreement or disagreement was expressed. Provided that the respondent agrees with item (b), he/she also should agree with item (a), and so on. The internal consistency of Guttman scales can be analyzed statistically (Babbie, 1990).

Other methods for data reduction and analysis used in survey research are the **Thurstone scale** and **factor analysis.** Although the Thurstone scale is designed to have equal-appearing intervals between response items, and is therefore statistically more powerful than a Likert or Guttman scale, it is seldom employed in present-day survey research because of the great difficulty and energy required in developing the items associated with its use (Babbie, 1990).

Factor analysis is a scaling procedure that has many statistical applications (see Chapter 12). The chief value of this method for survey research lies in its ability to reduce large sets of indicators to a limited number of composite scales (Chadwick et al., 1984). It, along with the other data reduction scaling techniques discussed above, is designed to combine responses from multiple items of a survey into a single score that can be used to represent the variable of interest.

Interviews

Because self-administered questionnaires are relatively economical to administer and are capable of sampling a large number of respondents, they are more widely used than interviews to obtain survey information. However, given the fixed structure of preformed questionnaires, respondents are often unable to elaborate on their feelings, attitudes, or beliefs. Interviews share many of the same characteristics as questionnaires but are more flexible in approach and capable of gathering more extensive information based on interactions with respondents. According to Chadwick et al. (1984), interviews have many advantages as survey instruments. Some of these include:

- Allowing the respondent to reveal otherwise concealed attitudes
- Revealing problems and their potential solution through discussion
- Encouraging free expression
- Allowing for observation and recording of nonverbal communication
- Discovery of personal information, attitudes, beliefs, and perceptions that a paper-and-pencil survey might not reveal
- Allowing interviewers to probe or follow up on survey items
- Facilitating the participation of individuals who are visually handicapped or who cannot read or write

For interviews to accomplish the goals of a survey, considerable training of interviewers is often required. Such training usually entails how to solicit the participation of respondents so as to maximize the number who agree to cooperate, how to instruct respondents to answer questions and interact with them in ways that will yield the desired information, how to avoid biasing the answers of respondents by "putting words in their mouth," and how to reliably interpret and record the information they provide.

Two major data-gathering methods are *personal interviews* and *telephone interviews*. Personal interviews involve face-to-face encounters in a variety of settings (home, work, school, clinic, etc.). Telephone interviews could potentially take place in any type of setting agreed to by a respondent. Whatever the method used to obtain information, the interview should be calm and as free from distractions as possible. Telephone respondents should be asked whether or not it is a convenient time to conduct an interview. If not, a more appropriate time should be scheduled. If a recording of the interview is to be made, for ethical and legal reasons the permission of respondents must be obtained.

Whether by personal contact or by telephone, the interviewer must establish rapport with the respondent from the outset. Beginning the interview by introducing him or herself, whom he or she represents, the purpose and importance of the interview, why and how the respondent was chosen, what the interview will require, and how long it will take, can accomplish this goal. The interviewer should convey the impression of being friendly and easy to talk with throughout the interview session and be prepared to respond to unanticipated questions. The research goals of an interview can best be met by the use of an **interview schedule.** Such a schedule contains explicit instructions to guide the interviewer in asking respondents a list of questions designed to obtain complete and honest answers. Such a schedule also contains instructions and reminders for the interviewer to facilitate this process.

The same principles that guide the construction of self-administered questionnaires to promote effective communication equally apply to interviews. The interviewer's questions should be stated simply so as to be understood by respondents. Lengthy, complex questions can be particularly troublesome when the time for the respondent to answer may be limited. As in the case of self-administered questionnaires, double-barreled questions, loaded questions, and leading questions also should be avoided. It is likewise important to consider the order of the questions to be asked. After establishing rapport with the respondent, the interview might begin with relatively nonthreatening questions that are relatively easy to answer before proceeding to probe issues that are likely to be more sensitive in nature.

The purpose of the survey will largely determine the type of questions asked during an interview. If the interviewer wishes to have very specific answers to questions with little or no deviation from a particular topic, a **structured interview** protocol will be followed in conjunction with closed-ended questions of the type discussed previously. In such a case, questions are often read verbatim to respondents and their answers recorded. On the other hand, if the interviewer wishes to probe a variety of topics while affording respondents considerable latitude in their answers, an **unstructured interview** that incorporated open-ended questions would be more suitable. The latter approach usually requires more ingenuity in planning the method for recording and coding answers into appropriate categories for analysis. As in the case of self-administered questionnaires, the data from interviews can be analyzed in a variety of ways. Descriptive statistics such as percentages, proportions, ratios, and the like can be used for analyzing responses that fall into predetermined categories of verbal behavior. Results can also be evaluated and reported using more sophisticated statistical techniques as discussed in Chapters 11 and 12. For additional information about interviewing methods employed in qualitative research, see Chapter 10.

EVALUATING DIAGNOSTIC TESTS

Another type of nonexperimental research relevant to the work of all clinicians involves the evaluation of diagnostic tests. Diagnostic test studies share several design features with other types of nonexperimental studies discussed in this chapter but differ with respect to their goals and the kinds of statistics applied for the analysis of data.

In the field of communication sciences and disorders, the results of diagnostic tests are used to:

1. Describe a client's current communication functioning and the degree to which such functioning might constitute:
   a. Impairment (loss or abnormality of structure or function that deviates from the norm)
   b. Disability (restricted or absent ability to perform an activity due to impairment)
   c. Handicap (social consequences of an impairment or disability that disadvantages an individual in performing a normal role) (World Health Organization, 1980)
2. Confirm or refute previous impressions or conclusions formed on the basis of informal observations—case histories, interviews, referral information, and the like
3. Aid in differential diagnosis
4. Estimate probable treatment benefits
5. Monitor treatment effectiveness over time and determine treatment outcomes
6. Reduce risks of legal and ethical violations

Accuracy of a Diagnostic Test

Despite the many applications of diagnostic test findings, the primary purpose of any such test is to detect a disorder or disease when present. A good diagnostic test is one that identifies people who have a particular disorder or disease and excludes people who do not. To assess the accuracy of a new test, results obtained from it are generally compared with some other established test(s) viewed as the **gold standard** in yielding valid results. Even though such tests may not prove to be 100% accurate, they serve as the standard against which the merit of new tests can be judged. A logical question to ask is "If a test judged as the gold standard is doing a good job in accurately diagnosing a particular disorder or disease, why not use it in all cases?" The answer is that the gold standard for diagnosis can be time consuming, expensive, and more difficult to perform. For this reason, a screening test is often used as an option during initial testing to decide who among people should be given a more definitive evaluation and who should not. Thus, an audiologist might give an audiometric screening test to decide when a more complete audiometric evaluation might be warranted. Four outcomes are possible in comparing the results of a new test with a gold standard in identifying people with and without a disorder or disease:

1. True positive (TP): People with the disorder or disease (D^+) are correctly identified as such (test positive, denoted by T^+). The results of the new test correspond with the results of the gold standard. Symbolically, TP is written as $P(D^+$ and $T^+)$.
2. False positive (FP): People without the disorder or disease (D^-) are falsely labeled as unhealthy (T^+). The results of the new test identify more people as disordered or diseased than the gold standard. Symbolically, FP is written as $P(D^-$ and $T^+)$.
3. True negative (TN): People without a disorder or disease are correctly identified as such (test negative, denoted by T^-). The results of the new test correspond with the gold standard. Symbolically TN is written as $P(D^-$ and $T^-)$.

TABLE 9-4   The Four Possible Outcomes in a Screening Test

		Disorders		
		D^+	D^-	Row Total
TEST	T^+	$P(D^+$ and $T^+)$	$P(D^-$ and $T^+)$	$P(T^+)$
	T^-	$P(D^+$ and $T^-)$	$P(D^-$ and $T^-)$	$P(T^-)$
				Grand Total
	Column Total	$P(D^+)$	$P(D^-)$	1

4. False negative (FN). People with a disorder or disease are falsely labeled as healthy. The results of the new test identifies fewer people with a disorder or disease than the gold standard. Symbolically, FN is written as $P(D^+$ and $T^-)$.

The four possible outcomes are summarized in Table 9-4.

Measures of Test Accuracy

In determining the accuracy of a diagnostic test, what a researcher or clinician wishes to determine is the extent to which normal as opposed to abnormal individuals can be distinguished on the basis of the test results. To accomplish this goal, a type of probability statistics called the Bayesian method is used (see Chapters 4 and 12). Essentially, the method allows for the determination of diagnostic test accuracy according to the proportion of all test results, both positive and negative, that are correct. Measures of diagnostic test accuracy used for this purpose are: (1) test sensitivity, (2) test specificity, and (3) predictive value.

Test Sensitivity

Generally speaking, **test sensitivity** can be defined as the probability that the test result is positive (T^+) given that the disorder actually exists (D^+). Symbolically, it is written as:

$$P(T^+ \text{given that } D^+) = \frac{P(T^+ \text{and } D^+)}{P(D^+)}$$

If a test has high sensitivity, it will have a low **false negative rate,** that is, the probability that a subject who tests out as negative but who is actually positive, denoted by $P(T^-$ given that $D^+)$. In such a case, the test result will seldom indicate that the disorder is not present when in fact it is present.

Test Specificity

Test specificity can be defined as the probability that the test result is negative (T^-) given that the disorder actually does not exist (D^-). Symbolically, this is written as

$$P(T^- \text{given that } D^-) = \frac{P(T^- \text{and } D^-)}{P(D^-)}$$

A test that has high specificity is one that has a low **false positive rate,** denoted by $P(T^+$ given that $D^-)$, meaning that it will seldom predict the presence of a disorder that does not exist.

Predictive Values of a Test

Although test sensitivity and specificity are important preliminary steps in constructing a diagnostic test, these indices alone have limited application to actual diagnosis and clinical decision making. More specifically, although these values may be used to estimate the accuracy of a particular diagnostic test, it is the predictive values of a test that actually have practical value in detecting a disorder or disease. In the case of measures of sensitivity and specificity, in contrast to predictive values, the disorder or disease status *is already known*. However, what a clinician and client really want to know is whether or not a disorder or disease *actually exists*. Only the predictive values allow for forecasting actual clinical outcomes based on test results.

There are two major components of predictive value of a diagnostic test. The first of these is **predictive value positive (PV$^+$),** which refers to the probability that a disorder or disease exists when the test result is positive. Symbolically, this is expressed as

$$PV^+ = P(D^+ \text{given that } T^+) = \frac{P(D^+ \text{ and } T^+)}{P(T^+)}$$

The second component of the predictive value of a diagnostic test is called **predictive value negative (PV$^-$),** which refers to the probability that a disorder or disease does not exist when the test result is negative. Like PV$^+$, PV$^-$ can be represented as follows:

$$PV^- = P(D^- \text{ given that } T^-) = \frac{P(D^- \text{ and } T^-)}{P(T^-)}$$

A Research Example

A study that is representative of how the above measures can be applied to evaluate the accuracy of a screening test was conducted by Klee, Pearce, and Carson (2000). As a part of their ongoing research, the general goal of the investigation was to develop ". . . accurate and economical ways of identifying children with language disorder as early in life as possible . . ." (p. 821). The study was based on a further analysis of data reported by Klee et al. (1998) in an earlier investigation that explored the feasibility and efficacy of screening children for language delay by sending the *Language Development Survey* (LDS) to parents of children turning two years old. The LDS, developed by Rescorla (1989), is a checklist of approximately 300 words on which the parent is asked to indicate all the words they have heard their child say. The screening questionnaire was mailed to the families of several hundred children.

The analysis of the data in this study was based on the results of the LDS supplemented by information from parents' written responses to questions on the screening questionnaire in an effort to improve the positive predictive value of the screening procedures. In order to calculate the various measures of test accuracy as discussed above, the screening test results were compared to a "gold standard" which, in the case of this study, was based on a clinical evaluation conducted by two independent examiners that included information from parent interviews, developmental testing, direct observation of the child's verbal interaction with parents, and conversational analysis of a sample of conversation during play. In addition, the child's performance on at least one of three standardized measures had to fall one standard deviation or more below the population mean.

TABLE-9-5   The sample data, projected to a hypothetical population with 13% prevalence of language delay (N = 1000), with positive and negative predictive values expected

	$N = 1000$		
	Cinical Outcome		
Screening	**LD (D^+)**	**LN (D^-)**	**Row Total**
Positive (T^+)	118	113	231
Negative (T^-)	12	757	769
Column Total	130	870	1000

Note: LD represents "Language Delayed"
       LN represents "Language Normal"

From "Improving the Positive Predictive Value of Screening for Developmental Language Disorder" by T. Klee, K. Pearce, and D.K. Carson, 2000, *Journal of Speech, Language, and Hearing Research, 43*, p. 823. © American Speech-Language-Hearing Association. Reprinted by permission.

Table 9-5 provides a summary of the results of this study. The table contains data based on the calculation of measures of test accuracy including sensitivity, specificity, and predictive values projected to a hypothetical population of 1000 children given the actual results of the study. We will now illustrate the calculations for the four measures of test accuracy, beginning with sensitivity.

Calculating test sensitivity.   As shown in Table 9-5, of the 130 language delayed children (D^+), 118 were found to test positive (T^+) on the screening test. Hence, the test sensitivity was equal to 118/130, or approximately 91%. Using the formula for calculating test sensitivity, we have:

$$P(T^+ \text{ given that } D^+) = \frac{\frac{118}{1000}}{\frac{130}{1000}} = \frac{118}{130} \text{ or } 91\%$$

$$\text{False negative rate} = P(T^- \text{ given that } D^+) = \frac{12}{130} \text{ or } 9\%$$

Calculating test specificity.   Of the 870 children with normal language (D^-), 757 were found to test negative (T^-). Hence, the test specificity was equal to $^{757}/_{870}$ or approximately 87%. Using the formula for calculating test specificity, we have:

$$P(T^- \text{ given that } D^-) = \frac{\frac{757}{1000}}{\frac{870}{1000}} = \frac{757}{870} \text{ or } 87\%$$

$$\text{False positive rate} = P(T^+ \text{ given that } D^-) = \frac{\frac{113}{1000}}{\frac{870}{1000}} = \frac{113}{870} \text{ or } 13\%$$

Calculating predictive values. Of the 231 children who had a positive result on the screening test (T^+), 118 were diagnosed as being language delayed (D^+) based on the results of the clinical evaluation. Hence, predictive value positive was equal to 118/231, or 51%. Using the formula for calculating predictive value positive, we have:

$$PV^+ = P(D^+ \text{ given that } T^+) = \frac{P(D^+ \text{ and } T^+)}{P(T^+)} = \frac{118}{231} = 51\%$$

The second component of the predictive value of a diagnostic test is predictive value negative (PV^-). Of the 769 children who had a negative result on the screening test (T^-), 757 children were found to have no language delay (D^-). Hence, predictive value was equal to 757/769 or 98.4%. Using the formula for calculating predictive value negative, we have:

$$PV^+ = P(D^- \text{ given that } T^-) = \frac{P(D^- \text{ and } T^-)}{P(T^-)} = \frac{757}{769} = 98\%$$

Whereas test sensitivity and test specificity are solely contingent on the characteristics of the screening test used in a research study, the predictive values of a test will fluctuate significantly based on the prevalence rate for a particular disorder or disease. Mathematically speaking, the higher the prevalence (D^+) rate for a particular disorder or disease is in the target population, the higher will be the PV^+ and the lower will be the PV^- of a diagnostic test. Thus, if a disorder or disease occurs infrequently in the target population, the screening may result in a high false positive rate (low PV^+). This point is important to remember when a new test is being constructed in a limited context, such as in a speech and hearing clinic where only a small number of cases having a particular disorder may be available for study.

For additional information about how to calculate other measures of test accuracy and to portray the relationship between such measures graphically on an instrument called a **nomogram,** see Appendix A-4.

SUMMARY

In this chapter we reviewed the general principles and procedures for conducting several types of nonexperimental research in the field of communication sciences and disorders. Such research is appropriate for many types of problems in which it is as yet impossible to perform an experiment through an active manipulation of an independent variable or where doing so would breach ethical standards of scientific conduct.

Case studies can involve the detailed reporting of clinical and laboratory findings for a single individual or a small number of individuals. A case study that entails the investigation of three or more persons is referred to as a case series. Because of their narrow focus on a selected number of cases and the absence of a comparison group, such studies are particularly subject to bias. The chief value of case studies and case series methods is their adaptability for the study of rare disorders or diseases when little is known about their causes or what interventions might prove helpful in their management. As noted, such methods should not be confused with more scientifically rigorous, valid, and reliable methodologies as reflected in single-subject designs.

Other nonexperimental approaches to research, on the basis of which causality is sometimes inferred yet cannot be validly demonstrated, are cohort, case-control, and causal-comparative (ex post facto) studies. Cohort and case-control studies are observational approaches to research that examine occurrences of disorders or diseases in relation to a specified time dimension. Cohort studies follow groups of subjects over a period of time. In prospective cohort studies, the status of currently healthy people is tracked to some point in the future to determine who among them will develop a disorder or disease based on their differing exposures to a risk factor(s) of interest. An advantage of this type of study is that it can yield a direct estimate of risk given the incidence of a particular disorder of disease. A disadvantage is that it requires a large number of subjects that must be tracked over an extended period of time.

In a retrospective cohort study, information about the risk of initially healthy people for developing a disorder or disease is assembled from past records. These people are then followed forward in time to determine the present incidence of a disorder or disease of interest. The advantage of this type of cohort study is that it can be carried out with existing data. However, the validity of the conclusions drawn depends on the accuracy and completeness of preexisting records.

In contrast to cohort studies, case-control studies look backward in time to examine the occurrence of disorders or diseases. The typical paradigm is to begin by identifying one group of subjects with a particular disorder or disease and another group that is healthy—the outcome is known at the outset of the study. The two groups are then compared on a particular risk factor thought related to the prevalence of the disorder or disease of interest. Although an advantage of case-control studies is that they can be conducted based on existing data, they are more vulnerable to bias than cohort studies for reasons we discussed in this chapter.

Another type of nonexperimental study that we reviewed, similar in perspective to a case-control study, examines between-group differences on some dependent variable in relation to a factor that has occurred in the past. Such a study, called a causal-comparative (ex post facto) study, is representative of investigative methods that proceed from effect to cause in an effort to explain a research outcome. While such studies sometimes attempt to derive causal conclusions based on associative relations between variables or the ability of one variable to predict another, they are inadequate in proving causality for reasons we discussed.

Still another type of nonexperimental research discussed in this chapter pertained to survey studies. Two broad categories of such studies, questionnaires and interviews, were reviewed including the steps involved in conducting such studies along with their relative advantages and disadvantages.

Finally, because clinical research often involves the evaluation of diagnostic tests, several measures of test accuracy including test sensitivity, test specificity, and predictive value were defined and discussed. The methods for calculating these indices of test accuracy were illustrated, along with the probabilities for drawing correct and incorrect conclusions from the test results.

KEY TERMS

case study	incidence rate
case series	prevalence rate
longitudinal study	causal-comparative study
cohort study	multiple regression
risk factor	multivariate analysis
prospective cohort study	units of analysis
retrospective cohort study	representativeness of the sample

cross-sectional design
double-barreled question
loaded question
leading question
open-ended question
closed-ended question
Likert scale
contingency question
internal consistency
Guttman scale
Thurstone scale
factor analysis

interview schedule
structured interview
unstructured interview
gold standard
test sensitivity
false negative rate
test specificity
false positive rate
predictive value positive (PV^+)
predictive value negative (PV^-)
nomogram

SELF-LEARNING REVIEW

1. The case study approach should not be confused with single-subject designs. Although case study observation may serve as a basis for forming a(n) _____ about the nature or treatment of a particular disorder, such cases are not often used to _____ a treatment _____.

2. Although there is no specific rule as to how many cases to include in a case report, three or more cases are often described as a(n) _____ _____.

3. Case series can be a(n) _____-_____ study, in which observations are made at a particular point in time, or they can be a(n) _____ study, in which repeated observations are made over an extended period of time.

4. Two observational strategies that permit stronger inferences about possible cause and effect relations than do case study methods are called _____ and _____-_____ studies. They entail the comparison of two or more groups based on their differing exposures to particular _____ _____ believed to be related to the occurrence of certain disorders.

5. In prospective cohort studies, the cohort is selected using _____ information about the people comprising it who are then tracked forward in time to determine their _____. Such studies are often expensive and inefficient designs for determining the risk for a particular disorder. This is especially true when the occurrence of the disorder is _____.

6. In a retrospective cohort study, individuals are selected for the study of factors that might explain their _____ status based on _____ records. An advantage of the study over a prospective cohort study is that the former can be completed _____ and more _____ because it is based on _____ data.

7. Whereas cohort studies explore the relations between variables by proceeding in the direction of the _____ _____ to the _____ _____, _____-_____ studies reverse this paradigm by proceeding from the _____ _____ to the _____ _____.

8. An advantage of case-control designs over _____ _____ designs is that the former are more practical for studying _____ disorders. Because cases are selected for study _____ the disorder has occurred, case-control studies are more subject to _____ than _____ _____ studies.

9. In mathematical terms, the conclusions drawn in cohort studies are based on the _____ _____, referring to the number of _____ cases that emerge in a defined population during the course of the study, whereas case-control studies draw conclusions based on the _____ _____, referring to the number of _____ cases in a defined sample at a particular point in time.

10. In _____-_____ studies, the dependent variable has already occurred so that its relationship to other variables can only be studied _____ _____ _____ of such an occurrence.

11. _____ _____ is a major scientific premise for determining causality—that is, the presumed cause must precede the effect.

12. In causal-comparative studies, investigators often examine the strength of association between variables thought to contribute to _____-_____ differences on some presumed criterion variable by using various _____ statistics.

13. A commonly used statistical procedure in causal-comparative studies is called _____ _____. This method allows for determining the relative power of the _____ variables as each contributes to the magnitude of the _____ variable under investigation.

14. In addition to _____ a distribution of traits for a sample of people believed to represent the larger population, the purpose of many survey studies is to explain or make assertions about the population based on _____ _____, that is, the simultaneous comparison of two or more variables believed to differentially influence some outcome.

15. The _____ _____ _____ is typically a person, and such _____ are aggregated into samples that as a whole are more or less _____ of a population of similar persons, depending on _____ the sample was drawn.

16. In considering the feasibility of a survey study, the adequacy of a sample must be considered both in terms of the _____ of the sample and the _____ _____ _____.

17. Based on Babbie's guidelines (1990), an adequate response rate requires at least _____%; you need at least _____% for a good response rate, and at least _____% for a very good response rate.

18. In cross-sectional surveys, the sample data is collected at a particular point in time for purposes of describing _____ and their patterns of _____. On the other hand, survey studies that collect the sample data over an extended period of time are called _____ surveys.

19. _____ survey studies can be used to evaluate one or more attributes in a population by sampling such attributes over an extended time period.

20. In _____ survey studies, the same people from one time period to the next are sampled, whereas in _____ survey studies, different people are usually sampled from one time period to another.

21. _____ can be calculated based on a fraction that shows the number of both new and previously diagnosed cases for a defined period (numerator) over the number of persons _____ _____ in the population for the disorder or disease of interest (denominator). _____ can also be expressed as a fraction in which the numerator represents the number of _____ cases during a specified time period while the denominator is the number of people _____ _____ during a specified time period.

22. _____ surveys are appropriate for longitudinal studies, whereas _____ surveys are more appropriate for cross-sectional surveys.

23. Two common tools used for collecting survey data are _____ and _____. Essentially, such instruments can be distinguished according to their manner of _____ and method for_____ data.

24. As compared to interviewing respondents face to face, questionnaires can be _____ saving.
25. When constructing a questionnaire, there are three types of questions that must be avoided. They are _____-_____ questions, _____ questions, and _____ questions.
26. _____-_____ questions ask respondents to answer questions in their own words. _____-_____ questions are generally the predominant type used on most self-administered surveys.
27. A(n) _____ _____ is often used in conjunction with a series of statements each followed by a number of alternative responses such as "strongly agree," "agree," "neutral," "disagree," or "strongly disagree." Scaling techniques of this kind allow a researcher to assess the _____ of _____ in the strength of people's attitudes or opinions in numerical terms.
28. Attention must also be paid to the _____ and _____ of the questionnaire used in a survey to avoid boredom, keep respondents' demographic information confidential, and maximize response rate. Another design strategy for maximizing response rate is by the use of _____ _____ that allow respondents to skip from one question to the next as appropriate.
29. _____ rate is calculated as the number of located respondents from the entire sample. _____ rate is the number of respondents contacted out of the number located. _____ rate is the proportion of respondents who begin a survey and complete all items. _____ _____ rate is the number of respondents who complete the questionnaire out of all possible respondents.
30. A(n) _____ scale is said to be _____ in character because if a respondent achieves a ranked score signifying agreement (disagreement) with an item at a certain level of intensity, the response will signify agreement (disagreement) with all other items ranked at a lower level of intensity.
31. Other methods for data reductions and analysis used in survey research are the _____ scale and _____ analysis. The chief value of the latter method lies in its ability to _____ large sets of indicators to a limited number of composite scales.
32. Two major data-gathering methods for interviews are _____ interviews and _____ interviews. The research goal of an interview can best be met by the use of an interview _____ that contains explicit instructions to guide the interviewer in asking respondents a list of questions designed to obtain complete and honest answers.
33. The purpose of the survey will largely determine the type of questions asked during an interview. If the interviewer wishes to have very specific answers to questions with little or no deviation from a particular topic, a(n) _____ interview protocol will be followed in conjunction with closed-ended questions. On the other hand, if the interviewer wishes to probe a variety of topics while affording respondents considerable latitude in their answers, a(n) _____ interview would be more suitable than incorporated open-ended questions.
34. A good diagnostic test is one that identifies people who have a particular disorder or disease and excludes people who do not. To assess the accuracy of a new test, results obtained from it are generally compared with some other established test(s) viewed as the _____ _____ in yielding valid results. There are four possible outcomes obtained from the diagnostic test, namely _____ _____, _____ _____, _____ _____, and _____ _____.

35. _____ _____ can be defined as the probability that the test result is positive given that the disorder actually exists. On the other hand, _____ _____ is defined as the probability that the test result is negative given that the disorder actually does not exist.

36. _____ _____ _____ refers to the probability that a disorder or disease exists when the test result is positive. Whereas _____ _____ _____ refers to the probability that a disorder or disease does not exist when the test result is negative.

37. The predictive values of a test will fluctuate significantly based on the _____ rate for a particular disorder or disease. Thus, if a disorder or disease occurs infrequently in the target population, the screening may result in a higher _____ _____ rate.

QUESTIONS AND EXERCISES FOR CLASSROOM DISCUSSION

1. Discuss the essential differences between nonexperimental and experimental research.

2. What is meant by the case study approach, and what are some of the data-gathering techniques used in this type of research?

3. Locate a current journal article in one of ASHA's publications that employed the case study method. What kinds of "case information" were reported?

4. Define the meaning of *index cases* and explain how such cases can advance understanding and clinical intervention.

5. Distinguish between retrospective and prospective cohort studies in relation to their time domains. Find a journal article representing each of these types of designs.

6. How do case-control studies and cohort studies differ in so far as the manner in which cases are selected for study? How does a case-control study differ from a retrospective cohort design?

7. Why do cohort studies draw conclusions based on incidence rates while the conclusions of case-control studies are based on prevalence rates?

8. Name and briefly describe two statistical procedures that are commonly used in causal-comparative studies.

9. Describe several goals of survey research.

10. Identify five major steps in developing a survey. Locate an article from an ASHA journal based on a survey and evaluate its content in relation to how each of these steps were followed.

11. What are some general guidelines for evaluating the adequacy of response rates to surveys?

12. Discuss three major types of survey designs and the circumstances that would lead you to select one of these as compared to another.

13. What are several factors to consider in developing the items and format for a questionnaire?

14. What are three types of questions that should be avoided? Provide an example of each.

15. When are open-ended versus closed-ended questions appropriate for use?

16. Discuss three types of scales that can be used in survey research.

17. How can response rate be maximized in survey research, and how can it be calculated?

18. Discuss when an interview survey might be more appropriate than one based on self-administered questionnaires.

19. Discuss two major data-gathering methods used in interviews and their relative advantages and disadvantages.

20. Why does the purpose of an interview determine the type of questions asked?
21. What are some purposes of diagnostic tests used in the field of communication sciences and disorders?
22. What is meant by a "gold standard," and what is the importance of this concept in assessing the accuracy of new tests?
23. Identify four outcomes that are possible in comparing the results of a new test with a gold standard in people with and without a disorder or disease.
24. Define *test sensitivity, test specificity,* and *predictive values.* Of these measures of test accuracy, which among them have the greatest clinical relevance and why?
25. Clinical Application Exercise:

    The following exercise involves the sample data compiled by Jerger et al. (1993) pertaining to the accuracy of acoustic reflex threshold measures in predicting audiometric status. In the original study, the authors presented their results in the form of several matrices that compared predictions of audiometric status (abnormal T^+ or normal T^-) with actual audiometric findings (abnormal D^+ or normal D^-) for a total of 1043 abnormal and normal ears. We have adapted and cross-tabulated the findings of their investigation in the form of a two-by-two (2×2) contingency table shown in Table 9-6. Given these data, calculate (1) test sensitivity; (2) test specificity; (3) predictive value positive; (4) predictive value negative; (5) true positive rate; (6) false positive rate; (7) true negative rate; and (8) false negative rate.

TABLE 9-6   **Two-by-Two Contingency Table for Predicting Audiometric Outcomes Based on Acoustic Reflex Thresholds**

Actual Audiometric Outcome	($N = 1043$)		
	Predicted Audiometric Outcome		
	Normal (T^-)	**Abnormal (T^+)**	**Row Total**
Normal (D^-)	349	241	590
Abnormal (D^+)	81	372	453
Column Total	430	613	1043

$-$ sign represents "normality"
$+$ sign represents "abnormality"

Qualitative Research Methods

CHAPTER 10

CHAPTER OUTLINE

LEARNING OBJECTIVES

After reading this chapter, you should be able to identify, describe, or define:

- The basis for distinguishing qualitative from quantitative research methods
- When the qualitative approach can be more applicable to problem solving than the quantitative approach

- Observational methods in qualitative research and ethical concerns
- Emic and etic perspectives of ethnography
- The nature and uses of qualitative research interviews
- Grounded theory and phenomenological perspectives of qualitative research
- Use of the case study method in qualitative research
- Discourse and conversational analysis
- Content analysis: recording units and measurement procedures
- Methods used for analyzing and interpreting qualitative findings
- How data analysis and interpretative procedures differ in qualitative and quantitative research

In the course of their everyday experiences, human beings use their specialized sensory organs in conjunction with their cognitive and linguistic competencies to process observations of the world. Before objects and events can be described, related, predicted, or controlled, they first must be observed. Oliver Sacks (2000) describes some of his early childhood observations of metals as follows:

> They stood out, conspicuous against the heterogeneousness of the world by their shining, gleaming quality, their silveriness, their smoothness and weight. They seemed cool to the touch, and they rang when they were struck. (p. 179)

Later in the same essay, he says:

> All these things . . . gave me a sense of invisible rays and forces, a sense that beneath the familiar world of colors and appearances lay a dark, hidden world of mysterious laws and phenomena. (p. 181)

This latter statement makes clear that we use our observational faculties not only to appreciate the world, but are driven to derive meaning from it.

How do our everyday observations of the physical, social, and psychological correlates of experience differ from scientific inquiry about the same phenomena? The answer to this question relates in part to the differences in the orientation that a "lay observer" versus a "scientific observer" brings to the object or event of interest. In the first case, one's observations are largely haphazard or accidental and generally lack the kinds of tactics and strategies that emerge from carefully formulated questions or hypotheses about the nature of the things observed. On the other hand, the scientific orientation, in what is often called the **logical positivist position,** typically begins with a definite set of questions or hypotheses that, through the use of explicit and sustained systematic methods, are intended to discover the characteristics, interrelatedness, or causes of phenomena. Because of their strict adherence to objectivity, logical positivists favor highly disciplined, quantitative methods for data collection and analysis.

Over the years, another type of research that is gaining popularity in a number of social, behavioral, and health related sciences employs what are called **qualitative methods.** Generally, this type of research results in findings that are not easily quantified using the techniques of statistical hypothesis testing. Instead, such research is geared toward describing peoples' lives, social relationships, cultural values, thought processes, personal likes and dislikes, feelings and emotions, or how they function within the structure of various groups, organizations, or nations. This is not to say that data gained through such inquiry cannot be quantified, but the primary emphasis in qualitative research is placed on attempts to understand the *meaning* underlying people's experience while rejecting the notion that the discovery of such meaning is dependent on the extent to which it can be interpreted in numerical terms. The goal of qualitative research is to determine *what* the experience was like rather than measuring the *intensity* of such experience or *how many times* it occurred. In this chapter, several commonly used qualitative research methods will be reviewed as appropriate for certain types of research problems. Before doing so, let us first attempt to distinguish more clearly between qualitative and quantitative approaches to research.

QUALITATIVE VERSUS QUANTITATIVE RESEARCH METHODS

There are three main perspectives about the nature of qualitative research. First, as noted above, some researchers attempt to distinguish it from quantitative research on mathematical or statistical grounds. According to some researchers, qualitative research entails the use of data comprised of words, picture descriptions, or narratives (Monett et al., 1998) as opposed to quantitative research that counts, calculates numbers, or measures the phenomenon of interest (Wakefield, 1995).

A second way to view qualitative methods is as a type of research consisting of essentially descriptive or exploratory efforts to understand a phenomenon when it is not yet possible to formally test hypotheses about the relations between operationally defined variables. Such research might be undertaken when one knows little about the possible relationship of one such variable to another.

Still a third distinction that is sometimes drawn between qualitative and quantitative research is that the former is aimed primarily toward investigating the subjective aspects of human experience—a realm of knowledge and understanding that is best captured by the study of people's personal problems and reactions thereto as these occur in natural settings or in everyday routines. For example, efforts to understand how disability or disease impacts the feelings, beliefs, and attitudes of the affected person and perhaps other family members is representative of a problem suited for qualitative research.

The use of operational definitions to specify the dependant variables under study can be helpful in distinguishing between the qualitative versus quantitative characteristics of such variables. For example, one goal of an audiological investigation could be to determine the *quality* of hearing loss that might exist in a sample of subjects—whether it is conductive, sensorineural, or mixed in nature. In mathematical terms, here the unit of analysis is essentially nominal (existing as a category in name only). However, it is likely that a second goal would be to *quantify* the precise level of hearing loss in decibels across a range of frequencies. As is the case in this example, sometimes it is difficult to draw a sharp line between qualitative and quantitative research because many studies entail the investigation of phenomena having both qualitative and quantitative characteristics. Prior to conducting a quantitative analysis of various behaviors within a laboratory or formal experimental setting, it is often necessary to observe, classify, and code the qualities of such behaviors in a manner that eventually might allow for their analysis using standardized or more rigorous measuring instruments.

WHEN IS THE QUALITATIVE APPROACH THE "BEST APPROACH"?

As noted previously, some types of questions may dictate the use of qualitative rather than quantitative methods in the search for answers. If we want to know how a child born with autism, deafness, or a craniofacial malformation impacts family relationships, then research strategies such as participant observation, in-depth interviewing, content analysis

of narratives or symbolic interactions, field-work, and so on may be more suited for generating such diverse and complex information than relying on numerical data collected
within the sterile confines of a laboratory setting.

Qualitative research may be thought of as more subjective or holistic in orientation, with
an ultimate goal of describing, understanding, and interpreting the phenomenon under
investigation—not controlling a behavior or determining its statistical probability as in the
case of quantitative research. To this end, like a good detective in an effort to solve the case,
the qualitative researcher must go beyond the "hard facts" to a study of the "suspect's" inner
experiences, feelings, emotions, and motives to reach a solution. So far as possible, qualitative researchers wish to see how people experience and interpret events in their own lives.
According to Filstead (1970),

> Qualitative research allows the researcher to "get close to the data" thereby developing the
> analytical, conceptual, and categorical components from the data itself—rather than from the
> preconceived, rigidly structured, and highly quantified techniques that pigeonhole the empir-
> ical social world into the operational definitions the researcher has constructed. (p. 6)

Many qualitative researchers take a similar position while emphasizing the need to
divest themselves of preconceived theories or ideas in favor of becoming as fully immersed in
the interactions of the research participants with their environment as possible. Jacobs
(1970) elaborates on this point further:

> . . . observation [by the researcher] is only a gate to . . . knowledge. What happens when one
> enters that gate depends upon his abilities and interrelationships as an observer. He must
> be able to see, to listen, and to feel sensitively the social interactions of which he becomes a
> part. (p. 7)

In this chapter, we will discuss several types of methodologies, perspectives, data analysis procedures and interpretative techniques applicable to qualitative research.

OBSERVATIONAL METHODS IN QUALITATIVE RESEARCH

Perhaps the most commonly used qualitative method, endemic to all forms of scientific
research, is observation. Indeed, humans in their everyday affairs make use of their observational faculties to comprehend the world. Yet, what differentiates the everyday observations
of the layman from the scientist is that the latter's are based on systematic and purposefully
designed strategies for advancing knowledge or theory. Before the researcher can hypothesize
about the attributes of a particular behavior, or the relation of such attributes to the conditions or settings in which the behavior occurs, the behavior first must be perceived and documented in a manner that will allow for drawing valid and reliable conclusions. For the
researcher, no matter his or her philosophical bent, the need to focus one's own eyes on the
phenomenon of interest is necessary in order to apprehend its qualities.

Several types of observational methods are used in the social and behavioral sciences with
the end goal of documenting and recording behavior. However, the means to this end may differ markedly among qualitative and quantitative researchers. The usual framework of the
quantitative paradigm provides for systematic observation of behavior under controlled conditions in which the independent and dependent variables are strictly defined (operationalized)
and measured. On the other hand, the qualitative research model is more likely to adopt
methods appropriate for observing behavior in the "field" or setting in which the behavior
naturally occurs. By studying behavior in the stream of everyday life, the researcher is able to

gain a better appreciation of the complexity of the behavior ". . . where connections, correlations, and causes can be witnessed and how they unfold" (Adler and Adler, 1998, p. 81).

Qualitative methodologies have not been as widely used in the field of communication sciences and disorders as quantitative methods, although they are often applied in the more informal context of the clinical setting. As an integral part of their work, clinicians routinely observe, interview, and empathize with their clients in matters that have clinical relevance. Unlike the presumably more objective observer—perhaps a student assistant behind a one-way mirror who has been assigned the task of charting and tallying minute elements of behavior within columns and rows—the clinician must bring a larger perspective to the analysis. To borrow a line from Pirsig (1974), who concluded about people who travel unmarked roads, ". . . we navigate mostly by dead reckoning, and deduction from what clues we find" (p. 6). These clues are often so subtle or obtuse as to lie outside the range of focus using objective measurement techniques. In such cases, we must extrapolate meaning from our observations based on larger "trends," "patterns," or "styles" of behavior. In other words, we must rely on our own subjective views and interpretations in place of what has been called "this detached and sterile view . . . rooted in the quantitative observational paradigm" (Adler & Adler, 1998, p. 81).

Participant Observation

A guiding principle for many qualitative researchers is that, in order to derive meaningful conclusions about human behavior, it is necessary to participate at some level in the world of the people under investigation. Unlike quantitative researchers, who may contrive various conditions for observing behavior or attempt to modify it through the use of various response contingencies, the methods of the participant observer are said to be more "naturalistic" in essence. In the latter case, no attempt is made to stimulate or alter the behavior under investigation. Instead, the observer attempts to enter into the field of study while provoking as little change as possible. The notion that human behavior is best studied unobtrusively in its natural state has its ideological counterpart in a branch of physics known as quantum mechanics. According to what has come to be known as the Heisenberg Uncertainty Principle, the very act of observing and applying measurements to an object changes its characteristics at a subatomic level, making it different from its condition before the measurement was taken (Kaku & Thompson, 1995).

Qualitative researchers believe that human beings do not respond in simple ways to environmental stimuli impinging upon them. Instead, they are complexly and dynamically involved in symbolically transforming experiences in ways that are meaningful within the natural context of their occurrence. Eschewing the use of standardized measuring instruments or formal questionnaires, the participant observer instead looks for categories of experience and the connections among them that appear most salient in the lives of their subjects. There are three predominant roles that a participant researcher might elect to play, depending on how deeply one might wish to become immersed in the phenomenon of interest. These roles are: the *complete-member researcher,* the *active-member researcher,* and the *peripheral-member researcher* (Adler & Adler, 1987).

Acting in the first of these roles, the complete-member researcher, the researcher pursues the deepest level of involvement and participation in the group. Such an observer participates as a genuine member of a particular group while collecting data given such an "insider perspective." As an example, a student known to one of the authors of this textbook was a member of a community support group for adults who stutter while he was simultaneously enrolled in a course in fluency disorders. As a person who stuttered himself, he was motivated initially to join the group to form bonds with others having a similar communication problem. In this context, he had hoped to share some of his own fears, failures, successes, and future hopes as a communicator. While taking the course in fluency disorders, he became interested in documenting the beliefs and opinions expressed by others within the group in relation to how these aligned or failed to align with accepted clinical values. After each meeting of the group, he wrote a *narrative account* of the problems discussed and the degree to which the content of the discussion corresponded to outcomes that could be evaluated as "favorable" or "unfavorable" in clinical terms—for example, did the discussion foster attitudes that might promote such positive changes as reducing avoidance and feelings of helplessness in social situations or did the opposite outcome prevail? Were suggestions about the use of certain fluency-enhancing techniques in accordance with accepted clinical practice or outside the realm of such practice? While simultaneously acting in the dual roles of participant and researcher, the student concealed his latter identity throughout the period of his involvement with the group.

In accordance with the typology of Adler and Adler (1987), the second type of role one can play in participant observation studies is that of an active-member researcher. This involves something less than full participation in the activities of the group, although an effort is made by the researcher to establish close and meaningful relationships with other group members. However, in this case, the researcher may attempt to assume a more active leadership or consultative role in the group but without necessarily adopting all of its values and goals as one's own. Using the example just given, the student might have articulated more explicit positions about matters pertaining to stuttering from the vantage point of his own clinical or theoretical knowledge, particularly if the views expressed within the group ran counter to such knowledge.

The third role that a researcher might assume in the naturalistic setting of a group is as a peripheral member researcher. While such a researcher might believe in the importance of observing the activities of a particular group from an insider's perspective, he or she may refrain from adopting the group's core values or from participating extensively in its central affairs. Again, given our running example, the student might have attended meetings of the group without contributing in meaningful ways to its discussions, operations, or social activities. By doing so, the student would have minimized his involvement by staying on the "sidelines" while collecting data from "within."

All of the roles just described are motivated by just how close the researcher wishes to approximate the phenomenon under investigation on a personal level. Ultimately, these roles can be viewed as falling along a continuum of participation (involvement) of a researcher with his or her subject matter. On one pole, we have full involvement, allowing for the forging of intimate and close friendships that spring from a genuine belief and investment in the core values of the group. At the other pole, we have a pragmatic, objective involvement that, while placing importance on establishing an insider's identity, remains personally aloof while appraising the group's activities. Located between these poles is the researcher who attempts to blend personal involvement with some degree of objectivity or what has been termed "closeness with distance" (Adler & Adler, 1987).

In the course of observation, the observer may assume either an **undisguised participant** (overt) or **disguised participant** (covert) role. The undisguised participant is one who makes no effort to conceal her or his intentions of observing the group for the purpose of collecting data. One problem with the undisguised role is that the researcher may be perceived as obtrusive. Such reactivity may affect the behavior of subjects and their natural patterns of interaction (see the *Hawthorne effect,* also known as *subject effects,* in Chapter 7).

A means of avoiding the potential confounding influence of the participant observer on behavior is through the use of *disguise*. In such a study, the other participants are unaware that their behavior is being observed for purposes beyond the goals and objectives of the group. By concealing one's identity, the researcher is able to observe behavior and derive conclusions without impeding or distorting the outcome due to subject reactivity. However, subject reactivity is only one of the factors that may bias the outcome of research observations. Of equal importance are *Rosenthal effects*, also known as *interpreter effects*, resulting from the subjective, biasing influence of the observer's opinions as to what the outcome ought to be given her or his own a priori beliefs (see Chapter 7). Such effects can result in either a self-fulfilling prophecy or a self-negating prophecy on the part of the investigator who must rely on his or her perceptions to draw conclusions (Kidder, 1981). Both kinds of prophecies can lead to invalid conclusions because one is likely to observe only what is consistent with one's preexisting mind-set—contradictory findings may be discounted or ignored. In addition, the reliability of the conclusions may be difficult to establish in the absence of statistical confirmation of the consistency of one's observations.

Ethical Concerns in Observational Research

As noted previously, a major goal of the qualitative researcher is to gain an understanding of research participants' lived experiences in the context of the natural setting in which these occur. To capture the subjective world of participants in this manner, the researcher and the technique he or she uses in gathering data must be as unobtrusive as possible. Although the ability to engage in such covert operations is viewed as a strength of several observational techniques, the researcher who adopts such methods must be aware of ethical concerns arising from the use of **deception.** There are at least two types of deception in research practice. According to Arellano-Galdames (1972), the first type, *deception by commission*, occurs as a result of actively misrepresenting the purpose of the research or the procedures to be used, lying about the identity of the researcher, or falsely promising some gain to the participants. The second type, *deception by omission*, entails a passive form of deceit. In such a case, the researcher may fail to tell subjects that they are being studied or that their behavior may be recorded in a clandestine manner. The researcher, who gains access to the private world of another person or group of such persons, in the absence of their knowledge or consent, walks a thin line between the need to gather valid and reliable data, on the one hand, and the possible abuse of human rights on the other.

Although there is a lack of agreement among researchers as to the circumstances under which such research practices can be justified, some may view deception as permissible in order to maintain the validity of the research conditions (Kimmel, 1988). As noted by Rosnow and Rosenthal (1996), deception is *sometimes* seen as permissible when:

1. It is necessary to the validity of the research
2. The research is worth doing
3. The physical and psychological risks to the participants are minimal
4. Adequate *debriefing* will be carried out (pp. 54–55)

The last condition, **debriefing,** entails disclosing to the subjects the purpose of the research in which they were asked to participate after their having done so. According to the *Code of Research Ethics of the American Psychological Association*, if subjects were misinformed as to the purpose of the experiment or otherwise supplied with false information that influenced their choices or behavior, they should be debriefed—that is, they should be informed of such deception as soon after their participation as possible. From an ethical standpoint, the purpose of such debriefing is to prevent or lessen the anger, hostility, or reduction in self-esteem that might otherwise result as a consequence of not being informed of the reason and purpose of the deception. From a practical standpoint, the researcher also might wish to assure that, during the course of the experiment, the participants did not misconstrue or "see through" the deception in such a way as to invalidate the experiment.

Perhaps the most important question to address in any research study, no matter the methods used, is whether or not the dignity of the research participants is protected. Especially in studies that involve concealment or deception, both researchers and institutional review boards (IRBs) must consider the pros and cons of doing such research while always keeping this question in mind (see Chapters 3 and 13).

ETHNOGRAPHY

Ethnography is a research tradition that may be viewed as a systematized form of participant observation where the focus of the researcher is on describing the patterns of behavior that characterize a particular culture as these patterns occur in the natural setting. As noted by Werner and Schoepfle (1987a) the stem of the word, *ethno* (folks), and its suffix, *graphy* (description), is an area of study concerned with the "description of folk." It is a favorite method among anthropologists, as well represented in the work of Margaret Mead, who lived among the Samoans and the natives of New Guinea in an effort to describe and understand the cultural meanings in their lives.

In more recent years, the term ethnography has come to signify various approaches now used by many disciplines to study symbolic patterns of interactions not only in entire cultures but also in certain segments of culture such as small groups, where the focus may be restricted to specific areas of inquiry. In fact, the ethnographic approach may be applied to any "isolatable human group" irrespective of its size (Werner & Schoepfle, 1987a).

As noted previously, fieldwork is the primary tool of ethnography. Unlike experimental approaches to research, where an investigator sets out to investigate a preconceived number of hypotheses under controlled conditions, the aim of the ethnographer is to observe, describe, and classify patterns of behavior in the natural setting of its occurrence. From the grist of such data, an effort is made to adopt at least one of two perspectives that can serve as the basis for deriving a holistic conception or theory pertaining to the group's meaning and purpose. The first view that the researcher strives to achieve is an **emic perspective**—one based on the way the members of a group see their world given their particular culture. This can be described as the "insider's framework" or the "participant observer's" view discussed earlier. The ability to adopt the emic perspective is important if one is to capture and accurately describe the group's own understanding of reality. Next, many ethnographers move on in an effort to achieve an **etic perspective,** also referred to as "cultural materialism" (Harris, 1979). Here the researcher attempts to gain an objective view or "outsider's framework" in order to make sense of one's own observations and derive theory based on a scientific explanation of reality. Some researchers would argue that by combining these perspectives, the ethnographer enriches both the validity of data collection and analysis.

Typically, three types of cultural information are of interest to ethnographers: (1) cultural behavior (how members of a culture act), (2) cultural artifacts (what members of the culture make or create), and (3) cultural speech (what members of the culture say to one another) (Polit et al., 2001). In the course of gathering data in one or more of these domains, ethnographers employ several types of data-gathering techniques including systematic observation, field notes and memos, transcribed interviews and such other evidence as might be contained in public or private documents, personal or family histories, letters, photographs, tape-recordings, films, newspapers, and so on. The researcher sorts through information obtained from these and related methods of data collection. Ultimately, the aim is to code, categorize, and interpret such data in the form of a narrative report or story that accurately reflects how certain social experiences are created and given meaning. Denzin and Lincoln (1998) note that this process of constructing and interpreting meaning progresses through the following stages:

- The researcher first creates a field text based on notes obtained from field observations.
- From this file of raw material, the researcher refines it further into a research text based on one's own interpretations of the field notes.
- This text continues to be reworked or recreated until the researcher is satisfied that "sense" has been made from what he or she has learned.
- Finally, the researcher publishes the text for public consumption.

An example of an ethnographic study completed by Hammer and Weiss (1999) entailed an effort to understand how African-American mothers of low and middle socioeconomic status (SES), living in a southern urban community, viewed their children's language development and structured their language-learning environment.

The mothers were interviewed using guided questions that covered such topics as the mothers' view of how children learned to talk, the parents' role in fostering communication development, the mothers' perception of their children's communication and language development, and so forth. The videotaped interviews were transcribed and coded according to the ideas that the researchers believed the mothers expressed.

In addition to questioning the mothers about aspects of their children's language development, they were observed at play with their children in a preschool classroom for two or three sessions, during which time information was gathered about their communication/interactional styles. Supplemental information was also gathered based on informal conversational interactions between one of the researchers and the mothers during various encounters such as home visits. The dyad observations and supplemental information were used to aid in interpreting the interview data and to support the conclusions drawn.

Generally, the findings of the study indicated that the two groups of mothers shared several similar views with regard to their children's language development (e.g., that they learned to talk by listening to and watching others, imitating others, etc.), but some mothers seemed to differ in the strategies they employed to foster language development. More of the middle-SES mothers reported employing extensive teaching agendas as compared to the low-SES mothers. In discussing these results, the authors noted that a subset of the mothers in the low-SES group appeared to believe that their children's language development occurred "naturally." They concluded that such a belief might have accounted for the tendencies of such mothers to provide less direct maternal teaching and to emphasize their children's nonverbal behavior instead of their verbal communication abilities. Speculating further, the authors suggested that such values and accompanying patterns of behavior among such mothers might have been related to their lower levels of education. An alternative explanation proposed was that the low-SES mothers, who were unemployed and at home with their children, may have felt less compelled to set aside time to teach language skills as compared to working mothers who may believe they must allocate play time more strategically for their children to have ample learning opportunities.

Qualitative researchers acknowledge that there is no single interpretative truth. Rather, how the "truth" of their interpretations is viewed is often dependent on the community that is doing the interpreting. To obtain the most objective and reliable results from ethnographic studies, it is important to carefully establish an **ethnographic record.** Depending on the nature of the study, such a record may take a variety of forms including tabulations of observed behavior, verbatim transcriptions of interviews or conversations, audio or video recordings, notes based on memory, archival material such as clinic files, journal articles, newspapers or magazines, and so on. These and many other materials may be used to establish the reliability and validity of the researcher's conclusions. Whatever the record used, to have value to others, its form and contents should be made patently clear and open to scrutiny.

QUALITATIVE RESEARCH INTERVIEWS

Just as a clinician may provide information, emotional support, and helpful suggestions during an interview, so too might a qualitative researcher provide such assistance. However, instead of focusing on a therapeutic outcome, the predominant goal of a qualitative research interview is to collect data through various methods in order to answer specific questions for scientific reasons—namely, understanding a particular phenomenon. Thus, when the researcher asks parents to describe their initial reactions to a child born with cleft lip and palate, the aim is perhaps to understand their feelings, perspectives, and ways of coping independent of achieving any therapeutic goal. The information gained from such an interview is sufficient in its own right, provided the researcher is able to comprehend and document the central themes or meanings of experience conveyed by a particular person or group of such persons.

For researchers or clinicians to be effective in their roles as interviewers, they must establish rapport with the interviewee, which, according to Ramhoj and de Oliveira (1991), means that the interviewer must "be present" during the interview and convey the sense of such presence to the interviewee. This is best accomplished by being attentive and responsive to the verbal and nonverbal communication of the interviewee. They further noted that the following three elements form the core of an effective interview:

1. A methodic consciousness of the form of the questioning
2. A dynamic consciousness of interaction
3. A critical consciousness of what is said, as well as one's own interpretations of what is said

The common principle uniting these elements is the need for a certain quality of "consciousness" on the part of the interviewer involving multiple modes of awareness including the unitary present (now), the just past (then), and the about to be (future). As the interview unfolds, the interviewer strives to be intentionally conscious of each of these time domains and to fuse them together to derive meaning from the experiences revealed by the participant. Over the span of the interview, a kind of internal dialog takes place continuously in the mind of the interviewer: "Given what I've heard thus far, what question should I ask next, how should the question be asked, what will be the effects of the question, will the answer advance my understanding?"

A basis for differentiating qualitative from quantitative research interviews is the *degree of structure* imposed by the interviewer. The degree of structure in an interview is largely the result of the style and content of the questions asked. In general, it can be said that a quantitative research approach favors the use of structured interviews as opposed to unstructured or semi-structured interviews. Conversely, the latter two types are favored in qualitative research. Each of these interview methods can be distinguished from one another on the basis of the kind of questions employed and according to their relative advantages and disadvantages.

As mentioned in the previous chapter, structured interviews often incorporate a series of specific *closed-ended questions,* predetermined to limit the range of possible answers, such as the following:

In your opinion, which *one* of the following items increases a child's risk for developing a stuttering problem?

[ ] genetic inheritance
[ ] psychological stress
[ ] delayed language development

Typically, the interviewer reads such questions to all respondents in the same order, and answers are recorded in the same manner on a standard form. Structured interviews that incorporate closed-ended questions have the advantage of being clear and organized by seeking explicit answers to questions. The techniques used facilitate "staying on track" and generating the type of data that generally can be easily tabulated, organized, and subjected to statistical analysis. Thus, such interview methods are generally the preferred choice of the quantitative researcher. On the other hand, such methods may not afford an opportunity for a respondent to expand on a topic or to provide alternative interpretations or explanations for an attitude, feeling, or behavior expressed during the interview.

In contrast to *structured interviews,* qualitative researchers generally prefer approaches that eschew the use of a prearranged formalized list of questions. In an *unstructured interview,* the interviewer typically begins by asking a single open-ended question decided, in advance of the interview, to be useful in probing a particular area of interest. Thereafter, the interviewee's train of discourse serves as the main basis for determining the direction the interview takes. As the interview proceeds, the interviewer adapts and formulates additional questions given the topic of discussion.

Recall from our discussion in the previous chapter that open-ended questions encourage a respondent to express a full repertoire of thoughts, experiences, images, and feelings that are self-generated and salient to their own life. Such questions often take the form of: "Why did you . . . ?", "How did you feel . . . ?", "What did you think. . . . ?", "What do you hope . . . ?", and the like. Such questions avoid problems associated with influencing respondents to slant their answers to questions in a particular direction or limit their responses to "yes" or "no" answers.

The advantage of an unstructured interview that uses open-ended questions is that it allows the interviewer the ability to explore the knowledge, attitudes, and feelings of people toward situations and events that might otherwise fail to emerge during a structured interview. A possible disadvantage is that the conversation may drift off track well beyond the interviewer's scope of interest. Still another possible disadvantage could arise from a lack of uniformity among the questions asked and the topics covered. Such lack of consistency might create difficulty in comparing one subject's responses to another.

A compromise between the extreme approaches of structured and unstructured interviews is the *semi-structured interview.* Although the questions to be asked may be predetermined and presented in a systematic order, the interviewer may decide to occasionally deviate from the plan of the interview in order to pursue a particular subject of interest. The ability to digress in this manner promotes greater fluidity in the exchange of information, allowing the interviewer to gain more knowledge from the respondent. At the same time, the ability to analyze information and systematically compare responses to a scheduled list of questions is preserved.

By using open-ended questions, both unstructured and semi-structured interviews allow for greater flexibility than structured interviews in exploring a *broader* range of topics while gaining an *in-depth* understanding of the respondents' own perspectives about a particular subject. For this reason, open-ended questions are the favored technique of qualitative researchers.

The type of methods employed by a qualitative researcher is usually guided by one of several research traditions. One of these, *ethnography,* was previously discussed. Other research traditions that guide the approach as well as the analysis and interpretation of data collected are *grounded theory* and *phenomenology.* Each of these traditions and their relevance to qualitative research is discussed below.

GROUNDED THEORY

Grounded theory is a commonly used approach to the study of social processes and social structures. First introduced by two social scientists (Glaser & Strauss, 1967), it is said to be the most widely used interpretative method in education, the health sciences, and communication (Denzin & Lincoln, 1998).

The term *grounded* is meant to imply an inductive approach to theorizing in which the researcher begins a study with no presuppositions as to the nature of the phenomenon of interest. The framework for the study is rooted in what has been described as symbolic interactionism (Blumer, 1969), wherein the investigator attempts to discover through observation and interview the manner in which a group constructs its social reality. Symbolic meaning is derived by the study of the artifacts, customs, behavior, and language of the group. An ever-deepening discovery of this reality is a process through which new questions continue to emerge.

Thus, the distinguishing feature of this approach is that the data precede and direct the development of theory—not vice versa. To this degree, the grounded theory method involves inductive analysis based on the researcher's observations or interview data. Instead of waiting until the end of a study to make "sense" of the data, as quantitative researchers typically do, a researcher using a grounded theory makes notes of and categorizes meaningful patterns in the data as soon as such patterns emerge. Ultimately, out of such patterns, a kind of "artful integration" is said to occur, as the researcher continues to check back and by so doing reveals the theory, and how all the parts fit together, as the theory develops (Stern, 1980). The theory is supported to the degree that the hypothesized patterns that emerge from the analysis correspond to the majority of the observations. To the extent this is found to be true, it can be said that the theory is "grounded" in the data.

An example of the use of the grounded theory approach to qualitative research is represented in a study by Globerman (1995) who used a qualitative *long-interview method* to examine how families decide "who does what" and " how they reach these decisions" in caring for relatives with Alzheimer's disease. The interview method employed in this study was based on an editing approach to text analysis developed by McCracken (1988) and used to explore family patterns, decision making, and the apportioning of care. This method of analysis has five stages:

1. *Stage one* begins by examining the original transcripts of the interview data merely "as utterances" that are treated independently of one another.
2. *Stage two* involves an attempt by the researcher to understand the meaning of such utterances based on a review of relevant literature, the researcher's own understanding

of the participants' cultural values, the researcher's own knowledge and values, and other relevant evidence in the transcript.

3. *Stage three* entails an examination of the researcher's observations in relation to one another in a search for themes, patterns, and interconnections among them.
4. *Stage four* continues to examine the data for consistencies among the themes as well as for inconsistencies among them.
5. *Stage five* involves comparisons within kin-groups and across kin-groups.

Open-ended questions were employed to interview the families of individuals having senile dementia of the Alzheimer type diagnosed within the last year. In collecting the interview data, a grounded theory method called **theoretical sampling** was used to uncover relevant categories and themes as they related to caregiving by their adult children. Such sampling is designed to build from and add to the findings that emerge from an interview in order to construct as many categories as possible as these relate to a wide range of pertinent areas (Strauss & Corbin, 1998). Interviewees were (1) individuals who considered themselves primary caregivers or individuals who had some caregiving responsibilities (encumbered kin) and (2) uninvolved family members (unencumbered kin).

The findings of the study suggested that the decisions about the care of relatives with Alzheimer's disease was largely based on "family legacies" pertaining to how childhood responsibilities had been delegated in the past. More specifically, the adult children who were unencumbered with providing care for their parents were those that had been excused from family responsibilities during childhood. Such adult children were described by themselves and other relatives as having been seen as a "spoiled child," "problem child," "flaky," "undependable," and the like. Furthermore, as unencumbered adults, they saw themselves as "justifiably unencumbered, and felt confused when confronted with messages from their siblings suggesting that they should do more" (p. 95). They also seemed to be more self-centered and had unrealistic notions about the disease (looked for a "magic pill"). On the other hand, the encumbered adult children were those seen by themselves and others as having behaved more responsibly during childhood. As current caregivers to their relatives, they felt the burden and sometimes the overwhelming demands that accompanied this role. Yet, they had a more realistic understanding than their unencumbered siblings of how things were or were not changing and took ownership of their involvement in making decisions and choices.

The grounded theory approach used in this study suggests that decisions about caregiving for relatives with Alzheimer's disease are a complex process. The author concluded that the way children are seen by other family members during childhood may explain why one child as an adult is called upon, chooses, or is chosen to be either a primary caregiver or one who is unencumbered with such responsibilities.

PHENOMENOLOGY

Another approach to qualitative research is guided by a research tradition known as phenomenology. Phenomenology has its roots in philosophy that has been long occupied with such questions as "What is being?" and "How do we know what we know?" (Ray, 1994). Although the term has been used inconsistently in a wide variety of contexts by qualitative researchers, the essence of the phenomenological approach is simply an effort to understand people's views of reality. According to Reeder (1989), the goal of the researcher is to gain an understanding of people's "sense of things" or of such phenomena as seeing, hearing, feeling, believing, judging, imagining, remembering, caring, willing, and the like.

An example of the phenomenological approach is a study by Yorkston, Klasner, and Swanson (2001), who examined "insider perspectives" of communication in multiple sclerosis (MS). Citing Colaizzi (1978), the authors noted that the phenomenological approach "uses guided interviews to engage participants in a dialogue with investigators to inductively describe their lived experience without constraint of theory or clinical perspective" (p. 127).

Seven participants having mild communication problems associated with MS were guided to answer several broad and open-ended questions. The authors stated that "loaded" questions such as "What communication strategies work for you?" were avoided because of the tendency of such questions to presuppose the existence of communication problems and the use of "strategies" to deal with them. Instead, more neutral questions such as "What's communication like for you?" were asked. Participants were encouraged to elaborate on the communication problems they happened to mention, the situations in which the problems occurred, how they felt, and how they coped with any identified barriers. The interview data was transcribed and coded to yield several themes and subthemes that emerged from the interview. Direct quotations from the interview were used to show how the messages reflected and restricted the communication experiences of individuals with MS. For example, speaking of her experiences with a store manager, one participant noted:

> And I remember stumbling . . . over my words talking very slowly, and she obviously was in a big hurry, and she wanted everything real quick and I couldn't do it. She just looked like I was driving her nuts, like I was really frustrating her. I ended up getting what I wanted which was good, but she really was cutting me short, and yeah, it was kind of unpleasant." (p. 134)

Based on the results of their study, Yorkston and her colleagues derived a model of the impairments and limitations associated with restrictions in communicative participation for the subjects in her study (see Figure 10-1). The authors noted that communicative participation was placed at the top of the pyramid because such a viewpoint appeared consonant with the "insider's perspective"—namely, that of the subjects who participated in the study. As the model indicates, the interviewees did not view limitations in their communicative participation as the sole result of impairments in speech and language but from many types of impairment.

The use of open-ended questions such as those used in the study by Yorkston and her colleagues demonstrates the value of such questions for investigating how individuals construct meaning from events or circumstances in their daily lives. Through such means, the interviewer hopes to gain a better understanding of the "lived experiences" of people given their own perceptions, suppositions, and judgments.

CASE STUDY METHOD

The term *case study* denotes diverse research strategies that typically have as their goal describing a condition, incident, or process (the case) believed to be relevant to one or more individuals. As noted in the previous chapter, cases may entail an in-depth study of a single person or groups of people found in businesses, health care organizations, educational institutions, urban or rural neighborhoods, ethnic or social communities, governmental agencies, or wherever. A variety of procedures are typically used for data collection over a lengthy period of time (Creswell, 2003).

Different perspectives and approaches to the use of the case method have evolved among various disciplines. The approach in the social sciences has focused largely on investigating the values and activities of groups of people as opposed to a single individual or a few

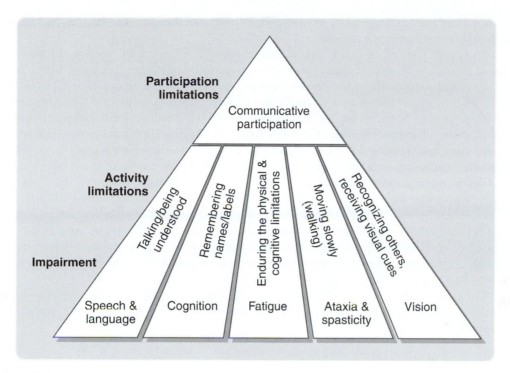

FIGURE 10-1   A schematic representation of the impairments and participation limitations associated with restrictions in communicative participation for individuals with mild MS.

Reprinted with permission from "Communication in Context: A Qualitative Study of the Experiences of Individuals With Multiple Sclerosis," by K. M. Yorkston, E. R. Klasner, and K. M. Swanson, 2001, American Journal of Speech-Language Pathology, 10, *p. 136.*

individuals. On the other hand, health professionals historically have taken the opposite approach by making an individual client or a small number of clients the main target for research, although the scope of interest has more recently broadened to include larger units of study (e.g., family dynamics, nursing home practices, managerial policies of insurance companies, etc.). Early acceptance of the case study method as a credible scientific approach for gaining knowledge and insight from the intensive, prolonged observation of unusual or unique persons is evident in the pioneering work of Sigmund Freud. His in-depth study of such individual patients as Anna O. led to an entirely new theory of neurosis and what was to become a widely accepted means for treating such illness—psychoanalysis.

A good example of the application of qualitative methodology to case study research is found in a study completed by Ruiz (1995). The study was an ethnographic investigation of a bilingual special education classroom using the case of Latino children in the United States who were labeled as language learning disabled (LLD). Citing literature which suggests that the abilities and disabilities of children in special education vary across different interactional contexts, the author set out to explore "optimal learning contexts" for Latino children identified as mildly handicapped. Ethnography was selected as the research methodology because, as stated by the author, it allows for "the extensive study of socio-cultural aspects of a group from the point of view of its members . . . produced through participant observation in regularly occurring cycles of events. . ." (p. 47).

The study took place in a bilingual special education classroom where emphasis was placed on the use of home language and home culture along with English for children identified as LLD. Over the course of several months, the author acted as a participant observer while making an audiotape recording of the students during the course of their classroom activities. In addition, careful *field notes* were kept that provided additional information about classroom interactions and the social structure shaping such interactions. Students' school files, individualized education plans (IEPs), and interviews with parents provided additional sources of data. From the analysis of such data, three distinct language learning profiles emerged: (a) children who had moderate to severe language learning difficulties, (b) children who were suspected of having a mild disability but possibly had no disability, and (c) children who had normal ability but who were misdiagnosed as disabled. Based on the results, the author concluded that the medical model involving formal test procedures as applied to children having special education needs, "over identifies children from diverse backgrounds as handicapped . . . even when the tests are in the child's dominant language" (p. 47).

The steps necessary for carrying out an ethnographic case study are much like those used in other qualitative research designs. Several guidelines for accomplishing such research are summarized in Figure 10-2.

- Select an appropriate case example (single person, group, event, etc.) that you believe will shed light on the problem of interest.

- Conduct the case study in a "naturalistic setting"–the real world conditions of the participant(s).

- Adopt an "insider's" point of view and interact with participants in accordance with their own terms and values.

- Spend considerable time gathering data from a wide variety of sources including information obtained through direct interactions with the participant(s) and from such secondary sources as interviews with significant others, preexisting records, etc.

- Analyze the data on a continuous basis to detect patterns or themes that will help direct or support future data collection activities.

- Evaluate the data as to the extent they may or may not support an existing or new proposition or theory.

- Communicate the findings as a narrative description that reconstructs the "reality" of the participants. Some researchers also emphasize the importance of making clear the "cultural context" of such reality (Wolcott, 1980).

FIGURE 10-2   Guidelines of conducting an ethnographic case study

DISCOURSE ANALYSIS

Discourse analysis is a hybrid field of inquiry that cuts across several disciplines including anthropology, sociology, psychology, and linguistics, among others. From a theoretical perspective, discourse analysis views language not merely as a neutral and passive symbolic system for reflecting personal and social realities but as the linguistic building blocks for *constructing* such realities. Essentially, the major focus of discourse analysis is on how people organize and express language in written texts or in conversational interactions to construct versions of their worlds (Potter & Wetherell, 1987). Although discourse analysis may be couched in different theories, it tends to focus on structures of text and talk that *express language* (sounds, gestures, images, word order, sentence structure, etc.) or *convey meaning* (organization of topics, sequence and coherence of propositions and the functions they serve, presuppositions, allusions, attributions, vague or detailed descriptions, etc.).

A methodology commonly used in conjunction with discourse analysis is called **conversational analysis.** Conversational analysis has its roots in the work of such researchers as Harvey Sacks (1992), whose pioneering efforts to develop this tool led to its widespread application in a number of fields. Conversational analysis is sometimes referred to as the study of the "rules for turn taking." It is perhaps better described as an account of "talk-in-interaction" (Potter, 1996). Sacks (1992) has argued that interactions during conversations are not just organized in a general way but are also organized according to particular details that require a fine grained analysis of the details of talk—that is, turns of talk and how they are responded to (questions, criticisms, invitations, etc.) or other particulars such as hesitations, repairs, or pauses. As the grist for analysis by a researcher, such details can be used to illuminate how talk makes things happen during conversational interactions.

A study by Leahy (2004) illustrates an application of *therapeutic discourse analysis,* a term which ". . . refers to the analysis of talk-in-interaction as a social practice in the speech clinic" (p. 71). The aim of the study was to highlight significant aspects of such "talk-in-interaction" between a speech-language pathologist and an adolescent girl who stuttered. The therapy session was videotaped to allow for recording not only what was said during conversational exchanges but also for revealing what aspects of nonverbal communication occurred during silent pauses of the interaction. Subsequently, the data were transcribed and the spoken interactions were analyzed and interpreted from the perspective of how the *sequential behavior* expressed by the clinician and client during speaking turns affected the overall quality of the talk. The recording was then listened to repeatedly and each line of the discourse was numbered.

Leahy's evaluative comments about the nature of the conversation that occurred between the client and clinician is typical of therapeutic discourse analysis. At the outset of the session, the author noted that the exchanges between the client and clinician were marked by an asymmetry in discourse with an authoritative role being assumed by the clinician and a subordinate role by the client. Further analysis of the conversation that occurred later in the session revealed an increased symmetry in the discourse. Apparently, this occurred as the client became more confident in her linguistic and social competence and began to shift her *sociorelational frame* from that of an "error maker" to a "competent communicator." The author noted that this would not have been possible had the clinician not recognized and complied with this shift by following the client's "conversational moves."

Upon completion, Leahy presented a report of her discourse analysis to the clinician, with whom she discussed the findings. According to the author, the clinician found the report to have value by increasing her awareness and "how issues of control and choice in therapy are negotiated." For example, the clinician said that she learned more about how the use of the inclusive pronoun "we" during conversations can increase collaboration in future sessions, how vocal dynamics, such as a soft vocal tone, can be used effectively to persuade or model behavior, and so forth. Leahy concluded her article by remarking that clinicians who are unfamiliar with discourse analysis may be reluctant to incorporate such methods for clinical purposes. The method can be time consuming and focused on what some might consider relatively insignificant details of conversation. Yet, she went on to say that "Although analyzing therapy talk will not demystify all the magical elements in the relationship . . . it will help to identify aspects of the relationship negotiated through talk and . . . develop awareness of factors that serve to influence therapeutic change" (p. 79).

CONTENT ANALYSIS

Content analysis is a general term referring to several types of methods that can be used for gathering and analyzing data obtained from **texts.** Texts can be constituted of any type of message designed for communicating information, including the content of spoken and written narratives, films, videotapes, photographs, music, artistic productions, and the like. According to Krippendorff (1980), sociologists were among the first to apply content analysis to the study of written forms of text such as newspapers. Later, the method was further refined as a method for measuring and assessing the message content of text according to metrically defined units of analysis. Krippendorff (1980) has identified five categories of **recording units.** One or more of these often serves as the focus for content analysis in research studies.

- *Physical units:* units that can be delineated according to their spatial or temporal characteristics. For example, these might be constituted of the separate pages of a book, frames of a motion picture film, or various time periods during the day for evaluating various media such as the types of television programs that occur during the morning, evening, or afternoon.
- *Syntactical units:* these serve as the grammatical basis for expressing a communication message. For example, in an oral or written narrative such units might be constituted of words, sentences, or paragraphs. In a film, the syntactical units are the scenes that result from the editing process. In a news broadcast, the syntactical unit could consist of a particular arrangement of news stories.
- *Referential units:* units that refer to particular objects, events, persons, ideas, organizations, countries, and so forth that serve as the focus of the analysis. For example, the focus might be on the messages and ideas communicated by fictional characters in books, by actors in films or stage plays, or by politicians in their public addresses.
- *Propositional units:* these entail a more complex level of analysis, requiring the examination of the relationship of one unit of analysis in relation to another. Thus, one might examine how powerful or weak certain characters in a book or film are in relation to other characters.
- *Thematic units:* the units that convey the major points of a communication message. For example, following the speeches or debates of politicians, news analyses typically summarize the themes that were emphasized (e.g., tax reform, improvements in health care or national defense, etc.).

The measurement procedures used in content analysis are based on systematic and careful observations in which the units of interest are recorded and coded according to one or more numerical characteristic(s) (Neuman, 2000). These characteristics include:

- *Frequency:* how often a recorded unit of the text message is observed to occur. For example, how many times a particular idea, feeling, or emotion is expressed in an oral or written text.
- *Direction:* the direction of the text message as evaluated along some continuum. For example, were the remarks or actions positive (friendly, supportive, considerate, etc.) or negative (antagonistic, accusatory, demeaning, etc.)?
- *Intensity:* how strongly or powerfully the text message is expressed in a particular direction. For example, during storytelling, the more relevant the content remembered is to the theme of the story, the more positive the text message; the less relevant the content remembered is to the theme of the story, the more negative the text message.
- *Space:* the size of the text message, or how much space or volume has been allocated to it. Given a page of a particular size, the space occupied by a written text message can be measured by counting the number of words, sentences, or paragraphs that appear on it. In the case of an audiovisual text, space can be measured according to how much time is allocated to the presentation of the message content. Thus, the "space" that ASHA allocates in educating the public about different forms of speech, language, and hearing disorders could be content analyzed by assessing the size of its text messages as these appear in official written publications or the time required for their presentation in films prepared for similar public relations purposes.

As noted previously, much of the research in content analysis has focused on the use of objective and systematic counting and recording procedures (Neuman, 2000). The emphasis in such quantitative research is on coding the message content based on what was readily manifested "on the surface" of the text. To use a simplified example, if a researcher wanted to study the emotional content of a written narrative, he or she might count how many times particular words were used that convey emotional meaning such as "happy," "sad," and so on. Because such *manifest coding procedures* are empirically based, they tend to yield data that are generally reliable. However, qualitative researchers typically wish to go "below the surface" of a text message to discover what latent meanings might lie beneath. For example, in evaluating the remarks of a politician, instead of merely tabulating certain written or spoken words, the researcher might examine entire paragraphs in an effort to derive themes or meanings otherwise hidden in the text. Such *latent coding procedures* tend ". . . to be less reliable than manifest coding because of their dependence on a researcher's knowledge of language and its social meaning . . . Yet, the validity of latent coding can exceed that of manifest coding because people communicate meaning in many implicit ways that depend on context, not just on specific words" (Neuman, 2000, p. 296).

Although counting the occurrences of things can improve precision in content analysis, qualitative researchers believe that it should not substitute for rich description and contextualization (Boyle, 1994). Whatever the type of content analysis performed, three elements common to any kind of such analysis should include: (a) deciding what the unit of the analysis will be, (b) borrowing or developing a set of categories, and (c) developing the rationale and illustrations to guide the coding of data into categories (Wilson, 1989).

An apt example of how content analysis can be usefully applied in the field of communication sciences and disorders is a study by Champion and colleagues (1999). In establishing the rationale for their study, the authors described some of the deficiencies in previous investigations that essentially entailed comparative descriptions of differences in the structure of narratives produced by African-American and Anglo-European children. More specifically, the authors noted that: "Narrative analysis must go beyond the structural coherence of a text . . . it is important that children's cultural and social practices be taken into account . . . An important educational question is 'how does the content of narratives reveal social and cultural practices?'" (p. 54).

To answer this question, the authors chose to use an approach to content analysis advocated by Spradley (1980) because of its ethnographic perspective focused on deriving cultural meanings from the data. As described by the authors, this approach to content analysis aims to determine how the parts or elements of the cultural meanings embedded in a narrative are organized. This involves creating cultural domains or categories of meaning within an organizational framework through which "things" of interest in culture can be identified and classified in accordance with the following three elements:

- *Cover term:* the name of the cultural domain subjected to analysis.
- *Included terms:* names of smaller categories of things inside the domain.
- *Semantic relationship:* elements that define and lend meaning to persons, objects, events, and activities. Spradley identified several semantic relationships that appear to be universal in every culture (e.g., inclusive, spatial, cause-effect). A single semantic relationship links together the cover term with the smaller categories and thereby aids understanding of bigger and smaller categories.

In the study by Champion et al. (1999), these three elements were applied to the written and oral narratives of children "until patterns emerged that made statements of relationships among features within and across social contexts" (p. 55). The participants in the study consisted of 20 African-Americans enrolled in a preschool classroom for 4 year olds. Children's narratives were elicited twice a week during a story telling period in which members of the research team would first tell or read a story to the children that focused on a variety of subjects related to African-American culture (folktales, stories from books about African-American life, personal stories told by African-American members of the research team). Subsequently, children were asked to write and draw their own stories. Shortly thereafter, the stories the children had written and drawn were read and told by them as they were audio-videotaped. The data from these tapes were transcribed verbatim for purposes of content analysis among other research goals related to the children's cultural and social practices.

The researchers identified several common cultural domains (themes) that emerged from the children's narratives. To illustrate the method of content analysis performed in their study, the researchers provided examples of the narrative transcripts used for this purpose. One common theme that emerged from the content analysis was labeled *identity*. For example, within the context of her written narrative, one of the children described herself as a "big girl," using this size reference to imply that she is capable of doing more things, such as going to kindergarten or first grade, if she "looks" big.

Based on the combined results of their study, the authors concluded that content analysis is a valuable supplement to more traditional forms of text analysis that can help teachers and speech-language pathologists gain valuable insights about particular social identities and social relationships of preschool children and how these can impact their language development. Several suggestions were offered as to how certain assessment and teaching strategies might best be used to facilitate emergent literacy skills within the classroom context.

ANALYZING QUALITATIVE DATA

Given the diversity of qualitative research methods, it is not surprising that the methods used for the analysis of qualitative data are similarly diverse. Despite this fact, Crabtree and Miller (1992) discussed four major approaches to data that fall along a continuum. At one end of the continuum, more objective, systematic, or standardized approaches to data analysis are employed. Techniques that are more subjective, intuitive, and interpretative in nature are found at the other end of the continuum. Four of these data analysis "styles" are discussed next.

Quasi-Statistical Analysis Style

This approach is consistent with *manifest coding procedures* used for data obtained from the *content analysis* of message texts previously discussed. To use this approach, the researcher must have some preconceived notions about the statistical analyses that he or she might wish to perform at the outset of the study. These ideas are then used to guide the researcher in the search for certain words, themes, or patterns in the text specified in advance that can be coded into categories. As defined by Lindlof and Taylor (2002), **codes** used for qualitative research purposes are short-hand devices for labeling or marking "the units of text as they relate meaningfully to categories (concepts, themes, constructs)" (p. 216). For purposes of content analysis, a **code book** (code sheet) containing precoded response categories is often used for assigning a range of numbers to the variables of interest. The actual coding process usually entails circling or checking a number corresponding to the appropriate response category that can be entered into a data file(s). For statistical purposes, the frequency of occurrence of certain words, themes, patterns, and the like can then be determined. Typically, the numerical data obtained through manifest coding procedures possess only *nominal measurement characteristics*. For reasons to be discussed in greater detail, the types of statistical analyses that can be performed on variables that only can be placed into response categories and counted are quite limited (see Chapter 12).

Because traditional methods of analyzing qualitative data can be very time consuming, a number of computer programs have been developed for this purpose. Such programs also allow for certain portions of an interview or text message to be retrieved and printed. Software packages for qualitative data analysis (QDA) are not used by researchers for the *interpretation* of such data, a job they must do alone. Instead QDA software is employed by the researcher for purposes of data storage, coding, retrieval, comparing, and linking various themes to one another, and so forth. Some QDA software packages are used for general purpose applications. Others are used for special purposes given the needs of a particular QDA researcher. A popular general purpose system is the *Ethnograph,* which is capable of not only retrieving and displaying coded data but also indexing data and performing statistical operations to expedite the analysis of prespecified portions of a text message. Other QDA software programs are shown in Figure 10-3.

As Richards and Richards (1998) point out, there are dangers associated with the use of any QDA software program. Specifically, they note that "a weak link will always be the adequacy of the coding process . . ." (p. 233). We would add that an ability to construct meaning from such codes is dependent on the skills of the researcher in deriving insights and understanding from patterns observed in the data.

Template Analysis Style

In place of using a code book, as is often done in a quasi-statistical analysis, a general template can be used to *guide* rather than to predetermine data analysis. Such a template often consists of several units (e.g., behaviors, events, linguistic units such as words) against which

ATLAS.ti
Developer: Thomas Muhr, Technische Universitat Berlin, Project Public Health A4
Address: Hardenbergstrasse 4-5, 10623 Berlin, Germany
Web site: www.atlasti.de/

Hyper RESEARCH
Developer: S. Hesse-Biber, Department of Sociology, Boston College
Address: Chestnut Hill, MA 02167, USA
Web site: www.researchware.com

QST.NUD*IST
Developer: Qualitative Solutions and Research
Address: Box 171, La Trobe University Post Office, Vic 3083, Australia
Web site: www.qsr-software.com

Ethnograph
Developer: Qualis Research Associates
Address: P.O. Box 460728, Denver, CO 80246
Web site: www.qualisresearch.com

FIGURE 10-3   Some selected QDA software programs

data obtained from a text such as a narrative can be compared. A template is more flexible than a code book because it is continuously refined throughout the data collection process. The data obtained from the use of such templates are not treated statistically. Instead, the researcher uses the template for *interpretive purposes* that are more aligned with the traditions of *ethnography* or *discourse analysis* than with content analysis.

Editing Analysis Style

Using this style of data analysis, the researcher listens to audiotapes repeatedly or rereads written transcripts extensively in an effort to identify meaningful segments. Once identified, the researcher develops a *categorization scheme* for coding, sorting and organizing the separate segments into larger categories or thematic structures. To accomplish this task, the researcher must have a keen ability to see patterns or *recurring regularities* in the data that can be developed into explanatory concepts. The first attempt by a researcher to adequately conceptualize the data may fail because of inadequacies in the categorization scheme. Therefore, it might be necessary to edit and revise the categorization scheme a number of times until salient concepts begin to emerge from the data. The edited analysis style is especially appropriate for *grounded theory methods* of qualitative research that use an inductive approach to theory development—that is to say again, the theory is generated from the "ground up" based on relationships observed in the process of coding data. Edited analysis is also relevant to the research tradition of *phenomenology* that attempts to inductively derive meaning from the "lived experiences" of people. Unlike grounded theory that seeks to derive theoretical propositions from the data, phenomenology is more focused on synthesizing or deriving common structures (themes) for the particular experience of interest through observation and reflection. The reflective process entails writing and rewriting the insights and understandings gained by the researcher in the process of observing and conversing with people about experiences encountered in their everyday lives.

Immersion/Crystallization Analysis Style

As stated previously, some qualitative researchers hold the opinion that the only valid approach to the study of many social phenomena is for an investigator to become totally immersed in the problem, believing that a true understanding can only come from an "insider perspective." Thus, to fully understand the life of a prisoner, the researcher would need to live the life of a prisoner—live in a cell, eat prison food, abide by prison rules, and on and on. A clinically relevant example that parallels this approach might be for a speech therapist to mimic the symptoms of a person who stutters for some period of time, hoping to crystallize the problems and feelings associated with speaking disfluently. While analysis of such experience through reflection and writing about its self-perceived essence might yield some valuable insights on occasion, it is rarely possible to fully understand experience as seen through the eyes of another person. To make this point, Patton (2002) quoted an exchange that occurred between a student assigned to do a participant observation exercise in a prison and an inmate. A portion of the conversation was as follows:

Inmate: "What are you in here for, man?"

Student: "I'm here for a while to find what it's like to be in prison . . . from the inside instead of just studying what it's like from out there."

Inmate: ". . .Shit, man, you can go home when you've had enough, can't you?"

Student: "Yeah."

Inmate: "Then you ain't never gonna know what it's like from the inside." (p. 266)

Whatever style of data analysis a researcher might use, Morse and Field (1995) have identified four cognitive processes that appear to be an integral part of all qualitative methods of data analysis:

- *Comprehension* is the process of "making sense of the data" that begins at the outset of the study and continues throughout its entirety. Data analysis, involving the transcription and coding of text materials, helps the researcher to uncover hidden meaning that gradually make clear the relationship of one pattern of experience to another. This process is repeated until the researcher feels that nothing more is to be learned. Having reached this so-called *saturation point*, a complete, detailed, and rich description is written.
- *Synthesizing:* is a process that entails aggregating data by comparing the transcripts of several participants and sorting experiences according to their commonalities. Data are fitted and linked together in order to see relationships, make conjectures, and verify findings.
- *Theorizing:* is a process in which segments of data are compared and contrasted while constructing alternative explanations to account for the findings. The theory that is finally chosen to explain the data is the one that does the most comprehensive job in linking seemingly diverse and unrelated facts in a useful way. Three aspects in theorizing are to (1) ask questions that will discover beliefs and values embedded in the data, (2) engage in *lateral thinking* by relating concepts to other settings or to other data sources that complement one's own conclusions, and (3) use inductive reasoning to infer causal links or sequences between certain behaviors and experiences to develop a theory that can be verified or refuted.
- *Recontextualizing:* is the process aimed at establishing the power and ultimate value of a developing theory. The theory is closely examined in relation to the established works

of other researchers in the published literature and existing theoretical models. By recontexualizing one's research findings and hypotheses within the framework of existing knowledge, the researcher is able to determine how applicable (generalizable) the emerging theory is to other settings and populations.

EVALUATING QUALITATIVE RESEARCH

In any research study, whether qualitative or quantitative in approach, questions pertaining to the reliability and validity of its finding must be addressed. In quantitative studies, the variables of interest are objectively defined at the outset of the investigation, followed by statistical testing of their relations as observed under highly controlled conditions. By contrast, qualitative researchers typically delay defining relevant variables and constructs until these are *discovered* during the course of the investigation. To a large degree, this discovery process is dependent on how well a researcher is able to see patterns in the data as they emerge, to code them into categories during data analysis, and to derive meaningful conclusions. As we have noted, just how deep and meaningful the conclusions are will be determined in part by the researcher's cognitive abilities and experiences (i.e., insight, judgment, knowledge, etc.). The outcome also will be affected by the quality of the evidence collected from other people—how reliable or biased their own perceptions and accounts of situations or events might be. For both of these reasons, qualitative research has been ". . . extensively criticized for the subjective nature of its methods" (Morse & Field, 1995, p. 140).

Let's examine further the traditional concepts of reliability and validity as applied by quantitative versus qualitative researchers. Within the tradition of quantitative research, reliability refers to the consistency of measuring instruments (whether human or mechanical in form) in yielding the same or highly similar results under similar conditions or circumstances (see Chapter 6). An abiding maxim of quantitative research is that establishing the reliability of a research finding is essential for determining its validity. If a research instrument fails to yield consistent results (is undependable for the intended purpose), the validity (accuracy) of the results cannot be presumed.

Because the measurements employed by qualitative researchers are generally more subjective in character than those used by quantitative researchers, reliability issues are often harder to address. Some qualitative methods are more amenable to establishing reliability estimates for research findings than others. For example, in many studies that employ conversational analysis or content analysis of message texts, **intercoder reliability** is often established by determining the consistency across coders. This can be accomplished by asking at least two people to code and classify the same material independently and then by examining the extent to which their judgments agree or disagree. In the absence of such a reliability check, the possibility that a given researcher has imposed his or her own views and interpretations on the material, which might differ substantially from those of other evaluators, cannot be ruled out. Should a research study extend over a lengthy time period, as is often the case in qualitative research, the researcher's internal consistency should also be evaluated. Such **intracoder reliability** can be established by comparing the coding judgments of text messages made by the same researcher on two or more occasions. Such an analysis can yield information as to whether a researcher's coding decisions are relatively stable or change over time. A statistical method that is often used for establishing coder reliability is Cohen's kappa coefficient (see Chapter 6).

As noted previously, reliability estimates can be difficult or not impossible to establish in some types of qualitative research. This is obviously the case in studies where the observations or measurements made by a researcher are not repeated. As Lindlof and Taylor (2002) point out, in many interview studies a given participant may be asked to answer a particular question only once. Furthermore, in interviews that involve the use of open-ended questions, the questions asked may vary widely across participants. Lindlof and Taylor point out that a more fundamental reason for the failure to establish reliability estimates is because they have little relevance to the fundamental belief held by qualitative researchers that the realities of the world are not static but are constantly changing. To the extent this is true, the researcher's own understanding must change accordingly so that "replication of results via independent assessment is neither practical nor possible" (p. 239).

What constitutes "good" interpretative practices in qualitative research in matters pertaining to validity is also debated (Hammersley, 1992). Whereas reliability refers to the consistency or stability of scientific findings, validity pertains to the accuracy or truth of such findings. As applied to qualitative research, Hammersley offered the following definition of validity: "An account is valid or true if it represents accurately those features of the phenomenon that it is intended to describe, explain or theorize" (p. 169). Not all qualitative researchers would find this definition acceptable, arguing that validity, like reliability, is not a static concept but is dynamically and reflexively linked to the assumptions, knowledge, cultural backgrounds, language, gender, location, and so on of "interpreters" who may hold very different views of reality (Altheide & Johnson, 1998).

To illustrate how different perspectives about truth and the nature of reality can vary among people viewing the same qualitative findings, Patton (2002) offers a humorous example from a story about three umpires discussing how they call balls and strikes:

"I call them as I see them," says the first.

"I call them as they are," says the second.

"They ain't nothing until I call them," says the third. (p. 553)

Evaluating Reliability and Validity

The paradigmatic differences in the criteria applied by qualitative and quantitative researchers in evaluating the reliability and validity of data extend well beyond "linguistic-hairsplitting" in their definitions of these terms. Indeed, many qualitative researchers contend that the standards used by quantitative researchers are inappropriate for judging the merit of qualitative research (Agar, 1986; Leininger, 1994; Lincoln and Guba, 1985; Merriam, 1995; Strauss and Corbin, 1998).

Acknowledging the paradigmatic differences in the evaluation criteria applied by qualitative and quantitative researchers, Leininger (1994) commented that it is inappropriate for qualitative researchers to simply "relabel" quantitative concepts of reliability and validity for adoption and use in qualitative evaluations. She argued that qualitative researchers should assert their autonomy by using evaluation criteria appropriate for their own research paradigm. Leininger identified six evaluation criteria that can be used in supporting and substantiating qualitative studies (see Box 10-1). She stated that each of these criteria are consistent with the goals of qualitative research. Furthermore, she emphasized the importance of a researcher understanding each of these criteria *prior* to initiating a qualitative study so that each criterion can be applied as the study proceeds rather than after the fact.

BOX 10-1

Six Evaluation Criteria of Qualitative Research Studies

1. **Credibility:** By observing and engaging participants over a prolonged period of time, a researcher accumulates knowledge of their lived-through experiences and how they think and feel about them. Credibility refers to the truthfulness, believability, and value of the researcher's findings in representing the "real world" as perceived by the participants.

2. **Confirmability:** A researcher seeks affirmation of his or her perceptions and ideas as these emerge throughout the study by periodically sharing findings with participants and seeking feedback to confirm that what the researcher has heard, seen, or experienced aligns with the views of the people being studied. Such *"feedback sessions"* or *"informant checks"* can help maximize the accuracy of findings by minimizing bias.

3. **Meaning-in-context:** This criterion focuses on the extent to which data make clear peoples' ideas, experiences, and understanding of life events within the holistic context of the environments or situations in which they live. This would include an effort to understand and interpret the actions, symbols, events, communication, and other human activities that take on meaning for people in the course of their lived experiences.

4. **Recurrent patterning:** This criterion refers to the extent to which repeated experiences, events, expressions, or activities that reflect identifiable patterns or sequences in people's lives have been documented. Numbers or percentages may be used for this purpose.

5. **Saturation:** Saturation refers a researcher becoming fully immersed in the phenomenon being studied in order to know and comprehend it as fully as possible. It implies that a researcher has performed what is sometimes called a "deep", "dense", or "thick" description in an exhaustive effort to extract as much meaning from the data as possible until no more can be said or told about the topic.

6. **Transferability:** This refers to the extent to which the finding from a qualitative study can be transferred to similar settings or circumstances without distorting the interpretations and inferences of the researcher. While the primary goal of qualitative research is not to produce generalizations but to advance "in-depth understanding" of phenomena, "It is the researcher's responsibility to establish whether this criterion can be met while preserving the original particular finds from a study." (Leininger, 1994) (p. 107).

Advancing Trustworthiness Through Triangulation

Ultimately, the underlying goals of qualitative research are not different from quantitative research. In both paradigms, researchers strive to achieve credible and verifiable results from their studies, although such studies might differ substantially in the means they employ to achieve these ends.

To advance the trustworthiness of their interpretations of data, qualitative researchers often use multiple observations, methods, and theories in an effort to "triangulate" their findings. *Triangulation* is a term adopted by qualitative researchers from the practices of land-surveyors to locate a particular point of interest at the intersection of the lines of two land-marks whose locations are known. The idea is that knowledge converging from two or more sources of data is more powerful in reducing bias than information gleaned from a single source. Patton (2002) identified several types of triangulation that researchers can use for verifying and enhancing the validity of their conclusions. The more relevant among these to our current discussion can be noted:

- *Methods triangulation* refers to procedures used for evaluating the consistency of findings obtained from different methods of data collection. For this purpose, a researcher can examine a variety of qualitative sources of data such as field notes, information from interviews, and the like in a search for converging meanings that might complement or support an explanation or theoretical interpretation. In addition to comparing one quali-tative method against another to boost the credibility of findings, data collected using qualitative methods can be triangulated with (compared to) data collected using quanti-tative methods. Patton notes that this is seldom a straightforward process because, as we have discussed, the methods of each paradigm are uniquely suited for asking some types of questions and not others. When these methods are combined in the same study, they are typically used in a ". . . complementary fashion to answer different questions that do not easily come together to provide a single, well-integrated picture of the situation" (p. 557). For examples of how this approach has been used in evaluating language and language intervention, see Culatta et al. (2003) and Brinton and Fujiki (2003).
- *Triangulation of sources* involves the comparison of data obtained from different sources within one data-gathering method to determine its consistency. For example, both a husband and wife might be interviewed independently to determine the extent of their agreement about aspects of their child's speech and language development. Their eval-uations also might be compared to a third party such as a teacher or a clinician. Still another application of this method includes checking the consistency of people's state-ments about the same thing over time.
- *Analyst triangulation* refers to efforts to reduce or overcome subjective bias and errors associated with an investigator working alone. Depending on the design of the study, instead of relying only on a single person, a team of observers might be deployed to work in the same field of study, or several interviewers might be used in the collection of data. Two or more researchers also might independently analyze and evaluate the collected data and compare their findings for purposes of verification. In some cases, where dependability of judgment is especially important, experts who are not associated with the study might be used to conduct an **external audit review.** When findings might be controversial or viewed with suspicion by one's professional peers, expert opin-ion sometimes can serve to increase the credibility of the results. Also, as we discussed, research findings can also be confirmed through collaborative efforts in which the peo-ple who served as the focus of the study are asked to review the research findings and provide their own perspectives about them. Cross-checking the interpretation of multi-ple assessors of the findings of a qualitative study is sometimes called **lamination.** Tetnowski and Franklin (2003) commented that the "layering on" of different levels of interpretation ". . . assists the assessor (as it does the qualitative researcher) in establish-ing a kind of 'disciplined subjectivity' " (p. 161).

Triangulation and other previously discussed evaluation criteria for qualitative research, provide essential tools for judging the reliability and validity of findings. The criteria are intended to ground such findings in ways that will be seen as fair, trustworthy, and sufficiently rigorous in implementation to promote credible new theories and understandings of people in the context of their daily lives. To the extent qualitative researchers are successful in achieving this goal, their methods will be increasingly adopted in a number of clinical fields including communication sciences and disorders.

RELEVANCE OF QUALITATIVE RESEARCH TO HUMAN COMMUNICATION

Simmons-Mackie and Damico (2003) review numerous qualitative studies from the social science literature and how such findings have helped to elucidate normal processes of human communication as well as the importance of such findings for clinical speech-language pathology. Damico and Simmons-Mackie (2003) and Tetnowski and Damico (2001) also cite a number of studies in which various therapeutic applications of such methods have been investigated. Tetnowski and Franklin (2003) identified several strengths of these methods, including their ability to:

- Promote holistic as opposed to fragmented approaches to assessment
- Focus on collecting "real data" in natural settings
- Engage in a rich description of the phenomenon of interest
- Adopt an open stance to data collection as opposed to allowing preconceived ideas to determine which behaviors to focus on and in what contexts
- Collect data from the perspective of the individual being assessed

The qualitative research principles discussed in this chapter complement each of these goals. In combination with or as an alternative to quantitative methodologies, they can help us to appreciate the rich substrate that underlies human communication skills (and how impairments in these skills can diminish the lives of people at many levels of operation—often in ways that cannot be numerically calculated. Apropos to this thought, while writing this chapter, the authors were reminded in a private communication from Professor Sally Maxwell of some comments by Albert Einstein:

> Not all things that matter can be counted . . . Not all things that can be counted matter.

SUMMARY

We began this chapter by describing qualitative research as an enterprise that is geared toward describing people's lives, social relationships, cultural values, thought processes, personal likes and dislikes, feelings and emotions, or how they function in various societal contexts. Unlike quantitative research methods that emphasize hypothesis testing and statistical testing under carefully controlled conditions, qualitative researchers are more concerned with deciphering the meaning underlying people experiences in the natural contexts in which they occur. Most often, the experiences they wish to investigate cannot be easily interpreted in numerical terms.

The methods commonly employed by qualitative researchers include such techniques as participant observation, interviews that employ open-ended questions, case studies, conversational analysis, and content analysis. Certain qualitative traditions or research perspectives that include ethnography, grounded theory, phenomenology, and discourse analysis guide these approaches. Examples from the literature were used to make clear how each of these traditions influence the approach taken to the collection, analysis, and interpretation of research findings.

We discussed the fact that the data analysis and interpretative techniques used in qualitative research are more subjective than in quantitative research and why this is a necessary outcome of their divergent philosophies and methods used in problem solving. The "styles" of data analysis used by qualitative researcher were reviewed as well as their methods for interpreting or "making sense" of data.

What constitutes "good interpretative practices" in qualitative research was discussed in relation to various criteria for evaluating the reliability and validity of findings. As noted, many qualitative researchers contend that the reliability and validity standards used by quantitative researchers are inappropriate for judging the merits of qualitative research. Several criteria appropriate for supporting and substantiating the findings of qualitative data were reviewed. The point was made that qualitative and quantitative researchers share the same goal of achieving credible and verifiable results from their studies, although the two methods differ substantially in the means they employ toward this end.

Finally, we commented that the qualitative methods discussed in this chapter are appropriate for the study of many problems that entail human communication, including communication disorders. Because of the versatility of qualitative methods in illuminating many aspects of people's lives in ways that cannot be understood through numerical calculations, the use of such methods is likely to increase in the future.

KEY TERMS

logical positivist position
qualitative methods
undisguised participant
disguised participant
deception
debriefing
emic perspective
etic perspective
ethnographic record
theoretical sampling

conversational analysis
texts
recording units
codes
code book
intercoder reliability
intracoder reliability
external audit review
lamination

SELF-LEARNING REVIEW

1. The _____ _____ _____ begins with a definite set of questions or hypotheses that, through the use of explicit and sustained systematic methods, are intended to discover the characteristics, interrelatedness, or causes of _____.

2. The primary emphasis in qualitative research is placed on attempts to understand the _____ underlying people's experience while rejecting the notion that the discovery of such meaning is dependent on the extent to which it can be interpreted in numerical terms.

3. The goal of qualitative research is to determine _____ the experience was like rather than measuring the _____ of such experience or _____ _____ _____ it occurred.

4. Qualitative research may be thought of as more _____ or holistic in orientation, with the ultimate goal of describing, understanding, and _____ the phenomenon under investigation.

5. Perhaps the most commonly used qualitative method, endemic to all forms of scientific research, is _____. The qualitative research model is more likely to adopt methods appropriate for _____ behavior in the _____ or setting in which the behavior naturally occurs.

6. Unlike quantitative researchers, who may contrive various conditions for observing behavior, the methods of the participant observer in qualitative research are said to be more _____ in essence.

7. The _____-_____ researcher pursues the deepest level of involvement and participation in the group. Such an observer participates as a genuine member of a particular group while collecting data given such a(n) _____ _____ .

8. The _____-_____ researcher pursues something less than full participation in the activities of the group, although an effort is made by the researcher to establish close and meaningful relationship with other group members.

9. While a(n) _____-_____ researcher might believe in the importance of observing the activities of a particular group from a(n) _____ perspective, he or she may refrain from adopting the group's core values or from participating extensively in its central affairs.

10. In the course of participant observation, the observer may assume either a(n) _____ or _____ role. One problem with the former role is that the researcher may be perceived as _____.

11. A means of avoiding the potential confounding influence of the participant observer on behavior is through the use of _____. In such a study, the other participants are unaware that their behavior is being observed for purposes beyond the goals and objectives of the group.

12. According to Rosnow and Rosenthal, deception is sometimes seen as permissible when (1) it is necessary to the _____ of the research; (2) the research is worth doing; (3) the physical and psychological risks to the participants are _____; and (4) adequate _____ will be carried out.

13. _____ is a research tradition that may be viewed as a systematized form of participant observation where the focus of the researcher is on describing the patterns of behavior that characterize a particular culture as these patterns occur in the natural setting.

14. A(n) _____ perspective is based on the way the members of a group see their world given their particular culture. A(n) _____ perspective is referred to as _____ _____. Adopting it, a researcher attempts to gain an objective view in order to make sense of one's own observations and derive theory based on a scientific explanation of reality.

15. Typically, three types of cultural information are of interest to ethnographers. Namely, (1) cultural _____ (how members of a culture act); (2) cultural _____ (what members of the culture make or create); and (3) cultural _____ (what members of the culture say to one another).

16. To obtain the most objective and reliable results from ethnographic studies, it is important to carefully establish a(n) _____ _____.

17. The predominant goal of a qualitative _____ _____ is to collect data through various methods in order to answer specific questions for scientific reasons. According to Ramhoj and de Oliveira, there are three elements that form the core of an effective

interview. They are (1) a(n) _____ consciousness of the form of the questioning; (2) a(n) _____ consciousness of interaction; and (3) a(n) _____ consciousness of what is said, as well as one's own interpretations of what is said.

18. A basis for differentiating qualitative from quantitative research interviews is the _____ _____ _____ imposed by the interviewer. It is largely the result of the _____ and _____ of the questions asked.

19. A possible disadvantage of a(n) _____ interview that uses _____-_____ questions is that the conversation may drift off track well beyond the interviewer's scope of interest.

20. A compromise between the extreme approaches of structured and unstructured interviews is the _____ interview. By using open-ended questions, both unstructured and _____ interviews allow for greater flexibility than structured interviews in exploring a(n) _____ range of topics while gaining a(n) _____ understanding of the respondents' own perspectives about a particular subject.

21. _____ theory is said to be the most widely used interpretative method in education, the health sciences, and communication. The term "_____" is meant to imply an inductive approach to theorizing in which the researcher begins a study with no presuppositions as to the nature of the phenomenon of interest.

22. The grounded theory method involves _____ analysis based on the researcher's observations or _____ data. A researcher using a grounded theory makes notes of and _____ meaningful patterns in the data as soon as such patterns emerge.

23. _____ sampling is designed to build from and add to the findings that emerge from an interview in order to construct as many categories as possible as these relate to a wide range of _____ areas.

24. _____ has its roots in philosophy that has been long occupied with such questions as "What is being?" and "How do we know what we know?"

25. The term _____ _____ denotes diverse research strategies that typically have as their goal describing a condition, incident, or process as believed to be relevant to one or more individuals.

26. From a theoretical perspective, _____ analysis views language not merely as a neutral and passive symbolic system for reflecting personal and social realities but as the linguistic building blocks for _____ such realities. The analysis tends to focus on structures of text and talk that _____ language or _____ meaning.

27. _____ analysis is sometimes referred to as the study of the "rules for turn taking"; it is perhaps better described as an account of "_____-_____-_____."

28. _____ analysis is a general term referring to several types of methods that can be used for gathering and analyzing data obtained from _____.

29. Krippendorff (1980) has identified five categories of _____ _____ that often serve as the focus for content analysis in research studies. They are _____ units, _____ units, _____ units, _____ units, and _____ units.

30. The four characteristics of content analysis include _____, _____, _____, and _____.

31. Because _____ coding procedures are empirically based, they tend to yield data that are generally reliable. On the other hand, _____ coding procedures tend to be less reliable because of their dependence on a researcher's knowledge of language and its social meanings.

32. Whatever the type of content analysis performed, three elements common to any kind of such analysis should include: (1) _____ what the unit of the analysis will be,

(2) _____ or developing a set of categories, and (3) _____ the rationale and illustrations to guide the coding of data into categories.

33. In content analysis, _____ term is the name of the cultural domain subjected to analysis, _____ terms are the names of smaller categories of things inside the domain, and _____ relationship includes the elements that define and lend meaning to persons, objects, events, and activities.

34. In analyzing qualitative data, a researcher commonly uses the following "styles" of data analysis. They are the _____ analysis style, _____ analysis style, _____ analysis style, and _____ analysis style. Whatever style of data analysis the researcher uses, Morse and Field have identified four key cognitive processes: _____, _____, _____, and _____.

35. In many studies that employ conversation analysis or content analysis of message texts, _____ _____ is often established by determining the consistency across coders. This can be accomplished by asking at least _____ people to code and classify the same material independently and then examining the extent to which their judgments agree or disagree.

36. _____ _____ can be established by comparing the coding judgements of text messages made by the _____ researcher on two or more occasions. A statistical method that is often used for establishing it is Cohen's _____ coefficient.

37. Leininger (1994) identified the six criteria that can be used in supporting and substantiating qualitative studies. They are _____, _____, _____, _____ patterning, _____, and _____ _____.

38. _____ _____ refers to procedures used for evaluating the consistency of findings obtained from different methods of data collection. _____ _____ _____ involves the comparison of data obtained from different sources within one data-gathering method to determine its consistency. _____ _____ refers to efforts to reduce or overcome subjective bias and errors associated with an investigator working alone.

39. Cross-checking the interpretations of multiple assessors of the findings of a qualitative study is called _____.

QUESTIONS AND EXERCISES FOR CLASSROOM DISCUSSION

1. Discuss three perspectives of qualitative research and how this approach is conceptually different from the logical positivist position of quantitative research.

2. Under what circumstances might qualitative research be a better option to problem solving than quantitative research? Provide an example of a clinically relevant problem.

3. Qualitative researchers talk about their desire to "get close to the data" by adopting an "insider perspective." What does this statement mean and why is their ability to achieve this goal critically important in meeting the standards and values of qualitative research?

4. Discuss three roles that a participant observer might play in relation to a qualitative research topic of your choosing. Which would be the "better" role given the problem you wish to investigate?

5. Why would a participant observer assume a disguised role as opposed to an undisguised role in a research study? What are the ethical considerations that should be evaluated in assuming such a role?

6. Under what conditions might the use of "deception" be justified, and what is the importance of "debriefing"?

7. Discuss the original meaning of the term "ethnography" and what it has come to signify in more recent years. What three types of cultural information are of interest to ethnographers?

8. Why do ethnographers believe that there is no single interpretative truth of culture? What is the value of an ethnographic record, and what forms might it take?

9. Describe three types of interview methods and the type most favored by qualitative researchers.

10. What three elements form the "core" of an effective interview? Describe your own understanding of each of these.

11. Describe the use of grounded theory as an interpretative method of qualitative research.

12. What form of logical analysis is employed in grounded theory, and how is it applied?

13. What field of study is the root of phenomenology, and how is this approach used by qualitative researchers?

14. Describe the case study method and the steps necessary for carrying out an ethnographic investigation using this design.

15. Describe the perspective of discourse analysis in qualitative research. What methodology is commonly used in conjunction with this approach, and what elements of interaction are its primary focus?

16. What kinds of texts can be "content analyzed"? Identify and describe five recording units. What measurement procedures can be used in conjunction with these units?

17. What "styles" of data analysis can be applied to qualitative research, and what cognitive processes underlie the use of these styles?

18. Why do quantitative researchers sometimes criticize qualitative researchers for their approach to data analysis and interpretation?

19. How do qualitative researchers justify their approach in accounting for the reliability and validity of findings?

20. Describe six criteria proposed by Leininger that can be used to support and substantiate qualitative studies.

21. What is the general purpose of "triangulation" in qualitative research, and what types of methods are used for this purpose?

22. What is the relevance of qualitative research to human communication and communication disorders?

23. Locate the following article on ASHA's Web site or through the resources of your library: Framework of Education: Perspective of Southeast Asian Parents and Head Start Staff, D. A. Hwa-Froelick and C. E. Westby, 2003, *Language, Speech, and Hearing Services in the Schools, 34:* 299–319.

   - Identify the qualitative research tradition or perspective of this study.
   - What research questions were pursued, and were the methods chosen to answer them appropriate within the context of the research tradition?
   - Was the research well designed and appropriate for the problem investigated? Justify your answer.
   - What methods were used to collect, analyze, and interpret the data? Were issues pertaining to reliability addressed in a thoughtful and appropriate manner?
   - What were the strengths and limitations of this study in your evaluation?

Analyzing Data: Descriptive Statistics

CHAPTER 11

CHAPTER OUTLINE

LEARNING OBJECTIVES

After reading this chapter, you should be able to identify, describe, or define:

- Various types of data and their measurement characteristics
- Organization of data values and how to construct a frequency distribution table
- Different shapes of frequency distributions
- The concept of central tendency and the methods for calculating the mean, median, and mode of a data set
- The meaning of statistical variability and the methods for calculating the range, variance, standard deviation, and skewness of a given data set
- The concepts and calculation of Tchebysheff's theorem and Pearsonian measures of skewness of a given distribution
- Characteristics of the standard normal distribution curve and how to calculate the percentile score and percentile rank of a given data set
- Methods used for calculating parametric and nonparametric correlation coefficients of a given data set
- Methods used for calculating the slope and y-intercept of a simple linear regression model
- Some of the clinical implication of correlation and regression methods

DESCRIPTIVE VERSUS INFERENTIAL STATISTICS

Two major categories of statistics are commonly identified as descriptive and inferential techniques. **Descriptive statistics** essentially involve what the term implies. They are used for classifying, organizing, and summarizing a particular set of observations in a manner convenient for numerically evaluating the attributes of *available* data. On the other hand, **inferential statistics** are designed to allow a researcher to generalize findings from a subset of subjects (sample) to a similar group (population) from which the subset was drawn. Making inferences about the probability of possible outcomes in the *future* is the main goal of inferential statistics. This chapter provides an overview of basic concepts and methods that underlie descriptive statistical techniques; this forms a preliminary basis for our discussion of probability theory and statistical inference in Chapter 12.

TYPES OF DATA

Before undertaking the analysis of a data set, it is important for a researcher to know the properties of the *measurement scale* used to represent the variables under study and the manner of their distribution. As we noted in Chapter 6, not all data collected share the same qualities. Enumerating the spoken opinions of jurors about "guilt" or "innocence" in a court of law is not the same as measuring the acoustic spectra of their various speech sounds. Data of the first type are best represented by *frequency counts*, whereas only the second type of data possesses properties amenable to formal mathematical operations.

Nominal and Ordinal Data

Frequency data are representative of the kind of distributions in which observations have been either (1) placed in certain categories or (2) arranged in a meaningful order.

As clinicians we may be interested in describing various individuals or groups within our work settings according to certain qualitative categories such as children/adults, male/female,

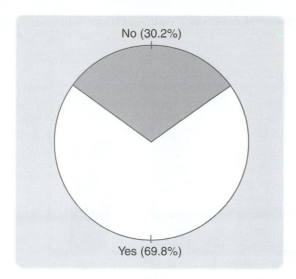

FIGURE 11-1

Desire to upgrade to AuD (*N* = 494)

Reprinted with permission from "Professional Education in Audiology," by D. Van Vilet, D. Berkey, M. Marion, and M. Robinson, 1992, ASHA, 34, p. 51.

normal/impaired, improvement/no improvement. Observations that can only be named and counted are called **nominal data.** Such data are sometimes described as **dichotomous** in nature because they involve "either/or" judgments about the presence or absence of a particular quality. Although such data may allow for some degree of numerical representation in terms of the frequency of the observations that fall within a given category, they have little or no quantitative meaning. For example, we can arbitrarily assign the number 1 to males and the number 2 to females as a means of designating the quality of gender. The reversal of the order of the two numbers would not make any difference in the type of gender involved.

Nominal data are commonly represented in various diagrams, charts, and graphs that illustrate the frequency or relative frequency (percentage) of observations that fall within certain categories or groups. For example, Figure 11-1 illustrates the use of a **pie chart** to summarize the results of a survey of audiologists in the state of California who were asked about their desire to upgrade their level of professional training to the Doctor of Audiology (AuD) degree. Data were coded simply in terms of the percentage of yes or no responses. The results of the study can be readily interpreted to mean that the most frequently expressed desire among the audiologists was to upgrade their level of professional competence through additional education.

To summarize the major characteristics of a nominal scale, it can be said that:

- It classifies without arranging data in a logical order.
- Data categories are mutually exclusive and exhaustive in that a numerical value can belong to one and only one category.

In addition to placing observations into particular categories, we often are interested in arranging them in relation to one another. Unlike the nominal scale, ordinal measurement involves the ranking or logical ordering of categories. For example, should one wish to explore factors contributing toward student decisions in selecting a particular graduate program, the study might be done by devising an appropriate questionnaire. Figure 11-2 illustrates the actual results of such a study completed by Lass and his associates (1995) in which students in communication disorders at several universities were asked to rank the importance of five factors in

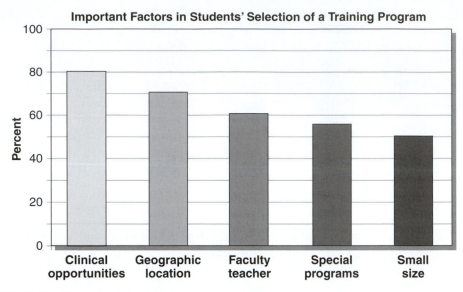

FIGURE 11-2   Illustration of a bar graph

Reprinted with permission from "Career Selection and Satisfaction in the Professions," by N. J. Lass, D. M. Ruscello, M. D. Pannbacker, G. F. Middleton, J. E. Schmitt, and J. E. Scheuerle, 1995, ASHA, 37, p. 50.

selecting a training program. A **bar graph** was used to depict the findings so that the percentage of students who considered a factor to be important was displayed on the vertical axis (ordinate), whereas the factors themselves were displayed along the horizontal axis (abscissa). Typically, in using a bar graph, the variable of interest (*X*) is scaled on the horizontal axis, whereas the tabulated results for the (*Y*) variable are depicted on the vertical axis. In terms of the results shown in Figure 11-2, the factor of clinical opportunities was ranked most important followed by geographic location, faculty/teachers, special programs, and small size, respectively.

Trend charts can also be used to illustrate frequencies or percentages of change in a data set arranged in a temporal or developmental order. In a study by Shriberg and his associates (1994) of speech sound normalization, ". . . the processes and behaviors by which speech becomes normally articulated over time," was examined in two groups of phonologically impaired children: those who "normalized" and those who failed to "normalize" sound productions over a one-year period. Figure 11-3 illustrates the results of this study for three categories of consonant comparisons from the *original* profiles of these children and ranked according to their developmental order of emergence (early, middle, or late). Visual inspection is suggestive of "intertwined trends" in the data for each category of sounds tested. The validity of this observation was supported by the failure of the researchers to uncover statistically significant differences between the normalized and nonnormalized groups so far as a specific profile of speech sound development that might otherwise have discriminated among them.

To summarize the features of an ordinal scale:

- Data are arranged in a distinctive order.
- Data categories are mutually exclusive and exhaustive.
- Data categories are logically ranked on the basis of the amount of the characteristic possessed.

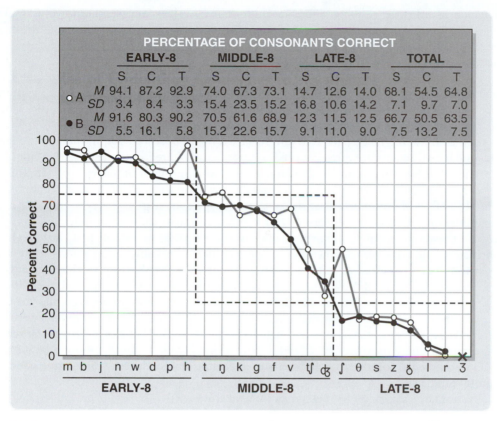

FIGURE 11-3   Consonants comparison for children who normalized (Group A) and for those who did not normalize (Group B)

Reprinted with permission from "Developmental Phonological Disorders II: Short-Term Speech-Sound Normalization," by L. D. Shriberg, J. Kwiatkowski, and F. A. Gruber, 1994, Journal of Speech Language Hearing Research, 37, p. 1139.

Interval and Ratio Data

An **interval scale** of measurement possesses two added features that are missing from the nominal and ordinal scale. Interval measurements are characterized by both equal intervals between data points and an arbitrary zero point. Whereas nominal and ordinal scales involve the measurement of **discrete variables,** those that can only be represented by integers (e.g., whole numbers 1, 2, 3, . . .), interval and ratio scales can represent **continuous variables** theoretically capable of taking on any value including fractional units of measurement (e.g., 1.2, 1.22, 1.23 . . .). In actual practice, continuous data are often rounded to the nearest appropriate value.

As noted in Chapter 6, interval scales contain an equal amount of distance between any two comparable points of measurement along the scale. Relating this fact to many tests involving psychological measurement, we could say, for example, that the difference between 90 and 100 points of intelligence is equal to the difference between 100 and 110 points of intelligence. Although some interval scales may contain an arbitrary zero point, such a designation is actually without meaning. Thus, in the same way that it would make no sense to conclude that the zero point on the Fahrenheit or Celsius scale means "no temperature," the idea of finding a living human without any measurable intelligence, personality, motivation, or language is equally implausible.

Nevertheless, it is often the case that both clinicians and researchers count the frequency of correct and incorrect responses without understanding whether or not the units of behavioral measurement are truly equal. For example, in the measurement of stuttering, one may not know the exact quantitative relation between one moment of stuttering and another, as these might be perceived and recorded by an observer. Yet, in many investigations, such disfluencies are often counted, averaged, and treated statistically as though they were the same. Similar dilemmas arise in the perceptual rating of other types of communication disorders where the assumption of equal intervals in the scale of measurement is tenuous. Too often, the summated ratings of a Likert-type scale (e.g., 1 = very mild, 2 = mild, 3 = moderate, 4 = severe, 5 = very severe) are treated statistically as though the intervals between these numerical values are equal when there may be no established basis for this conclusion. The principle to remember is that, so much as possible, assumptions about the applicability of any measurement scale should be consistent with the characteristics of the variables being measured. Unless equality between intervals can be determined, there is no basis for determining mathematical relations in a data set. Furthermore, regardless of the type of mathematical operations that might be permissible, good judgment must always be exercised in the interpretation of a data set. To conclude on the basis of a general test score that a person with a measured IQ of 100 is twice as intelligent as another individual having an IQ of 50 would do little to enlighten our understanding of specific differences in their cognitive abilities.

In summary, the major features of an interval scale are:

- It has distinctive and logically ordered data categories.
- Data categories are mutually exclusive and exhaustive.
- Comparable differences between any two points on the scale are equal regardless of their position along the line of data points.
- An arbitrary zero point in the scale denotes neither the presence of a starting point for measurement nor the absence of the quality being measured.

A ratio scale not only allows numbers to be classified, ordered, and linearly specified at equal intervals, but also contains an absolute zero starting point. Measurements of length or weight are examples of physical attributes that can be interpreted using the ratio scale. Starting at zero, we can say that four inches is exactly twice two inches; the same could be said for four pounds as compared to two pounds. Thus, ratio scales permit not only the addition and subtraction of measurement units but also their division and multiplication both as whole numbers or fractions. Although infrequently used in the study of most psychological phenomenon (Stevens, 1960), certain psychophysical procedures, as in the **method of constant stimuli,** do incorporate ratio scales of measurement. This particular method requires that several comparison stimuli be paired at random with a fixed standard. The observer is required to judge whether each comparison is greater or less than the fixed standard. Relevant examples of this procedure might include studies of loudness or pitch in which listeners have scaled these perceptions according to fractional units of measurement called the *sone* and *mel,* respectively.

ORGANIZING AND PORTRAYING DATA

A convenient way to begin summarizing an unorganized set of data is with a frequency table. Suppose we wish to determine the vocabulary comprehension of first-grade students in a particular elementary class using the Peabody Picture Vocabulary Test-Revised (PPVT-R) (Dunn & Dunn, 1981). The following is a sample of scores that might be found:

Peabody Picture Vocabulary Scores
(30 First-Grade Students)

100 87 84 100 98 89 67 115 80 76
72 70 91 110 94 79 86 91 93 105
83 89 92 84 100 81 105 86 95 80

As these scores are presently arranged, they provide the reader with little useful information. In order to make better sense out of this **ungrouped data,** the first step is to arrange the scores into a frequency table. Such a table provides a convenient format for summarizing and presenting data within a series of predetermined **class intervals** along with a tally of the number of observations that fall within each class interval.

An illustration of a frequency table and tally of the data shown above is provided in Table 11-1. Also illustrated are the class intervals into which the data are grouped. In deciding the size and number of class intervals to be used in an investigation, chief among the factors to consider is the *degree of detail* that is desired. Greater detail in describing data is provided by smaller class intervals, whereas larger **interval sizes** are useful should the investigator wish to achieve greater condensation of data. Thus, the selection of a particular class interval depends on the goals of the investigation and the purposes that the data will serve.

Generally, 10 to 20 class intervals are used to portray data in research studies. A convenient method for determining the size of a class interval is based on the following:

$$\text{Interval size} = \frac{\text{Highest score} - \text{lowest score}}{\text{Number of class intervals}}$$

Using this method, the **range** of scores (highest minus lowest) is simply divided by the number of class intervals selected for use. Given the raw ungrouped data that we listed previously, we note that the high score achieved on the PPVT was 115 and the low score was 67.

To find the interval size for about 10 class intervals, we would calculate the following:

$$\frac{115 - 67}{10} = 4.8$$

Rounding the decimal to the nearest place, the class interval size is 5.

In some cases, a researcher may wish to transform the data of a grouped frequency distribution into a **relative frequency distribution.** Such a distribution shows the percentage of scores that fall within each class interval. This can be determined by dividing the frequency of scores falling within each interval by the size of the sample (n) and multiplying the result by 100. For example, in the case of the frequency data found in Table 11-1, the results indicate that 6.67% of the cases achieved language scores falling within the 109.5 − 114.5 class interval.

TABLE 11-1   Frequency Distribution of Hypothetical Test Scores Obtained on the Peabody Picture Vocabulary Test-Revised (PPVT-R)

Class Interval	Midpoint	Tally	Frequency	Cumulative Frequency	Relative Frequency (in %)
114.5–119.5	117	I	1	1	3.33
109.5–114.5	112	I	1	2	3.33
104.5–109.5	107	II	2	4	6.67
99.5–104.5	102	III	3	7	10.00
94.5–99.5	97	II	2	9	6.67
89.5–94.5	92	IIIII	5	14	16.67
84.5–89.5	87	IIIII	5	19	16.67
79.5–84.5	82	IIIIII	6	25	20.00
74.5–79.5	77	II	2	27	6.67
69.5–74.5	72	II	2	29	6.67
64.5–69.5	67	I	1	30	3.33
59.5–64.5	62		0	30	0.00
			$n = 30$		100.00

Graphic Displays of Frequency Distributions

Previously, we noted that numerically discrete data, as found on nominal or ordinal scales, are often presented graphically by means of a bar chart with spaces between the horizontal bars to depict separate categories or different ranks. Continuous data, on the other hand, are often displayed as **histograms** that are much like bar charts in their visual appearance, except the data are partitioned along the abscissa (horizontal or x axis) so as to fall within several equal class intervals. As in the case of the bar graph, the frequencies of occurrence are shown on the ordinate (vertical or y axis).

Figure 11-4 is a histogram of the grouped data shown in Table 11-1. Scores are depicted in terms of the percentages of cases falling within a particular interval. The same data are also graphically portrayed in the form of a **frequency polygon.** The latter figure is a line graph that can be used in portraying all types of scaled measurements with the exception of nominal data. Such a graph is formed by connecting the midpoint of each class interval with straight lines.

Although graphs can be useful in providing a visual and readily interpretable summary of data, they can also convey a misleading impression if not thoughtfully constructed. Figure 11-5 contains two line graphs that represent an identical data set. Both reflect a decrement in the relative frequency of stuttering that might occur during the repeated oral reading of the same passage (adaptation effect) by a hypothetical group of stutterers. However, as can be seen, by extending the length of the ordinate and shortening the length of the abscissa in the second graph, the impression of a greater decline in the frequency of stuttering is thereby conveyed. Although there are no specific standards for constructing a graph according to a uniform size or scale, the graph should convey an impression that accurately reflects the data it is intended to represent. The following additional guidelines are offered for preparing and evaluating the utility of tables, charts, and graphs:

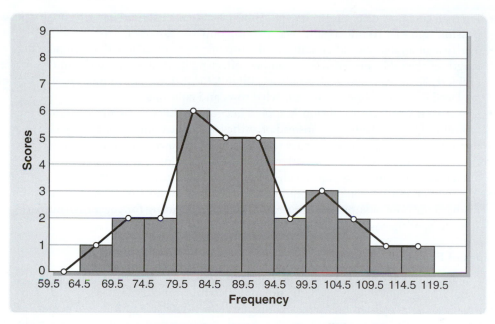

FIGURE 11-4   Histogram of hypothetical test scores on the Peabody Picture Vocabulary Test-Revised (PPVT-R)

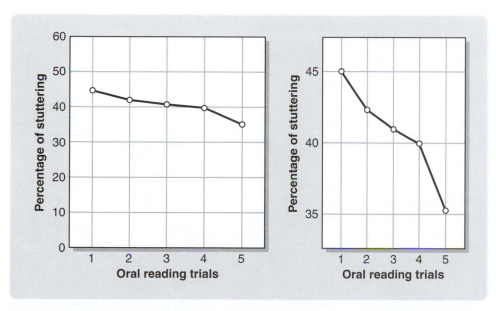

FIGURE 11-5   Two line graphs depicting the same hypothetical data: the percentage of stuttering during five oral reading trials

- First, all such means of displaying and summarizing data should be made as simple as possible and easy to understand by conveying only the essential facts.
- The title of a table should be stated at the top of a horizontal line that extends the length of the table, preceded by a number reflecting its consecutive order in the article (Table 1, 2, 3, etc.) or book chapter (e.g., Table 1.1, 1.2, 1.3, etc.). Numerical information is placed below this line in clearly labeled rows and columns.
- The same need for clarity obviously applies in constructing graphs, in which titles are typically placed at the bottom instead of at the top of the figure. This is a logical placement because, unlike tables that are read from the top down, graphs are usually read from the bottom to the top. As with tables, figures should be consecutively numbered, and all variables depicted must be identified using distinctive symbols, legends, and keys.
- All such methods of data presentation should be self-explanatory, while serving the primary purpose of supplementing rather than substituting for cogent narrative descriptions of the research findings.

Shapes of Frequency Distribution Scores

Histograms and polygons are used, in part, to gain some idea of the shape of a frequency distribution. As shown in Figure 11-6, the **normal distribution curve** is bell shaped with data points symmetrically distributed along a horizontal line to the left and right of center. Several departures from this normal shape are also shown. Asymmetrical distributions are said to be **skewed.** A **negatively skewed distribution** is one in which the tail points to the left (negative)

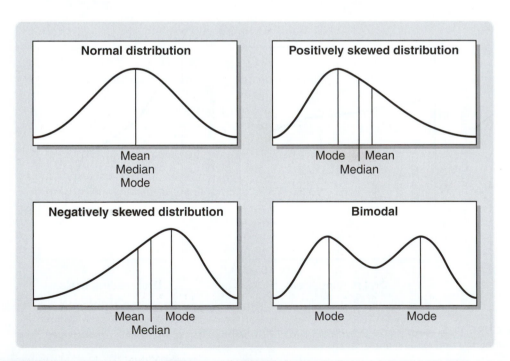

FIGURE 11-6 Various shapes of frequency distribution curves depicting relationships among different measures of central tendency

side of the curve, signifying that the proportion of high scores in the distribution is greater than for low scores. Conversely, a **positively skewed distribution** is found in cases in which the tail points to the right (positive) side because the frequency of low scores greatly outnumbers that of high scores in the distribution. A **bimodal distribution** curve characterized by the presence of two modes is suggestive of two distinct populations. In cases in which a distribution is not homogeneous, serious misinterpretations of data are possible. For example, if we set out to test the knowledge of graduate students at a particular college or university about certain communication disorders, and this population was made up partly of students with an undergraduate background in that field and partly of students having no academic preparation, a bimodal curve might result.

As we shall see in Chapter 12, populations that lack homogeneity in a distribution can limit or contra-indicate the application of some types of inferential statistical procedures to the analysis of data sets.

CENTRAL TENDENCY OF DATA

In representing frequency distributions numerically, researchers are commonly interested in the extent to which scores cluster around the center of a distribution.

Measures of the Center

Measures of central tendency that represent the average size of a frequency distribution include the **mean** (the arithmetic average value), the **median** (the midscore value), and the **mode** (the most frequently occurring value).

Suppose a researcher is interested in comparing the performance of five groups of subjects (A, B, C, D, E) on a test of auditory sequential memory (ASM). Assume that the following scores were obtained (higher scores indicate better memory performance).

```
A    7,   5,   4,    4
B    6,   8,   10,   4,   9,   5,   8,   6
C    3,   7,   9,    5,   6
D    9,   10,  8
E    1,   0,   4,    4
```

To answer such questions as "Does Group A have better memory than Group B?" or "Which group shows the lowest score?" data values representing the performance of each group would be needed. This one numerical measure, called a measure of **central tendency,** can be used to represent where a particular group of scores in a distribution "stands out." As mentioned previously, there are three different measures of central tendency (mean, median, and mode) that can be used to represent what is sometimes called the "center of gravity" in a data set. The most important thing to determine is which measure can *best be used* for this purpose.

The Mean

The mean is known as the arithmetic average of a set of data values. The formula for calculating the mean is simply the ratio of the total sum of data values to the total number of subjects, denoted by N (population size) or n (sample size). Symbolically, the general formula for the mean is:

$\mu = \Sigma X / N$ (population mean)
$\bar{X} = \Sigma X / n$ (sample mean)

where Σ (sigma)   represents "the total sum of"
     X represents "score" or "data value"
     μ (mu)   specifies the mean from the population of scores or data values
     $\bar{X}$ (X bar)   specifies the mean from the sample of scores or data values

For purposes of calculation, there is no difference between μ and $\bar{X}$. Thus, the mean for Group D is given by $(9 + 10 + 8) / 3 = 27 / 3 = 9$.

The mean can also be calculated from *grouped* data by dividing the product of the midpoint of the class interval and its corresponding frequency by the sample size (n). Let us now illustrate this particular calculation using the midpoint values for PPVT-R scores shown in Table 11-2. The steps in calculating the mean of our grouped data are as follows:

Step 1.   Construct a table to include the midpoint (X), frequency (f), cumulative frequency (cf), and the product of X and f ($X \cdot f$) (see Table 11-2).

Step 2.   Enter the appropriate values into the standard formula for calculating the mean of grouped data. The formula is given by:

$$\bar{X} = \frac{\sum (X \cdot f)}{n}$$

Hence, after entering the appropriate values, i.e., 1 and 2695 ($\Sigma X \cdot f = 2695$) and $n = 30$, into the above formula,

$$\bar{X} = \frac{2695}{30} = 89.83 \text{ (rounded)}$$

As a general rule, the mean is preferred over other measures of central tendency because of its greater accuracy and reliability in representing a data set and its suitability for a wider range of arithmetic computations. However, two qualifications to this statement are important to consider in the evaluation of any data set. First, the *normal* shape of the distribution about its center ought to be *symmetrical* so that the mean closely approximates the values obtained for other measures of central tendency as discussed below. As noted previously, if the distribution is relatively *skewed* in either a positive or negative direction, the mean may not be a good reflection of central tendency because of the biasing effects of extreme scores. Second, it is important to consider the scale of measurement as appropriate for a particular data set. The mean is best applied in cases where the data can be assumed to have at least interval characteristics that are subject to quantitative manipulation.

The Median

The median is the midvalue in a distribution of scores. The easiest way to identify the median is to rearrange all data values in order of magnitude (from smallest to largest). One must be sure to list all data values even though some values may repeat more than once. Ordering Group C's scores gives:

     3,   5,   6,   7,   9

Next, one must determine whether or not n is odd. When n is odd, there exists a single value in the middle of the distribution. Symbolically, the location of the median is given by the $((n + 1) / 2)$ number from the left. Therefore, $(5 + 1) / 2 = 6 / 2 = 3$rd number from the left, or the median of 6 for this distribution. When n is even, the location of the median is expressed as half way between the $(n / 2)$ number and the $((n/2) + 1)$ number from the left.

TABLE 11-2   The Product of Hypothetical Midpoint Values and Their Corresponding
Frequencies on the Peabody Picture Vocabulary Test-Revised (PPVT-R)

X	f	cf	Xf
117	1	1	117
112	1	2	112
107	2	4	214
102	3	7	306
97	2	9	194
92	5	14	460
87	5	19	435
82	6	25	492
77	2	27	154
72	2	29	144
67	1	30	67
Σ	30		2695

For example, should we wish to calculate the median of Group A's distribution, all data values must first be arranged from smallest to largest, yielding:

4,   4,   5,   7

Next, we determine two numbers that correspond to the $(n / 2) = (4 / 2) = $ 2nd and the $((n / 2) + 1) = $ 3rd from the left. They are 4 and 5, respectively. Next, we average 4 and 5, or $(4 + 5) / 2 = 4.5$. The median is 4.5, although 4.5 did not appear in the original data set.

As in the case of the mean, it is also possible to calculate the median from grouped scores shown in Table 11-1. The steps for this calculation are as follows:

Step 1.   Find: (1) the higher exact limit of the interval containing $n \cdot (.50)$, denoted by II, (2) the cumulative frequency of the interval containing $n \cdot (.50)$, denoted by cf_b, (3) the frequency of the interval above the one containing $n \cdot (.50)$, denoted by f_i, and (4) the width of the class interval, denoted by w. In our case, $n \cdot (.50) = 30 \cdot (.50) = 15$, II $= 89.5$, $cf_b = 19$, $f_i = 5$, and $w = 5$ were found.

Step 2.   Enter the appropriate values shown in step 1 into the standard formula for calculating the median of grouped data. The formula is given by:

$$\text{Median} = \text{II} + \left[\frac{cf_b - n \cdot (.50)}{f_i} \right] \cdot w$$

Thus, after entering the appropriate values in step 1 into the above formula, the median is given by:

$$\text{Median} = 89.5 + \left[\frac{19 - 15}{5} \right] \cdot 5 = 93.5$$

Because the median is less sensitive than the mean to the biasing influence of extreme scores in a data set, it is best used when a distribution is known to be asymmetrical or when its shape is otherwise unknown. The median is particularly suitable for scales of measurement having ordinal characteristics and when the validity of assumptions about equality in the size of the intervals between data points is questionable.

The Mode

The mode is constituted by the data value in a set of scores that occurs most frequently. By definition, the mode is represented by a number that must occur more than once. The mode could represent more than one data value if (1) there is a tie, and (2) each value occurs at least twice. Referring to the ASM scores previously listed for Group A, the data value 4 occurred most frequently (twice). Therefore, 4 is the modal score for this distribution. On the other hand, there is a tie for the most frequently occurring value in the distribution of scores of Group B. Two values, 6 and 8, occurred equally often and, in this case, both values are identified as modes. Thus, although it is common for most distributions to contain exactly one mode, it is possible for more than one mode to exist. A distribution having one mode is called **unimodal.** A distribution having two modes is called **bimodal.** For groups C and D, no mode can be said to exist because no value occurred more than once in either case.

As an index of central tendency, the mode often provides a crude and limited representation of the characteristics of a distribution as compared to the mean and median. This is true because, in some cases, the mode may be the lowest or highest value in a distribution. For example, the following three distributions have the exact same mode, namely 6.

Group F	6,	6,	7,	8,	9,	10
Group G	0,	1,	2,	3,	6,	6
Group H	6,	6,	25,	26,	27,	28

As can be seen, the differences in the magnitude of the scores in each group are quite large and not well represented by the mode. Furthermore, because the mode is extremely sensitive to fluctuations in the distribution, different samples from the same population can have widely divergent modes. For example, in the case of Group H, if one of the 6's is changed to 28, the mode likewise becomes 28, swinging from the extreme low end to the high end of the distribution.

As the weakest measure of central tendency, the use of the mode is restricted to nominal scales of measurement and is seldom reported except in association with other indices of central tendency.

VARIABILITY OF DATA

In the nineteenth century, the German mathematician Carl Gauss formulated the **"law of errors,"** which holds that the majority of repeated measurements made on the same subject *normally* cluster about the center of a distribution to form a bell-shaped curve with progressively fewer values dispersed symmetrically toward the tail ends on the left and right of center. A distribution that conforms to this shape is suggestive of good measurement reliability. If measurements are made on a number of individuals, they can be said to constitute a homogeneous group provided there is little variability among scores. More specifically, the scores should follow a predictable bell-shaped pattern of distribution with the majority of values clustering in the center.

Measures of Variability

Three important measures of variability that describe the shape of the distribution include (1) the range (the difference between the highest value and the lowest value), (2) the **variance** (the mean of the squared deviation from the mean), and (3) the **standard deviation** (the square root of the variance). The range is the difference (span) between the lowest and highest value in a distribution. However, like the mode, the range is extremely sensitive to fluctuations in a data set because, with the exception of the two extreme scores (lowest and the highest values), all other scores in the distribution are completely neglected. Therefore, another measure of dispersion is needed that can take into account the magnitude of *every* value of a distribution, not just the two extremes.

Mathematically, this measure of variance must calculate the *deviation* (the difference between each data value and the mean) and the *mean of the deviations*. For a population, the mean of these deviation scores is expressed as $\Sigma(X - \mu) / N$. For Group D, $\Sigma(X - \mu) / N$ is given by:

$$\frac{(9-9)+(10-9)+(8-9)}{3} = 0 \text{ (because } \mu = \frac{9+10+8}{3} = 9)$$

In fact, the sum of the deviations from the mean is always equal to zero. This is because the values above the mean must have positive deviations and the values below the mean must have negative deviations, resulting in a kind of mathematical cancellation effect. This problem surely affects the status of the mean as the "center of gravity" for the distribution. As a result, a solution is required to deal with this zero-sum deviation to confirm the fact that: *The more spread out the distribution, the larger the mean deviation from the mean.*

A solution is found in squaring each deviation from the mean and summing these squared deviation scores. The result is called the *mean squared deviation from the mean,* symbolically expressed as $\Sigma (X - \mu)^2 / N$, or simply called *variance* (denoted by σ^2). Therefore, with the data values of Group D,

$$\sigma^2 = \Sigma(X - \mu)^2 / N = \frac{(9-9)^2 + (10-9)^2 + (8-9)^2}{3} = \frac{2}{3} = .67$$

where σ^2 represents *population variance* and is pronounced as "sigma square."

The formula for sample variance, denoted by s^2, is given by:

$$s^2 = \frac{\Sigma(X - \bar{X})^2}{n-1} \text{ when } n \leq 30 \text{ and } s^2 = \frac{\Sigma(X - \bar{X})^2}{n} \text{ when } n > 30.$$

The variance is quite useful for ratio measures but has one disadvantage. Large deviations in values furthest from the mean may outscore small deviations in values nearest to the mean. Squaring a large deviation would result in a disproportionately greater value than squaring a small deviation. It is possible to overcome (or compensate for) the disadvantage associated with the use of variance as a measure of dispersion by simply taking the square root. The resulting value is called the *standard deviation,* denoted by σ (for a population) or s (for a sample). The standard deviation is sometimes denoted by the symbols SD in describing the spread among a set of measurements about the mean. The standard deviation for the population and sample is calculated by one of the following formulas:

$$\sigma = \sqrt{\Sigma(X - \mu)^2 / N} = \sqrt{\sigma^2} \text{ (population } SD)$$

$$s = \sqrt{\frac{\sum(X - \bar{X})^2}{n-1}} \quad \text{(sample } SD \text{ when } n \leq 30)$$

$$s = \sqrt{\frac{\sum(x - \bar{x})^2}{n}} \quad \text{(sample } SD \text{ when } n > 30)$$

The standard deviation is useful in indicating the position of data values that are this "mean distance" away from the mean μ or $\bar{X}$. However, the most practical use of the standard deviation can be observed in relation to a **normal distribution curve,** which has a characteristic bell shape (see Figure 11-7). In such a distribution, approximately 68.26% of the data values lie within one standard deviation from the mean, denoted by $(\mu - \sigma, \mu + \sigma) = .68$, 95.44% of the data values lie $\pm 2\sigma$ from the mean μ, denoted by $(\mu - 2\sigma, \mu + 2\sigma) = .9544$, and 99.74% of the data values lie $(\mu - 3\sigma, \mu + 3\sigma)$.

In general, regardless of the shape of the distribution, the standard deviation is the key measure of dispersion.

Tchebysheff's Theorem

According to **Tchebysheff's theorem,** for any set of data, at least $100 \cdot [(1 - (1 / K^2)]\%$ of the data values are lying within K standard deviations of the mean, where $K > 1$.

Although many frequency distributions have different patterns of variation, it is true of all sets of data values that at least $100 \cdot [(1 - (1/2)^2)]\% = 75\%$ are lying within 2 standard deviations and at least $100 \cdot [(1 - (1/3)^2)]\% = 88.89\%$ are lying within 3 standard deviations from the mean. The importance of Tchebysheff's theorem is that it helps guide us to where the major portion of the data values are located and how much variation there is in a set of data. A small standard deviation indicates that the data values are clustered near the mean. A large standard deviation indicates that the data values are widely dispersed about the mean.

Coefficient of Variation

To determine whether a set of data values has much variation (spread) or whether a number of measurements are precise, the ratio of the mean to the standard deviation is calculated. This value, called the **coefficient of variation,** is determined by the following:

$$\text{Coefficient of variation} = 100 \cdot (S/\bar{X})\%$$

For example, the coefficient of variation of the set $\bar{X} = 10$ and $S = 0.3$ is $100 \cdot (0.3/10) = 3\%$. This data set has very little variation. On the other hand, for the set $\bar{X} = 10$ and $S = 3$, the coefficient of variation is determined to be $100 \cdot (3/10) = 30\%$, suggesting that this latter data set is relatively varied.

Pearsonian Measure of Skewness

Previously, four different shapes of frequency distribution curves were shown in Figure 11-6. In a *normal* distribution, the mean, median, and mode are all equal. In a *positively skewed* distribution, the mean is the largest of the three measures of central tendency. This distribution occurs when the extreme items are large in value compared to the vast majority of other data values. A distribution called a *negatively skewed* distribution contains some data values that are significantly smaller than the vast majority of all data values, that is, the mean is the smallest of the three measures of central tendency; the mode is the point of largest frequency because it is unaffected by extreme data values, and the

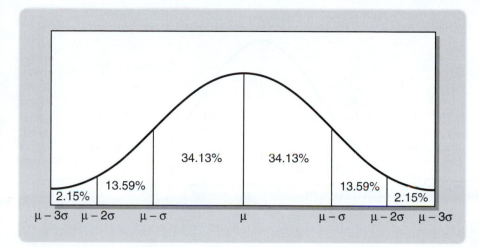

FIGURE 11-7

Areas under the standard normal curve

median, less affected by extreme data values, is located between the mode and mean. Karl Pearson, a notable statistician in the mid nineteenth century to early twentieth century, found that the median is generally located about two-thirds of the distance from the mode to the mean in moderately skewed frequency distributions. Mathematically, such a measure, called the **Pearsonian measure of skewness** (denoted by S_k), is calculated as follows:

$$S_k = \frac{3(\bar{X} - M_d)}{S}$$

where S_k = Pearsonian measure of skewness
$\bar{X}$ = the mean from the sample
M_d = the median
S = the standard deviation from the sample

If $S_k > 0$, then the distribution is positively skewed, whereas it is negatively skewed if $S_k < 0$. When $S_k = 0$, the distribution is normal. Generally, S_k is used to (1) describe the shape of a frequency distribution, (2) select the most representative measure of central tendency, and (3) measure the lack of normality in a given frequency distribution. In our example of the distribution of the hypothetical data values on PPVT-R, we can derive the value of S_k as follows:

$$S_k = \frac{3(89.83 - 85.5)}{15} = .866$$

where $\bar{X} = 89.83$, $M_d = 85.5$, and $S = 15$.

Therefore, we can conclude that the distribution shown in Figure 11-4 is positively skewed.

Calculating Standard Scores and Percentile Ranks

The standard score, denoted by z, refers to the number of standard deviation units away from the mean that its raw-score (X) equivalent lies. Standard scores are very useful in comparing raw scores in different distributions of the same shape. Raw scores (X) can be converted into

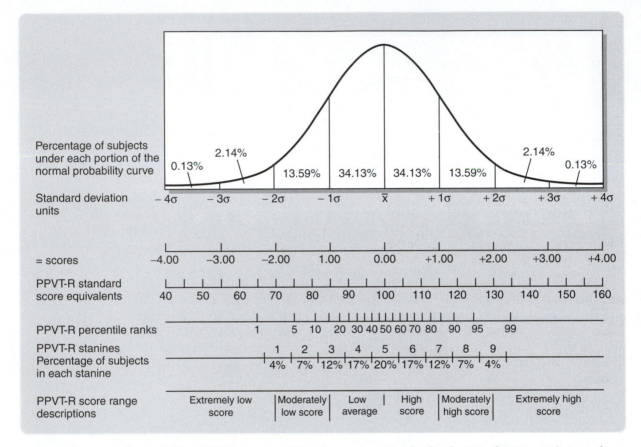

FIGURE 11-8   Interchangeability of different types of deviation norms when the distribution of raw scores is normal, or has been normalized, as in the case of the PPVT-R

Reprinted with permission from Peabody Picture Vocabulary Test-Revised, *by L. Dunn, and L. Dunn, 1981, Circle Pines, MN: American Guidance Service, p. 21.*

standard scores (*z*) and expressed as the number of standard deviation units away from the mean through the following formula:

$$z = (X - \mu) / \sigma$$

A positive *z*-score indicates that the raw score is above the mean, and a negative *z*-score indicates that the raw score is below the mean. For example, given the standardization data of the PPVT-R, it is known that the national mean score (μ) for this test is 100 and the standard deviation (σ) is 15 (see Figure 11-8).

Suppose a randomly selected subject has a PPVT-R score *above* the mean of 100, with a score of 124. What is his/her *z*-score? Such a score can be calculated as follows:

$$z = (124 - 100) / 15 = 1.6$$

The result indicates that the subject's score is 1.6 standard deviations above the mean. For ease of interpretation, it is common practice in the standardization of tests to convert standard scores into **percentile ranks.** A percentile rank is simply a number on a particular measurement scale at or below which a given percentage of the remaining distribution of scores can be found. Percentiles range from 0 to 100 with 50 being the median score in the distribution. For example, the 45th percentile in a distribution of scores would be interpreted as the score at or below which 45% of all scores in the distribution falls. Percentile ranks are highly useful in interpreting the results of many clinical tests and measuring instruments because they are readily interpretable indices of an individual's performance.

How do we determine the percentile rank for a raw score on the PPVT-R of 124, when the corresponding $z = 1.6$? To answer this question, three important properties of a normal distribution must be understood. These are as follows:

1. The entire area under the curve is 100%.
2. The normal distribution curve is symmetrical around the center: $z = 0$.
3. The percentage of data values between the mean and any given z-score in a normal distribution can be derived through a z-table like that found in Appendix A-1-1. Such a table consists of two major components, namely a z-score and the percentage of a distribution that falls between $z = 0$ and some specific positive value for z. This area is called a **table area** as described more fully in relation to our example.

As we can see in Figure 11-9 (A), a z-score of 1.6 appears on the positive side of a normal curve. The shaded area of the graph is the percentage of data values derived from the table for z. This was determined by consulting Appendix A-1. A portion of a z-table applicable to our example is shown in Figure 11-9 (B). More specifically, the percentage of the distribution that falls between $z = 0$ and $z = 1.6$ was derived by locating:

1. The number in the left-hand column of the z-table that contains the same units and tenth's digits as 1.60 (1.6).
2. The number that has the same hundredth's digit which, in the case of our example, is .00.
3. The intersection of the row containing 1.6 and the column .00. This number is .4452, or 44.52%.

In order to determine the percentile rank for the z-score in question, we then add 50% of the area to the left of $z = 0$, yielding 44.52% + 50% = 94.52%. The result of our example can be interpreted to mean that approximately 94.52% of all PPVT-R scores fell at or below a score of 124.

To use another example, suppose we wish to determine the percentile rank for a PPVT-R score falling *below* the mean of 100, say a score of 85. First, we must convert the raw score X of 85 into the corresponding z-score by the formula:

$$z = (85 - 100) / 15 = -1$$

Second, we draw the diagram of $z = -1$ in order to better conceptualize the data in graphic terms (see Figure 11-10).

Third, we find the table area. As noted previously, this area is defined as the percentage of a distribution that falls between $z = 0$ and a given z-score. In the case of our example, the table area is the percentage of the distribution that falls between the mean ($z = 0$) and ($z = -1$). We subtract it from 50% with the following result:

$$50\% - 34.13\% = 15.87\%$$

From this example, we can conclude that 15.87% of all PPVT-R scores fell at or below the score of 85.

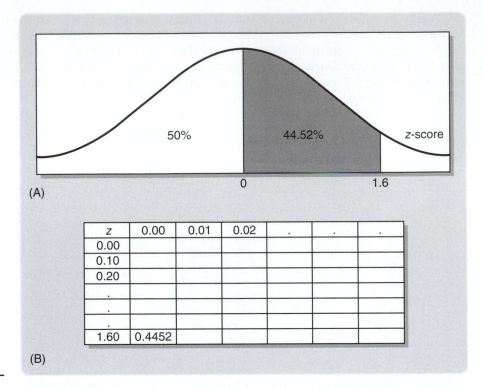

FIGURE 11-9

(A) Interpreting a z-score under the normal curve, and (B) finding the corresponding area from a portion of a z-table

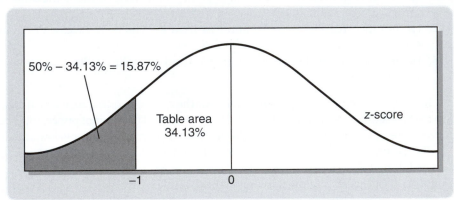

FIGURE 11-10

The area under the normal curve that falls at or below $z = -1$

Calculating Proportions from Two Standard Scores

Suppose we wish to calculate the percentage of all PPVT-R scores falling between two raw scores in a distribution. In illustrating how to accomplish this task, we will use two examples.

Case 1.   In the first case, imagine that we have two raw scores, with one score, say a score of 85, falling below the mean of 100 and the other, say a score of 130, falling above the mean. Initially, in order to solve this problem, we must calculate the corresponding z-scores of 85 and 130, namely -1 and 2, respectively. When two z-scores are on *different* sides of the mean, such as the area between $z = -1.0$ and $z = 2.0$, we add the two table areas (34.13% for $z = 0$

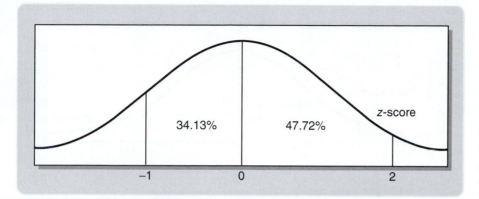

FIGURE 11-11

The area of the normal curve that falls between $z = -1$ and $z = 2$

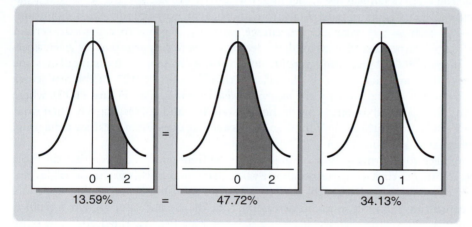

FIGURE 11-12

The area of the normal curve that falls between $z = 1$ and $z = 2$

and $z = -1.0$; 47.72% for $z = 0$ and $z = 2.0$). (See Figure 11-11.) The area between $z = -1$ and $z = 2$ can be calculated as follows:

$$34.13\% + 47.72\% = 81.85\%$$

Hence, we can see that 81.85% of all PPVT-R scores fall within the interval of 85 and 130.

Case 2.   Suppose that we have two raw scores, let us say that one of these scores is 115 and the second score is 130. In this case, both of these scores are *above* the mean of 100. First, we must calculate the corresponding z-scores of 115 and 130. This results in z-scores of 1 and 2, respectively. When two z-scores are on the same side of the mean, we subtract the smaller table area from the larger table area. For example, in order to determine the percentages of $z = 1.0$ and $z = 2.0$, we must first consult the z-table in Appendix A-1-1 to find the table area of $z = 1.0$ (34.13%) and the table area of $z = 2.0$ (47.72%). Next, we subtract 34.13% from 47.72% to find the percentage. The results of this calculation are graphically displayed in Figure 11-12.

It can be seen that 13.59% of all PPVT-R scores fall within the interval of 115 and 130. Note that the same technique is used in determining the percentage of data values between two negative z-scores.

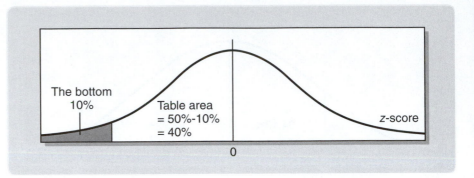

FIGURE 11-13

The area under the normal curve that represents the bottom 10% of the distribution

Calculating Raw Scores from Proportions

In constructing a test, a clinical researcher might wish to know the specific score that separates or "cuts off" a category of individuals from another category of individuals. For example, we might wish to use a certain percentage as a cutoff score to categorize certain speech-language-hearing disorders as mild, moderate, or severe. Suppose you are given a certain percentage of PPVT-R scores and asked to solve for the raw score that distinguishes one such category from another. Given our knowledge that the bottom 10% of the test scores obtained on the PPVT-R falls within the *moderately low score range* (see Figure 11-13), where the mean (μ) and standard deviation (σ) of the test were 100 and 15, respectively, then what is the cutoff raw score for this range? In order to answer this question, first draw a diagram, like that illustrated in Figure 11-13.

Next, we need to determine the table area. From the figure, it can be seen that the table area is 40%. In order to find the corresponding z value that contains this particular table area, we will need to look up the closest table area to 40% in a z-table like that found in Appendix A-1-1. By consulting the table, one can determine that the closest value to 40% (.4000) is .3997, or 39.97%. This value corresponds to a z-score of 1.28. Because the desired raw score appears on the negative side, $z = 1.28$ must be interpreted as $z = -1.28$. Next, substitute all numbers into the appropriate places of a z-score formula and solve for X:

$$-1.28 = (X - 100) / 15$$
$$X = (-1.28) \cdot 15 + 100$$
$$= 80.8$$

Therefore, given these data, the hypothetical cutoff score for the *moderately low score range* of the PPVT-R is 80.8. It is noteworthy that this particular value closely approximates the actual cutoff score for the identical range on the PPVT-R test.

DESCRIBING RELATIONSHIPS AND PREDICTING OUTCOMES: CORRELATION AND REGRESSION

Thus far, several descriptive statistical methods have been reviewed that are useful in summarizing observations on a single variable, or *univariate* characteristic of a sample. However, it is often the case that a researcher wishes to describe or predict the relationship between two variables (**bivariate relationship**) or more (**multivariate relationship**). This can be accomplished by means of correlation and regression techniques.

Although the overall goals of correlation and regression methods bear close resemblance, these techniques must be distinguished as they apply to different types of sampling procedures and to the definition of variables in an experiment. Generally, we can say that if the main goal of an experiment is to simply examine the association between two or more variables without regard to distinguishing between the independent and dependent variable, then correlational methods are used. If the specific goal is to predict one variable from another, then regression analysis methods are the better choice.

To illustrate some of the distinguishing features of correlation and regression more clearly, suppose we obtain two sets of observations on a group of children, in which values of X represent scores on a language comprehension measure, such as hearing vocabulary, and Y reflects their performance on some standardized test of intelligence. Suppose further that we have no preconceived idea about the causal relations among these variables such that X is believed to influence the direction of Y or vice versa. In other words, for any individual in our sample, values of X and Y are merely assumed to represent joint or "coexisting" events that are in no way controlled or manipulated by the experimenter. In such a case, values of X and Y are *not* selected in advance of an experiment but are allowed to vary freely as inherently found in a sample of n individuals drawn from some population.

In contrast to correlational problems of the type just described, the use of regression techniques requires that the independent variable be selected and defined *prior to* an experiment. If the question asked concerns the degree to which Y (the dependent or criterion variable) can be predicted from X (the independent or predictor variable), then **simple linear regression** analysis can be used. Thus, in the case of our example just noted, we might inquire about the extent to which certain measured levels of vocabulary comprehension are predictive of IQ. Had additional language measures been used as predictor variables, **multiple regression** methods (see Appendix A-2) might also be incorporated given the aims of a more comprehensive analysis. The concepts and statistical applications underlying correlation and regression problems are discussed in greater detail in the following sections.

Correlation

Correlational problems pertain to observations made under conditions in which an observed change in one variable appears to be associated with a concomitant change in another. Such variables form a joint distribution of data sets that are said to be *mutually dependent* or related. The following properties of correlational statistics are important to understand as a basis for their application.

1. *Linearity of correlations.* When two variables are plotted alongside one another in such a way that they follow a straight line, they are said to be linearly related. The correlation coefficient, denoted by r, describes a **linear relationship** between two variables. This means that a straight line can be drawn through the number of given points when a scatterplot of the joint variables is constructed. As shown in Figure 11-14, three main types of r can be observed indicative of (1) a positive relationship, (2) a negative relationship, or (3) no relationship.

2. *Magnitude of correlations.* A quantitative index of the degree of dependence (relatedness) between variables is the *correlation coefficient*. The range of a correlation coefficient falls between -1 ($r = -1$, absolute negative) and $+1$ ($r = 1$, absolute positive). Very often, r can be translated into the shape of a linear equation. For example, $r = .50$ means that Y increases by .50 unit while X increases 1 unit. And $r = -.33$ means that Y de-

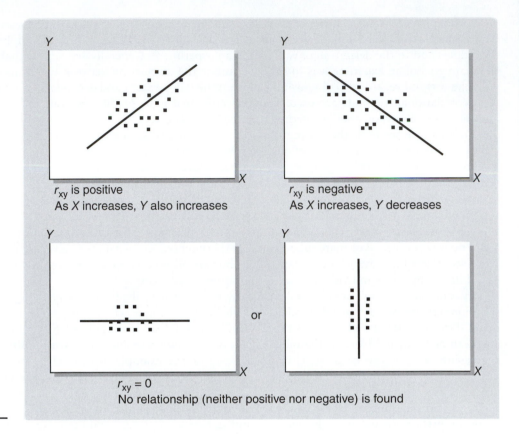

FIGURE 11-14

Three main types of correlational relationships

creases .33 unit while X increases 1 unit. If the absolute value of r, denoted by $|r|$, is greater than .80, then it is said to be a *strong correlation*. If $|r|$ is less than .40, then it is said to be a *weak correlation*. If $|r|$ falls between .4 and .8, then it is said to be a *moderate correlation*. Lastly, as mentioned before, there is *no correlation* if $|r| = 0$. The closer the correlation is to 0, the weaker the relationship. The closer the correlation is to -1 or $+1$, the stronger the relationship between the variables.

3. *Correlations versus causation.* As we have emphasized in previous chapters, correlation coefficients can only be interpreted as indices of *association* between variables—not as evidence that one such variable is *causative* of the other. An amusing example might help the reader to keep this important fact in mind. Students in a research class taught by one of the authors of this text were once asked to list two variables on *separate* slips of paper that they would like to study using correlational methods. After making their choices, the slips were collated, placed in a hat, then two slips were randomly selected by each student, resulting in an interesting assortment of paired variables. One student had by chance selected two seemingly unrelated variables for study involving the number of passenger's arriving on planes during a particular time of day at Boston's Logan International Airport and the number of births occurring around the same time in the city's hospitals. Subsequently, the results of the student's correlational study turned up a Pearson r of approximately .60, suggestive of a moderate association between the two variables. Perhaps the results reflected the ef-

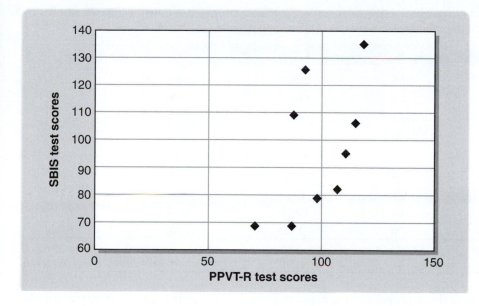

FIGURE 11-15

Scatterplot showing the relationship between hypothetical test scores obtained on the Stanford-Binet Intelligence Scale (SBIS) and the Peabody Picture Vocabulary Test-Revised (PPVT-R)

forts of anxious dads scampering home as quickly as possible to meet their newborns. More likely, because both variables involved time-related events, the results were merely indicative of a spurious association between them. In thinking about the meaning of correlations, remember the adage, "If you wait long enough, almost anything can happen."

Calculation of the Pearson Product-Moment Correlation

Let us now illustrate an application of correlational methods in the analysis of a hypothetical data set involving the association between hearing vocabulary and IQ scores. For this purpose, imagine that we have randomly selected a group of nine subjects for whom scores on the Peabody Picture Vocabulary Test-Revised (PPVT-R) and the Stanford-Binet Intelligence Scale (SBIS) were obtained. Given both of these data sets consisting of X and Y, respectively, we assume that the test scores for each instrument forms a continuous distribution. It will be recalled that the values of such a distribution possess fractional numerical properties as measured on an interval or ratio scale. For data of this kind, the **Pearson product-moment correlation** is a suitable technique for calculating the correlation of interest. The formula and steps involved in the computation of our example are given below:

Step 1.   Draw a scatterplot like that shown in Figure 11-15 to verify X and Y are linearly related.

Step 2.   Construct a table as illustrated in Table 11-3 to include:

$$X = \text{PPVT-R test scores} \qquad \Sigma X = \text{Sum of } X \text{ values}$$
$$Y = \text{SBIS test scores} \qquad \Sigma Y = \text{Sum of } Y \text{ values}$$
$$X^2 = \text{Square of } X \text{ values} \qquad \Sigma X^2 = \text{Sum of square of } X$$
$$Y^2 = \text{Square of } Y \text{ values} \qquad \Sigma Y^2 = \text{Sum of square of } Y$$
$$XY = \text{Product of } X \text{ and } Y \text{ values} \qquad \Sigma XY = \text{Sum of } XY$$

TABLE 11-3 Calculation of the Pearson Product-Moment Correlation Coefficient Based on Hypothetical Data for PPVT-R Test Scores (*X*) and SBIS Test Scores (*Y*)

X	Y	X²	Y²	XY
115	105	13225	11025	12075
105	90	11025	8100	9450
110	94	12100	8836	10340
95	120	9025	14400	11400
89	104	7921	10816	9256
126	135	15876	18225	17010
77	70	5929	4900	5390
100	80	10000	6400	8000
90	70	8100	4900	6300
$\Sigma X = 907$	$\Sigma Y = 868$	$\Sigma X^2 = 93201$	$\Sigma Y^2 = 87602$	$\Sigma XY = 89221$

Step 3.   Enter the appropriate values into the standard formula for calculating the correlation coefficient. The formula for the Pearson product-moment correlation coefficient, denoted by *r*, is given by:

$$r = \frac{N(\Sigma XY) - (\Sigma X)(\Sigma Y)}{\sqrt{[N(\Sigma X^2) - (\Sigma X)^2] \cdot [N(\Sigma Y^2) - (\Sigma Y)^2]}}$$

After entering the appropriate values into the above formula, $r = .66$ (verify this number if desired).

As we noted above, a correlation in this range is indicative of a moderate relationship between two variables. Based on the analysis of our hypothetical data, the resulting coefficient is very close to the results of actual studies that have collectively yielded a median correlation of .62 between the PPVT and SBIS (Dunn & Dunn, 1981).

Correlation as an Index of Common Variance

As we noted earlier, a correlation coefficient is simply an index of the relationship between variables. It does not express the amount of variance that *X* and *Y* share. However, when *r* is squared (r^2), it can be interpreted as the proportion of variability in *Y* that can be predicted based on a knowledge of *X* or vice versa. The actual percentage of variance in *Y* accounted for by *X* can be found by the following formula:

$$\text{\% of variance in } Y \text{ accounted for by knowing } X = r^2 \cdot 100$$

Therefore, based on our previous example, with a correlation of .66, the proportion of variance in *Y* (SBIS) predictable from *X* (PPVT-R) is 43.56% since $(.66)^2 \cdot 100 = 43.56$. The common variance shared by *X* and *Y* variables is illustrated graphically in Figure 11-16.

Other Correlation Techniques

The basic assumption underlying the use of the Pearson *r* is that both variables reflect a continuous distribution that is normally distributed. More specifically, the shape of the distribution for both variables should conform to the bell curve, lacking skewness. If this

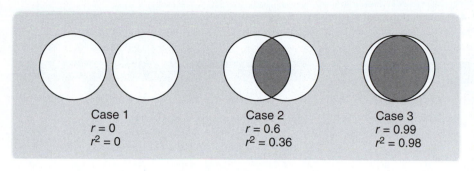

FIGURE 11-16

Illustration of the degree of the common variance shared by three cases

assumption is violated, a nonparametric correlation technique should be used as an alternative to the Pearson r.

When the level of measurement for both data sets is ordinal, the **Spearman rank (rho, denoted by ρ) correlation** coefficient may be employed. Let us illustrate the application of this particular technique as it might be used in determining the relationship between two components of stuttering severity as defined on the Stuttering Severity Instrument (SSI) (Riley, 1986). Specifically, we will determine the correlation between two parameters of the SSI, namely (1) the physical concomitants of stuttering, such as distracting sounds, facial grimaces, and (2) the frequency of stuttering occurrences. The following steps are outlined to illustrate the actual calculation of the Spearman correlation coefficient based on some fictitious SSI results.

Step 1.   Construct a table, as shown in Table 11-4 , to include:

$$X = \text{physical concomitant test scores, as defined}$$
$$Y = \text{frequency of stuttering, as defined}$$
$$X_r = \text{rank of } X$$
$$Y_r = \text{rank of } Y$$
$$d = X_r - Y_r$$
$$d^2 = \text{square of } d$$
$$\Sigma d^2 = \text{total sum of } d^2$$
$$N = \text{number of pairs of ranks}$$

Step 2.   Enter the appropriate values into the standard formula for calculating the correlation coefficient. The formula for the Spearman rank correlation coefficient is given by:

$$\rho = 1 - \frac{6 \cdot (\Sigma d^2)}{N \cdot (N^2 - 1)}$$

Thus, after substituting the appropriate values into the formula above, ρ is equal to 0.33. This coefficient indicates that there is a weak positive correlation between X (physical concomitants) and Y (frequency of stuttering). This correlation is identical in magnitude to that actually found in the standardization of the SSI.

A number of alternative correlation techniques are available as appropriate for a particular scale of measurement. Some of the commonly used correlational techniques are listed in Table 11-5.

TABLE 11-4   Calculation of the Spearman Rank Correlation Coefficient Based on Hypothetical Data for Physical Concomitants of Stuttering as Measured (X) and Frequency of Stuttering Occurences (Y)

X	X_r	Y	Y_r	d	d^2
3	5	14	8	−3	9
2	3	10	5	−2	4
1	1.5	8	3	−1.5	2.25
5	10	12	6	4	16
3	5	4	1	4	16
1	1.5	9	4	−2.5	6.25
4	8	6	2	6	36
4	8	18	10	−2	4
3	5	16	9	−4	16
4	8	13	7	1	1
N = 10					$\Sigma d^2 = 110.5$

TABLE 11-5   Types of Correlation and Their Statistical Applications

Type of Correlation	Statistical Application
Pearson product-moment (r):	Two continuous or normally distributed variables on an interval or ratio scale.
Spearman rank, or rho (ρ):	Two discrete variables on an ordinal (rank order) scale. Nonparametric equivalent of the Pearson r.
Contingency coefficient:	Two dichotomous variables on a nominal (categorical) scale.
Point biserial r:	Two variables when one is on an interval scale and the second is on an ordinal scale.
Multiple correlation:	One single variable and some combination of two or more other variables. Applications for parametric and nonparametric statistics.
Partial correlation:	Two variables are studied while holding constant the influence of a third or several other variables.

Regression

As noted previously, when the main goal of an investigation is to quantify the relationship between variables, correlation coefficients are the most useful tool for this purpose. However, provided that the correlation observed between two data sets is reasonably high, next we might want to estimate individual scores on one of two correlated variables from scores obtained on the other. Such an estimate is made possible by the use of a *regression equation* to calculate what is called "the best fit" of the data points of the X and Y variables as they are scattered about a **regression line.**

The general equation for a regression line consists of the following three major components: (1) the slope, (2) the Y-intercept, and (3) the predicted score of Y. The sloping line shown in Figure 11-17 approximates the general configuration of a regression line. Each of the components of such a line is described below.

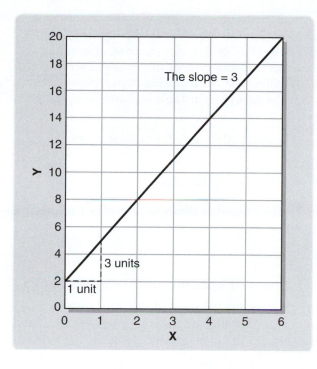

FIGURE 11-17

Graphic illustration of a linear equation when the slope equals 3

Slope. The slope of a line is sometimes called "average rate of change" or "the average ratio of Y to X," which means the amount of change in Y that corresponds to a change of one unit in X. For example, given the regression line shown in Figure 11-17, the statement "the slope equals 3" indicates that, on the average, a gain of 3 units in Y corresponds to a gain of 1 unit in X. The mathematical formula for determining the value of the slope (b) is given as

$$b = \frac{N(\sum XY) - (\sum X)(\sum Y)}{N(\sum X^2) - (\sum X)^2}$$

Y-intercept. The intercept of a line is defined as the value of Y when X equals 0. In other words, the Y intercept is the value of Y where the line intercepts (crosses) the Y axis. Thus, as shown in Figure 11-17, the average gain of 2 units along the Y axis, when X is equal to 0, corresponds to the term "Y intercept is equal to 2." The mathematical formula for determining the value of the Y intercept is given by: $a = \bar{Y} - b\bar{X}$

Predicted score of Y. The regression line is used to estimate the value of Y for a given value of X. The mathematical equation of a regression line expresses a *functional relationship* between two variables X and Y. In predicting the value of Y from the value of X, we can say that "Y is a function of X." This equation is given by:

$\hat{Y} = bX + a$

where $\hat{Y}$ = predicted value of Y
$\quad b$ = slope of the regression line
$\quad a$ = Y-intercept of the regression line

Clinical Application of Regression

Let us now illustrate the use of linear regression techniques in predicting an individual's SBIS score from a test score obtained on the PPVT-R. For this purpose, assume that the PPVT-R score was found to be 103. Given this knowledge, how can we use this score to estimate the SBIS score obtained by the same individual? The following steps represent the calculation of the slope and Y-intercept using the data given in Table 11-3 and the appropriate formula for each parameter as noted above.

Step 1.   Enter the appropriate values into the standard formula for calculating the slope and Y-intercept.

$$b = 0.97 \text{ and } a = -1.32 \text{ (verify the values)}$$

Therefore, the general equation of the regression line that allows us to predict Y from X can be written as

$$\hat{Y} = 0.97 \, X - 1.32$$

A graphic representation of the results from the above equation is shown in Figure 11-18.

Step 2.   Replace X in the equation above by the PPVT-R score of 103. This yields the predicted SBIS score (approximately 99). Given these hypothetical results, we can conclude that hearing vocabulary, as assessed by the PPVT-R, was a good predictor of intelligence as measured by the SBIS.

In conclusion, there are many types of regression techniques in addition to simple linear regression that have application to a variety of clinical and research problems. In this chapter, we have illustrated the application of simple linear regression to estimate a criterion variable from a single predictor variable. However, there are several clinical and research problems that necessitate the use of more comprehensive regression techniques. As noted earlier, one of these methods, called multiple regression, permits the simultaneous estimation of a criterion variable from several predictor variables. Thus, instead of using only the scores obtained on the PPVT-R to predict IQ, we might have incorporated such other semantic language measures as found on the Clinical Evaluation of Language Fundamentals (CELF-R) and the Woodcock-Johnson Psycho-Educational Battery (WJ-R), among many others.

There are a number of *multivariate* techniques that can be used to predict a binary dependent variable from a set of independent variables. Among these, multiple regression techniques have numerous applications in answering a variety of clinical and research questions, such as: What factors in a client's history best predict a certain speech-language-hearing disorder? What clinical and laboratory data best identify patients with such disorders? What therapy procedures are most likely to predict favorable clinical outcomes? On the other hand, such techniques have major limitations when the dependent variable has dichotomous values—for example, an event either occurs or does not occur. In this situation, the assumptions required for performing multiple regression analysis, such as normality in the distribution of data, will be violated.

Another difficulty is that the predicted values cannot be calculated as *probabilities* falling in the interval between 0 and 1 (see Chapter 12). In this situation, another multivariate technique called **logistic regression** might be used instead. The mathematical

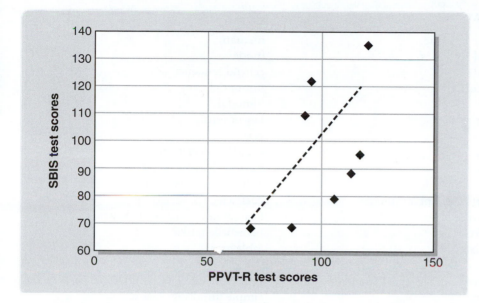

FIGURE 11-18

Scatterplot illustrating the line of best fit between hypothetical test scores obtained on the Stanford-Binet Intelligence Scale (SBIS) and the Peabody Picture Vocabulary Test-Revised (PPVT-R)

derivation and illustration of the latter technique is beyond the scope of this chapter. Generally, it can be said that logistic regression is useful in estimating the probability that an event will occur when the independent variables in an experiment include both quantitative and nonquantitative measures and the criterion or outcome variable is dichotomous.

SUMMARY

In this chapter, the theory of measurement was discussed in relation to four numerical scales. As noted, data can be classified according to its nominal, ordinal, interval, and/or ratio characteristics. The method for calculating class intervals of an appropriate size for grouping raw data and the graphical means for displaying such data were described. Several measures of central tendency were discussed including the mean, median, and mode and the methods for their calculation. Furthermore, measures of dispersion such as the range, variance, and standard deviation were reviewed.

The characteristics of a standard normal distribution curve were discussed, along with measures of skewness for such a curve. We also discussed Tchebysheff's theorem, which is useful in determining whether or not a distribution of scores is normally distributed, and the coefficient of variation, which determines the variation (spread) of data values in a distribution. Pearsonian measures for determining the type of skewness (positive, negative, bimodal) were described and illustrated.

Correlational measures of the association between two variables were discussed, and calculation examples were provided. Also, a measure of simple linear regression was described as a tool for predicting the magnitude of a dependent variable from an independent variable.

KEY TERMS

descriptive statistics	median
inferential statistics	mode
nominal data	central tendency
dichotomous	unimodal
pie chart	bimodal
bar graph	law of errors
trend chart	variance
interval scale	standard deviation
discrete variable	normal distribution curve
continuous variable	Tchebysheff's theorem
method of constant stimuli	coefficient of variation
ungrouped data	Pearsonian measure of skewness
class interval	percentile ranks
interval size	table area
range	bivariate relationship
relative frequency distribution	multivariate relationship
histogram	simple linear regression
frequency polygon	multiple regression
normal distribution curve	linear relationship
skewed curve	Pearson product-moment correlation
negatively skewed distribution	Spearman rank correlation
positively skewed distribution	regression line
bimodal distribution	logistic regression
mean	

SELF-LEARNING REVIEW

1. Two major categories of statistics are commonly identified as _____ and _____ techniques. _____ statistics are used for classifying, organizing, and summarizing a particular data set.

2. _____ data are representative of the kinds of distributions in which observations have been placed in certain _____ or arranged in a meaningful _____.

3. Observations that can only be named and counted are called _____ data. Such data are sometimes described as _____ "either/or" judgments about the _____ or _____ of a particular quality.

4. A nominal scale _____ without arranging data in a logical order. Its data categories are said to be _____ _____ in that a numerical value can belong to one and only one category.

5. Unlike the nominal scale, _____ measurement involves the _____ or logical _____ of data categories.

6. A _____ _____ can be used to graphically depict the percentage of subjects who consider a certain factor to be important. Such a percentage is typically displayed on the vertical axis, or _____, whereas the factors themselves are displayed along the horizontal axis, or _____.

7. Three characteristics of an ordinal scale are: (1) data categories are arranged in a distinctive _____; (2) data categories are _____ _____; and (3) data categories are logically ranked on the basis of the _____ of the characteristic possessed.

8. An interval scale contains two added features missing from a nominal scale. These are (1)_____ intervals and (2) an arbitrary _____ point.

9. A _____ scale not only allows numbers to be classified, ordered, and linearly specified at equal intervals, but also contains an _____ zero point.

10. Although nominal and ordinal scales involve the measurement of _____ or _____ variables, both interval and ratio scales can represent _____ variables.

11. In order to organize ungrouped data in a logical manner, the first step is to arrange the scores within a _____ table. Such a table provides a convenient format for summarizing the data within a series of predetermined _____ _____. The number of observations that fall within each class interval is called a frequency _____.

12. In deciding the size and number of _____ _____ to be used in an investigation, chief among the factors to consider is the degree of _____ desired.

13. A convenient method for determining the size of a class interval is to _____ the _____ of scores by the number of class intervals.

14. A _____ frequency distribution shows the percentage of scores that fall within each class interval. This can be determined simply by dividing the _____ of scores falling within each interval by the size of the _____ and multiplying the result by _____.

15. Continuous data are often presented graphically as a _____ that is much like a _____ chart except the data are partitioned along the abscissa so as to fall within _____ intervals.

16. A line graph that is useful in portraying all types of scaled measurements except nominal data is a _____ _____. Such a graph is formed by connecting the _____ of the class intervals with a straight line.

17. The normal distribution curve is _____ shaped with data symmetrically distributed to the _____ and _____ of _____.

18. A _____ skewed distribution is one in which the tail points to the _____ side of the curve. This signifies that the proportion of _____ scores in the distribution is greater than for _____ scores.

19. A _____ skewed distribution is found in cases where the tail points to the _____ side of the curve because the frequency of _____ scores greatly outnumber _____ scores in the distribution.

20. Two characteristics of frequency distributions that commonly are of interest to researchers relate to (1) the tendency for the scores to cluster around the _____ and (2) their degree of _____ or spread. The first characteristic is often summarized by measure of _____ _____ and the second by measures of _____.

21. Measures of central tendency include the _____ (arithmetic average), _____ (midscore value), and the _____ (most frequently occurring value).

22. In using mean scores, two important qualifications are important to consider. First, the shape of the distribution should be _____ so as to approximate the values for other measures of _____ _____. Second, the data should have _____ measurement characteristics that are subject to _____ manipulation.

23. The median is the _____ value in a distribution of scores. Symbolically, the location of the median is given by _____.

24. In order to calculate the median from grouped scores, we must find (1) the exact _____ of the interval containing $n \cdot (.50)$; (2) the _____ frequency of the interval containing $n \cdot (.50)$; and (3) the width of the _____ _____.

25. As an alternative to the mean, the _____ can best be used when the shape of a distribution is known to be _____ or when its shape is otherwise _____.

26. The _____ is simply the score that occurs most frequently. It is the weakest measure of central tendency because, in some cases, it may be the _____ or _____ value in a distribution.

27. The mode could represent more than one data value if (1) there is a _____ and (2) each value occurs at least _____. The mode is restricted to _____ data.

28. A distribution having one mode is called _____, whereas a distribution having two modes is called _____. The use of the mode is restricted to _____ scales of measurement and is seldom reported unless in association with other measures of _____ _____.

29. In the nineteenth century, the German mathematician Carl Gauss formulated the _____, which holds that the majority of repeated measurements made on the same subject _____ cluster about the center of distribution to form a _____-shaped curve.

30. If measurements are made on a number of individuals, they can be said to constitute a _____ group provided there is little _____ among scores.

31. The range is the _____ between the lowest and highest value in a distribution. Like the mode, the range is extremely sensitive to _____ in a data set.

32. Mathematically, the measure of variance must calculate the _____ and the _____ of the deviations of a data set.

33. The rule of zero-sum deviation confirms the fact "the _____ spread out the distribution, the larger the _____ _____ from the mean."

34. The population mean squared deviation from the mean is symbolically expressed as _____, or the _____.

35. The disadvantage of using variance as a measure of _____ can be repaired by simply taking the _____ _____. The resulting value is called the standard deviation.

36. The standard deviation is useful for indicating the _____ of data values that are this _____ _____ away from the _____.

37. The most practical use of the standard deviation can be observed in relation to what is called a _____ _____ curve that has a characteristic bell _____.

38. In a normal distribution, approximately _____ % of the data values lie within one standard deviation from the mean, _____ % of the data values lie within two standard deviations from the mean, and _____ % of the data values lie within three standard deviations from the mean.

39. The standard deviation is a key measure of _____ that can be used to determine the _____ _____ of an individual's score in relation to other group members'.

40. According to Tchebysheff's theorem, at least _____ % of the data values normally lie within 1.5 standard deviations from the mean.

41. The coefficient of variation of the set $\bar{X} = 20$ and $S = 5$ is _____ %, suggesting that the data set is relatively _____.

42. The _____ measure of skewness, denoted by S_k, is calculated as _____. For instance, $S_k =$ _____ if $\bar{X} = 50$, $M_d = 48$, and $S = 5$ are given. Then the distribution is _____ skewed.

43. The standard score, denoted by _____, expresses the number of _____ _____ units away from the mean.

44. A percentile rank is a number on a particular measurement scale _____ or _____ which a given _____ of the remaining distribution of scores can be found.

45. The normal distribution curve is _____ around the center, and the entire area under the curve is _____ %.

46. The percentage of all PPVT-R scores falling between 76 and 94 is approximately _____ %. The cutoff score for the bottom 20% of the test scores obtained on the PPVT-R is _____. (Given $\mu = 100$ and $\sigma = 15$.)

47. In correlational studies, the variable Y is called the dependent or _____ variable and X is called the independent or _____ variable.

48. Correlational problems pertain to observations made under conditions where an observed change in one variable appears to be associated with a concomitant change in another. Such variables form a joint distribution of data sets that are said to be _____ _____ or _____.

49. The correlation coefficient, denoted by _____, describes a _____ relationship between _____ variables. If the absolute value of r, denoted by $|r|$, is greater than _____, then it is said to be a strong correlation. If $|r|$ is less than _____, then it is said to be a weak correlation.

50. When r is squared (r^2), it can be interpreted as the proportion of _____ in Y that can be _____ based on a knowledge of X.

51. The general equation for a regression line consists of the following major components, namely (1) the _____, sometimes called the "average rate of change"; (2) the _____, defined as the value of Y when $X = 0$; and (3) the _____ score of Y for a given value of X.

52. Generally, it can be said that _____ regression is useful in estimating the _____ than an event will occur when the independent variables in an experiment include both quantitative and nonquantitative measures and the criterion or outcome variable is _____.

QUESTIONS AND EXERCISES FOR CLASSROOM DISCUSSION

PART 1

Calculation Question 1
Suppose a clinician or researcher is interested in examining the relationship between some measure of receptive language ability (X) and a measure of reading achievement (Y). Some hypothetical results for such a study are given after the table:

X	Y
100	110
95	85
105	105
125	111
90	107
118	99

For the receptive language ability scores, the mean $\bar{X}$ is _____, the median is _____, the mode is _____, the variance S^2 is _____, and the standard deviation S is _____.

The Pearson product-moment correlation coefficient r between X and Y is calculated as _____ and the coefficient of determination is _____. Therefore, the actual percentage of variance in Y accounted for by X is _____ %.

If the Spearman rank correlation technique was used for this hypothetical study, then the correlation coefficient ρ is _____.

The linear regression equation for predicting Y from X yields the slope of _____ and Y intercept of _____. The predicted Y score for a given X score of 110 is _____.

Calculation Question 2

The following study investigated relationships between working memory (WM) and reading comprehension skill (RC) among younger and older healthy African-American adults. All participants were required to complete two WM tests (The Size Judgment Span Test and The Alphabet Span Test) and a reading ability test, (The Nelson-Denny Reading Tests). Selected results of the WM (Alphabet Span Test) and RC (Vocabulary) tests for ten younger adults and ten older adults are summarized as follows:

	Younger			Older	
Subject	WM (Alphabet Span Test)	RC (Vocabulary)	Subject	WM (Alphabet Span Test)	RC (Vocabulary)
1	21	44	1	25	83
2	38	58	2	20	61
3	14	40	3	30	79
4	29	49	4	18	55
5	45	70	5	16	51
6	33	55	6	19	48
7	38	55	7	9	17
8	53	80	8	20	69
9	31	43	9	5	21
10	40	56	10	17	34

Reprinted from "Age, Working Memory, Figurative Language Type, and Reading Ability: Influencing Factors in African American Adults' Comprehension of Figurative Language," by C. D. Qualls and J. L. Harris, February, 2003, American Journal of Speech-Language Pathology, 12, pp. 92–102.

a. Find the mean, median, mode, range, variance, and standard deviation of the WM and RC test scores for each group.

b. Which correlational method, Pearson or Spearman, is more appropriate for the study? Explain briefly and calculate the appropriate correlation coefficients of (1) Younger adults versus Older adults on the WM test, (2) Younger adults versus Older adults on the RC test, (3) the WM test scores versus the RC test scores for younger adults, and (4) the WM test scores versus the RC test scores for older adults.

Calculation Question 3

The following table summarizes demographic information for patients with Alzheimer's disease (AD) and normal controls (NC), including severity of dementia as gauged by performance on the Mini-Mental State Examination (MMSE, total possible = 30) (Almor et al., 1999).

AD ($n = 30$) Mean = 17.9 Median = 22.5 *SD* = 5.0
NC ($n = 23$) Mean = 28.4 Median = 20.0 *SD* = 1.5

  a. Find the Pearsonian measures of skewness for both groups.
  b. Discuss the type of shapes of distributions for both groups.

PART 2

1. What are two major categories of statistics? Explain the nature of each type.
2. Identify four categories of data and their statistical characteristics.
3. What can a bar graph illustrate?
4. Explain how the size of a class interval can be determined.
5. List all guidelines that were offered in this chapter for use in preparing and evaluating the utility of tables, charts, and graphs.
6. Describe the major characteristics of a normal distribution, a positively skewed distribution, a negatively skewed distribution, and a bimodal distribution.
7. What is the meaning of the term *homogeneity*? Give at least two examples of homogeneous distributions.
8. Name three measures of the central tendency of data in a frequency distribution and provide a clinical example of each.
9. What is the difference between a unimodal distribution and a bimodal distribution?
10. Explain the "law of errors."
11. What are two of the main measures of variability of data in a frequency distribution? Describe each of these measures using clinical examples.
12. Explain Tchebysheff's theorem.
13. What do Pearsonian measures of skewness say about the shape of a frequency distribution? Give a clinically relevant example.
14. What is the main difference between correlation and regression? Give a clinical example to illustrate the difference between the two methods.
15. Identify and describe three major components of a regression line.

Analyzing Data: Inferential Statistics

CHAPTER OUTLINE

LEARNING OBJECTIVES

After reading this chapter, you should be able to identify, describe, or define:

- Two views of probability and their relation to hypothesis testing
- The central limit theorem and how to construct a confidence interval for μ
- The general steps in performing hypothesis testing by means of the classical approach
- Statistical inference concerning means and proportions for one and two population parameter(s)
- Errors and power of the test in statistical inference
- A z distribution and Student's t distribution and their characteristics
- Logic behind several nonparametric statistical methods and calculations
- Statistical inference concerning means for three or more groups
- Logic and calculation of one-way analysis of variance
- Various types of multiple comparison statistical methods
- The p value approach in hypothesis testing
- Various types of more advanced statistical methods
- Several computer software packages in statistics
- Demonstrations of solutions to problems using MINITAB® and SPSS computer software

---

PROBABILITY: THE BASIS FOR STATISTICAL INFERENCE

In previous chapters, we discussed the concept of the normal distribution curve and the calculation of standard scores. These can be quite useful in estimating the probability that the measured performance of a randomly sampled individual from a normally distributed population will be above or below a certain value. However, most research studies are concerned with the opposite problem of making inferences about a larger target population based on representative sample cases drawn from that population. Quantities used to describe characteristics of populations are termed **parameters.** On the other hand, quantities derived from samples that are used in estimating population parameters are called **statistics.** This chapter discusses several methods for making inferences about the **significance** of sample statistics in conjunction with hypothesis testing. The basis for statistical inference and hypothesis testing is the theory of probability.

The word **probability** is an elusive concept that is difficult to define. In the vernacular of everyday language, we commonly use the term *probably* to express the notion that some event is likely to happen or that a particular observation is likely to be true. Indeed, the manner in which we make most routine decisions throughout the day is predicated on the likelihood for certain outcomes. For example, we either carry an umbrella or leave it at home based on our personal reactions to the weather forecast. Some might make the decision to carry the umbrella only if the likelihood for rain is 90%. Based on a more conservative view, even a 50% probability of rain might lead some individuals to take it along "just in case."

In a clinical sense, probability is akin to the clinical concept of **prognosis.** According to Emerick and Hattten (1979), prognosis involves:

> prediction of the outcome of a proposed course of treatment for a given client: how effective treatment will be, how far we can expect the client to progress, and perhaps, how long it will take . . . accurate prognosis can help establish our credibility . . . the ability to predict with reasonable precision is the highest form of scientific achievement. (pp. 67–68)

Like clinicians, researchers attempt to make good decisions based on the findings of their studies. From a statistical perspective, there are several meanings of probability. Perhaps the best known of these is the classical view also called the "frequentist," "objectivist," or "a posteriori" view of probability. The classical view is based on a principle first developed by James Bernoulli in the eighteenth century. According to the so-called **Bernoulli theorem,** the relative frequency of an observed event will approximate its probable frequency of future occurrence if observed over an indefinitely long series of trials.

To understand the Bernoulli theorem in more concrete terms, imagine that you are asked to determine the probability of a tossed coin turning up heads. In theory, provided that the coin is fair (unbiased), the probability of its turning up heads is 50%. Furthermore, the mathematical likelihood of the coin turning up heads will get closer and closer to 50% as the number of tosses increases. Thus, five tosses will typically yield results that conform with the expected outcome more often than one toss, ten tosses more often than five, and so forth. (See Figure 5-2.) Nevertheless, it is important to understand that such outcomes can be predicted with only relative degrees of confidence. Although improbable, it is still possible that 100 tosses may yield a more equal distribution of heads and tails than, let's say, 500 or more tosses of the same coin.

Just as chance can account for why a coin does not turn up heads or tails exactly 50% of the time when tossed, the same random variation must be considered when assessing the truth of our clinical observations and research findings. The fact that the future occurrence of an event can only be stated in relative terms is the basis for statistical inference.

Typically, the researcher begins with a theoretical proposition or hypothesis about the *expected* relative frequency of a particular observation or event as it might exist in a sample drawn from a population. For example, we might hypothesize about the degree to which an observed sample mean ($\bar{X}$) is representative of the population mean (μ) based on the probability of comparable findings in a long sequence of repeated trials or experiments. In fact, the sample mean might be greater or smaller than the population mean; it may be almost equal to, or quite different from the population mean.

To determine the fairness of a coin toss in absolute mathematical terms, it would have to be tossed an infinite number of times—an obvious impossibility. Because of the same constraints, a theory or hypothesis can never be proved to be true in absolute terms. Nevertheless, the confidence that we can place in our data increases in proportion to sample size or the number (n) of observations made by the experimenter. The larger the sample n, the more confidence we can have in the credibility of our findings.

Probabilities and Level of Confidence

As noted above, data can never be interpreted as having "proved" a hypothesis. For this reason, decisions about the statistical significance of data are most commonly formulated as probability statements like those found in Table 12-1. As the table makes clear, there is an inverse relationship between the probability for a chance error due to random factors and the level of confidence that can be placed in a systematic experimental effect. More specifically, it can be seen that relatively small alpha (α) values such as $p \leq .001$, are interpreted as statements of greater confidence in the data (less chance for error) than are relatively large α values such as $p \leq .05$ (more chance for error). As statements of probability, the intermediate α values in the table reflect moderate positions relative to acceptable risks for error versus levels of confidence in experimental findings based on statistical outcomes.

TABLE 12-1 Common Qualifying Probabilities and Levels of Confidence

Qualifying Probability	Probability of Chance Error (Chance Differences)	Level of Nonchance Confidence (Nonchance Differences)
$p \leq .05$	5% or less	95.0%
$p \leq .025$	2.5% or less	97.5%
$p \leq .01$	1% or less	99.0%
$p \leq .001$	.1% or less	99.9%

The Bayesian View of Probability

Although the most popular view of probability is founded on the classical school of statistical inference, as developed by Sir Ronald Fisher and by E. S. Pearson in the early 1900s, not all researchers and statisticians believe that frequentist methods are suitable for all problems. Indeed, some might say that so far as clinical practice, as in our assessment of everyday events, we rarely attempt to forecast the future by sampling the relative frequency of past occurrences. In other words, we do not actually state a null hypothesis that the population percentage equals, say, 50%, then use sample data to decide whether or not to reject the hypothesis based on the probability of achieving similar results over a long sequence of trials. Instead, we typically cast our predictions based on experiential beliefs or personal opinions. This so-called **subjective view** of probability, based on the "degree of belief" that one happens to hold, is summarized well by Good:

> Various authorities have attempted to eliminate the necessity for subjective probability judgments. . . . It is maintained here that judgments should be given a recognized place from the start . . . it is helpful if something is stated about the subjective initial probability of the hypothesis. . . . To omit such a statement gives only the superficial appearance of objectivity. (Good, 1950)

A mathematical basis for assessing probability in terms of the subjective views of individuals was first introduced by a Presbyterian minister by the name of **Thomas Bayes** in 1763. Classical statisticians have often criticized the Bayesian view, as it has come to be known, based on the fact that subjective probabilities for a particular event may vary widely among individuals. The rejoinder of Bayesian statisticians has been that the ability to take such individual differences into account and to assess changes in subjective views as new information emerges is a strength rather than a weakness of the Bayesian approach. To the extent that this is true, Bayesian methods have obvious application to many clinical situations where we must depend on personal experience or that elusive quality called "intuition" to guide our decision making.

The clinical utility of Bayesian methods for inferring the consequences of certain diagnostic and management decisions (a priori) and for evaluating the validity of a clinician's views given new data (a posteriori) is increasingly recognized in the field of medicine. Such methods have not yet been used extensively in the behavioral fields even though they would appear to have numerous applications. In Chapter 9, we discussed some important applications of this method in relation to determining the diagnostic accuracy of a screening test.

In general, we can say that statistical inference, regardless of the point of view held by the researcher, requires an extrapolation from the given sample (explained portion) to the larger unknown population (unexplained portion). Since we are extrapolating in this manner, there always exists uncertainty about our conclusions. This uncertainty may be dealt with using probabilities such as significance level (α), confidence interval, or Bayesian subjective probabilities.

For purposes of this chapter, we shall limit our discussion to the classical view of probability and statistical hypothesis testing since it is currently the more widely used approach by researchers in the field of communication sciences and disorders.

SAMPLING VARIABILITY

Fundamental to the understanding of statistical inference is the notion that the amount of trust that can be placed in any measure obtained from a sample is directly contingent upon its reliability as an estimate of the true measure of the population. Whether it be the sample mean, the standard deviation, or some other measure, all such measures should be stable—that is, should express little variability. A highly useful measure of the degree of variability in a sampling distribution is called the **standard error of the mean,** variously denoted by $\sigma_{\bar{x}}$, *SEM,* or simply *SE.* The *SE* is an estimate of the expected amount of deviation of sample means from the true population mean that is a result of chance or measurement errors. Stated more simply, *SE* is merely the standard deviation of a set of sample means. However, it is important to distinguish between the *SE* and the standard deviation (σ or *SD*). Whereas the *SD* is a measure of the degree of variability that *currently* exists among individuals in a population, the *SE* is an estimate of how much variability to expect in the means of *future* samples when the complete population parameter is unknown. On practical grounds, the *SE* has great value because it eliminates the need of repeatedly sampling the same distribution, thereby relieving investigators of what might otherwise be a highly onerous burden.

Consider a population of three individuals with the following raw scores on a digit span test: 5, 9, and 7. We consider two parameters, the mean and standard deviation, from this distribution. Suppose we select two scores randomly from this population. With this sampling procedure, there are three equally likely possible samples of two raw scores that can be drawn from the population. They are as follows:

Sample	$\bar{X}$
(5, 9)	7
(5, 7)	6
(9, 7)	8

where $\bar{X}$ represents the sample mean of each outcome.

The mean of all possible sample means from the original population is referred to as the *sampling distribution of the mean of samples of size n.* Two parameters for sampling distributions are as follows:

a. The mean = Mean of sample means = $\mu_{\bar{x}}$
b. The standard deviation = Standard deviation of sample means = $\sigma_{\bar{x}}$

In the original population ($N = 3$), we find μ (the population mean) to be 7. Let us calculate $\mu_{\bar{x}}$ given by the arithmetic average of three sample means 7, 6, and 8:

$$\mu_{\bar{X}} = \frac{7 + 6 + 8}{3} = 7 \text{ as well}$$

Therefore, keep in mind that:

a. The mean of the sampling distribution for the sample mean is *always* the population mean $\mu_{\bar{x}} = \mu$

By using the same mathematical procedure, we can compare the standard deviations for the original population $\bar{X}$ and the sampling distributions for the mean ($\sigma_{\bar{x}}$) in the sample above. Because the mathematical derivation for accomplishing this is relatively complex, only the result is given below. Furthermore, the standard deviation, as we already know, is sensitive to sample size so that the value of $\sigma_{\bar{x}}$ changes as n changes. Thus, it can be said that:

b. For random samples from a large population, the standard deviation of the sampling distribution for the mean of sample size n approaches $\sigma_{\bar{x}} = \sigma/\sqrt{n}$ as n increases.

Combining the results of (a) and (b) above, we can state the characteristics of the sampling distribution for the mean of sample size n. More specifically, if the original population of the distribution of the raw scores is normal, then the sampling distribution for $\bar{X}$ will yield the following properties:

1. normality
2. $\mu_{\bar{x}} = \mu$
3. $\sigma_{\bar{x}} = \sigma/\sqrt{n}$
4. $Z = (\bar{X} - \mu_{\bar{x}})/\sigma_{\bar{x}}$ for a large n ($n > 30$)

The combined properties as noted above are often referred to as the **central limit theorem,** which provides the foundation for much of modern statistical inference. This theorem makes possible the ability to calculate the standard error as an estimate of the degree of dispersion present in any group of sampling means provided that the sample is random.

Confidence Intervals

As noted in earlier chapters, investigators are ultimately interested in determining the significance of their research findings. The statistical meaning of significance pertains to the probability that an observed result is truly the consequence of a systematic influence under investigation rather than the unlikely consequence of chance alone. Typically, in determining the significance of a single sample mean, its probable position in relation to the population mean is estimated to lie within the boundaries of certain **confidence intervals,** as they are sometimes called.

To illustrate the role of the standard error in statistical inference, suppose that we wish to estimate the probable mean intelligence of the current population of graduate students in the field of communication sciences and disorders. Using appropriate random sampling techniques, we first select a sample of 144 students (note that the sample is large, therefore, a z distribution will be used) for our study. Assume further that the mean ($\bar{X}$) IQ of this sample is determined to be 110 with a population standard deviation (σ) of 12. What can be inferred about the probable position of the true population mean within one standard deviation from the mean? To answer this question, we must first calculate the standard error accordingly:

$$SE = \frac{12}{\sqrt{144}} = \frac{12}{12} = 1.0$$

Based on a standard error of this size, the true mean of graduate student IQ can be estimated to lie between $\bar{X} - 1 \cdot SE$ (109) and $\bar{X} + 1 \cdot SE$ (111). This assertion can be made with a limited degree of confidence. More specifically, if we were to randomly select numerous repeated samples from the same population, we could expect the same or highly similar findings about 68% of the time (see Figure 11-7). Should we wish to take a conservative position, we could assert that the true mean lies between $\bar{X} - 2 \cdot SE$ (108) and $\bar{X} + 1 \cdot SE$ (112) about 95% of the time. An ultraconservative assertion might be that μ is located between the limits $\bar{X} - 3 \cdot SE$ (107) and $\bar{X} + 3 \cdot SE$ (113). In the latter case, we could be confident of the relative truth of our assertion in about 99 cases out of 100.

Remember that the larger the confidence interval, the more confident one can be that the true population mean is included within that interval. The resultant tradeoff is less precise information about the exact value of the population mean.

In general, there are two different types of questions that researchers ask. The first type of question determines whether or not a *single sample* belongs to some defined population (or a target population). The second question asks whether or not two or more *different samples* come from the same population.

The general steps in performing hypothesis testing are as follows:

1. Form the hypothesis in statistical terms (H_0 and H_1).
2. Select an appropriate statistical test.
3. Choose a significance level and criterion for rejecting H_0.
4. Calculate the test statistic by computing what is variously termed the *observed* or *calculated* value.
5. Draw conclusions.

ONE-SAMPLE CASE: TESTING HYPOTHESES FOR A SINGLE GROUP

The simplest type of hypothesis testing involves the one-sample case, also known as the **single-group design.** Such a design allows for asking if the mean of a single sample is comparable to the population mean.

In order to understand the application of this test, imagine that we are interested in investigating the intelligence of school-age children born with clefts of the palate and testing the claim that their intelligence is different from the norm. To do so, we will randomly select a hypothetical group of 36 subjects from the population of children with this type of cleft who are being followed by a certain group of craniofacial clinics. Assume that we administer the Wechsler Intelligence Scale for Children (WISC-III) to our sample with the following results:

$$\bar{X} = 89, \sigma = 15, \mu = 100, \text{ and } SE = \frac{15}{\sqrt{36}} = 2.5$$

The steps necessary for hypothesis testing are outlined below:

Step 1.   Form the hypothesis in statistical terms.

Null hypothesis: (H_0): $\mu = 100$

Alternative hypothesis (H_1): $\mu \neq 100$

If the null hypothesis (H_0) is rejected, the alternative hypothesis (H_1) is supported. In the absence of a significant finding, the null hypothesis is retained pending the outcome of future experiments. Remember that the null hypothesis cannot be accepted because it is always possible that it will be disproved in some future investigation.

The alternative hypothesis as stated above signifies that the result will be evaluated by means of a **two-tailed test.** Such a test is selected when the *direction* of the difference cannot be predicted on the basis of preexisting knowledge. In the case of our example, the research findings from previous studies that bear on this problem are equivocal, leading to the selection of a two-tailed test. If we had wished to predict the research outcome on the basis of prior knowledge, the alternative hypothesis would have been directional; that is, it would have been stated as $\mu > 100$ or $\mu < 100$. A **one-tailed test** of this kind is said to be "less stringent" than a two-tailed test because a smaller amount of variance between mean scores is needed to be considered a significant finding.

The direction of the sign contained in H_1 identifies the area within the normal curve for rejecting H_0. More specifically, the basis for deciding where to look within the curve for a significance difference is summarized below:

If H_1 Contains	$\neq$	$<$	$>$
Perform:	two-tail	one-tail (left-sided)	one-tail (right-sided)

Step 2.   Select an appropriate statistical test.

Given our hypothetical problem, the appropriate test for evaluating the null hypothesis is based on the z distribution. The major criterion for using the z test is that the population standard deviation (σ) must be known. In studies of intelligence based on the WISC-III, the population mean is known to be 100 with a σ of 15.

When the population standard deviation (σ) is unknown, the appropriate statistical test for evaluating the null hypothesis is the *t* **test.** Furthermore, a *t* distribution is designed for testing hypotheses when the sample size is small ($n \leq 30$).

Step 3.   Choose the significance level and criterion for rejecting H_0.

A two-tailed test will be performed at $\alpha = .05$ because the alternative hypothesis (H_1) is nondirectional ($\mu \neq 100$). Recall that the significance level must be established *before* the study is conducted. The decision rule for a two-tailed test at $\alpha = .05$ involves the following considerations:

1. Reject H_0 if the magnitude of the observed value is greater than or equal to a critical value of 1.96, that is

$$\text{Observed } z \geq \text{Critical } z = 1.96$$

2. Do not reject H_0, otherwise.

Step 4.   Calculate the test statistic.

Given the data provided in our hypothetical study, we will now calculate the test statistic. The formula for calculating z is as follows:

$$z = \frac{\bar{X} - \mu}{SE}$$

Entering the appropriate values into the formula above, we find that

$$z = \frac{89 - 100}{2.5} = -4.4 \text{ (Observed } z = -4.4)$$

Step 5. Draw conclusions on the basis of critical value(s).

Because the magnitude of the observed z value exceeded the critical value of 1.96 (see Figure 12-1), a decision is made to reject the null hypothesis. More specifically, even though the mean IQ of the sample (89) was in the range of low average intelligence, our fictitious data indicate that their scores on the WISC-III were significantly different from (lower than) the population mean IQ of 100.

Although the z test is highly useful in testing hypotheses when the population standard deviation (σ) is known, in reality, this is rarely the case. In most research studies, the standard error must be estimated based on the sample data alone. In place of z scores, t scores are used to make estimates about the values of sample means in relation to their population values.

The distribution for t scores was first described by the English statistician William Gossett in 1908. As an employee of the Guinness Brewery, he was required to publish his findings anonymously in order to protect the secrets of a beer-making process. Because he chose to sign his name merely as "A Student," Gossett's statistical distribution subsequently became widely known as the **Student t test.**

The formula for t is:

$$t = \frac{\bar{X} - \mu}{SE}$$

where $\bar{X}$ = mean of sampling distribution
  μ = population mean
  SE = standard error of the mean = $S/\sqrt{n}$

As can be seen in this formula, the t test is actually a ratio wherein the numerator is the difference between two means. The denominator (standard error) is an estimate of the degree of variance between the means. Generally, a t distribution somewhat resembles the standard z distribution curve in shape. Its curve is symmetric with respect to a vertical line through the origin 0, and the curve extends indefinitely in both negative and positive directions. The mean value of t is 0 and it is more spread out than a z curve; that is, a t distribution has a greater standard deviation. Furthermore, as n gets larger and larger, a t distribution will get closer and closer to a z distribution in shape. In fact, for $n > 30$, a t distribution is approximately a normal z distribution.

As noted previously, in addition to the relevance of the t test in cases in which σ is unknown, its use is also applicable to circumstances in which the sample size $n < 30$. We will now demonstrate the application of this test based on the previous example. However, in testing H_0 and H_1, the sample size in this case will be 9 instead of 36. Furthermore, assuming the σ is unknown, we will replace it by the estimated sample standard deviation (S).

Based on our example, the following values are given: $\bar{X} = 89$, $S = 16$, $\mu = 100$, and $SE = 16/\sqrt{9} = 5.33$. Substituting these values into the appropriate formula below, we find the value of t:

$$t = \frac{\bar{X} - \mu}{SE} = \frac{89 - 100}{5.33} = -2.064 \text{ (observed } t = -2.064)$$

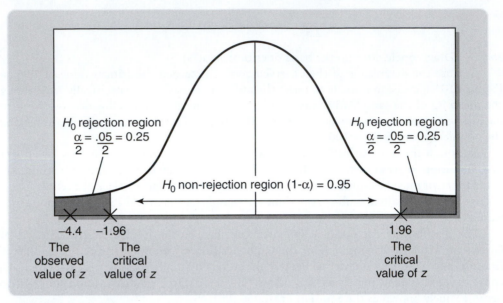

H_0 rejection region
$\alpha = \dfrac{.05}{2} = \dfrac{.05}{2} = 0.25$

H_0 rejection region
$\alpha = \dfrac{.05}{2} = \dfrac{.05}{2} = 0.25$

H_0 non-rejection region $(1-\alpha) = 0.95$

−4.4   −1.96

1.96

The
observed
value of z

The
critical
value of z

The
critical
value of z

FIGURE 12-1   The critical z values (± 1.96) associated with $\alpha/2 = .025$ and a nondirectional, two-tailed test of the null hypothesis

The decision rule for a two-tailed t test at $\alpha = .05$ involves the same considerations as stated previously for a two-tailed z test. However, the critical value of t in the former case depends in part on the number of **degrees of freedom (df)** allowed. Df is best viewed as an "index number" for the purpose of identifying the appropriate distribution to be used given a specific sample size. The value of df for a one-sample t test is $n-1$. Referring to the table for t values found in Appendix A-1-2, it can be seen that the critical value for our hypothetical study is 2.306 for $df = 9 - 1 = 8$. We will not get into the mathematical rationale and derivation involved in degrees of freedom here. We will simply follow the custom of using this notion to appropriately identify the particular t distribution with which we are working.

Because the magnitude of the observed t value does not exceed the critical value (see Figure 12-2), the decision is made to retain the null hypothesis. More specifically, in contrast to the significant finding for the z test based on the same example, the nonsignificant t test result indicates that the IQ scores of children with cleft palates are equivalent to (not significantly different from) the population mean at $\alpha = .05$.

The reader may wonder why the z and t tests in this example produced disparate outcomes so that the first value was associated with a statistically significant result in contrast to the second value. Generally, researchers can expect the results of z and t tests to reflect comparable results because their distributions are highly similar. However, our hypothetical t test results are predicated on an n of only 9 subjects. For small n's of this size, t values may differ significantly from z values based on larger n's. On the other hand, as noted earlier, with successive increments in sample size, the obtained t value becomes closer and closer to the obtained z value. As a rule of thumb, most practitioners prefer to use a t distribution when n is small ($n \leq 30$). However, it may be used for large samples as well ($n > 30$). In this case, the assumption of normality is no longer our major concern because a t distribution will

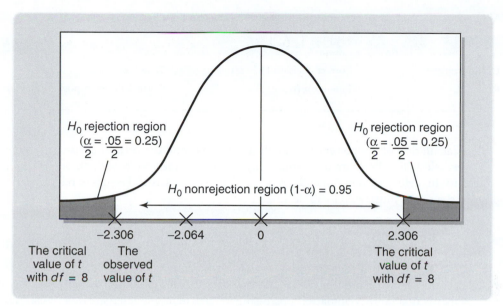

FIGURE 12-2   The critical t values ($\pm$2.306) associated with $\alpha/2 = .025$, 8 df, and a nondirectional, two-tailed test of the null hypothesis

eventually become or at least get closer to a z distribution when n gets larger than 30. Indeed, many statisticians use a t distribution whenever σ (the population standard deviation) is known. They prefer to use large-sample methods, like the z test, only when σ is known, regardless of n, whereas when we use such large-sample methods, we must estimate the value of an unknown σ by the sample standard deviation S. The two approaches are equally effective and popular because, again, a t distribution and a z distribution are approximately the same when $n > 30$.

Errors and Power in Statistical Inference

As discussed in previous chapters, there are two major types of errors a researcher can commit when making statistical inferences. The first type of error is called a type I error (denoted by α). Recall that this error is the result of rejecting the null hypothesis when it is true. The second type of error, called a type II error (denoted by β), is the consequence of retaining the null hypothesis when it is false.

Ideally, the goal of research is to avoid or minimize the probability of both type I and type II errors. However, the unfortunate reality is that these errors are interactive to the degree that when one type decreases, the other type increases. In most cases, researchers in the communication sciences and disorders are more concerned about making a type II error than a type I error because the former type primarily determines the power of a statistical test, denoted by $1 - \beta$.

The **power of the test** can be defined as the probability of rejecting a *false* null hypothesis— that is, the probability of reaching a correct decision. Determining the power of the test is an important goal in research because an investigator wishes to make valid conclusions based on *true* differences rather than chance occurrences.

TABLE 12-2   Possible Correct and Incorrect Decisions in Hypothesis Testing

	H_0 **is True**	H_0 **is False**
Do not reject H_0	Correct decision $(1 - \alpha)$	Type II error (β)
Reject H_0	Type error (α)	Correct decision power $(1 - \beta)$

The calculation of the power of a statistical test is beyond the present aims of this chapter. Nevertheless, for the more mathematically inclined reader, we have included the steps involved in this calculation in Appendix A-3. A summary of statistical errors in relation to the power of the test is illustrated in Table 12-2.

ONE-SAMPLE PROPORTION TEST: INFERENCE CONCERNING A SINGLE PROPORTION

In this section, we discuss the method of estimating a true population proportion (p) of those elements in a target population possessing a particular characteristic of a researcher's interest. For example, a clinician wishes to estimate the proportion of all clients in a city clinic who have a particular communication disorder. In this scenario, the set of all subjects in the city clinic constitute a target population. A subject possesses the characteristic of interest; that is, he or she possesses the disorder, and the proportion of all subjects possessing that disorder is a population proportion p. Suppose the clinician collects a random sample of 100 subjects from the target population and finds that 45 of them possess the disorder. A **point estimate** (or a sample proportion), denoted by $\hat{p}$, is calculated as follows:

$$\hat{p} = \frac{45}{100} = .45$$

In general, we define

trial = a subject who is randomly selected
success = S = a randomly selected subject who possesses the disorder
failure = F = a randomly selected subject does not possess disorder
p = proportion of all subjects who possess the particular disorder
$q = 1 - p$ = proportion of all subjects who do not possess the particular disorder
n = number of trials (the number of subjects in the sample)
x = number of successes (the number of subjects in the sample who possess the particular disorder)
$\hat{p} = x/n$ = a point estimate for p (a sample proportion that will estimate p)

As all readers are already aware, in order to hold the assumption of normality, n must be sufficiently large. Here is a rule of thumb to assure the normality: the normal approximation is held if both $n\hat{p}$ and $n\hat{q}$ are at least 5. The calculation of an observed z value is given by

$$\text{Observed } z = \frac{\hat{p} - p}{\sqrt{\dfrac{pq}{n}}}$$

where mean $= p$ and standard deviation $= \sqrt{pq/n}$.

Because the mathematical derivation for constructing a $(1 - \alpha)$ confidence interval for p is extremely complex, only the results can be given here.

A point estimate for p is the sample proportion $\hat{p} = \dfrac{x}{n}$. When n is large enough, a $(1 - \alpha)$ confidence interval is given by

$$\hat{p} - z_{\alpha/2} \cdot \sqrt{\frac{\hat{p}\hat{q}}{n}} < p < \hat{p} + z_{\alpha/2} \cdot \sqrt{\frac{\hat{p}\hat{q}}{n}}$$

and if we replace p by $\hat{p}$ for estimation, the maximum error of the estimate E with a $(1 - \alpha)$ confidence is

$$E = z_{\alpha/2} \cdot \sqrt{\frac{\hat{p}\hat{q}}{n}}$$

where $z_{\alpha/2} =$ the critical z value such that the area under the standard normal z curve to the right of it is $\alpha/2$.

When we also estimate p by $\hat{p}$, if we wish the maximum error E to be some given value, we must choose the sample size n to be at least (or conservatively)

$$n = \left(\frac{z_{\alpha/2}}{E} \right) \frac{1}{4}$$

The calculation of the maximum error of the estimate E is beyond the present aim of this chapter. Nevertheless, for the more mathematically inclined reader, we have included the steps involved in this calculation in Appendix A-5.

TWO-SAMPLE CASE: TESTING HYPOTHESES FOR TWO GROUPS

In the behavioral sciences, researchers are interested in testing the significance of difference between two means reflecting the scores of two randomly assigned groups. One of these groups receives an experimental treatment (experimental group) and another group is given no treatment or a different form of treatment (control group). The mean scores of the two groups are then compared to determine the probability that a particular finding is statistically significant.

We noted earlier that in cases where the standard deviation of a population (σ) is unknown and $n \leq 30$, a z distribution cannot be used. Thus, the standard error must be estimated based on the sample data alone. We printed out that, in place of z scores, t scores are used to make estimates about the values of sample means in relation to their population values.

The calculation of t is similar to z except that t is calculated by estimating the number of standard errors that a sample mean lies above or below the population mean. On the other hand, z is derived by finding the actual population parameter. As noted previously, for large samples ($n > 30$), the value of t and z scores become increasingly comparable.

In order to determine whether two or more means come from the same population, researchers employ the strategy of testing the statistical significance of the null hypothesis, which is a proposition that no significant difference between mean scores will be found. If the results of such testing reveal that the probability for the sample means to reflect a common mean is less than 5 percent (p < .05), the null hypothesis is usually rejected in favor of a significant finding.

In testing the differences between two means, several methods may be used depending on the type of research design employed by the investigator. Two common statistics used for this purpose are: (1) the unpaired t test for independent samples and (2) the paired t test for dependent samples.

Unpaired t Test for Independent Samples

In cases in which the data arising from separate and unrelated groups of subjects are independent of one another, the unpaired t test is an appropriate statistic to use.

Suppose we are interested in evaluating the effectiveness of "therapy approach X" as compared to "therapy approach Y." Assume further that, from a common pool of available subjects, 14 subjects are randomly assigned to Group X and 11 subjects to Group Y. We wish to know whether the performance of Group X will differ from Group Y under two different sets of treatment circumstances. More specifically, we wish to determine whether the mean score (μ_X) of Group X will differ from the mean score (μ_Y) of Group Y based on the results of statistical testing. Assume further that there is no basis for predicting, prior to the experiment, whether one therapy approach is more effective than the other.

The actual steps involved in testing the significance of the difference between the means using the unpaired t test are outlined below:

Step 1. Form the hypothesis in statistical terms.

$$\text{Null hypothesis } (H_0)\text{: } \mu_X = \mu_Y$$
$$\text{Alternative hypothesis } (H_1)\text{: } \mu_X \neq \mu_Y$$

Stating the null hypothesis as $\mu_X = \mu_Y$ is the same as saying that μ_X and μ_Y will be assumed not to differ unless a difference is found in a subsequent experiment. If the null hypothesis is rejected, the alternative hypothesis is supported. In the absence of a significant finding, the null hypothesis is retained pending the outcome of future experiments. Remember that the null hypothesis cannot be accepted because it is always possible that it will be disproved in some future investigation. The alternative hypothesis as previously stated above signifies that the result will be evaluated by a two-tailed test. Such a test is selected when the direction of the difference is not predicted because no prior expectation is held by the investigator about the outcome. If the investigator had expected that one treatment would be more effective than the other treatment, the alternative hypothesis would have been stated as either $\mu_X > \mu_Y$ or $\mu_X < \mu_Y$. A one-tailed test is said to be less stringent than a two-tailed test because a smaller amount of variance between mean scores is needed to be considered a significant finding.

Step 2. Select an appropriate statistical test.

As noted previously, the most commonly selected statistics used for evaluating the significance of difference between two means are the z and t tests. The z test may be used in cases in which the conditions of the *central limit theorem* are satisfied; that is, the distributions are presumed to be normal and the population standard deviation (σ) is known. However, in the field of communication sciences and disorders, research often involves the use of small samples of individuals having relatively unique problems so that population standard deviation

(σ) is unknown. Given such limitations, as in the case of our experiment, the t test often is the more appropriate choice for the statistical analysis of data.

Step 3. Select the level of significance.

In order to evaluate a null hypothesis, it must be decided *before* the investigation begins the point at which a difference between the means will be considered significant, that is, not a result of chance as the null hypothesis claims. This decision requires the establishment of an alpha value (α) as the criterion for rejecting the null hypothesis. In conjunction with this decision, the alpha is typically set at .05 as the highest cutoff value for rejecting the null hypothesis. Although lower alpha values (e.g., .01 or .001) may be used for determining statistical significance, they rarely are set higher than the .05 level. Because α is a type I error, it quantifies the risk of an error when H_0 is rejected. Generally speaking, determining the severity or seriousness of a type I error in a particular situation is subjective; that is, it is a decision made by an investigator prior to an experiment. However, it is known to be true that we would feel more confident about our decision if we reject H_0 as α gets smaller and smaller. Some readers may ask why we would settle for a value of .05 for α when we could choose a smaller value (for instance, a value of .01 for α instead) to minimize the risk associated with a type I error. The answer lies in the fact that when we decrease the value of α there will be an increase in the value of a type II error (β) that leads to a smaller value of a statistical power and our decision would be "less credible." Therefore, even though a value of β is unknown, we could have some influence on its size by our choice of α. For a fixed sample size, the smaller the value of α, the larger the value of β. The larger the value of α, the smaller the value of β. In some cases, if a researcher believes that a type I error is more serious than a type II error in terms of his or her final decision, a smaller value of α (say, .01 or .025) should be chosen. On the other hand, if a researcher is very concerned about committing a type II error, a larger value of α (.10) should be chosen. One technique that can often be used by a researcher to minimize a type II error (β) while retaining a smaller value of α is to simply increase the sample size. The larger the sample size, the more likely it is that a test will detect an even smaller significant difference that exists between the population mean and the hypothesized value in H_0 and H_1.

Step 4. Calculate the test statistic.

The calculation of the t test for independent (unpaired) samples is as follows:

a. First calculate the means for the two distributions. These are given here as: $\overline{X} = 100$, $\overline{Y} = 88$.

b. Calculate the standard deviations for the two distributions. Again, these are given as $S_X = 12$, $S_Y = 15$.

c. Calculate the pooled standard deviation of the means. In order to do this, the values of n for each mean are also needed. They are given here as

$$S_P = \sqrt{\frac{(n_X - 1)S_X^2 + (n_Y - 1)S_Y^2}{n_1 + n_2 - 2}}$$

$$= \sqrt{\frac{(14 - 1)(12)^2 + (11 - 1)(15)^2}{14 + 11 - 2}}$$

$$= \sqrt{\frac{4122}{23}}$$

$$= 13.39$$

d. Calculate the standard error of the mean difference

$$SE(\bar{X} - \bar{Y}) = S_p \sqrt{\frac{1}{n_X} + \frac{1}{n_Y}}$$

$$= 13.38 \sqrt{\frac{1}{14} + \frac{1}{11}}$$

$$= 5.39$$

e. Determine the value of t. This score constitutes the ratio of the difference between two means to the standard error of the difference. In our investigation, it is given by

$$t = \frac{\bar{X} - \bar{Y}}{SE(\bar{X} - \bar{Y})}$$

$$= \frac{100 - 88}{5.39}$$

$$= 2.23$$

Step 5.   Draw conclusions on the basis of critical value(s).

Having completed the t test, the next step is to determine the probability that a t score as large or larger than the value obtained might have resulted as the consequence of chance. This can be accomplished by consulting a probability table, like that in Appendix A-1-2, that lists the **critical values** for the t distribution. Determining the significance of a critical value is possible by examining the areas for acceptance and rejection under the normal curve. The t distribution conforms closely to the shape of the normal curve for large sample sizes.

The critical value of t depends in part on the number of degrees of freedom (df) allowed. In the case of testing the difference between two means, as in the above study, this is defined as $N_1 + N_2 - 2$. The critical value of t also depends on whether the test is one tailed or two tailed and on the significance level selected (.05, .01, etc.).

Referring to the table for t in Appendix A-1-2, we note that the calculated value (observed value) of t (2.23) for 23 degrees of freedom exceeds the critical value of t (2.069) located under the column designating the 0.05 significance level for a two-tailed test. These results are shown graphically in Figure 12-3.

Thus, we are able to reject the null hypothesis in favor of the alternative hypothesis. More specifically, we are able to conclude that there was a significant difference between the two therapy approaches, with therapy approach X appearing to have been more effective than therapy approach Y. Had the calculated t score exceeded the critical value of 2.807 listed in the table under the area of the upper tail of the curve, the result would have reached an even higher level of significance ($p < .01$). However, recall from our previous discussion that the choice of a particular alpha value (α) should be made before the test is performed. The actual probability value (p) or calculated (observed) t value is determined on the basis of statistical

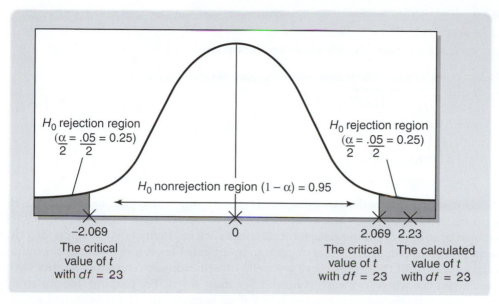

FIGURE 12-3   The critical t values ($\pm$2.069) associated with $\alpha/2 = .025$, 23 df, and a nondirectional, two-tailed test of the null hypothesis

testing. If the absolute value of the calculated (observed) t value is greater than the critical value shown in the table, the null hypothesis is rejected.

To say that $p < .01$ is *more* significant than $p < .05$ may be statistically correct but has little substantive importance in evaluating possible outcomes of an experiment. Based on the statistical evidence, either the null hypothesis is rejected, indicating a significant outcome, or retained, indicating a nonsignificant outcome. In the former case, the significant difference is considered to result from the systematic influence of the independent variable rather than from chance alone. On the other hand, in the instance of a nonsignificant finding, the amount of difference found is considered to be the result of chance factors rather than the consequence of systematic influences known to the investigator.

Paired t Test for Dependent Samples

In our discussion we have outlined the steps required for testing the significance of difference between the means of two independent random samples. However, certain hypotheses can be better evaluated using what are variously called *dependent, correlated,* or *related* samples. Such samples can result from certain matching procedures to form matched pairs or the same group can be measured twice in a *pairing-design* where each subject is used in both conditions. Sampling procedures that entail matching subjects on factors that might influence the outcome of an experiment, other than the independent variable, were considered in Chapter 5. The so-called pairing design involves the use of subjects as their own control. This type of design is also known as a *within-subject, self-control,* or *repeated measurements* design.

The formula for this test is given by

$$t = \frac{\overline{d}}{S_d / \sqrt{n}} \text{ with } df = n - 1$$

where

$$\bar{d} = \text{the mean of the difference scores for the sample pair} = \frac{\Sigma d}{n}$$

S_d = the standard deviation of the sample difference calculated by

$$S_d = \sqrt{\frac{\Sigma d^2 - \frac{(\Sigma d)^2}{n}}{n-1}}$$

n = The number of pairs in the sample

μ_d = a testing mean difference = 0 (the numerator is actually written as $\bar{d} - \mu_d$)

Let us now illustrate the use of the paired t test as it might be applied to a clinical problem in the area of stuttering. There is evidence that the adrenergic blocking agent propranolol is useful in controlling certain neuromotor disorders such as essential tremor and tardive dyskinesia. Hypothetically, assume that we want to investigate the potential effect of the minimal therapeutic dose of this drug against a placebo on self-ratings of stuttering severity using a Likert-type scale where 1 = least severe and 5 = most severe. For purposes for our study, a *cross-over design* is selected for use in which half of ten subjects initially will be treated with propranolol and the other half with placebo for a two-week period, at the end of which they will provide self-ratings of stuttering severity. A six-week "wash out period" will separate the two treatments before crossing over to the alternate form. At the end of the second two-week treatment period, self-ratings of stuttering severity will be made again.

The actual steps involved in testing the significance of the difference between the means of the drug and placebo conditions using the paired t test are outlined below:

Step 1.   Form the hypothesis in statistical terms.

The null hypothesis that we wish to evaluate statistically is $H_0{:}\mu_d = 0$ (the mean difference in the paired observation is zero).
The alternative hypothesis can be stated as $H_1{:}\mu_d < 0$ (the mean difference in the paired observations is less than zero).

Step 2.   Select an appropriate statistical test.

The statistical test for comparing the differences between two means of dependent samples is the t test for paired observations, or simply the **paired t test**. This test statistic is comparable to the previously discussed test for unpaired samples. However, the calculations for the means and the standard deviations are replaced by difference scores (ds).

Step 3.   Choose the significance level.

In order to evaluate the null hypothesis, the significance level will be set at .05 for a one-tailed test. More specifically, because we are predicting that stuttering will be rated as less severe under the propranolol condition than under the placebo condition, we will look for a significant difference in the left tail of the curve.

Step 4.   Construct a table to include n, d, d^2, Σd, $\bar{d}$, Σd^2, and $(\Sigma d)^2$ and calculate the test statistic (see Table 12-3).

TABLE 12-3 Paired t Test Results for the Self-Rating of Stuttering Under Two Treatment Conditions (1 = least severe and 5 = most severe)

Subject	Propranolol	Placebo	Difference d	Difference Squared d^2
1	4	5	−1	1
2	0	1	−1	1
3	0	0	0	0
4	2	4	−2	4
5	1	4	−3	9
6	3	5	−2	4
7	3	3	0	0
8	1	3	−2	4
9	2	2	0	0
10	1	4	−3	9
Σ(sum)			−14	32

$n = 10$, $\Sigma d = -14$, $\bar{d} = -1.4$, $\Sigma d^2 = 32$, $(\Sigma d)^2 = 196$

The calculation of the paired t-test proceeds as follows:

a. Calculate S_d: Based on the data in Table 12-3, it is equal to 1.17.

b. Calculate the observed t value: $t = \dfrac{-1.4}{\dfrac{1.17}{\sqrt{10}}} = -3.78$

Step 5. Draw conclusions on the basis of critical value(s).

Referring to Appendix A-1-2, we can determine the critical value of t for $df = 9$, which is −1.833. The observed value of t, −3.78, falls into the H_0 rejection region ($\alpha = .05$). These results are shown graphically in Figure 12-4. Hence, the null hypothesis that the two treatments are equivalent can be rejected in favor of a significant finding in support of H_1. In other words, we can conclude on the basis of our hypothetical results that the self-rating of stuttering severity was lower under the propranolol condition than under the control condition at $\alpha = .05$.

So far, our approach enables us to determine whether or not there is sufficient evidence to prove the alternate hypothesis (H_1) but not the null hypothesis (H_0). So, you may say that we would actually accept H_1 if we reject H_0. In this case, we always know the risk associated with a type I error (α), and it is chosen to be small. However, if we do not reject H_0, we would possibly have a type II error (β), which is usually unknown. In some instances, β can be large enough to make our conclusion "less credible" because the statistical power of a test will decrease as β increases. Hence, if we do not reject H_0, we are not confident enough to say that the null hypothesis has been established, because we do not know our chance of being wrong. This is the main reason why we avoid using terms such as "accept H_0" or "accept H_1." The basic idea is to state the hypothesis you wish to prove as the alternate hypothesis H_1. Then, hopefully, a test will lead you to rejection of H_0. You may place some confidence (faith) in the

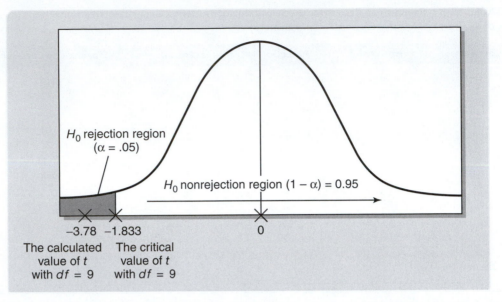

FIGURE 12-4   The critical *t* values (-1.833) associated with $\alpha = .05$, 9 *df* and a directional, one-tailed test of the null hypothesis

truth of H_1 because you established the chance associated with a type I error (α) prior to an experiment.

NONPARAMETRIC ALTERNATIVES TO PARAMETRIC STATISTICS

Thus far, our discussion of statistical inference has focused on the use of parametric tests of significance, which generally include the following assumptions:

1. *Normality.* The population distribution is normal.
2. *Homogeneity of variances.* When two populations are being compared, especially in the case of independent observations, their distribution values should have relatively equal variances.
3. *Randomness.* Subjects should be chosen randomly.
4. *Interval/ratio data.* The data should be quantifiable on a numerical scale when common arithmetic is appropriate.

When these assumptions cannot be met, then the use of such parametric statistics as the mean, standard deviation, and *t* test may be inappropriate and may lead to invalid conclusions. Three **nonparametric statistics** that do not make these assumptions are discussed next.

Chi-Square Test (χ^2)

A test that is useful in evaluating hypotheses about the relationship between nominal variables having two or more independent categories is the χ^2 statistic or chi- (pronounced "kai") square. The inventor of this test, Karl Pearson, also developed a well-known method for computing correlation coefficients as discussed in Chapter 11. Throughout his career, this acknowledged founder of modern statistics was interested in studying the relations among variables. One of the most modern thinkers of his time, Pearson rejected the search for causality in favor of studying the association or *contingency* of phenomenon. Pearson's fervent interest in the topic of association also extended into the social realm, to such matters as the relations between the sexes. In 1885 he founded a "Men and Women's Club" in England to promote the discussion of such relations, where he met his future wife (Peters, 1987). Apparently, their interests were indeed contingent—that is, a "good fit!"

In essence, the chi-square test provides a means of determining the *independence* between two or more nominal variables by calculating the discrepancy between the *observed frequencies* (actual counts) for a set of categories and the *expected frequencies* for the same categories (probability estimates). Suppose we wish to determine whether graduate students preparing for clinical careers in either speech-language pathology *or* audiology have different preferences for the type of setting in which they might choose to work, say, a medical versus nonmedical setting. Imagine further that our two-sample case is based on the job preferences expressed by 50 students who wish to be certified as speech-language pathologists and an equal number who desires certification in audiology. Let us now illustrate the steps involved in testing to see whether the variables of interest are independent or in some way associated. Before we begin, it is important for us to understand some of the important characteristics about a chi-square distribution. So, we first will introduce the properties of a chi-square distribution.

A chi-square distribution has the following properties:

1. There are an infinite number of chi-square distributions. Each one has a number (or index number) with it called its *degrees of freedom*. We use the degrees of freedom to specify which chi-square distribution we are using.
2. The shape of a chi-square distribution curve is not symmetric but is skewed to the right (positively skewed). It begins at 0 and extends indefinitely in a positive direction. The total area under the curve is 1.
3. The mean value of χ^2 is the degrees of freedom.

With that background, to perform a chi-square test do the following:

Step 1. Form the hypothesis in statistical terms.

H_0: The proportion of subjects from each sample selecting a particular preference category will be independent (unrelated).
H_1: The proportion of subjects from each sample selecting a particular preference category will *not* be independent (somehow related).

Step 2. Select an appropriate statistical test.

The chi-square test is appropriate for our problem because two samples of subjects are being compared on a nominal variable that has two categories.

Step 3. Choose the significance level.

We will set the significance level (α) at .05 for a one-tailed test. A one-tailed test is employed for interpreting the statistical significance of χ^2 because the result is used to evaluate whether the discrepancy between the observed and expected frequencies is *greater* than can be accounted for by chance.

Step 4. Organize the data in a 2 × 2 contingency table and calculate the test statistic.

The data are organized into a contingency table, like that shown in Table 12-4 in order to compare the frequency of responses in each cell that actually occurred (observed frequency)

TABLE 12-4   Hypothetical Survey of Work Preferences Among Speech-Language Pathology Students and Audiology Students.

| | WORK PREFERENCE | | | |
	Medical	Nonmedical	Row Sum	N = 100
Sp-lang. path.	18	32	50	
Audiology	31	19	50	
Column sum	49	51	100	

with the number of responses estimated to occur (expected frequency). The latter proportion can be calculated with the following formula:

$$E = \frac{\text{Row total} \times \text{Column total}}{\text{Grand total}}$$

For example, the expected frequency of speech-language pathology students preferring to work in a medical setting is the computational result of 50 (first row sum) times 49 (first column sum) divided by 100 (grand sum), which is equal to 24.5. The same computation is performed for the remaining cells to yield an expected frequency for each category.

Once the observed values have been entered into a 2 × 2 contingency table, we can perform the chi-square test in accordance with one of the following formulas, depending on the number of degrees of freedom:

a. $\chi^2 = \sum \frac{(O - E)^2}{E}$ for degrees of freedom greater than 1, where O = the observed frequency (actual counts), and E = the expected frequency (probability estimates)

b. $\chi^2 = \frac{N(ad - bc)^2}{(a + b)(c + d)(a + c)(b + d)}$ for degrees of freedom = 1

where N = the total number of subjects
a = the observed frequency of the first row and first column
b = the observed frequency of the first row and second column
c = the observed frequency of the second row and first column
d = the observed frequency of the second row and second column

For degrees of freedom equal to 1, the second formula, called **Yates' correction for continuity,** should be used instead of the first formula. Generally, Yates' formula deals with the inconsistency between the theoretical chi-square distribution and the actual sampling distribution having 1 degree of freedom. Based on our example, it can be seen that Yates' correction must be used because $df = (r - 1)(c - 1) = (2 - 1)(2 - 1) = 1$ where r represents the total number of rows and c represents the total number of columns. Next, enter the appropriate values into the formula to calculate the χ^2 value.

$$\chi^2 \text{ (observed)} = \frac{100(18 \cdot 19 - 32 \cdot 31)^2}{(18 + 32)(31 + 19)(18 + 31)(32 + 19)} = 6.76$$

Step 5.   Draw conclusions on the basis of critical value(s).

For a 2×2 contingency table, like the one in our example, there are two rows and two columns, so the degrees of freedom $(df) = (2 - 1) \cdot (2 - 1) = 1$. Chi-square tables have been constructed that allow the statistical significance of χ^2 to be assessed directly. By referring to such a table, as that found in Appendix A-1-3, we note that with $df = 1$, the critical value that must be exceeded to achieve a .05 level of significance is 3.841 for a one-tailed test. Because the calculated (observed) value of χ^2 obtained from our sample exceeds the critical value of 3.841, we would reject the null hypothesis of independence. Given the fictitious results of our example, we are able to conclude that there is a significant relationship between emphasis in graduate training and preferences for future employment. More specifically, it appears that there is a difference in job setting preferences between students of speech-language pathology and audiology. Whereas the majority of the former group in our sample preferred a nonmedical as opposed to medical work setting, the opposite was true for the latter group.

Because of its wide range of applications, the chi-square test is useful for many problems involving the comparison of proportions. The example we used involved only two groups and two categories of variables. However, the number of rows and columns can be extended for the study of relationships among multiple groups and variables depending on the nature of the research question.

The chi-square test is often referred to as a "goodness-of-fit" test when the question pertains to whether distributions of scores fall into certain categories according to an investigator's expectation. Other uses include testing to see whether an obtained distribution drawn by random sampling reflects a normally distributed population. A nonsignificant chi-square would indicate that the shape of the obtained distribution fits the shape of the normal curve. On the other hand, a significant chi-square would be interpreted as a lack of fit between the obtained and normal distribution.

Unfortunately, the chi-square test is often applied inappropriately to statistical problems for which it is not intended. Remember that it is most suited for categorical data in which each case falling within a category or cell is independent of every other case. This is necessary to determine the true relationship between column and row variables—whether they are indeed independent of one another. In the case of our example, had we inadvertently mixed among our categories graduate students pursing certification in *both* speech-language pathology and audiology, such a linkage would have violated the assumption of independence. In the use of the chi-square, the best policy is to have only one frequency count per subject and to have the subjects as unrelated to one another as possible.

Nonparametric Rank-Order Methods

There are two highly useful alternative methods to the *t* test that were developed by Wilcoxon and are said to be "distribution free" for two reasons. First, like the chi-square, they are free of assumptions about the shape of the underlying population distribution. Second, they both entail *transforming* scores to ranks. Such tests are well suited for ordinal scales of measurement when the scores in a distribution can be logically arranged from most to least frequent but the intervals between the data points are either unknown or skewed.

The **Wilcoxon matched-pairs signed ranks test** is a commonly used nonparametric analog of the paired *t* test that utilizes information about both the *magnitude* and *direction* of differences for pairs of scores. Within the behavioral sciences, it is the most commonly used nonparametric test of the significance of difference between dependent samples. This test is appropriate for studies involving repeated measures, as in pretest–posttest designs in which the same subjects serve as their own control, or in cases that use matched pairs of subjects. The ranking procedures used by the Wilcoxon test allow for (1) determining which member of a pair of scores is larger or smaller than the other, as denoted by the sign of the difference (+ or −, respectively), and (2) the ranking of such size differences. The null hypothesis under this test is that the median difference among pairs of ranked scores is zero.

Let us illustrate the steps in hypothesis testing using the Wilcoxon test in conjunction with some hypothetical data that might be generated in a study of the relationship between grammatical complexity and phonological production. More specifically, suppose we wish to determine whether preschool children with impairments in both grammar and phonology will make more speech sound errors when imitating grammatically complex sentences than when imitating relatively simple sentences that are comparable in length. We can proceed as follows:

Step 1.   Form the hypothesis in statistical terms.

H_0: There is no difference in the occurrence of phonologic errors when subjects imitate complex and simple sentences of the same length.

H_1: Phonologic errors will occur more often in the production of complex sentences than in that of simple sentences of the same length.

Step 2.   Select an appropriate statistical test.

As an alternative to the paired *t* test, the Wilcoxon test has been selected because it also is an appropriate test for the analysis of dependent or correlated samples. With respect to its overall *power* (probability for rejecting a false null hypothesis), the Wilcoxon test closely approximates the efficiency of the parametric *t* for large *n*'s. For small *n*'s, the power efficiency of the Wilcoxon test is approximately 95% of its counterpart (Siegel, 1956). For data that are not normally distributed, the Wilcoxon test is more powerful than the *t* test. The likelihood of skewness increases as *n* becomes small as in the case of our sample.

Step 3.   Choose the significance level.

The significance level (α) is set at .05 in a one-tailed test. We have chosen a one-tailed test in view of some preexisting evidence that phonological errors occur more often in the production of complex sentences than simple sentence (Menyuk & Looney, 1972; Panagos & Prelock, 1982).

Step 4.   Organize the paired-scores into a table and calculate the test statistic (see Table 12-5).

The difference score is positive if the first number of a pair is larger than the second or, conversely, carries a negative sign if the second number is larger than the first. The sign of a number has no real mathematical significance in the Wilcoxon test, but serves to mark the direction of difference between the pairs of scores. The next step is to rank the difference scores according to their relative magnitude, assigning an average rank score to each tie irrespective of whether the sign is positive or negative. Zero difference scores between pairs ($d = 0$) are dropped from the analysis. Therefore, the total number of signed ranks (*n*) in determining the criterion for rejecting H_0 is 9. Finally, in the last column of the table, sum the absolute value of the ranked difference scores having the *least* frequent sign. This last operation yields *T*: the smaller sum of the least frequent ranks.

Step 5.   Draw conclusions of the basis of critical value(s).

Critical values for one-tailed and two-tailed tests have been developed for *T*, which has its own sampling distribution developed by Wilcoxon. Recall that in the case of the

TABLE 12-5 Hypothetical Study of Speech Sound Errors for Preschool Children During Imitation of Complex and Simple Sentences

Subject	Complex	Simple	d	Rank	Less Frequent Rank
1	17	18	−1	−1.5	1.5
2	14	11	3	4.5	
3	16	13	3	4.5	
4	11	11	0	0	
5	13	7	6	8	
6	31	29	2	3	
7	12	7	5	6.5	
8	29	21	8	9	
9	17	12	5	6.5	
10	9	10	−1	−1.5	1.5
					$T = 3$
					$n = 9$

parametric t, values of t *larger* than the critical values listed in the probability table under the chosen significance level serve as a basis for rejecting the null hypothesis in favor of a significant finding. However, in the case of the Wilcoxon T, values *smaller* than the listed table values under a particular α for the *total number of signed ranks* (n) is the basis for rejecting the null hypothesis. Turning to Appendix A-1-5, we find that the critical value for an n of 9 is 8. Because our observed T value is less than the critical value of 8, we would reject H_0 in favor of H_1. More specifically, we can conclude that the complexity of imitated sentences seems to have a direct bearing on phonological productions. Thus, the outcome of our hypothetical study is consistent with the results of previous investigations that have found more phonological errors in children occurring during imitation of complex sentences than of simple sentences.

The **Mann-Whitney U test** is a highly useful test for determining the probability that two independent samples came from the same population. It is variously called the Mann-Whitney U or Wilcoxon-rank sum test. In contrast to its parametric equivalent, the unpaired t test for independent samples, the Mann-Whitney U test is concerned with the equality of medians rather than means.

Suppose we are interested in knowing whether the physical status of newborns is related to their subsequent development of receptive language. For this purpose, we conduct a prospective study in which Apgar scores are collected on a random sample. Such scores are used to denote the general condition of an infant shortly after birth based on five physical indices including skin color, heart rate, respiratory effort, muscle tone, and reflex irritability. The maximum score of 10 is indicative of excellent physical condition. Using these numerical values as our independent variable, we divide our sample into two groups: (1) 10 children with high Apgar scores (greater than 6) and (2) 8 children with low Apgar scores (less than 4). Composite receptive language scores, obtained for these same children at ages 3 to 3.5 years on the appropriate subtests of the Clinical

Evaluation of Language Functions-Preschool (CELF-P) (Wiig et al., 1992), serve as the dependent variable.

We will now use some fictitious data in order to illustrate an application of the Mann-Whitney U test. The steps for calculating the Mann-Whitney U statistic are shown below:

Step 1.   Form the hypothesis in statistical terms.

> H_0: There is no difference in the receptive language ability of children who scored high on the Apgar scale versus those who scored low.
> H_1: There is a difference in the receptive language ability of children who scored high on the Apgar scale versus those who scored low.

Step 2.   Select an appropriate statistical test.

As an alternative to the unpaired t test, the Mann-Whitney U is chosen because it is an appropriate test for detecting differences between two independent groups. It is commonly used when the parametric t-test's assumptions of normality and homogeneity of variance are violated.

Step 3.   Choose the significance level.

The significance level (α) is set at .05 in a two-tailed test. In the case of our problem, a two-tailed test is appropriate because we are assuming that no prior knowledge is available that can be used as a basis for predicting the outcome of our study.

Step 4.   Organize a table to include test scores, their ranks, and the sum of their ranks, and calculate the test statistic (see Table 12-6).

Table 12-6 shows the results for our hypothetical study including CELF-P scores for the two groups, their corresponding ranks, and the sum of their ranks. The Mann-Whitney U is calculated as the smaller of U_1 and U_2, where

$$U_1 = (n_L)(n_S) + \frac{n_L(n_L + 1)}{2} - T_L$$

$$U_2 = (n_L)(n_S) - U_1$$

where n_L = the number of subjects in the group with the larger sum of ranks (denoted by n_1) and n_S = the number of subjects in the other group (denoted by n_2) See Appendix A-1-6.

Given our hypothetical data, U_1 and U_2 are found to be 15 and 65, respectively. Thus, the value of the Mann-Whitney U is 15.

Step 5.   Draw conclusions on the basis of the critical value(s).

By consulting a special table for Mann-Whitney critical values like that found in Appendix A-1-6, we can observe that the obtained U of 15 is less than the table value of 17 (n_L = 10, n_S = 8 for a two-tailed test at α = .05). In the table shown, n_L is labeled as n_1 and n_S is labeled as n_2. The criterion rule for rejecting the null hypothesis (H_0) indicates that we reject H_0 when the observed value of U *is less than or equal to* the critical value of U. Therefore, because the observed value of U is less than the critical value, we conclude that the receptive language abilities of the two groups as distinguished on the basis of their Apgar scores are significantly different.

TABLE 12-6 Receptive Language Scores for Children with High and Low Apgars (Fabricated Data)

Language Scores (High Apgar Group)	Rank	Language Scores (Low Apgar Group)	Rank
37	14.5	22	1
32	11.5	23	2
34	13	30	9.5
28	6.5	37	14.5
32	11.5	24	3
47	18	27	5
29	8	30	9.5
45	17	28	6.5
39	16		
26	4		
	Sum = 120		Sum = 51

T_L = Larger sum of the ranks = 120
N_L = number of subjects in the group with the larger sum of ranks = 10
N_S = number of subjects in the other group = 8

MULTIGROUP DESIGNS: TESTING HYPOTHESES FOR THREE OR MORE GROUPS

In previous sections of this chapter we discussed a variety of parametric and nonparametric tests for analyzing data from two different experimental conditions or from two different groups of subjects in order to test hypotheses. However, researchers often wish to set up experiments in which a single independent variable (factor) may be represented by more than two treatments (levels) and/or two or more factors may be manipulated consecutively.

Analysis of Variance (ANOVA)

More complex designs than the *t* test are often necessary for answering questions that go beyond the two-sample case—such as, "Is treatment *A* more effective than treatment *B*?" In some cases we might want to compare the treatment effectiveness of approaches (*A, B, C,* etc.) or the performance of several groups on a particular dependent variable. It is also possible to study combined treatment effects as might result from the interactions of treatment (*A* × *B*, *A* × *C, B* × *C,* etc.).

One could ask, "Why not perform a single *t* test for each statistical comparison of mean scores that might need to be made?" There are two main answers to this question. First, if no significant differences exist among any of the comparisons, then conducting numerous *t* tests in order to make this "dry gulch" determination is a needless waste of time. If this could be achieved by a single omnibus test, the goal of research efficiency is better served. Such a test, called the *analysis of variance (ANOVA),* invented by the British statistician Sir Ronald Fisher, accomplishes this very goal. Although the ANOVA can be used for the analysis of two means, its greater utility lies in testing variation among three or more means.

A second problem relating to the use of multiple t tests is the probability of one or more of them reaching significance merely by chance. Because multiple t tests typically are not independent of one another, the probability of a type I error becomes greater with the number of tests performed. For example, assuming that three t tests are performed where $\alpha = .05$, the actual probability of obtaining a significant result by chance from any of the three tests (there are three different t tests that can be performed when we compare three group means simultaneously, such as A versus B, A versus C, and B versus C) is not .05. Rather, the true probability is given by:

$$p \text{ (type I error)} = 1 - (1 - \alpha)^n$$

where n represents the number of the tests performed. Thus, the true probability is $1 - (1 - .05)^3 = .14$, not .05.

Logic of ANOVA

The use of ANOVA for hypothesis testing is somewhat analogous to a familiar problem encountered in studies involving the electronic transmission of signals called the "signal to noise ratio." For example, a "good" tape recorder is one that allows for the input of signals at high sound pressure levels with as little as possible distortion owing to extraneous noise. No doubt, we have all experienced the unpleasant "hum" that occurs on playback when the capacity of the recording unit has been exceeded. Thus, a good recording device is one in which the ratio of the signal to the noise is large—that is, one that is able to maximize the transmission of salient information (the signal) while minimizing the transmission of artifacts (noise). In designing instrumentation, an oscilloscope can be helpful to electronic engineers in the computation of the signal-to-noise ratio. Similarly, the main goal in using the ANOVA is to "scope the data" in an effort to isolate systematic treatment effects intended by the experimenter (the signal) from sources of error (noise).

In Chapter 6, we discussed the conceptual basis of systematic variance versus error variance in accounting for the results of an experiment. The main goal of ANOVA is to compute the ratio of systematic variance (the amount of variation owing to a treatment effect) to the degree of error variance that may involve both sampling errors and measurement errors. Recall that a statistical term for systematic variance is *between-group variance*, whereas the statistical moniker for error variance is *within-group variance*. As we also noted, the difference between these types of variance can be expressed symbolically as an F ratio, or

$$F = \frac{V_b}{V_e}$$

where the denominator in the equation is error variance and the numerator is systematic variance.

In reality, the degree of systematic variance in any experiment is the consequence of not only treatment effects but some chance fluctuations as well. Therefore, the *total variability* in data sets can also be expressed as:

$$S^2 \text{ within groups} = \text{error variance}$$

$$S^2 \text{ between groups} = \text{error variance} + \text{treatment effects}$$

ANOVA provides a convenient method of calculating whether the variability between group means is greater than the variability within group means. This is accomplished by dividing up sources of variance into two major components: (1) the variation of the score of each subject from the mean of their group and (2) the variation between each group mean and the grand mean for the sample. If there are large differences between the group means, the variation between them and the grand mean will be large compared to the amount of variation within each group. If this is found to be true on the basis of an **F test,** then the null hypothesis of equivalence between groups is rejected. On the other hand, if the group means are similar in size, their variation from the grand mean should not differ substantially from the variation among the subjects within each group beyond chance expectations. In such a case, the null hypothesis is retained.

Calculation of ANOVA

In order to illustrate the use of ANOVA in hypothesis testing, let us examine its application in estimating the significance of difference among three independent means. For this purpose, the simplest of the ANOVA designs involving the analysis of a single factor will be used. This method, called a *one-way ANOVA,* may be viewed as an extension of the unpaired t test for two independent means discussed previously in this chapter.

Suppose we are interested in exploring the relationship between auditory processing abilities and phonological disorders. We will model our hypothetical study, in part, after the investigation of Thayer and Dodd (1996), who evaluated the auditory perceptual abilities of children whose speech sound errors consisted of either *delayed* phonologic acquisition or *disordered* phonology against a control group.

For purposes of our example, we will fabricate some data for three groups of children: Control group (A), Consistent group (B), and Delayed group (C). The Consistent group are children who display consistent phonologic errors that are atypical of normal phonologic development. On the other hand, the Delayed group is constituted of those subjects whose speech sound errors are inappropriate for age but typical of earlier stages of phonologic development. Assume that there are 10 children in each of the three groups. As in the study by Thayer and Dodd, the Pediatric Speech Intelligibility (PSI) Test will be used for the assessment of the subjects' auditory processing abilities. This test involves assessment of the ability to process messages in the presence of competing but semantically related sentences presented either contralaterally (one sentence to each ear) or ipsilaterally (both sentences to the same ear). For purposes of simplifying the analysis, we will limit our discussion to some hypothetical outcomes for the right ear results under contralateral testing conditions.

Let us now illustrate the steps in testing the hypotheses associated with this problem and the procedures necessary for their evaluation based on a one-way ANOVA.

Step 1. Form the hypothesis in statistical terms.

H_0: There is no difference in the auditory processing ability among the three groups. Symbolically, we can also state that $\mu_A = \mu_B = \mu_C$.
H_1: There is a difference in the auditory processing ability among the three groups. Symbolically, we can also state that at least one μ is different from other μ's.

Step 2. Select an appropriate statistical test.

The use of a one-way ANOVA is predicated on the following three assumptions: (1) there is independence among the groups; (2) the sampling distribution of the groups follows a normal curve; and (3) the variances of the scores in each group are equal. Symbolically, we can state that the σ's of all groups are equal (homogeneity of variance). The first two assumptions are also necessary for the use of the *t* test for two independent groups, as previously described. However, the third assumption is an additional component underlying the use of any parametric ANOVA. In cases in which the homogeneity of variance among groups is questionable, the **Bartlett test** should be used for making this determination. An application of this test as it is used as a prerequisite to the ANOVA is illustrated in Appendix A-2.

When each group is constituted by an equal number of subjects or scores, the assumptions of homogeneity of variance are better met. Thus, the one-way ANOVA design is appropriate for hypothesis testing given our hypothetical research problem.

Step 3.   Organize a table to include the necessary numerical values and calculate the test statistic (see Table 12-7).

The mathematical formula for the one-way ANOVA F value is given by

$$F = \frac{\left[\Sigma n_j(\bar{Y}_j - \bar{Y})^2\right] \div (J-1)}{\left[\Sigma(Y_{ij} - \bar{Y}_j)^2\right] \div (N-J)}$$

$$= \frac{\text{Between-group variance}}{\text{Within-group variance}}$$

with df (between) $= J - 1$ and df (within) $= N - J$.

The actual calculation of an observed F value involves the following substeps:

a. Calculate the between-group variance (numerator).

$$\text{Between-group} = \frac{10[(2.33)^2 + (0.33)^2 + (-2.67)^2]}{3-1} = 63.34$$

b. Calculate the within-group variance (denominator).

$$\text{Within-group} = \frac{628 + 840 + 888}{30 - 3} = 87.26$$

c. Calculate the observed F value.

$$F = \frac{63.34}{87.46} = 0.73 \text{ with } df \text{ (numerator)} = 2 \text{ and } df \text{ (denominator)} = 27$$

Step 4.   Draw conclusions on the basis of critical value(s).

By consulting the table for F in Appendix A-1-3, we can observe that the critical value of the test statistic at $\alpha = .05$ for df (numerator) $= 2$ and df (denominator) $= 27$ is 3.35. Because the calculated (observed) F value does not exceed the critical F value, we must retain H_0 in rejection of H_1. More specifically, as in the case of the actual study by Thayer and Dodd, our hypothetical findings indicate that the consistent and delayed groups did not perform differently from one another nor from the control group. Therefore, we can conclude that auditory processing abilities as operationally defined in our investigation do not appear to provide a basis for determining the risk for phonologic disorders.

Two-Way ANOVA

In cases in which an investigator is interested in the effect of two independent variables on one dependent variable involving two or more groups, a two-way analysis of variance (two-way ANOVA) may be performed. For example, if we are interested in comparing the effect of individual therapy (factor 1) versus group therapy (factor 2) on some specific measure of

TABLE 12-7   PSI Scores for the Right Ear Under Contralateral Testing Conditions for Three Groups of Children Classified According to Pattern of Phonologic Development (Fabricated Data)

Control (A)	Consistent (B)	Delayed (C)
73	74	86
98	100	76
100	100	90
99	100	88
99	96	99
100	78	74
100	100	100
98	95	98
100	97	100
93	100	99

$n_A = 10$ $\qquad n_B = 10$ $\qquad n_C = 10$

$\bar{Y}_A = 96$ $\qquad \bar{Y}_B = 94$ $\qquad \bar{Y}_C = 91$

$\Sigma(Y_{ij} - \bar{Y}_A)^2 = 628$ $\quad \Sigma(Y_{ij} - \bar{Y}_B)^2 = 850$ $\quad \Sigma(Y_{ij} - \bar{Y}_C)^2 = 888$

$\bar{Y}_A - \bar{Y} = 2.33$ $\qquad \bar{Y}_B - \bar{Y} = .33$ $\qquad \bar{Y}_C - \bar{Y} = -2.67$

where $\bar{Y}$ = Overall mean $= \dfrac{96 + 94 + 91}{3} = 93.67$

J = Total number of groups = 3

N = Total number of subjects in all groups combined = 30

j = Group identification where j = A, B, C

nj = Number of subjects in each group where $n_A = 10$, $n_B = 10$, and $n_C = 10$

$\bar{Y}_j$ = Sample mean of each group such as $\bar{Y}_A = 96$, $\bar{Y}_B = 94$, $\bar{Y}_C = 91$

$\bar{Y}_{ij}$ = Sample scores in rows (i) by group (j), e.g., $\bar{Y}_{1A}$ is the score of the first row in the control group (A) or 73

$\Sigma(\bar{Y}_{ij} - \bar{Y}_j)^2$ = Sum of the squares of between-group differences

$\bar{Y}_j - \bar{Y}$ = Between-group differences

language performance (dependent variable), this statistical method would be suitable for data analysis. Based on a hypothetical problem of this kind, there are three different ways to measure the relative effect of the individual variables under investigation. These are (1) the main effect owing to factor 1, (2) the main effect owing to factor 2, and (3) the interaction effect owing to factor 1 and factor 2 (denoted by factor 1 × 2). The **main effect** can be defined as the average effect of an independent variable across levels of the dependent variable—for instance, how each *separate* therapy factor will contribute to the outcome measure of language performance. The **interaction effect** can be defined as the *joint* effect of the two independent variables—for instance, how the two therapies combine or interact to influence measured language performance. The latter effect is extremely important in many clinical studies because clinicians often combine treatment modalities instead of using a single treatment approach. Figure 12-5 illustrates the three possible types of interaction patterns

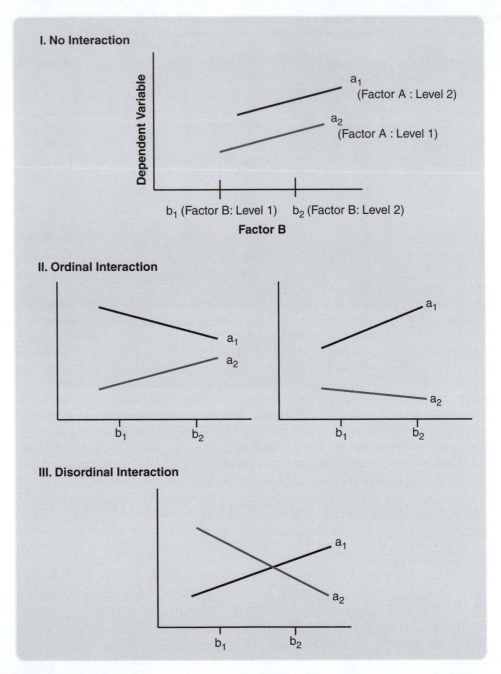

FIGURE 12-5 Illustrations of three possible types of interaction patterns. (I) No interaction exists between Factor A and Factor B. It indicates that, regardless of the level of treatment (Factor A), there is a constant difference between the means at each level of the other factor (Factor B). (II) Ordinal interaction exists between Factor A and Factor B. It indicates a greater difference between groups at one level of Factor A than at the other levels of the same factor. (III) Disordinal interaction exists between Factor A and Factor B. It shows that the effects of the levels of one factor reverse themselves as the levels of the other factor change.

that can be identified for each pair of lines indicating two factors, 1 and 2, when the two-way ANOVA is performed. The conceptual basis for computing the two-way ANOVA is illustrated below:

Total variability of effects = variability owing to main effect of factor 1

+ variability owing to main effect of factor 2

+ variability owing to interaction effect (1 × 2)

+ variability within groups (error variance)

A clinical example from an actual research study and the mathematical calculations associated with performing a two-way ANOVA are illustrated in Appendix A-2.

MULTIPLE COMPARISON METHODS

As noted previously, in cases in which three or more group comparisons are to be made, ANOVA is typically performed as the first step in statistical testing. If the result of the F test indicates that the null hypothesis should be rejected, we conclude that at least one of the group means is different from the other group means. However, we are unable to know on the basis of the F test alone which *specific* group means among the various comparisons are significantly different from others. In order to make this determination, several so-called post hoc multiple comparison tests are available, such as **Scheffe's method** or **Tukey's method.**

In the case of an unequal sample size among the comparison groups, Scheffe's test is highly useful for calculating the significance of the observed F and t values for each combination of two group means. For instance, having found a significant F value among three groups (say groups A, B, C) based on calculation of an ANOVA, the null hypothesis for Scheffe's test can be stated as:

$$H_0: \mu_A = \mu_B, \mu_A = \mu_C, \mu_B = \mu_C$$

In a statistical sense, this procedure is considered to be somewhat conservative; that is, the α level is generally set at .10 if the α level of the ANOVA was previously set at .05. Scheffe's method is used to control a type I error, entailing the rejection of the null hypothesis when it is correct.

When the sample sizes among comparison groups are equal, then the Tukey test (sometimes called *HSD—Tukey's honestly significant difference*) may be performed instead of the Scheffe's test. Tukey's method is less conservative than Scheffe's test and is designed to make all possible pairwise comparisons among group means while maintaining the type I error rate at the same α as set in the ANOVA. The null hypothesis is identical to that of the Sheffe's test.

Finally, we will briefly mention three **planned** (a priori) **comparison** procedures used in cases in which an investigator wishes to accomplish the analysis of a limited number of pairwise comparisons in lieu of performing a more comprehensive and time-consuming ANOVA. Such procedures are used when prior theory leads to specific hypotheses about where significant differences between means might be found. For this purpose, we might use a revised version of the t test. The revised t procedure is accomplished by means of the following formula:

$$t = \frac{(\bar{X}_i - \bar{X}_j)}{\sqrt{2MS_E/n}} \text{ with } df = N - J \text{ as defined above}$$

where subscripts i and j represent group identifications and

$$MS_{\mathrm{E}} = \sqrt{\left(\frac{S_i^2}{n_i} + \frac{S_j^2}{n_j} \right)}$$

Thus, rather than using the pooled standard deviation in the denominator, we use MS_{E} (the error mean square) instead.

Another planned comparison method designed to reduce the probability of making a type I error is to shift the α (significance level) downward. For example, given the probability that approximately one t test in four will be significant as the consequence of chance alone ($4 \times .05 = .20$), an option is to shift the α downward by dividing it by the number of comparisons to be made. Thus, $.05/4 = .0125$—a more stringent significance level.

Another approach to making an a priori pairwise comparisons of group means is called the **Bonferroni t procedure,** also termed *Dunn's multiple-comparison procedure*. This method increases the critical value (table value) of an F needed for reaching statistical significance, depending on the number of comparisons to be made and the sample size. It is used in cases in which the researcher wishes to avoid a type I error (rejecting the null hypothesis when it is true).

OTHER ANOVA DESIGNS AND METHODS

Numerous variations of ANOVA designs and methods are available for special types of research applications. The following sections will summarize some of the more widely used techniques.

Randomized-Blocks Analysis of Variance (RBANOVA)

This test is especially appropriate for within-subject designs in which the data comes from repeated measures on the same subject. According to Shavelson (1988), "the RBANOVA is to the t test for dependent samples what the one-way ANOVA is to the t test for two independent samples" (p. 487). Its primary purpose is to determine whether or not the differences between two or more groups may be due to chance or to systematic differences among the groups. Although RBANOVA is similar to ANOVA, the former method also takes into account the fact that two or more observations can be made on the same subject, as opposed to a single observation as in the case of the latter. This is accomplished by (1) partitioning subjects into homogeneous blocks and (2) randomly assigning subjects to different levels within each treatment. For example, this design would be appropriate if we were interested in studying the relative influence of three conditions (A, B, C) as these interact with three different severity levels (1, 2, 3) on some element of measured performance.

In many research studies, a *Latin square* is used in conjunction with a block design when order effects may otherwise confound the influence of two or more treatment conditions. To control for the unwanted influence of confounding factors, a contingency table can be used to form a Latin square in which the confounding factors are assigned to rows and columns and the cells within the table are used to denote the observations (treatments) of interest. The objective of this procedure is to arrange the order of treatment conditions so that each condition precedes and follows each treatment condition. The number of ordinal arrangements should equal the number of treatment conditions, and each treatment (letter) should appear only once within a cell of each column and row. For example, in a study of treatment efficacy in aphasia, suppose we wish to control for the possible confounding influences of language severity and time post-onset, as these nuisance variables might interact with three levels of an independent variable, say, the number of therapy sessions per week. In accordance with the blocking principle of the Latin square, the levels of the confounding factors could be assigned to columns and rows of a square, with the cells of the square then used to identify the levels of treatment. Given this arrangement, there are three blocks of severity, three blocks of time post-onset, and three treatment levels (A, B, C) forming a Latin square consisting of nine cells for analysis. This hypothetical design is illustrated below:

		Time Post-Onset (in months)		
		1	**2**	**3**
Severity	≤35	A	B	C
based on	36–55	B	C	A
percentile rank	>55	C	A	B

An example of a clinical research study that used a RBANOVA in conjunction with a Latin square design can be found in Appendix A-2.

Analysis of Covariance (ANCOVA)

The major purpose of the analysis of covariance is to allow for an adjustment in factors that might potentially influence the results of an experiment *before* the experiment begins. More specifically, this test, abbreviated ANCOVA, allows for the statistical adjustment of data values of a dependent variable in accordance with known quantities of a variable that the investigator might wish to control (control variable). In effect, this adjustment removes from a dependent variable the degree of variability that otherwise could be attributed to the control variable.

Mathematically, the calculation of such variance is made possible by the use of the linear regression line, discussed previously in Chapter 6, to specify the slope of the relationship between a dependent variable and control variable. By using the regression line, scores on the dependent variable can be predicted based on a knowledge of corresponding scores on the control variable. Residual deviation scores are used to specify the degree of variability in the dependent variable that is not associated with the control variable.

Suppose we wish to measure the maintenance of clinical gains in response to some treatment for three groups of subjects following the termination of therapy. Group A will be evaluated 6 months after therapy, Group B after 12 months, and Group C after 18 months. There are several within-group and between-group variables besides the independent variable that might potentially influence the outcome of such a study. For example, the researcher may wish to control for the degree of improvement that occurred during the course of therapy. It is possible that subjects who made more progress in therapy will be the same individuals who best maintain clinical gains through time. Although this is an interesting question in its own right, it is not the purpose of our study, which seeks only to determine the degree of maintenance across different spans of time. Thus, we might wish to control for within- and between-group differences for the *degree* of progress that occurred during therapy by factoring these *gain scores* into the analysis of the dependent variable. The intelligence and the motivation of subjects are examples of other control variables that might need to be considered. Because the mathematical calculation of ANCOVA is highly complex, we refer the reader to

Appendix A-2 where the necessary computational steps are outlined in relation to an actual research study along with a discussion of the relative advantages and disadvantages of ANCOVA as compared to ANOVA.

Nonparametric Tests for Multigroup Designs

There are several nonparametric tests that can serve as alternative methods to ANOVA for testing hypotheses for multigroup designs. As an alternative to the two-way ANOVA, one of the most commonly used of these is the **Friedman two-way analysis of variance by ranks.** Remember that nonparametric tests of this kind should be chosen when the assumption of homogeneity of variance is questionable or has been violated.

Just as the Wilcoxon matched-pairs signed ranks test is a useful distribution-free method for detecting a significant difference between two matched or related groups, the Friedman two-way analysis of variance by ranks test is also useful with a randomized block design when a block consists of three or more repeated measures obtained from the same subject. As an example application of the Friedman test, let us consider a question in the aural rehabilitation of profoundly hearing-impaired children related to the effectiveness of various communication methods in facilitating the accuracy of speech reception. More specifically, imagine that we wish to evaluate the use of a training system known as *cued speech* in association with other training modalities. Cued speech involves the use of a set of hand cues to reduce or resolve ambiguities in speech reception (Cornett, 1967). In our hypothetical study, this system will be examined as it might be used in conjunction with three other conditions, namely (1) audition (AC), (2) lip reading (LC), and (3) audition and lip reading (ALC). For this purpose, a group of 10 profoundly hearing-impaired adolescents will serve as subjects. Assume that a speech recognition task is designed that requires subjects in each of the groups to identify key words embedded in sentences. Subjects' responses to the stimulus items are recorded in terms of the percentage of correct identifications made. Let us now illustrate the steps in conducting the Friedman test in the context of our example.

Step 1.   Form the hypothesis in statistical terms.

   H_0: There is no difference in the subjects' speech recognition scores under the three conditions.

   H_1: There is a difference in the subjects' speech recognition scores under the three conditions.

Step 2.   Select an appropriate statistical test.

   As noted above, the Friedman test is an appropriate statistic for data involving repeated measures of subjects tested on three or more conditions when scores are to be ranked. The specific goal of the test is to determine whether the sums of the ranks for the various conditions differ significantly.

Step 3.   Choose the significance level.

   An α level of .05 will be used to test the null hypothesis in a one-tailed test. A one-tailed test is always applied in testing the significance of three or more treatment conditions or groups.

Step 4.   Organize a table to include test scores, their ranks, and the sum of their ranks, and calculate the test statistic (see Table 12-8).

TABLE 12-8 Hypothetical Results for a Study of Cued Speech Training in Association with Audition, Lip-reading, and Audition and Lip-reading

Subjects	AC	LC	ALC	AC	Ranks (R) LC	ALC
1	31	83	63	1	3	2
2	42	77	81	1	2	3
3	44	81	76	1	3	2
4	33	69	65	1	3	2
5	37	69	74	1	2	3
6	32	70	72	1	2	3
7	35	87	82	1	3	2
8	39	88	73	1	3	2
9	46	95	96	1	2	3
10	35	81	79	1	3	2
n = 10				Sum = 10	26	24

The test scores for the subjects in the three conditions of our hypothetical experiment are cast in a two-way table of n rows (subjects) and k columns (conditions). It can be seen that:

n = total number of subjects = 10
k = total number of conditions = 3
ΣR = a column sum of ranks such as AC-10, LC-26, and ALC-24

The observed value of the Friedman test statistic approximates the chi-square distribution with $df = k - 1$. Therefore, the general formula for the Friedman test statistic is given by:

$$\chi^2 = \frac{12(\Sigma R^2)}{nk(k+1)} - 3n(k+1) \text{ with } df = k-1$$

Entering the appropriate values into the formula above,

$$\chi^2 = \frac{12[10^2 + 26^2 + 24^2]}{10 \cdot 3 \cdot (3+1)} - 3 \cdot 10 \cdot (3+1) = 15.2$$

Step 5. Draw conclusions on the basis of critical value(s).

Appendix A-1=3 lists critical values of the chi-square distribution. For a critical value of 5.991 where α = .05 and df = 3 − 1 = 2, it can be seen that the observed value of χ^2 is greater than the critical value of 5.991 listed in the table. Thus, we would reject the null hypothesis and conclude that there was a difference in the speech recognition abilities of subjects among the three conditions. Our hypothetical results are compatible with the findings of an actual experiment concerned with a similar problem (Nicholls & Ling, 1982).

Another nonparametric alternative to the ANOVA is the **Kruskal-Wallis one-way analysis of variance by ranks (KWANOVA).** This test, a nonparametric version of the one-way ANOVA and extension of the Mann-Whitney U test, is useful for deciding whether the distribution of scores in the populations underlying each group are identical. Instead of using actual test scores, ranks are substituted in order to represent the dependent variable. As in the case of the Friedman, scores are entered into a table and rank ordered from lowest to highest without regard to group membership. After summing the ranks of each group, if their respective sums are similar, then the null hypothesis is retained. Otherwise, H_0 is rejected. An application of KWANOVA based on data from an actual study is included in Appendix A-2.

The *p*-value Approach in Testing Hypotheses

The approach to testing hypotheses we have discussed so far is called the **classical approach** to hypothesis testing. However, current widespread use of computers and statistical software packages make another approach called the ***p*-value approach** an important method in drawing the final conclusion, because many scholastic journal articles in the field of communication sciences and disorders report the final results in a *p*-value form. The general definition of a *p*-value is the probability of obtaining a value of the sample test statistic as favorable or more favorable to the alternative hypothesis (H_1) than the null hypothesis (H_0), if H_0 were true, A *p*-value measures how credible your alternative hypothesis is (or how confident you are in rejecting the null hypothesis), whereas the classical approach simply reports the conclusion by stating "reject or fail to reject the null hypothesis," and it does not calculate the amount of confidence when you reject the null hypothesis. Conversion from the classical approach to the *p*-value approach and mathematical derivation of the *p*-value are as follows:

- *Reject* the null hypothesis if the *p*-value is less than or equal to the predetermined value of α.
- *Fail to reject* the null hypothesis if the *p*-value is greater than α.
- In a one-tailed test, the *p*-value is the area to the right (if H_1 contains >) of an observed value or the area to the left (if H_1 contains <) of an observed value. In a two-tailed test, the *p*-value is twice the area to the right or left of an observed value.

If the conclusion is reported solely by the *p*-value, many researchers will use the following guide to determine the significance of their test results based on the sample test statistic.

$p < .01$	the result is highly significant—very strong evidence against H_0
$.01 \leq p < .05$	the result is significant—sufficient evidence against H_0
$p \geq .05$	the result is not significant—insufficient evidence against H_0

Figure 12-6 summarizes the general procedure of hypothesis testing and how to formulate the correct wording of the conclusion by both classical approach and *p*-value approach. As noted earlier, the *p*-value approach has become more common and important in research because a vast majority of commonly used statistical software packages, like MINITAB, SPSS, and the like, always display only *p*-value with output in determining the significance of the final test result.

Meta-Analysis

An increasingly popular methodology for statistically combining the results from two or more independent studies is called **meta-analysis**—a term introduced by Glass (1977) to describe a kind of higher-order level of data synthesis. Meta-analytic techniques should not be confused with traditional reviews of literature in which the findings of separate but related studies are summarized in an effort to "make sense out of the data." However, the underlying concern of meta-analysis is focused on the same problem, namely, the tendency

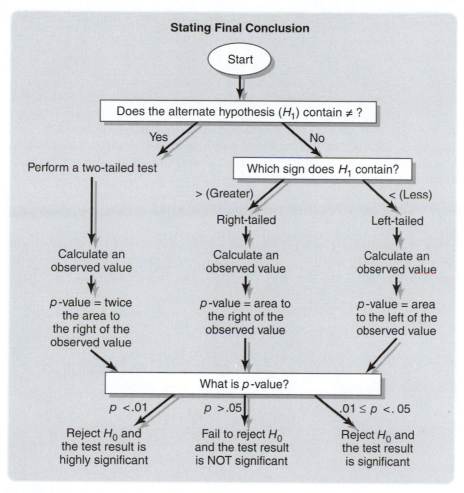

FIGURE 12-6   Flowchart of classical and *p*-value approaches in testing hypothesis

of many research studies, designed to answer the same or a highly similar question, to yield conflicting results.

According to Sachs et al. (1987), meta-analysis has four main objectives:

1. Increasing statistical power by enlarging the size of the sample
2. Resolving the uncertainty associated with conflicting results
3. Improving estimates of effect size
4. Answering questions not posed at the beginning of the study

Among these aims, number 3, relating to effect size, is a key concept underlying the application of many meta-analysis techniques. **Effect size** is an index of the degree to which the phenomenon of interest exists in the population (Cohen, 1977). There are several methods of determining effect size, depending on the unit of analysis. In the case of mean scores, effect size is the difference between the means divided by the averaged standard deviations between the groups.

As noted above, effect size relates to the *power of the test* to yield a significant finding if the research hypothesis is true. The greater the difference between means, and the smaller the population variance, the larger will be the effect size. Criteria for interpreting effect sizes have been established by Cohen (1977). An effect size of .2 (interpreted as small) indicates that the means of two groups are separated by .2 standard deviations. Effect sizes of .5 (moderate) and .8 (large) indicate that the means are separated by .5 and .8 standard deviations, respectively. Meta-analytic technique can be used to combine effect sizes from independent studies into an overall average effect size and probability value based on the pooled results.

As an example of the use of effect size in conjunction with meta-analysis, a study by Nye and Turner (1990) is noteworthy. Using a data base of 65 studies to evaluate the effectiveness of articulation therapy, the authors reported a mean effect size (ES) of .892, "indicating that articulation treated subjects moved from the 50th to the 81st percentile as a result of intervention . . ." Several variables where sorted out that appeared to have the greatest influence on articulation improvement.

In the field of communication sciences and disorders, some researchers have held that statistical significance testing has been overly emphasized (Attansio, 1994; Maxwell & Satake, 1993) or should be supplemented by additional tests (Young, 1993; Maxwell & Satake, 1993; Attansio, 1994). Although the authors of this text firmly believe that statistical significance testing has value, the calculation of effect size can be of equal importance, particularly in the context of applied research as demonstrated in studies like those of Nye and Turner and others as completed by Andrews et al. (1980) in assessing the effects of stuttering treatment. In discussing the future role of meta-analysis, Attanasio (1994) noted that its importance lies in providing ". . . an estimate of the practical significance of a statistically significant finding" (p. 758). For a more detailed discussion of meta-analysis, see Pillemer and Light, 1980; Cooper and Lemke, 1991; and Wolf, 1986, as well as many advanced statistical textbooks that provide a review of the subject. Also, for the more mathematically inclined reader, we have included the fundamental concepts and some applications of meta-analysis involved in the calculations of sample size and effect size in Appendix A-4.

COMPLEX STATISTICAL METHODS

Several other complex statistical techniques are frequently encountered in the reading of research literature. Although demonstrating the steps involved in calculating these statistics exceeds the purpose of this textbook, we will briefly mention three of the more commonly used multivariate methods that involve the analysis of more than one dependent variable, including: (1) **multivariate analysis of variance (MANOVA),** (2) **discriminant analysis,** and (3) **factor analysis.**

Multivariate Analysis of Variance (MANOVA)

This method is designed for problems in which there are more than one dependent variable under investigation. In general, two or more different measures of approximately the same characteristic (related variables) are taken, and a question is asked regarding the degree to which these dependent variables serve to separate two or more groups. Hypothetically, suppose we wish to determine whether or not children classified according to three levels of socioeconomic strata (low, mid, high) show different profiles on three types of language processing measures (phonologic, syntactic, semantic). In this case, our independent variables are constituted of the three levels of random group assignment, whereas our dependent variables consists of the three language measures. One option would be to conduct a univariate ANOVA for each of the dependent variables and calculate the significance of three separate F tests. However, this would be akin to conducting three separate experiments. As an alternative, we can use the MANOVA to accomplish the same goal more efficiently and in a manner in which the main effects and their interactions on the combinations of all the dependent variables can be evaluated simultaneously. Just as performing an ANOVA often eliminates the need for numerous t tests, so too can the MANOVA eliminate the need for numerous ANOVAs, thereby reducing the likelihood of a type I error. In cases in which the value of F for MANOVA is significant, leading to a rejection of the null hypothesis of no differences, post hoc ANOVAs are performed to determine where such differences can be found. The same statistical assumptions for performing ANOVA apply to MANOVA as well.

Discriminant Analysis

A statistical procedure whose purpose is somewhat similar to MANOVA is called *discriminant analysis*. The name of the test is appropriate because it is often employed to identify which dependent variables in a set of such variables are *most* responsible for discriminating among groups. Thus, whereas both MANOVA and discriminate analysis are concerned with identifying which variables contribute to group separation, only the latter evaluates the *magnitude* of the contribution of each variable toward this end. Discriminant analysis can be useful in identifying factors that distinguish among subtypes of communication disorders such as stuttering—for example, Van Riper's (1982) four developmental tracks that he distinguished on the basis of different combinations of factors including age of stuttering onset, manner of onset, symptoms, and general speech skills. Whereas Van Riper's approach to subtyping developmental stuttering was largely based on the methods of clinical observation and description, discrimant analysis has obvious applications to problems of this kind.

Although mathematically complex, the method essentially involves identifying which variables or combination of variables are most powerful in discriminating among groups. In addition to its primary use in studies concerned with describing or identifying factors that discriminate groups, the method also has utility in predicting group membership of an individual. For example, based on a prior knowledge of certain factors in a client's history, we might calculate the probability that he or she belongs to a particular category or subtype of disorder within the population of people who stutter. The accuracy of discriminant analysis is based on the percentage of cases that are classified correctly. Some of the basic assumptions of the discriminanat analysis are that (1) there are two or more groups; (2) there are at least two cases per group; and (3) discriminating variables have nominal characteristics for dependent variables and continuous characteristics for independent variables.

Factor Analysis

A major goal of scientific research is to organize data in such a way that existing relationships among variables can be more readily comprehended. An important statistical method for accomplishing this goal is termed *factor analysis*. Some of the earliest work on factor analysis was carried out by Thurstone (1947), who believed it to be a powerful tool for exploring "vectors of the mind." Its primary aim is to reduce or condense a large number of observations into a small number of key indicators of underlying constructs (factors). Over the years, factor analysis has found many theoretical and practical applications. It is especially useful in the development of clinical tests and rating scales by summarizing the relationships among variables in a concise way.

TABLE 12-9   Factor Analysis Study of Intelligence Based on Thirteen Items

1. Arithmetic	6. Information	11. Similarities
2. Block design	7. Mazes	12. Symbol search
3. Coding	8. Object assembly	13. Vocabulary
4. Comprehension	9. Picture arrangement	
5. Digit span	10. Picture completion	

Adapted from Wechsler Intelligence Scale for Children, by Wechsler, D., 1991, 3rd ed. (p. 39), San Antonio: Harcourt, Brace, Jovanovich, Inc.

Suppose we are interested in uncovering some of the principle dimensions of intelligence in children. Assume further that we do not know what these dimensions are and therefore decide to collect several types of measures on a large number of subjects. We select our measures given the presumption that some of them ought to be related to intelligence, but we are unsure how or to what degree this is true. After administering a large array of tests as shown in Table 12-9, the second step is to calculate correlations among each and every one of them. The result of correlating each test item with all other test items in the list results in a very large number of *intercorrelations*. The third step is to see how the measures tend to *cluster* or condense based on their intercorrelations. This can be done by constructing a matrix that displays the correlations between each possible variable, or, more conveniently, by the use of a computer. Some measures will be correlated with each other but not with other measures. Measures that are found to be correlated are called *factors*. The fourth step is to determine the *factor loadings* for the various measures. The mathematical basis for such loading is beyond the scope of this book. Generally, this is done by determining the degree to which the measure correlates with a certain factor. Like other correlations, factor loads can range from -1 to $+1$. Although a measure may load onto more than one factor, it is generally the case that it will load *highly* on only one. The fifth step in factor analysis is to name or label the factors based on our theoretical understanding of their nature.

The results of the factor analysis are displayed in Table 12-10. As can be seen from such an analysis, four factors emerged which have been named: (1) Verbal Comprehension; (2) Perceptual Organization; (3)Freedom from Distractibility; and (4) Processing Speed. Of course, the knowledgeable reader will recognize that the factors named and their associated test measures constitute a well-known intelligence test—the Wechsler Intelligence Scale for Children-Third Edition (WISC-III) (Wechsler, 1991).

Although we have illustrated the use of factor analysis based on 13 subtests of a standardized test instrument, it is common for dozens or even hundreds of measures to be included at the outset of factor analytic studies. Over the years, factor analysis has led to the refinement of the theoretical foundations of the WISC as it has gone through several revisions. A major strength of factor analysis is that it advances conceptualization of the quality being studied. On the other hand, in the absence of some theoretical approach designed to integrate data toward a meaningful end, it probably should not be done. Such "fishing expeditions" rarely advance our conceptual understanding of complex phenomena. For additional information on the theory and methods of factor analysis, see Gorsuch (1983) and Child (1990).

TABLE 12-10   Four Named Factor of an Intelligence Test and the Subtests of Each Factor

Factor 1: Verbal Comprehension

- Comprehension
- Information
- Similarities
- Vocabulary

Factor 2: Perceptual Organization

- Block design
- Mazes
- Object assembly
- Picture arrangement
- Picture completion

Factor 3: Freedom from Distractibility

- Arithmetic
- Digit span

Factor 4: Processing Speed

- Coding
- Symbol search

Adapted from Wechsler Intelligence Scale for Children, by Wechsler, D., 1991, 3rd ed. (p. 192), San Antonio: Harcourt, Brace, Jovanovich, Inc.

COMPUTER APPLICATIONS IN STATISTICS

Undoubtedly, the use of computers and statistical software packages has eased the work of researchers in analyzing data. Before the development of modern computer systems, such data analysis was laboriously performed by hand perhaps with the assistance of a handheld pocket calculator.

Calculations were extremely time consuming and often fraught with human error. Because of this fact, many researchers and statisticians expended much effort in devising short-cut formulas for analyzing data more efficiently. Nevertheless, until the computer became available, many of the complex statistical designs that currently exist for data analysis exceeded the statistical abilities of researchers to answer certain questions. Access to high-speed computers and the software that run them presently allow researchers to expend their energies more creatively in designing and conducting scientific studies. Brief descriptions of several commonly used software packages follow.

- **MINITAB:** This software package is easy to use and is often incorporated within the curriculum of introductory computer/statistics courses. It is especially appropriate for descriptive statistical applications such as calculations of measures of central tendency, variability, simple linear regression, and correlation. Some limited number of inferential statistics, such as the z or t test for univariate calculations, also can be performed. This software stores the data values in rows and columns, like a spreadsheet, allowing for various types of elementary analyses. After inputting the data into the appropriate cells, the computer can be instructed to perform the desired calculation. Although this is a good introductory program for students, it is less capable, compared to competitors, in performing more advanced multivariate statistical calculations as required by many complex research designs.

- **Biomedical Computer Programs *P*-Series (BMDP):** The BMDP is one of the most sophisticated packages for statistical analysis. It is especially suitable for many applications in the medical and biological sciences such as in clinical trial studies, pharmaceutical research, prevalence/incidence studies, and the like. The data management programs contained within this software are well organized and flexible so as to allow for different types of analyses on the same data with only minor changes in the coding operations. Among the operations that the BMDP can perform are data description, frequency tables, regression analysis, ANOVA, MANOVA, and so forth.

- **Statistical Package for the Social Sciences (SPSS):** SPSS programs are widely used in the educational, social, and behavioral sciences because of their simplicity and the complete labeling of statistical analyses on data printouts. The SPSS program is capable of performing a wide range of graphical and data analysis operations as appropriate for descriptive statistics, categorical, univariate and multivariate ANOVA, correlation/regression, discriminant analysis, log-linear models, factor analysis, and so on. Among the three software packages that we have mentioned, SPSS is the most comprehensive. Another system called *Statistical Analysis System (SAS)* performs statistical functions in a manner comparable to SPSS.

- **JMP Version 5 (JMP):** The JMP program is widely used in the behavioral, natural, and social sciences. The program possesses all capabilities that MINITAB, BMDP, and SPSS have. In addition, JMP can perform more complex probabilistic designs such as Bayesian design and survival analysis for actuarial sciences.

The majority of the computer programs described above are on the mainframes of academic computing services in colleges and universities so that data management operations can occur online from the desktop or laboratory through links to one's own personal computer. Although fluency in a computer language such as BASIC (Beginner's All-purpose Symbolic Instruction Code) may prove useful, this is no longer a requirement for using the technology successfully for a myriad of research applications. Software packages have detailed instructional manuals and many have "tutorials" that help the user find and correct errors as they occur. Programming assistance is typically available in academic computer centers to help the researcher to design an operation for a specialized need. For more limited graphic and data analysis applications, there are many commercial software packages for personal computers available through computer stores. We will now use the printouts from MINITAB and SPSS computer programs to illustrate the calculations of (1) a paired *t* test, (2) the Mann-Whitney *U* test, and (3) a one-way ANOVA, respectively, given the examples provided in this chapter.

Referring to Table 12-3, the actual steps involved in a paired *t* test using MINITAB and SPSS are outlined below:

MINITAB

Step 1.   Enter the data into a MINITAB worksheet.

All data values must be entered into the worksheet; the data for propranolol are entered in column C1 and for the placebo in column C2 (see Figure 12-7).

Step 2.   Click on *Stat – Basic Stat – Paired T.*

This pull-down menu, shown in Figure 12-8, asks for data to be supplied (see Figure 12-8). In MINITAB, a paired *t* test always evaluates the first sample data value (C1) minus the second sample data value (C2); therefore, the difference is symbolically written as C1 − C2.

	C1	C2
	Propranolol	Placebo
1	4	5
2	0	1
3	0	0
4	2	4
5	1	4
6	3	5
7	3	3
8	1	3
9	2	2
10	1	4

FIGURE 12-7

Illustration of data entry on MINITAB worksheet for an example of a paired *t* test

Portions of the input and output contained in this book are printed with permission of Minitab Inc.

 Paired t

overview   how to   example   data   see also

Stat > Basic Statistics > Paired t

Performs a paired t-test. This is appropriate for testing the mean difference between paired observations when the paired differences follow a normal distribution.

Use the Paired t command to compute a confidence interval and perform a hypothesis test of the mean difference between paired observations in the population. A paired t-procedure matches responses that are dependent or related in a pairwise manner. The matching allows you to account for variability between the pairs usually resulting in a smaller error term, thus increasing the sensitivity of the hypothesis test or confidence interval.

Typical examples of paired data include measurements on twins of before-and-after measurements. For a paired t-test:

$H_0: \mu d = \mu 0$ versus $H_t: \mu d \neq \mu 0$

where μd is the population mean of the differences and $\mu 0$ is the hypothesized mean of the differences.

When the samples are drawn independently from two populations, use the two-sample t-procedure.

Dialog box items

First sample: Enter the column containing the first sample

Second sample: Enter the column containing the second sample

<Graphs>

<Options>

FIGURE 12-8   Illustration of MINITAB pull-down menu for a paired *t* test

Portions of the input and output contained in this book are printed with permission of Minitab Inc.

```
──────── 6/24/2004 8:35:27 AM ────────

Welcome to Minitab, press F1 for help.

Paired T-Test and CI: C1, C2

Paired T for C1 - C2

                    N       Mean      StDev     SE Mean
C1                  10      1.700     1.337     0.423
C2                  10      3.100     1.663     0.526
Difference          10     −1.400     1.174     0.371

95% upper bound for mean difference: −0.720
T-Test of mean difference = 0 (vs < 0): T-Value = −3.77  P-Value = 0.002
```

FIGURE 12-9 Illustration of MINITAB output containing the final result for an example of a paired t test

Portions of the input and output contained in this book are printed with permission of Minitab Inc.

Step 3. Click *OK*.

This command allows MINITAB to (1) calculate the observed t value and corresponding p-value for our dependent sample, and (2) produce the output containing the final result shown in Figure 12-9.

Step 4. Interpret the final result.

The output shows a left-tailed t test with the observed t value (T-Value) $= -3.77$ and p-value $= 0.002$. Because the p-value falls below 0.01, we would reject the null hypothesis (H_0). In other words, there exists strong evidence against the null hypothesis—the result is found to be highly significant. We conclude that the self-rating of stuttering severity was significantly lower under the propranolol condition than under the placebo condition.

SPSS

Step 1. Enter the data into an SPSS worksheet.

All data values must be entered into the worksheet; the data for propranolol in column VAR00001 and for the placebo in column VAR00002 (see Figure 12-10).

Step 2. Click on *Analyze – Compare means – Paired-Sample t test*.

This produces the pull-down menu shown in Figure12-11, which asks you to make certain choices as shown (see Figure 12-11). In SPSS, a paired t test always evaluates the first sample data value (VAR00001) minus the second sample data value (VAR00002), therefore, the difference is symbolically written as VAR00001 − VAR00002.

Step 3. Click *OK*.

This command allows SPSS to (1) calculate the observed t value and corresponding p-value for our dependent sample, and (2) produce the output containing the final result shown in Figure 12-12.

	VAR00001	VAR00002
1	4.00	5.00
2	.00	1.00
3	.00	.00
4	2.00	4.00
5	1.00	4.00
6	3.00	5.00
7	3.00	3.00
8	1.00	3.00
9	2.00	2.00
10	1.00	4.00

FIGURE 12-10

Illustration of data entry on SPSS worksheet for an example of a paired *t* test

From SPSS for Windows®, Rel. 13.0.1. Copyright 2004 by SPSS Inc. Used with permission.

To Obtain a Paired-Samples T Test

▶ From the menus choose:

    Analyze
      Compare Means
        Paired-Samples T Test...

▶ Select a pair of variables, as follows:

  • Click each of two variables. The first variable appears in the Current Selections group as *Variable 1*, and the second appears as *Variable 2*.

  • After you have selected a pair of variables, click the arrow button to move the pair into the Paired Variables list. You may select more pairs of variables. To remove a pair of variables from the analysis, select a pair in the Paired Variables list and click the arrow button.

Optionally, you can click Options to control the treatment of missing data and the level of the confidence interval.

Related Topics

Paired-Samples T Test
Paired-Samples T Test Data Considerations
Paired-Samples T Test Options
Paired-Samples T Test: Related Procedures

FIGURE 12-11   Illustration of SPSS pull-down menu for a paired *t* test

Paired Samples Statistics

		Mean	N	Standard Deviation	Standard Error Mean
Pair 1	VAR00001	1.7000	10	1.33749	.42295
	VAR00002	3.1000	10	1.66333	.52599

Paired Samples Correlations

		N	Correlation	Sig.
Pair 1	VAR00001 & VAR00002	10	.714	.020

Paired Samples Test

		Paired Differences					
		Mean	Standard Deviation	Standard Error Mean	95% confidence interval of the difference		t
					Lower	Upper	
Pair 1	VAR00001 - VAR00002	−1.40000	1.17379	.37118	−2.23968	−.56032	−3.772

Paired Samples Test

		df	Sig. (2-tailed)
Pair 1	VAR00001 - VAR00002	9	.004

FIGURE 12-12   Illustration of SPSS output containing the final result for an example of a paired t test

Step 4.   Interpret the final result.

The output shows the observed t value $= -3.772$ and p-value $= 0.004$ for a two-tailed test. After we convert the two-tailed test to the left-tailed test, we would obtain one-half of the p-value: that is the p-value for a left-tailed test is 0.002. Because the p-value falls below 0.01, we would reject the null hypothesis. Therefore, there exists strong evidence against the null hypothesis (the result is found to be highly significant). We can conclude that the self-rating of stuttering severity was significantly lower under the propranolol condition than under the placebo condition.

Next, referring to Table 12-6, we will illustrate the steps involved in performing a Mann-Whitney U test using MINITAB and SPSS.

MINITAB

Step 1.   Enter the data into a MINITAB worksheet.

All data values must be entered into the worksheet—the data for the High Apgar Group in column C1 and for the Low Apgar Group in column C2 (see Figure 12-13).

Step 2.   Click on *Stat – Nonparametric – Mann-Whitney.*

The pull-down menu shown in Figure 12-14 displays the statistical procedure of the Mann-Whitney U test, which asks for certain selections to be made (see Figure 12-14). Note that

	C1	C2
	High Apgar	Low Apgar
1	37	22
2	32	23
3	34	30
4	28	37
5	32	24
6	47	27
7	29	30
8	45	28
9	39	
10	26	

FIGURE 12-13

Illustration of data entry on MINITAB worksheet for an example of the Mann-Whitney U test

Portions of the input and output contained in this book are printed with permission of Minitab Inc.

 Mann-Whitney

overview   how to   example   data   see also

Stat > Nonparametrics > Mann-Whitney

You can perform a two-sample rank test (also called the Mann-Whitney test, or the two-sample Wilcoxon rank sum test) of the equality of two population medians, and calculate the corresponding point estimate and confidence interval. The hypotheses are

    Ho: $\eta_1 = \eta_2$ versus H1: $\eta_1 \neq \eta_2$, where η is the population median.

An assumption for the Mann-Whitney test is that the data are independent random samples from two populations that have the same shape (hence the same variance) and a scale that is continuous or ordinal (possesses natural ordering) if discrete. The two-sample rank test is slightly less powerful (the confidence interval is wider on the average) than the two-sample test with pooled sample variance when the populations are normal, and considerably more powerful (confidence interval is narrower, on the average) for many other populations. If the populations have different shapes or different standard deviations, a 2-sample t without pooling variances may be more appropriate.

Dialog box items

First sample: Select the column containing the sample data from one population.

Second sample: Select the column containing the sample data from the other population.

Confidence level: Specify the level of confidence desired between 0 and 100; the attained level will be as close as possible.

Alternative: Click the arrow to choose the kind of test performed by selecting less than (lower-tailed), not equal (two-tailed), or greater than (upper-tailed) from the drop-down box.

FIGURE 12-14   Illustration of MINITAB pull-down menu for the Mann-Whitney U test

---
6/24/2004 8:43:50 AM

Welcome to Minitab, press F1 for help.

Mann-Whitney Test and CI: C1, C2

```
C1              N = 10     Median =        33.00
C2              N =  8     Median =        27.50
Point estimate for ETA1-ETA2 is            7.00
95.4 Percent CI for ETA1-ETA2 is (1.00, 15.00)
W = 120.0
Test of ETA1 = ETA2 vs ETA1 not = ETA2 is significant at 0.0295
The test is significant at 0.0292 (adjusted for ties)
```

FIGURE 12-15   Illustration of MINITAB output containing the final result for an example of the Mann-Whitney U test

Portions of the input and output contained in this book are printed with permission of Minitab Inc.

the goal of the Mann-Whitney U test is comparable to that of the Wilcoxon rank sum test. Both are used to determine whether a significant difference exists between two independent groups' medians when the assumptions of normality and homogeneity of variances are violated.

Step 3.   Click *OK*.

This command allows MINITAB to (1) calculate the observed value and corresponding *p*-value for our sample data, and (2) produce the output containing the final result shown in Figure 12-15.

Step 4.   Interpret the final result.

The output shows the *p*-value = 0.0295 for a two-tailed test. Because this *p*-value of 0.0295 is less than 0.05 but greater than 0.01, we would reject the null hypothesis at $\alpha = 0.05$ (the result is found to be significant—there exists sufficient evidence against the null hypothesis). In other words, the observed U of 15 is less than 0.05 but greater than 0.01. Hence, the receptive language abilities of the two groups, as distinguished on the basis of their Apgar scores, are significantly different.

SPSS

Step 1.   Enter the data into an SPSS worksheet.

All data values must be entered into the worksheet; the data for the High Apgar Group and the Low Apgar Group in column VAR00001 and the random variables representing their membership (High Apgar = 1, Low Apgar = 2) in column VAR00002 (see Figure 12-16).

Step 2.   Click on *Analyze – Nonparametric Tests – 2 Independent Samples – Mann-Whitney U*.

The pull-down menu that appears resembles Figure 12-17, and asks that choices be made as shown (see Figure 12-17). In SPSS, we separate all data values (Test Variable List) from group membership (Grouping Variable), and we will assign 1 to the High Apgar Group and 2 to the Low Apgar Group.

	VAR00001	VAR00002
1	37.00	1.00
2	32.00	1.00
3	34.00	1.00
4	28.00	1.00
5	32.00	1.00
6	47.00	1.00
7	29.00	1.00
8	45.00	1.00
9	39.00	1.00
10	26.00	1.00
11	22.00	2.00
12	23.00	2.00
13	30.00	2.00
14	37.00	2.00
15	24.00	2.00
16	27.00	2.00
17	30.00	2.00
18	28.00	2.00

FIGURE 12-16

Illustration of data entry on SPSS worksheet for an example of the Mann-Whitney U test

From SPSS for Windows®, Rel. 13.0.1. Copyright 2004 by SPSS Inc. Used with permission.

Step 3. Click *OK*.

This command allows SPSS to (1) calculate the observed value and corresponding *p*-value, and (2) produce the output containing the final result shown in Figure 12-18.

Step 4. Interpret the final result.

The output shows the *p*-value = 0.026 for a two-tailed test. Because this *p*-value is less than 0.05 but greater than 0.01, we would reject the null hypothesis at $\alpha = 0.05$ (the result is found to be significant—there exists sufficient evidence against the null hypothesis). In other words, the observed U of 15 is less than 0.05 but greater than 0.01. Hence, the receptive language abilities of the two groups, as distinguished on the basis of their Apgar scores, are significantly different.

Next, referring to Table 12-7, we will show the actual steps involved in performing a one-way ANOVA using MINITAB and SPSS.

MINITAB

Step 1. Enter the data into a MINITAB worksheet.

All data values must be entered into the worksheet; all data values are entered in column C1 (Response) and the corresponding group membership number (Factor) in column C2. We assign 1 to Control group, 2 to Consistent group, and 3 to Delayed group (see Figure 12-19).

To Obtain Two-Independent-Samples Tests

From the menus choose:

Analyze
  Nonparametric Tests
    2 Independent Samples...

▸ Select one or more numeric variables.

▸ Select a grouping variable and click **Define Groups** to split the file into two groups or samples.

Related Topics

Two-Independent-Samples Tests
Two-Independent-Samples Tests Data Considerations
Two-Independent-Samples Test Types
Two-Independent-Samples Tests Define Groups
Two-Independent-Samples Tests Options
Two-Independent-Samples Tests: Related Procedures

FIGURE 12-17   Illustration of SPSS pull-down menu for the Mann-Whitney U test

From SPSS for Windows®, Rel. 13.0.1. Copyright 2004 by SPSS Inc. Used with permission.

Ranks

	VAR00002	N	Mean Rank	Sum of Ranks
VAR00001	1.00	10	12.00	120.00
	2.00	8	6.38	51.00
	Total	18		

Test Statistics[b]

	VAR00001
Mann-Whitney U	15.000
Wilcoxon W	51.000
Z	−2.226
Asymp. sig. (2-tailed)	.026
Exact sig. [2*(1-tailed Sig.)]	.027 [a]

a. Not corrected for ties.   b. Grouping variable: VAR00002

FIGURE 12-18   Illustration of SPSS output containing the final result for an example of the Mann-Whitney U test

From SPSS for Windows®, Rel. 13.0.1. Copyright 2004 by SPSS Inc. Used with permission.

	C1	C2
	PSI Scores (Response)	Group (Factor)
1	73	1
2	98	1
3	100	1
4	99	1
5	99	1
6	100	1
7	100	1
8	98	1
9	100	1
10	93	1
11	74	2
12	100	2
13	100	2
14	100	2
15	96	2
16	78	2
17	100	2
18	95	2
19	97	2
20	100	2
21	86	3
22	76	3
23	90	3
24	88	3
25	99	3
26	74	3
27	100	3
28	98	3
29	100	3
30	99	3

FIGURE 12-19

Illustration of data entry on MINITAB worksheet for an example of one-way ANOVA

Portions of the input and output contained in this book are printed with permission of Minitab Inc.

Step 2.   Click on *Stat – ANOVA – ONE-WAY.*

A pull-down menu such as that shown in Figure 12-20 appears. It asks for your choices as illustrated (see Figure 12-20). To determine whether the assumption of homogeneity of variances is violated, MINITAB can perform hypothesis testing for equality or homogeneity of variances using Bartlett's *F* test or Levene's *F* test. As a rule of thumb, the ANOVA test is only slightly affected by homogeneity of variances if the ANOVA model contains fixed factors only and has equal sample sizes. More specifically, the ANOVA is relatively insensitive to the violation of homogeneity of variance if (1) all samples have the same or similar sizes, (2) the sample size is large (all groups $n > 30$), and (3) the largest sample standard deviation is no more than twice as large as the smallest sample standard deviation. If any one of the three conditions fails to be met, then we must apply Bartlett's *F* test or Levene's *F* test for homogeneity of variance to determine whether to use a nonparametric version of the ANOVA such as the Kruskal-Wallis test. Nevertheless, for the more statistically inclined reader, you may perform such tests by clicking on *Stat – ANOVA – Test for Equal Variances.*

Step 3.   Click *OK.*

This command allows MINITAB to (1) calculate the observed *F* value and corresponding *p*-value for our sample data, and (2) produce the output containing the final result shown in Figure 12-21.

Step 4.   Interpret the results.

The output shows an observed *F* value = 0.72 and *p* value = 0.495 for an ANOVA. Because this *p*-value exceeds 0.05, we would fail to reject the null hypothesis (the result is found to be nonsignificant—the evidence against the null hypothesis is insufficient). Therefore, we conclude that auditory processing abilities as operationally defined in our investigation do not appear to provide a basis for determining the risk for phonologic disorders.

SPSS

Step 1.   Enter the data into an SPSS worksheet.

All data values must be entered into the worksheet (see Figure 12-22). All data values for the three groups (called *dependent lists* in SPSS language) are entered in column VAR00001 and the random variables representing group membership (Control = 1, Consistent = 2, and Delayed = 3) are entered in column VAR00002.

Step 2.   Click on *Analyze – Compare Means – One-Way ANOVA.*

A pull-down menu appears, like Figure 12-23. It needs choices made as shown (see Figure 12-23). You may also click the *Options* menu and choose *Homogeneity of variance test* to perform the test of equal variances as shown in Figure 12-24. That screen will show that the *p*-value that is derived from Levene's *F* test is greater than .05—that is, the evidence for rejecting the null hypothesis is insufficient. In other words, all groups have relatively equal variances, so the parametric one-way ANOVA is justified.

Step 3.   Click *OK.*

This command allows SPSS to (1) calculate the observed *F* value and corresponding *p*-value, and (2) produce the output containing the final result shown in Figure 12-25.

Step 4.   Interpret the result.

The output shows an observed *F* value = .723 and *p*-value = .495 for an ANOVA test. Because this *p*-value exceeds 0.05, we would reject the null hypothesis (the result is found to

Test for Equal Variances

overview   how to   example   data   see also

Stat > ANOVA > Test for Equal Variances

Use variance test to perform hypothesis tests for equality or homogeneity of variance using Bartlett's and Levene's tests. An F Test replaces Bartlett's test when you have just two levels.

Many statistical procedures, including analysis of variance, assume that although different samples may come from populations with different means, they have the same variance. The effect of unequal variances upon inferences depends in part upon whether your model includes fixed or random effects, disparities in sample sizes, and the choice of multiple comparison procedure. The ANOVA F-test is only slightly affected by inequality of variance if the model contains fixed factors only and has equal or nearly equal sample sizes. F-tests involving random effects may be substantially affected, however [18]. Use the variance test procedure to test the validity of the equal variance assumption.

Dialog box items

Response: Select the column containing the response variable.

Factors: Select the column(s) containing the factors in the model.

Confidence level: Specify a value from 0 to 100 for the level of confidence desired for the confidence intervals displayed on the graph. The default level is 95. The confidence intervals use a Bonferroni method of achieving an overall confidence level.

Title: To replace the default title with your own custom title, type the desired text in this box.

<Storage>

One-way Analysis of Variances

overview   how to   example   data   see also

Stat > ANOVA > One-way

Performs a one-way analysis of variance, with the dependent variable in one column, subscripts in another. If each group is entered in its own column, use Stat > ANOVA > One-way [Unstacked].

One-way also performs multiple comparisons.

Dialog box items

Response: Select the column containing the response.

Factor: Select the column containing the factor levels.

Store residuals: Check to store residuals in the next available column.

Store fits: Check to store the fitted values in the next available column. For a one-way analysis of variance, the fits are the level means.

<Comparisons>

<Graphs>

FIGURE 12-20   Illustration of MINITAB pull-down menu for test of equal variances and one-way ANOVA

Test for Equal Variances

Response   C1
Factors   C2
ConfLvi   95.000

Bonferroni confidence intervals for standard deviations

| | | | | Factor |
Lower	Sigma	Upper	N	Levels
5.32138	8.35331	17.7765	10	1
6.19090	9.71825	20.6812	10	2
6.32777	9.93311	21.1385	10	3

Bartlett's Test (normal distribution)

Test Statistic: 0.294
P-Value   : 0.863

Levene's Test (any continuous distribution)

Test Statistic: 0.831
P-Value   : 0.446

One-way ANOVA: C1 versus C2

Analysis of Variance for C1

Source	DF	SS	MS	F	P
C2	2	126.7	63.3	0.72	0.495
Error	27	2366.0	87.6		
Total	29	2492.7			

Individual 95% CIs for mean
based on pooled StDev

Level	N	Mean	StDev
1	10	96.00	8.35
2	10	94.00	9.72
3	10	91.00	9.93

```
                                 -+---------+---------+---------+-----
 1                                        (-----------*-----------)
 2                                   (-----------*-----------)
 3                              (-----------*-----------)
                                 -+---------+---------+---------+-----
Pooled StDev =     9.36          85.0      90.0      95.0      100.0
```

FIGURE 12-21   Illustration of MINITAB output containing the final result for an example of one-way ANOVA

Portions of the input and output contained in this book are printed with permission of Minitab Inc.

	VAR00001	VAR00002
1	73.00	1.00
2	98.00	1.00
3	100.00	1.00
4	99.00	1.00
5	99.00	1.00
6	100.00	1.00
7	100.00	1.00
8	98.00	1.00
9	100.00	1.00
10	93.00	1.00
11	74.00	2.00
12	100.00	2.00
13	100.00	2.00
14	100.00	2.00
15	96.00	2.00
16	78.00	2.00
17	100.00	2.00
18	95.00	2.00
19	97.00	2.00
20	100.00	2.00
21	86.00	3.00
22	76.00	3.00
23	90.00	3.00
24	88.00	3.00
25	99.00	3.00
26	74.00	3.00
27	100.00	3.00
28	98.00	3.00
29	100.00	3.00
30	99.00	3.00
31		
32		
33		
34		
35		
36		
37		
38		
39		

FIGURE 12-22

Illustration of data entry on SPSS worksheet for an example of one-way ANOVA

From SPSS for Windows®, Rel. 13.0.1. Copyright 2004 by SPSS Inc. Used with permission.

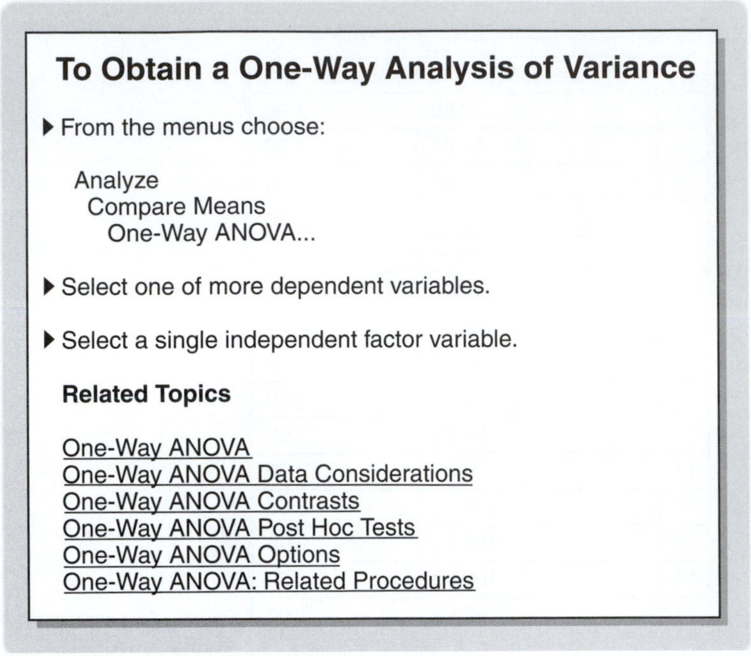

FIGURE 12-23

Illustration of SPSS pull-down menu for one-way ANOVA

From SPSS for Windows®, Rel. 13.0.1. Copyright 2004 by SPSS Inc. Used with permission.

be nonsignificant—the evidence against the null hypothesis is insufficient). Therefore, we can conclude that auditory processing abilities as operationally defined in our investigation do not appear to provide a basis for determining the risk for phonologic disorders.

SUMMARY

In this chapter, we discussed the classical and Bayesian views of probability and their importance in hypothesis testing. The classical view of probability is based on the assumption that the relative frequency of an observed event will approximate its probable frequency of future occurrence if observed over a long series of trials. We briefly mentioned a second view of probability based on the degrees of subjective belief that a researcher might hold for the future occurrence of a particular event (Bayesian view). Because classical statistics is the primary method of inference used in the field of communication sciences and disorders, this particular approach was the focus of the chapter.

The concept of variability within a sampling distribution and its relation to testing hypotheses for a one-sample case and two-sample case were reviewed. The theory of the parametric z test and t test for independent and dependent samples was discussed, and step-by-step illustrations for each method were provided. Nonparametric alternatives to these statistical methods such as the chi-square test were also discussed, and their methods were illustrated.

We also discussed the rationales and methods of various multigroup statistical techniques such as the parametric one-way and two-way ANOVA, RBANOVA, and ANCOVA. Other complex statistical methods such as the MANOVA, discriminant analysis, and factor analysis were also reviewed. Step-by-step computer applications for the calculation of selected statistical tests were provided.

One-Way ANOVA Options

Statistics. Choose one or more of the following:

- **Descriptive**. Calculates the number of cases, mean, standard deviation, standard error of the mean, minimum, maximum, and 95% confidence intervals for each dependent variable for each group.

- **Fixed and random effects**. Displays the standard deviation, standard error, and 95% confidence interval for the fixed-effects model, and the standard error, 95% confidence interval, and estimate of between-components variance for the random-effects model.

- **Homogeneity of variance test**. Calculates the Levene statistic to test for the equality of group variances. This test is not dependent on the assumption of normality.

- **Brown-Forsythe**. Calculates the Brown-Forsythe statistic to test for the equality of group means. This statistic is preferable to the F statistic when the assumption of equal variances does not hold.

- **Welch**. Calculates the Welch statistic to test for the equality of group means. This statistic is preferable to the F statistic when the assumption of equal variances does not hold.

Means plot. Displays a chart that plots the subgroup means (the means for each group defined by values of the factor variable).

Missing Values. Controls the treatment of missing values.

- **Exclude cases analysis by analysis**. A case with a missing value for either the dependent or the factor variable for a given analysis is not used in that analysis. Also, a case outside the range specified for the factor variable is not used.

- **Exclude cases listwise**. Cases with missing values for the factor variable or for any dependent variable included on the dependent list in the main dialog box are excluded from all analyses. If you have not specified multiple dependent variables, this has no effect.

Related Topics

Specifying Options for One-Way ANOVA
One-Way ANOVA
One-Way ANOVA Data Considerations
To Obtain a One-Way Analysis of Variance
One-Way ANOVA Contrasts
One-Way ANOVA Post Hoc Tests
One-Way ANOVA: Related Procedures

FIGURE 12-24   Illustration of SPSS pull-down menu for one-way ANOVA option containing homogeneity of variance test

From SPSS for Windows®, Rel. 13.0.1. Copyright 2004 by SPSS Inc. Used with permission.

One Way

Test of Homogeneity of Variances

VAR00001

Levene Statistic	df1	df2	Sig.
.696	2	27	.507

ANOVA

VAR00001

	Sum of Squares	df	Mean Square	F	Sig.
Between Groups	126.667	2	63.333	.723	.495
Within Groups	2366.000	27	87.630		
Total	2492.667	29			

FIGURE 12-25   Illustration of SPSS output containing the final result for an example of one-way ANOVA along with the final result of homogeneity of variance test

From SPSS for Windows®, Rel. 13.0.1. Copyright 2004 by SPSS Inc. Used with permission.

KEY TERMS

parameters
statistics
significance
prognosis
Bernoulli theorem
probability
subjective view
Thomas Bayes
standard error of the mean
central limit theorem
confidence interval
single-group design
two-tailed test
one-tailed test
Student *t* test
degrees of freedom
power of the test
point estimate
critical values
paired *t* test
nonparametric statistics
Yates' correction for continuity

Wilcoxon matched-pairs signed-ranks
    test
Mann-Whitney *U* test
F test
Bartlett test
main effect
interaction effect
Scheffe's method
Tukey's method
planned comparisons
Bonferroni *t* procedure
Friedman two-way analysis of variance
    by ranks
Kruskal-Wallis one-way analysis of variance
    by ranks
classical approach
p-value approach
meta-analysis
effect size
MANOVA
discriminant analysis
factor analysis

SELF-LEARNING REVIEW

1. In the vernacular of everyday language, we commonly use the term _____ to express the likelihood of a future event.

2. Clinically speaking the term *probability* is akin to the concept of _____.

3. According to the _____ theorem, the relative frequency of an observed event will approximate its _____ frequency of occurrence if observed over an indefinitely _____ series of trials or experiments.

4. The mathematical likelihood of a coin turning up heads will get closer and closer to _____ 50% as the number of tosses _____.

5. The classical view of probability is also called the _____, or _____ view.

6. Quantities used to describe characteristics of populations are termed _____. On the other hand, quantities derived from samples that are used in estimating population parameters are called _____.

7. Relatively small _____ values such as $p \leq .001$ are interpreted with _____ confidence than are larger alpha values such as $p \leq .05$.

8. A mathematical basis for assessing probability in terms of the subjective views of individuals was introduced by Thomas _____ in 1763.

9. A highly useful measure of the degree of variability in a sampling distribution is called the _____ error of the _____, denoted by $\sigma_{\bar{x}}$ or SE. The SE is an estimate of the expected amount of _____ of sample means from the true population mean as a result of chance or _____ errors.

10. While the SD is a measure of the degree of _____ that currently exists among individuals in a population, SE is an estimate of how much _____ to expect in the means of _____ samples when the complete population parameter is unknown.

11. The central limit theorem states that: (a) the mean of the sampling distribution for the sample mean is always equal to the _____ mean, and (b) the standard deviation of the sampling distribution for the mean of sample size n approaches _____ as n increases.

12. The statistical meaning of significance pertains to the _____ that an observed result is truly the consequence of a _____ influence under investigation.

13. Assuming that the mean IQ score is 100 with a standard deviation of 15, the true mean for a sample of 225 subjects can be estimated to lie between 98 and _____ about 95% of the time.

14. The simplest type of hypothesis testing involves the one-sample case, also known as a _____-group design. In essence, we are asking if the sample mean of one group is comparable to the _____ mean.

15. An alternative hypothesis containing an unequal sign will be evaluated by means of a _____-tailed test. Such a test is selected when the _____ of the difference cannot be predicted on the basis of preexisting knowledge.

16. An alternative hypothesis containing either $>$ or $<$ is called a _____-tailed test. Such a test is said to be _____ stringent than a _____-tailed test since a smaller amount of _____ between mean scores is needed to be considered a significant finding.

17. When σ is unknown, the appropriate statistical test for evaluating H_0 is the _____ test. Furthermore, such a distribution is designed for testing hypotheses when the sample size is less than or equal to _____.

18. When a two-tailed test z test is performed at $\alpha = .05$, H_0 will be _____ if the magnitude of the observed value is _____ or equal to a critical value of _____.

19. In a sampling distribution, the formula for calculating a z score can be written symbolically as $z =$ _____.

20. In a t distribution, the standard error of the mean (SE) is equal to _____.

21. The critical value of t depends on the number of degrees of _____ allowed. The value of df for a one-sample t test is _____.

22. A type I error, denoted by _____, is the result of _____ the null hypothesis when it is _____.

23. A type II error, denoted by _____, is the consequence of _____ the null hypothesis when it is _____.

24. In most cases, researchers are more concerned about making a type _____ error because it is the one that primarily determines the _____ of a statistical test.

25. In cases where the data arising from separate and unrelated groups of subjects are independent of one another, the _____ t test is an appropriate statistic to use.

26. In the case of testing the difference between two independent group means, the number of degrees of freedom is defined as _____.

27. When we test the significance between the means of two dependent groups, the _____ t test is used with $df =$ _____.

28. Dependent samples can result from certain correlating procedures to form _____ pairs, or the same group can be measured twice in a _____ design.

29. A pairing design is also called a _____-subject, self-control, or _____ measures design.

30. The formula for the paired t test is written symbolically as $t = \dfrac{\bar{d}}{S_d / \sqrt{n}}$, in which $\bar{d}$ represents the mean of the _____ scores for the sample pair, S_d represents the _____ _____ of the sample difference, and n represents the number of _____ in the sample.

31. The four basic assumptions underlying the use of parametric tests of significance include _____ of variance, _____ or _____ data, a _____ curve, and _____.

32. If one or more of the assumptions are violated or remain questionable, a _____ statistic should be used.

33. A test that is useful in evaluating hypotheses about the relationship between nominal variables having two or more independent categories is the _____-square, denoted symbolically as _____. This test calculates the discrepancy between observed frequencies and _____ frequencies.

34. The chi-square test is most suited for _____ data where each case falling within a cell is _____ of every other case. When the question pertains to whether distributions of scores fall equally into certain categories, χ^2 is called the "goodness of _____" test.

35. The Wilcoxon matched-pairs signed ranks test is a nonparametric version of the _____ t test.

36. For small n's, the power efficiency of the Wilcoxon test is approximated _____ of its parametric equivalent.
37. The Mann-Whitney U test, as a nonparametric equivalent of the _____ t test, is concerned with the equality of _____.
38. The use of multiple t tests increases the probability of a type _____ error.
39. The main goal of ANOVA is to find the ratio of systematic variance, also called _____-group variance, to the degree of error variance, also termed _____-group variance.
40. The two-way ANOVA consists of main effect and _____ effect.
41. In the case of an unequal sample size among comparison groups, _____ test is highly useful for post hoc multiple comparisons. On the other hand, if the sample sizes are equal, then the _____ test may be performed.
42. The Bonferroni t procedure _____ the critical value of an F needed for reaching statistical significance. This procedure is used in cases where the researcher wishes to increase the _____ of the test.
43. RBANOVA is appropriate for _____-subject designs where the data comes from repeated measures on the same subject. The primary purpose of this method is to determine whether or not the differences between two or more groups may be due to chance or to _____ differences among the groups.
44. ANCOVA allows for an adjustment in factors _____ the experiment begins that might potentially influence the results of an experiment.
45. The observed value of the Friedman test statistic approximates the _____ distribution.
46. The KWANOVA test is a nonparametric equivalent of the one-way _____ and is an extension of the Mann-Whitney _____ test.
47. An increasing popular methodology for statistically combining the results from two or more independent studies is called _____.
48. MANOVA is designed for problems in which there are more than _____ dependent variable under investigation.
49. Discriminant analysis has utility in predicting _____ membership of an individual.
50. In performing factor analysis, researchers must see how the measures tend to cluster based on the test items' _____. Measures that are found to be correlated are called_____.
51. _____ is an introductory computer software package that stores the data values in columns and rows like a spreadsheet.
52. BMDP is used in medical sciences and allows for different types of analyses on the same data to be performed with only minor changes in the _____ operations.
53. _____ is suitable for the behavioral and social sciences and widely used because of its simplicity and complete labeling of statistical analyses on data printout.
54. _____ program possesses all capabilities that other software programs have. In addition, it can perform more complex probabilistic designs like Bayesian design and survival analysis.
55. _____ the null hypothesis if the p-value is less than or equal to α. If the p-value is less than _____, then the result is highly significant and there exists very strong evidence against the _____ hypothesis.

QUESTIONS AND EXERCISES FOR CLASSROOM DISCUSSION

PART 1

Calculation Question 1

Referring to our previously cited hypothetical study of the effect of propranolol on self-ratings of stuttering severity, perform a paired t test to evaluate the significance of the difference between the mean scores for the drug and placebo conditions at $\alpha = .05$. Use the data in the table to perform your calculations.

	Self-Ratings of Severity	
Subject	Propranolol	Placebo
1	3	5
2	0	1
3	2	4
4	1	3
5	3	3
6	1	4
7	2	3
8	4	5

The null hypothesis should be stated as:

H_0: The mean difference is _____.

The formula for the paired t test is given by $t = \dfrac{\bar{d}}{S_d / n}$ with $df =$ _____, where $\bar{d}$ represents the mean _____, S_d represents the standard deviation of the sample difference, and n represents the number of _____ in the sample.

In order to calculate $\bar{d}$ and S_d we must first find the sum of d, denoted by _____, and the sum of the square of d, denoted by _____. The sum of d is _____ and the sum of the square of d is _____. Similarly, $\bar{d} =$ _____ and $S_d =$ _____. Finally, the observed value of t is _____ with $df =$ _____. The absolute critical value of t at $\alpha = .05$ is _____. Therefore, the null hypothesis is _____.

Lastly, use one of the software packages to calculate the p-value and draw the proper conclusion from it.

Calculation Question 2

Based on our previously cited study of work preferences among speech-language pathology versus audiology students, conduct a chi-square test at $\alpha = .05$ to determine whether or not the membership of the two groups and their work preference are independent. Use the hypothetical data given here:

Work Preference N = 100

	Medical	Nonmedical	Row Sum
Sp-Lang. Path.	16	34	50
Audiology	32	18	50
Column Sum	48	52	100

The null hypothesis can be stated as:

H₀: The two categories are _____.

For this study, a _____-tailed test will be used and _____ correction for continuity should be used since $df =$ _____.

The observed chi-square value is found to be _____ and the critical χ^2 is found to be _____. Hence, the null hypothesis is _____.

Calculations Question 3

Recalling our hypothetical study concerning the auditory processing abilities of three groups of children with different phonological skills—Control Group (A), Consistent Group (B), and Delayed Group (C)—perform a one-way ANOVA to determine the significance of difference among them.

The table shown below summarizes the data you need to complete the calculations.

Control (A)	Consistent (B)	Delayed (C)
78	72	88
98	100	78
100	98	91
97	99	87
96	94	100
100	85	76
100	90	98
94	100	96
95	100	100
92	92	96

The _____ _____ can be symbolically stated as $\mu_A = \mu_B = \mu_C$.

The three basic assumptions of the one-way ANOVA are (1) _____ among the groups, (2) the sampling distribution of the group follows a _____ curve, and (3) the _____ of the scores in each group are equal. This assumption is also referred to as _____ of variance.

Assuming these assumptions have been met, calculate the necessary numerical values to obtain the F value for the scores in the table. These values are found to be as follows:

$n_A =$ _____ $n_B =$ _____ $n_C =$ _____

$\bar{Y}_A =$ _____ $\bar{Y}_B =$ _____ $\bar{Y}_C =$ _____

$\bar{Y} =$ _____ $J =$ _____ $N =$ _____ ,

Between-group variance = _____   Within-group variance = _____
df (between) = _____, df (within) = _____

Finally, the observed F value is _____. By consulting the F-table in Appendix 1-4-1, the critical F value at $\alpha = .05$ is found to be _____. Therefore, we must _____ H_0.

Absolutely finally, using one of the software packages to perform a test of homogeneity of variances and a one-way ANOVA, calculate the p-value, and conclude from it.

PART 2

1. Explain the central limit theorem, and list all properties of the theorem symbolically.
2. List the general steps in performing hypothesis testing using the classical approach.
3. What is the meaning of the term *degrees of freedom*?
4. Explain what distinguishes a z distribution from a t distribution?
5. Explain the relationship between a type I error, a type II error, and the power of a test.
6. What is the difference between a paired t test and an unpaired t test?
7. List all assumptions for parametric statistics.
8. When do we use nonparametric statistics? Give at least two nonparametric alternatives to parametric statistics.
9. What is the purpose of the Mann-Whitney U test? When employing it, how do we state H_0 and H_1?
10. List the assumptions of the analysis of variance.
11. Explain why the use of multiple t tests cannot be used instead of ANOVA.
12. Illustrate the conceptual basis for computing the two-way ANOVA.
13. What is the main difference between Scheffe's method and Tukey's method?
14. What is the logic behind RBANOVA? How does RBANOVA differ from ANOVA?
15. Explain how the p-value is calculated. List all guidelines for the p-value approach in hypothesis testing.
16. What are the purposes of meta-analysis, MANOVA, discriminant analysis, and factor analysis?

Reading, Writing, and Presenting Research

CHAPTER 13

CHAPTER OUTLINE

LEARNING OBJECTIVES

After reading this chapter, you should be able to identify, describe, or define:

- The difference between "catabolic" and "anabolic" thinking as these terms have been used in reference to reading and writing scientific research papers, and the value of each process
- Questions to ask in evaluating the various sections of a scientific research article
- The components of a scientific research proposal
- Ethical guidelines in the use of humans and animals in scientific research
- Sources of funding for scientific research
- What to consider in writing a plan (prospectus) for a thesis or dissertation
- Some principles for efficient and effective writing and helpful manuals and handbooks

■ The advantages of oral presentations of scientific research in the form of technical papers and poster sessions, and some tips for presenters

According to one dictionary definition, a *profession* is the "faith in which one is professed." To a large degree, "faith" in any scientific discipline is based on the quality of its research and the manner in which new knowledge is communicated. Good reading, writing, and oral communication skills are essential tools for interpreting and professing thoughts, opinions, ideas, and conclusions about new findings as they emerge.

THE VALUE OF CRITICAL THINKING

In earlier chapters, the point was made that different people may differ widely in their perceptions of truth based on a wealth of accumulated information. The same can be said for professionals working in scientific fields who are frequently critical of the research of their colleagues. Among scientists, *critical thinking* is a highly regarded means of exercising judgment in the search for truth. Evidence of this fact can be found in the "letters to the editor" section of many scientific journals, where space is provided for thoughtful analyses and commentaries by the readers of articles. Such letters are often geared toward uncovering methodological problems in a research study or providing alternative interpretations of the data. Sometimes, letters may include brief summaries of other research findings that bear on the problem. Authors of articles are typically given the opportunity to reply to criticisms of their work. This frequently results in a lively and useful interchange of opinion about the validity and implications of the research outcome. Much can be learned from a careful review of the articles that initially stimulated such commentaries as well as from the debate subsequently highlighted in letters written to the editor. Of course, we must keep in mind that critical thinking is not only usefully applied in the analysis of the work of others but also in the design and evaluation of one's own work.

By being critical in the course of reading and writing research literature, we ultimately build a rational foundation for decision making, or "quasi-faith" in what is professed. In essence, we construct a kind of temporary reality by seeking and finding empirical evidence for hypotheses, knowing that their ultimate proof will always remain questionable to some degree. Because critical reading and writing are the best tools available for evaluating and communicating such evidence, these skills are important to learn.

CATABOLIC THINKING IN READING RESEARCH

As an integral part of a course in research and statistical methods, the authors of this text require that students engage in two kinds of critical-thinking exercises akin to two well-known processes in the field of biochemistry. The first of these exercises is designed to foster what we choose to call **catabolic thinking** in evaluating research articles. Catabolism is actually a metabolic process of breaking food particles down into smaller parts to facilitate digestion. Therefore, in a figurative sense, we ask that students thoroughly "digest" the various components of a research article by critically evaluating each of its subcomponents. To guide this process, students are asked to provide a detailed evaluation of a selected research article according to the research questionnaire shown in Figure 13-1. A research article questionnaire of the kind shown can help to make the reading of scientific literature an important scientific

I. Title and Abstract
    A. Did the title of the article clearly and accurately represent the topic or overall purpose of the study? Were words used that should have been omitted or substituted for by better words? Could the words in the title be readily adopted as "key words" in reference guides and computer-based information services to accurately identify the content of the article? Was the title condensed and abbreviated appropriately to provide a running header at the top of the article's pages?

    B. Did the abstract provide a concise yet adequate description of the problem? Generally, did the author(s) make clear the questions or hypotheses investigated, the methods employed, the statistical results obtained, and the conclusions drawn?

II. Introduction
    A. Did the introduction provide an objective and balanced survey of the literature that progressed smoothly and logically to culminate in a summary statement of the problem?

    B. Was the rationale (need) for the study firmly established based on a paucity of previous research or observed limitations in other studies--i.e., inadequacies in sampling, design errors, inappropriate choice of statistics, mistakes in the analysis, or interpretation of data, etc.?

    C. Was the theoretical and practical importance of the findings adequately addressed?

    D. What specific research questions of hypotheses were raised? What independent and dependent variables were incorporated within these questions or hypotheses and were the variables operationally defined?

III. Methods
    A. Were the characteristics of the sample fully described in terms of the population to which the results were generalized; the number of subjects used; the criteria for their inclusion or exclusion; their physical, psychosocial, and educational attributes; the manner of their selection and assignment to various treatment conditions; and the attrition of subjects from the control and experimental groups during the course of the experiment?

    B. Were all known variables in the study specified and their validity established? Could these be replicated in future research? What instruments, test measures, or recording devices were used to operationally define the parameters of the dependent and independent variables? Were specific brand names, model numbers or other kinds of identifying information listed? If a noncommercial specialized apparatus was used, were descriptive diagrams or sketches provided to explain its various components, their electrical/mechanical operation, and the manner of calibration and reliability?

    C. What type of design was used in the study? Was a rational basis for its selection made known? Were the controls (e.g. randomization, counterbalancing, blinding, etc.) appropriate for eliminating threats to internal and external validity? Were the test environment and testing conditions adequately described? What instructions were given to the subjects? Were the procedures for manipulating the independent variable and recording the dependent variable clearly specified, and was their reliability established?

continues

FIGURE 13-1   Example of research journal article questionnaire

IV. Results
   A. Were the data qualitative or quantitative in nature? What types of statistical methods were selected to test the research questions or hypotheses? Were the methods chosen appropriate for this task? Were all relevant results reported including those running counter to the hypotheses? Were any findings presented that seemed tangential to the stated goals of the investigation?

   B. Were the data well organized and logically presented using suitable tables and figures? Were there clear legends and captions? Were averages and standard deviation reported in addition to probability values, degrees of freedom, and the direction of the effect? Did the data appear to come from a normal distribution or did the distribution appear skewed (e.g., containing an inordinate number of scores higher or lower than the mean)?
   Was the power of the test evaluated in relation to the likelihood for a type II error? How many statistical comparisons were made on the groups? Was the probability that some of these tests might yield statistically significant findings as a result of chance alone taken into account?

   C. Were the data assessed in an objective and straightforward manner while avoiding theoretical speculation?

V. Discussion
   A. Did the discussion provide a brief summary of the study in view of the questions or hypotheses posed in the introduction and the data presented in the results section? If hypotheses were stated in the introduction, was every one of them evaluated and its validity interpreted based on the results of the present study as well as the findings of similar investigations? If new hypotheses were advanced, were these consistent with the present findings, or did the authors extrapolate beyond the limits of their statistical analyses?

   B. Were the strengths and weaknesses of the study thoroughly evaluated? To what degree did possible design problems or the failure to control for extraneous or confounding influences hamper the generalization of findings?

   C. Were both positive and negative results discussed in view of their theoretical or practical implications? What suggestions were offered for future research, and did the suggestions appear to be logical and justifiable given the results of the current study?

VI. References and Appendices
   A. Were all references used in the text of the article included in an alphabetical list at the end of the article? Was an appropriate bibliographical style used? In the case of journal publications of the American Speech-Language-Hearing Association, the style of reference should conform with the format recommended in the current *Publication Manual of the American Psychological Association*

   B. Was any supplementary information included in alphabetically arranged appendices, such as additional statistical data, questionnaires, technical notes or equipment diagrams, instructions for subjects, and details of clinical treatments or training programs? Did this material facilitate understanding? Was certain material omitted that should have been included, particularly in reference to its judged importance for replication of the study.

VII. Overall Assessment
   Imagine that as an editorial consultant for a journal you had been asked to peer review and evaluate the publication merit of the same article you selected for this exercise. Would you have judged the article acceptable for publication, perhaps with some revisions, or recommended that it be rejected?

   Provide a concise rationale for your decision in either case. If revisions had been recommended, what constructive advice might you have offered? If the investigation was so flawed as to have been rejected, what practical steps might be taken in future studies to correct the problems you identified?

FIGURE 13-1   *continued*

activity in its own right. In essence, it serves as an analytical tool for *investigating an investigation* in order to judge its worth. Although no questionnaire should be expected to provide universal coverage for all types of research problems, we have found ours to be a useful guide for the systematic dissection of most articles, as one of our students said, "right down to the bones."

ANABOLIC THINKING IN WRITING RESEARCH

Earlier, we noted that the term catabolism is a useful metaphor for describing the process of breaking down the separate elements of a research article so that the validity of its contents can be digested and logically appraised. Of equal importance to the development of critical thinking skills is the notion of anabolism—a process that entails building up or assembling complex structures from more elementary components. What we call **anabolic thinking** is reflected in the type of scientific work that culminates in a written research proposal. Such a proposal requires not only a critical review of the separate elements of many previous studies, but also a well crafted and integrated plan for addressing current deficiencies in knowledge uncovered in the literature review.

The format for writing a research proposal will vary depending on its use. Students enrolled in the course we teach are asked at the beginning of the semester to form a designated number of "research teams." Each team is required to develop a research proposal as outlined below. A well written proposal shares many of the same features as a good research article. In addition, it must address important administrative, ethical, and financial concerns if the project is to succeed.

Research Proposal Outline

I. Title

The title should be effective in conveying what the study is about. Avoid the use of unnecessary words that lead to cumbersome and confusing titles such as, "*A Study to Investigate* Physiological *Measures of* Anxiety and *Their Relation to* Stuttering Adaptation *During Oral Reading Trials* Under Two Levels of Audience Complexity." A shorter, neater version of this title would be: "Physiological Anxiety and Stuttering Adaptation Under Two Levels of Audience Complexity." The improved version is achieved by simply omitting the italicized words. Paring down verbiage in the titles of articles generally achieves the dual goals of brevity and increased clarity. Of course, a title that is too short may also cause ambiguity. For example, the following title meets the criterion of brevity but conveys little information: "Stuttering and Anxiety." A good rule to follow in constructing titles is to include *key words* that concisely identify the variables under investigation and the conditions for testing their relationships.

The title page should also include the following identifying information under the title:

- The first name, middle initial, and last name of each investigator, their highest academic degree, and institutional affiliation(s)
- The name of the institutional unit, review board, or agency to whom the proposal is being submitted
- The name, address, and telephone number of the individual who is to serve as the principal investigator or coordinator of the project

II. Abstract

As a comprehensive summary of the content of the proposed research study, an abstract should be approximately 100 to 200 words in length. Because the abstract provides a succinct summary of the problem, the subjects and methods to be used, and the importance of the findings, it should be written after the components of the proposal are assembled in final form. According to the APA's publication manual, a good abstract is one that is accurate, self-contained, concise and specific, nonevaluative, coherent, and readable.

III. Table of Contents

A table of contents should be included on a separate page to provide a convenient means of locating specific information contained in the proposal by page number. Pages preceding the table of contents are typically paginated using lowercase roman numerals (i, ii, iii, etc.). Consecutive arabic numbers are used for pagination following the table of contents.

IV. Budget

A budget should be included to cover anticipated expenses over the time frame of the study. A detailed budget should be provided for the first year and a summary budget for each subsequent year. Such costs might be incurred because of the need to

- Purchase, fabricate, or maintain equipment and supplies
- Compensate subjects for their participation
- Pay salaries and fringe benefits of individual investigators and support staff based on the percentage of their time allocated to the project
- Reimburse travel expenses
- Cover consultant costs, fee for service contracts, or expenses connected with physical alterations or renovations
- Pay for administrative and overhead costs, such as telephone and utility bills, mailing, photocopying, computer use, rental fees, and the like

A good budget is realistic to the degree that it (1) truly reflects the estimated funds needed for completing the research study within a given time frame and (2) complies with the funding guidelines of the institution or granting agency from which support will be requested. A rationale must be provided for each budget need accompanied by documented evidence for all estimated costs (manufacturer's quotes, catalog prices, etc.).

V. Other Support and Resources

Be sure to describe any other sources of funds, whether federal, nonfederal, or institutional, that will be used to support the project. Such funds might include training grants, cooperative agreements, contracts, fellowships, gifts, prizes, or other awards specifically related to the study.

The available resources for completing the study are also important to describe. This might include a description of the space allocated for testing subjects, special laboratory equipment, and computer facilities. Formal agreements with other institutions to provide needed resources for the study and related administrative details are typically included in an appendix. Confirming letters of all institutional agreements must be included and signed by authorized officials. In the case of complex arrangements with other institutions or the need to coordinate the activities of multiple investigators, such documentation is important for clarifying administrative authority and responsibility in overseeing various operations of the project.

VI. Biographical Sketches

Institutional review boards and funding agencies will want to know about the education and special abilities of the investigator(s) to complete the proposed investigation as well as all consultants. Therefore, a resume summarizing the academic training, academic degrees, and relevant professional accomplishments of each investigator should be included with the research proposal. It is especially important that the resumes of investigators highlight those pilot studies, completed investigations, or former grant support for projects most relevant to the proposed topic of research. This may not be necessary for certain types of internal reviews (e.g., reviews of master's theses or doctoral dissertation proposals). However, virtually all *external reviews* of research proposals conducted by outside institutions, government agencies, corporations, or foundations require an evaluation of the credentials of the applicant investigator(s).

VII. Research Protocol (Study Plan)

A protocol is a detailed narrative of the research study that one wishes to perform. It should include the following elements: (1) specific aims; (2) background and significance; (3) methods; and (4) ethical considerations.

A. Specific aims.   The objectives of the study, what the investigator intends to accomplish, should be stated clearly and include the rationale for the research questions or hypotheses upon which the study is based. An example of a specific aims statement, excerpted from a funded NIH proposal that meets these requirements, is quoted below:

> Many studies have shown a higher frequency of language impairments and reading disabilities in children with socially disadvantaged backgrounds . . . However, most definitions of language and reading disorders exclude socially disadvantaged children because of the *implicit* assumption that cultural and sociological deprivation "causes" the disability. Consistent with our emphasis on validation of definitional criteria, we propose to study explicitly the influence of social disadvantage on language and reading disability. This study will permit clarification of the role of social disadvantage on disability definitions and the more general issue of the influence of social disadvantage on developmental reading disabilities. We hypothesize that language impairment and social disadvantage will exercise joint but independent influences on reading disability consistent with a main effects model (i.e., no interaction effect). (Aram et al., 1994, pp. 5–6).

The point at which the specific aims should be addressed within the sequence of the various sections of a research proposal is a matter for debate. Logically, it might be contended that a statement of the aims should follow a background review of the salient literature after establishing a well grounded need for further investigation. On the other hand, an equal if not better argument is that the specific aims should be stated at the beginning of the protocol so that reviewers can determine from the outset just what the research is about. As noted by Colton (1974), "effective critical appraisal hinges on the reader's initial understanding of the aim of the investigation" (p. 317). Ultimately, the "formula" for structuring a research proposal must be based on the requirements stipulated by the reviewers who will read and decide on its merit.

B. Background and significance.   The background and significance section of the protocol provides a critical review of the literature relevant to the problem to be investigated. In effect, it marshals the facts about what is presently known and unknown and states the importance of learning more. Any preliminary work by an investigator related to the proposed study should receive special emphasis because it may strengthen the investigator's credibility for continuing studies in a particular research area in which certain types or levels of expertise may be desirable or required. It is particularly important to state clearly the theoretical and practical importance of the findings. As much as possible, one should describe how the results of the study might alter understanding, influence clinical procedures, resolve theoretical debates, and so forth.

C. Methods.   The methods section should be written to allow the reviewers to assess the appropriateness of your sampling techniques, measurements, experimental procedures, design for executing the study, and plans for data analysis. Any anticipated difficulties with proposed procedures along with alternative approaches to achieve the aims should likewise be discussed.

The organization and content of the narrative in the methods section is much like the format found in a research article (see Chapter 2). In essence, you should describe in specific terms:

- Who you plan to use for subjects
- What you wish to do to them
- How it will be done
- The means for assessing outcomes

The methods section of the protocol is also a convenient place for the inclusion of a timetable that specifies when each stage of the investigation will start and be completed. The specification of such deadlines is important for assuring the accountability of the investigator(s) to the goals stated in the research proposal. Furthermore, institutional sponsors of research, review boards, and government agencies typically mandate adherence to certain calendar deadlines for submitting research applications, progress reports, and the renewal of funding for projects.

As noted in Chapter 2, the methods section serves as the blueprint for conducting the investigation. If this section of a research protocol is flawed or written poorly, the study will likely be rejected.

D. Ethical considerations.   Ethical considerations *must* be addressed in protecting the rights and welfare of subjects. As discussed previously in Chapter 4, if human subjects are to participate in an investigation, the research proposal must be evaluated and given approval by an institutional review board (IRB). Federal regulations pertaining to the composition and duties of an IRB have been specified in the *Federal Register,* June 18, 1991. The Department of Agriculture and Public Health Service have also published guidelines related to the use and care of laboratory animals in research. Institutions that use animals for such purposes must also have an institutional animal care committee (IACC) consisting of a veterinarian, a scientist, and an individual who is not a member of the institution. The American Speech-Language-Hearing Association (ASHA) has also established publication guidelines for approval of articles in its journals related to the use of humans and animals in research (see Figure 13-2).

Because IRB approval is necessary *prior to* implementing most research studies, it is wise to seek such approval early in the process of planning the investigation. This is particularly important if the *ratio of potential risks to potential benefits* is estimated to be high. Although the majority of studies in the field of communication disorders involve minimal risk of harm or discomfort to subjects, this is not always the case. The use of certain drugs, the surgical removal of tissue, implantation of foreign devices or materials, radiographic imaging techniques, and aversive conditioning procedures are examples of the kinds of experimental methods that may carry a high level of risk.

An IRB will look carefully at the written consent form that subjects will be asked to sign as well as the research protocol. It is particularly important that the consent form be written in a manner that can be easily comprehended by the subjects or parents or legal guardians for whom its use is intended. An example of a well written consent form is shown

Humans in Research

All research to be submitted for publication in journals of the American Speech-Language-Hearing Association in which human subjects are used must adhere to the basic ethical considerations for the protection of human subjects in research. Where applicable by law or institutional affiliation, authors must provide assurance of approval by an appropriate institutional review board or equivalent review process. The basis for these considerations can be found in The Belmont Report: Ethical Principles and Guidelines for the Protection of Human Subjects (1979), which can be found at http://ohrp.osophs.dhhs.gov.

Animals in Research

All research to be submitted for publication in journals of the American Speech-Language-Hearing Association in which animal subjects are used must ensure that animals have been treated humanely with appropriate consideration of their comfort and health. Where applicable by law or institutional affiliation, authors must provide assurance of approval by an appropriate institutional animal care and use committee. The basis for these considerations can be found in the statement of the American Physiological Society regarding use and care of animals in research which can be found by searching their web site at http://www.the-aps.org.

FIGURE 13-2   ASHA's publication guidelines for research in which human or animal subjects are used

Adapted from "Information for Authors," by American Speech-Language-Hearing Association, 2004, Journal of Speech Language Hearing Research, 47, (3).

in Figure 13-3. An IRB protocol and consent form written in a precise and organized style will be of great help in gaining approval for your study and assuring its ultimate success.

VIII. References

All names cited in the proposal should be properly referenced. In the text of the proposal, names that are directly cited in the context of a sentence should be referenced by listing the last name of the author(s) followed by the date of the publication enclosed in parentheses: *"Boberg and Kully (1996) reported . . ."*

When there are multiple authors of a single research study, list all of their last names in the initial reference but only the name of the first author in subsequent references to the same study: *"The results of a study by Conture, Colton, and Gleason (1986) indicated . . .",* and subsequently, *"As the results of the study by Conture et al. indicated . . ."*

If an author's name is not directly used in the sentence but his or her work is cited, the following format is appropriate: *"In a review of the research literature on child language disorders it was noted that . . . (Miller, 1991)."* Multiple references of this kind should be listed alphabetically and separated by a semicolon: *(Green & Kuhl, 1989; MacDonald & McGurk, 1978; Massaro, 1987).*

Complete references also should be listed alphabetically in a "Reference" section at the end of the text. The following examples illustrate the style recommended by the APA for referencing several types of published and unpublished resources:

Book (single author):
Emmorey, K. *Language, cognition, and the brain: Insights from sign language research.* (2002). Mahwah, NJ: Lawrence Erlbaum Associates.

Participant's Name _____   Date _____

Participant Investigator: (Name), (Institution), (Address)

Informed Consent
  1. Title of Study: Proper Name Recall in Younger and Older Adults: The Contributions of Word Uniqueness and Reported Strategies.
  2. Purpose of Study: The purpose of this study is to investigate the effects of aging on the learning and retrieval of proper names and occupations assigned to pictures of unfamiliar faces.
  3. Procedures: I will be asked to look at some pictures of people and learn their names and occupations so that I can recall them later. I will also be asked to complete a brief questionnaire related to my recall of these items and to complete a rating scale of the names and occupations. In addition, there will be some tests to test my memory and attention. The testing will take approximately 1 to 2 hours. All testing will be scheduled at my convenience.
  4. Risks and Discomforts: There are no known medical risks or discomforts associated with this project, although I may experience fatigue and/or stress when taking these tests. I will be given as many breaks as I want during the testing session.
  5. Benefits: I understand there are no known direct medical benefits to me for participating in this study. However, the results of the study may help researchers gain a better understanding of how we learn and recall information about other people.
  6. Participant's Rights: I may withdraw from participating in the study at any time.
  7. Financial Compensation: I will be reimbursed $ _____ per hour for my participation and $ _____ for any travel expenses.
  8. Confidentiality: In order to record exactly what I say in the tests, a tape recorder will be used. The tape will be listened to only by the Principal Investigator and authorized members of the research team at _____ . I understand that the results of testing will be kept confidential unless I ask that they be released. The results of this study may be published in professional journals or presented at professional conferences, but my records or identity will not be revealed unless required by law.
  9. If I have any questions or concerns, I can call _____ at (000) 000-0000 at any time during the day or night.

I understand my rights as a research subject, and I voluntarily consent to participation in this study. I understand what the study is about and how and why it is being done. I will receive a signed copy of this consent form.

_____   _____

Subject's Signature   Date

_____

Signature of Investigator

FIGURE 13-3   Example of a written consent form

Book (multiple authors):
Peterson-Falzone, S. J., Hardin-Jones, M. A., & Karnell, M. P. (2001). *Cleft palate speech* (3rd ed.). St. Louis: Mosby.

Chapter in edited book:
Maxwell, S. E. & Wallach, G. P. (1984). The language-learning disabilities connection: Symptoms of early language disability change over time. In G. P. Wallach & K. G. Butler (Eds.), *Language learning disabilities in school-age children* (pp. 15–340). Baltimore: Williams and Wilkins.

Journal article (multiple authors):
Grievink, E., Peters, S., van Bon, W., & Schilder, A. (1993). The effects of early bilateral otitis media with effusion on language ability: A prospective cohort study. *Journal of Speech and Hearing Research, 36,* 1004–1012.

Thesis or dissertation:
Miller, S. M. *Predicting the complexity of generative syntax from measures of working memory in younger and older adults.* (2001). Unpublished doctoral dissertation, Emerson College.

Conference paper:
Solomon, N. P., Robin, D. A., & Luschei, E. S. (1994, March). *Strength, endurance and sense of effort: Studies of the tongue and hand in people with Parkinson's disease and accompanying dysarthria.* Paper presented at the Conference on Motor Speech, Sedona, AZ.

IX. Appendices

Technical descriptions of instrumentation, photographs, test questionnaires, documentation of IRB approval if already obtained, and other relevant information that supplements the proposal is included within alphabetically arranged appendices (A, B, C, etc.).

Funding Research

Research proposals are often motivated by the need to obtain financial support for new or continuing research projects. Funds for such support are available through a variety of sources including department or institutional funds, government agencies, foundations, and corporations.

Institutional Funds

Many colleges and universities allocate "seed money" for getting new research projects started. At the authors' own institution, applications for *intramural research funds,* as they are called, are made through the office of the Graduate Dean. A faculty research committee is appointed each year to evaluate the proposals, which must be structured and written according to uniform guidelines. The awards are made through a competitive process in which the merit of each proposal is evaluated according to well-defined criteria. As in many institutions, the amount of money available for the support of individual faculty projects is relatively small, consisting of a few thousand dollars. Nevertheless, these funds are often crucial for collecting preliminary data or laying the groundwork for more extensive studies. The appeal of an *extramural grant application* (beyond the institution) often can be greatly enhanced by providing tangible evidence that an investigator is not only motivated but also competent to complete the proposed study. Intramural research awards can assist in marshaling such evidence, particularly for young faculty members at the start of their careers. Such awards to faculty can also serve the interests of graduate students who may receive stipends and gain experience as research assistants by working on such projects. Students might also be afforded data collection opportunities that facilitate their own plans for completing theses and dissertations in related areas of research.

NIH Grants and Contracts

A major source of research funds is through the federal government with the *National Institutes of Health (NIH)* serving as the primary agency for the support of projects in biomedical and behavioral fields. The most common type of research application that is self-initiated by an investigator is called an **RO-1 proposal.** The proposal must be written strictly in accordance with the instructions provided in *Grant Application Form PHS 398*. NIH will mail this form to applicants on request, or a copy can usually be obtained through the grants or development office of one's own institution. This and other types of grant application forms can be downloaded from the *NIH Office of Extramural Research* Web site: http://grants1.nih.gov/grants/oer.htm or from the *Center for Scientific Review (CSR)* Web site: http://csr.nih.gov/. These Web sites also provide information about funding opportunities, deadline dates for submitting applications, helpful guidelines for preparing them, and policies and procedures for reviewing applications. All competing grant applications for NIH are received by CSR, and it reviews the majority of them. Between 1998 and 2003 the number of applications received by CSR increased greatly (55%) to 41,899.

The review of a research proposal by CSR is a complex process structured to assure that each grant application is given a fair, independent, expert, and timely review. As they arrive, a CSR referral officer examines applications and assigns them to an NIH institute for review by an appropriate *Integrated Review Group (IRG)*. Some of the institutes whose scientific interests most closely align with research in the field of communication sciences and disorders are listed in Figure 13-4.

Committee members decide which among the total number of applications received are in the upper half and lower half based on an evaluation of their scientific merit. Typically, only applications identified in the upper half during this initial review process will be considered by the entire review group. The members of this committee, called a study section, typically consists of 20 productive researchers whose combined expertise spans a particular scientific field of study and who are the principle investigators on projects comparable to those being reviewed. Research grant applications in communication sciences and disorders are commonly reviewed by the:

- Cognition and Perception Study Section (CP)
- Cognitive Neuroscience Study Section (COG)
- Child Psychopathology and Developmental Disabilities Study Section (CPDD)
- Adult Psychopathology and Disorders of Ageing Study Section (APDA)
- Motor Function, Speech and Rehabilitation Study Section (MFSR)
- Auditory System Study Section (AUD)
- Language and Communication Study Section (LCOM)

Such study sections are said to conduct **peer reviews** because working scientists review proposals in the research field of their own expertise.

Study section members usually convene for about two days. During this time, they will discuss and further evaluate the applications and assign a numerical rating *(priority score)* to each. A few days after the meeting, a computer-generated letter is forwarded to applicants listing their priority scores and percentile rankings, the written critiques of the assigned reviewers, and the study section recommendations. The study section's recommendations

National Institute on Aging (NIA): Leads a national program of research on the biomedical, social, and behavioral aspects of the aging process; the prevention of age-related diseases and disabilities; and the promotion of a better quality of life for all older Americans. http://www.nia.nih.gov

National Cancer Institute (NCI): Leads a national effort to eliminate the suffering and death due to cancer. Through basic and clinical biomedical research that will lead to a future in which we can prevent cancer before it starts, identify cancers that do develop at the earliest stage, eliminate cancers through innovative treatment interventions, and biologically control those cancers that we cannot eliminate so they become manageable. http://www.nci.nih.gov

National Institute of Child Health and Human Development (NICHD): NICHD research on fertility, pregnancy, growth, development, and medical rehabilitation strives to ensure that every child born healthy and wanted grows up free from disease and disability. http://www.nichd.nih.gov

National Institute on Deafness and Other Communication Disorders (NIDCD): Conducts and supports biomedical research and research training on normal mechanisms as well as diseases and disorders of hearing, balance, smell, taste, voice, speech, and language that affect 45 million Americans. http://www.nimh.nih.gov

National Institute of Dental and Craniofacial Research (NIDCR): Provides leadership for a national research program designed to understand, treat, and ultimately prevent the infectious and inherited craniofacial-oral-dental diseases and disorders that compromise millions of human lives. http://www.nidr.nih.gov

National Institute of Mental Health (NIMH): Provides national leadership dedicated to understanding, treating, and preventing mental illnesses through basic research on the brain and behavior, and through clinical, epidemiological, and services research. http://www.nimh.nih.gov

National Institute of Neurological Disorders and Stroke (NINDS): The mission is to reduce the burden of neurological diseases—a burden borne by every age group, every segment of society, and people all over the world. To accomplish this goal the NINDS supports and conducts research, both basic and clinical, on the normal and diseased nervous system, fosters the training of investigators in the basic and clinical neurosciences, and seeks better understanding, diagnosis, treatment, and prevention of neurological disorders. http://www.ninds.nih.gov

FIGURE 13-4   Some NIH institutes that support research in the field of communication sciences and disorders

are also forwarded to the *advisory council* for an institute who decides priorities for funding based on public health needs. Not all approved applications are funded. Approximately 20% are being funded at the present time for periods of 2–5 years.

In addition to funding self-initiated research grants of the type described above, NIH also makes efforts to stimulate and support research in various areas designated by its own advisory committees. Applications under this program, called *P0-1 applications,* are made either in response to a **Request for Proposal (RFP)** or a **Request for Application (RFA).** Essentially, investigators who respond to an RFP may be awarded a contract to conduct research as determined by NIH. On the other hand, although a grant awarded under an RFA also addresses a topic of interest to NIH, the research plan used for this purpose is the creation of the investigator. Program announcements *(PAs)* are published regularly in the *NIH Guide for Grants and Contracts* and the *Federal Register* (see their Web sites at http://grants.nih.gov and http://www.gpoaccess.gov, respectively). Appendix C contains the summary pages of a representative NIH application that was recently funded.

For additional information about federal sources of funding in speech, language, voice, and hearing, see ASHA's Web site: http://www.asha.org.

Foundation and Corporate Grants

Thousands of nongovernmental, nonprofit foundations in the United States give money to assist worthy projects of special interest to them. Although the total giving of foundations amounts to billions of dollars each year, only a small percentage of this money is allocated for research in the behavioral, educational, and health science fields. Nevertheless, research projects that require a modest level of funding and that have goals closely related to the mission of a particular foundation are strong candidates for support.

An excellent resource that describes the goals and objectives of major foundations and the kinds of projects they fund is the **Foundation Grants Directory** maintained by a national organization called the *Foundation Center*. The Foundation Center is an independent agency that gathers and disseminates factual information on the philanthropic foundations through programs of library service, publication, and research. It has organized a nationwide network of foundation reference collections in all 50 states. *The Centers for Cooperating Collections* offer a number of free publications and provides a trained staff to assist patrons in locating resources on funding information. The Foundation Center also maintains a database of more than 40,000 grant-making foundations and direct corporate giving programs. The center staff will provide assistance in searching its database for foundations whose interests align with the individual or institution seeking support for a particular project, or it will recommend the best online and other sources of regional and national information. For addition information about the Foundation Center, see its Web site: http://fdncenter.org.

Once an appropriate foundation has been identified, a three- to five-page letter should be written to the grants officer describing the objectives of the research plan. The qualifications of the investigator(s) to carry out the research, the anticipated time period for the project, and the amount of money needed for its completion should also be described. Depending on the level of interest in the applicant's letter, the grants officer of the foundation may respond by requesting additional information. Some foundations will only make awards under certain cost-sharing arrangements with the applicant's own institution or in conjunction with another philanthropic organization.

The American Speech-Language-Hearing Foundation (ASHF) also invites applications for funding that promote scientific research in the field of communication sciences and disorders. A number of New Investigator Research Grants are available each year to individuals who have received their latest degree (master's or doctoral level) in communication sciences and disorders within the last five years and who are starting their research careers. As funds allow, ASHF offers other funding opportunities that, in the past, have included the support of treatment outcome research in speech-language pathology and audiology. ASHF also supports student research grants each year, one of these for a one-year study in Early Childhood Language Development and another for a one-year study in Clinical or Rehabilitative Audiology. Another recent initiative of ASHF is the New Century Scholars Program. Two components of the program include a doctoral scholarship competition that supports students accepted and enrolled in a research/teaching PhD or equivalent program, and a research grant competition to support individuals committed to teacher-investigator careers in the university or college academic environment or in external institutes or laboratories. Box 13-1 highlights a doctoral candidate in communicative disorders who was a recent recipient of a

BOX 13-1

Spotlight on New Century Scholars: Nathan Welham

Not many people would turn down a Fulbright Scholarship—but Nathan V. Welham did. A current doctoral candidate in the communicative disorders program at the University of Wisconsin-Madison, and international student from New Zealand, Nathan needed the money. But accepting the prestigious award would have restricted his career options following graduation—a requirement that was unacceptable to this talented individual studying speech-language pathology.

But all things happen for a reason, and this was no exception. Late in 2003, Nathan received word that he had been named one of the first New Century Scholars, awarded a $10,000 doctoral scholarship from the American Speech-Language-Hearing Foundation. "Being recognized in that way is unbelievable," says Nathan. "It's a significant financial contribution to the cost of pursuing a PhD, and it's amazing to be one of the first people to receive the award. It is honoring, overwhelming, and also encouraging that I am on the right track."

Nathan's track is an interesting one: His major area of interest is voice, coupled with a minor study in genetics. As a doctoral student, he works in a number of different areas, including conducting nontraditional research studies in voice and genetics. He has studied vocal fatigue in professional voice users; worked with biomedical engineers on the development and evaluation of new synthesized speech technologies for augmentative and alternative communication applications; and is now focused on studying the genetic mechanisms that potentially underlie differences in laryngeal structure and function, susceptibility to disease, and responses to treatment.

He also works at the University of Wisconsin-Madison's Voice Clinic, where he assesses and treats patients with voice disorders. "It's a well-known facility, and for the past 18 months, I have worked toward completing my clinical fellowship year (CFY) in conjunction with my PhD studies," Nathan explains. "It keeps me clinically grounded. As someone who does research, the kind of questions I ask and the work I do have to be clinically relevant."

Nathan also holds a position as a teaching assistant to professor Diane Bless, PhD, in her voice disorders class. He has been instrumental in bringing new teaching methods to the class, introducing a pilot program using online multimedia technology for distance learning. "We have online lectures with narrated PowerPoint slides and notes, movie clips, audio clips—students can hear me talking about what they are seeing onscreen," he says. "We asked the on-campus students to spend time going through these lectures so that we could move most of our didactic content material online and then spend our class time with students on application, case-based problem solving, and hands-on use of technology. In this way, we have attempted to accelerate students' development, clinical problem solving, and analytical thinking."

These opportunities were not available to Nathan in New Zealand. "The U.S. is foremost in terms of research programs and progression," he explains. "The field started here, so there is more tradition, and most of the people I wanted to study

continues

BOX 13-1 *continued*

with were here. A more important consideration when choosing a program, however, more than the country or the institution, is the individual who will mentor you through your PhD and guide how you will begin your career in the field."

And Nathan is someone who carefully considers his future. Even in high school, he chose speech-language pathology as his career goal after evaluating all of his interests—science, music, the arts, interacting with and helping people. He also had some personal experience with communication disorders through an uncle, who is profoundly deaf, and his mother, a sign language interpreter.

As he has pursued his career, he says, "I can think of numerous clinical situations and occasions during which I have felt that speech-language pathology, and particularly the subspecialty of voice, is the right place for me. First, possessing a body of clinical and scientific knowledge and a set of clinical skills, and being able to use this knowledge and these skills to help one of my patients obtain an understanding of their condition, move towards a diagnosis, or make progress in treatment or recovery, is a very satisfying thing. Second, encountering patients with difficult and challenging problems that break the clinical mold, are confusing to diagnose and understand, and sometimes are resistant to treatment spurs my research interest even further. Both reinforce my feeling that this is the field for me."

The New Century Scholars doctoral scholarship offers Nathan some security as he continues his studies. In the short term, he plans to replace a "very old computer with a bad hard drive and a permanent green band on the screen" with one that will allow him to run analyses for his research. "I can use this award as I need to throughout the remainder of my program, and so an unexpected cost will not be so terrifying."

The award also allows Nathan to think about his future post-graduation, which he hopes ultimately will lead to a professorship in the United States. He is also considering taking a post-doctoral fellowship, continuing nontraditional and crossdisciplinary research "as a bridge to becoming a professor." "I enjoy all aspects of what I do. I love teaching and interacting with the students, and I love research, discovering new knowledge and asking questions and trying to answer them."

Best of all about being a professor says Nathan, in the true spirit of a teacher-investigator, "is you are paid to track down answers to questions that you choose to ask!"

New Century Scholars Award. For more information about funding opportunities, visit the foundation Web site at www.ASHFoundation.org.

Some businesses and corporations are also interested in funding research or providing needed equipment, particularly if the anticipated outcome is consistent with their own advertising and marketing objectives or is expected to enhance their public image. Manufacturers of hearing aids, augmentative communication devices, diagnostic equipment, or computer software are examples of the kinds of enterprises that may be interested in cooperative research ventures. In considering such partnerships, it is imperative that the researcher be able to conduct an independent and impartial research study untainted by the biasing influences of certain expectations that might otherwise operate, even in subtle ways. The use of blinding control procedures in both the collection and analysis of data may be highly useful in assuring valid results (see Chapter 6).

THESES AND DISSERTATIONS

In numerous fields of graduate study, a written thesis (master's level) or dissertation (doctoral level) is required to demonstrate mastery of the thinking processes and tools of research.

The majority of graduate programs in communication sciences and communication disorders no longer require the completion of a formal thesis project. The reasons underlying the lack of such a requirement are complex. Perhaps the most important of these are the market forces that have led to a rapidly expanding demand for trained clinicians. Such growth has placed great strain on the educational resources of many college and university programs. Furthermore, the corpus of knowledge pertaining to speech, language, and hearing disorders has also grown immensely requiring additional course work and clinical training to meet the increased requirements for certification.

Whether or not all students who plan to work professionally in the field of communication sciences and disorders should have formal research training is a matter for debate. Some might argue, as Jerger (1963) did in an often-cited editorial that stirred up much debate in the field, that the practical realities of the profession are such that research cannot be done well by everyone and is best left to those who are trained to do it well. Research, Jerger said, "is the province of trained researchers, just as diagnosis and therapy are the province of trained clinicians" (p. 3). A counterargument to the Jerger position is that the meaning of the term "research" should not be restricted to carrying out a set of narrowly defined procedures. As we discussed in Chapter 1, research also should be thought of as those antecedent scientific thinking processes that *lead* to the application of certain methods in problem solving. In extending this line of logic, it could be said that the primary value of thesis and dissertation research is not so much in the research outcome but in the development of the scientific thinking processes that make the outcome possible.

Although a thesis may not be required, many academic programs often give students the option of pursuing this experience. Assuredly, the demands associated with writing a thesis will help prepare students for an even more rigorous level of advanced scholarship—the doctoral dissertation. To gain approval for either a thesis or dissertation, a **prospectus** must be written. Such a prospectus is a detailed outline of the plan for research. Although there is no universally acceptable format for writing a prospectus, it will share many of the same elements of any research proposal.

Prior to writing a prospectus, you should ask a professor to serve as your thesis or dissertation advisor. The choice of a particular advisor is usually based on her or his expertise in the area related to the topic that you would like to pursue. Based on a review of salient literature and discussions with your advisor, you will gradually refine the subject matter of your research into testable questions or hypotheses backed up by well-grounded rationales. Important considerations in selecting and defining a research problem were discussed previously in Chapter 3. The type of question or hypothesis that is finally selected for study may be a component of a larger ongoing research program being pursued by your advisor or may be of your own invention. In either case, the problem should be intellectually challenging and judged worthy of investigation by both you and your advisor. Working together, you will also decide on the methods to be employed in the investigation, and a plan for data analysis.

You should also ask your advisor to help you develop a realistic timetable for completing your thesis or dissertation. Despite unforeseen obstacles that might hinder your progress, such a timetable can serve as a highly useful plan for guiding and disciplining the course of your actions as you work toward the goal of successfully completing your project. While most colleges and universities stipulate that theses and dissertations *must* be completed within a specific time period, both you and your advisor will prefer adhering as closely as possible to a reasonable schedule for finishing the project well within the strictures of such deadlines.

Your advisor will also assist you in selecting and assembling a thesis or dissertation advisory committee. Such a committee typically consists of three or more faculty members. A common practice is to select at least one member of the committee from a related discipline outside one's major department who can represent and uphold the overall academic standards of the college or university in evaluating the proposed research.

When you have completed a clearly written and well organized plan for your research, your advisor will distribute it to all members of the advisory committee, who will critically evaluate its quality using the same standards as they would apply to any research protocol as previously discussed. Subsequently, your advisor will schedule a prospectus meeting during which time you will be asked to summarize your plans for the proposed research and answer all questions raised by the advisory committee. Changes in the prospectus may be recommended by one or more committee members. Sometimes, disputes about recommended changes will need to be reconciled by your research advisor. Once the prospectus has been formally approved, it serves as a kind of "contract of agreement" between all the involved parties that the study will be carried out precisely as stated. Any variance in the written plan of research must be reflected in a revised prospectus that meets with the approval of the advisory committee.

In addition to providing an action plan for the proposed research, an approved prospectus safeguards against future criticisms of the research protocol by committee members *provided that* the research was conducted carefully and competently as originally proposed. This assurance is important because the content of a thesis or dissertation when completed must be approved by the advisory committee that reviewed the original plan. Generally, such approval is contingent on an evaluation of the written document in addition to a successful oral defense by the student. While a well-written research prospectus is no guarantee of a successful outcome, one that is ambiguous or lacking in sufficient details can lead to shoddy results accompanied by a negative evaluation.

WRITING WELL

Whether writing a research proposal, thesis or dissertation, or an article for publication, it is important to attend closely not only to the content but also to the mechanics of the written result. Unfortunately, this principle is often ignored by researchers. Indeed, as a study by Armstrong (1980) made clear, obscure and pedantic writing with a high frequency of polysyllabic sentences can sometimes be more highly esteemed by college professors than prose characterized by simple straightforward sentence structures. Commenting on the obscurity and awkwardness of prose in many medical science areas, Crichton (1975) noted that the preferred "stance of authors seems designed to astound and mystify the reader with a dazzling display of knowledge and scientific acumen . . ." (p. 1297). This "stance" also commonly prevails in many applied behavioral science areas to the detriment of clarity in written communication.

In addition to conforming to grammatical rules, good writing possesses the properties of *efficiency* and *effectiveness*. Efficient writing is constituted of concise sentences that state the point directly. Don't say: "*On the basis of the results of this study, it is possible to form a tentative hypothesis of a possible relationship between anxiety and stuttering.*" Instead, simply state, "*The results are indicative of a relationship between . . .*" or, better still "*A relationship was found between . . .*" Efficient writing conveys meaning using a minimal number of words.

Effective writing also possesses the property of clarity. Imprecise or vague words should be avoided whenever possible. Consider the following:

> The results of the study indicated that when faced with hyperactive children with short attention spans (AD-HD) who were clearly unmotivated and who eventually became unresponsive to test stimuli because of their distractibility, clinicians were prone to modify their instructional techniques by terminating reinforcement followed by the introduction of a "time out" phase, during which time the training program was suspended for a period of a few minutes or more.

The above sentence not only contains superfluous words, but creates unnecessary ambiguity by the use of many vague, abstract words and professional jargon. Clarity is achieved by the use of precise, concrete, specific words that convey quantitative meaning whenever possible. Thus, the above sentence might be improved by the following revision:

> When the rate of the response being trained decreased by 10%, the clinicians suspended the training program for 5 to 10 minutes.

The readers of scientific articles often complain of difficulty in comprehending the content of such articles. Most often, the fault lies in the obscure verbiage of the writer—not because of inadequacies in the readers' comprehension abilities. As the professional writer Michael Alley (1987) said, "In scientific writing, precision is the most important goal of the language. If your writing does not communicate exactly what you did, then you have changed your research" (p. 28).

Many manuals and handbooks are available to help writers improve the efficiency and effectiveness of their writing style. Some of the more useful of these aids to scientific writing include

- *Publication Manual of the American Psychological Association* (5th ed.), Washington, DC: APA, 2001. Contributors of research papers to ASHA's major journals are expected to follow this style. An electronic version of the manual is available by subscription online at: http://www.apastyle.org/stylehelper. Free tips on how to write in APA style are provided.
- *A Manual for Writers of Term Papers, Theses, and Dissertations* (6th ed.), by Kate Turabian. Chicago: University of Chicago Press, 1996.
- *The MLA Handbook for Writers of Research Papers*, New York: Modern Language Association of America, 2003.
- *The Chicago Manual of Style* (15th ed.), Chicago: University of Chicago Press, 2004.
- *Science and Technical Writing: a Manual of Style*. Edited by Philip Rueben. New York: Routledge, 2001.

PROFESSIONAL PRESENTATIONS

An important channel for communicating current research findings is that of oral presentations. The conveyance of information to professional audiences "by word of mouth" allows the speaker to communicate directly with her or his peers and to receive immediate feedback.

Such feedback can be particularly useful in exploratory studies or pilot investigations, when refinements in one or more components of the research protocol may need to be made before submitting an article to a journal for peer review. Critical comments and constructive advice offered by audience members during question and answer periods, especially from those whose expertise is in the subject matter presented, may be highly useful in evaluating the validity of the findings and in uncovering potential pitfalls that might jeopardize publication of the work. In this sense, an oral presentation can sometimes serve as a kind of "testing ground" in considering the publication merit of a research study. Generally, opportunities for orally presenting one's research findings exceed the prospects for a journal publication. Such opportunities can be found within the colloquia of colleges and universities, in the "grand rounds" of clinics and hospitals, and through the sponsored institutes or research seminars and the professional programs of state, regional, or national conferences of scholarly organizations.

Program committees for conferences will typically require that proposals for oral presentations be written in a standard format in accordance with the submission guidelines of the organization. In the case of conventions sponsored by ASHA, submission requirements include the completion of cover sheets, a narrative summary, and a proposal rating form. The cover sheets include the title of the proposal, the content area to be covered (fluency/fluency disorder, voice/voice disorder, language science, etc.), the session type requested (brief presentation, poster presentation, experimental seminar, etc.), any special equipment requests, the names and professional affiliations of the presenters, and a brief abstract.

The abstract serves two major purposes. First, it provides a basis for the program committee to determine the overall suitability of the research for the intended scholarly aims of the conference and the degree to which it is likely to align with the interest of the audience. Second, because all abstracts of accepted presentations are usually published in a program bulletin of the conference proceedings, audience participants can quickly review the key elements of the research paper(s) to be presented within a particular session and decide whether or not they wish to attend. As in the case of abstracts prepared for journal publications, the abstract for an oral presentation should be well-written because it too may be selected for inclusion within certain indexing services and databases. Because of space limitations in program bulletins, abstracts may have to be condensed to an even greater degree than required for article publications. Abstracts of research studies proposed for presentation at ASHA's convention currently are required not to exceed 100 words. The following is an example of an abstract that the first author of this text submitted to ASHA's convention program review committee in response to a "call for papers."

> The California Verbal Learning Test (CVLT) was used to investigate a number of interrelated components of verbal memory in a group of dyslexic readers and matched control subjects. Several between-group differences were observed on measures of verbal learning ability, immediate recall, and recognition measures. The CVLT was found to be a reliable instrument for differentiating several cognitive processes and mnemonic strategies used by impaired versus normal readers in learning and remembering verbal material.

In addition to a written abstract, the program committee often will require a narrative summary of the research paper that describes the background, methods, and results of the research study in greater detail. ASHA specifies that the summary of the proposal should, in 1000 words or less, give the program committee a clear understanding of the proposal's content. The proposal should also describe learner outcomes. For the proposal described above, the following learner outcomes were appended to the summary:

> Session participants will learn about:
> * The general utility of the California Verbal Learning Test as it is designed to assess multiple components of verbal memory.
> * The way the CVLT was used in this particular study to assess memory operations in adult dyslexics as compared to normal readers.
> * The predominant types of errors found in the recall and recognition measures based on a statistical analysis of within- and between-group differences.
> * Theoretical and clinical implications of the results, particularly in reference to the finding that dyslexics appeared to rely more heavily on the semantic than phonologic memory route during word retrieval.

An increasingly popular medium for presenting research at professional conferences consists of *poster presentations*. As opposed to brief technical sessions or research papers, where the allotted time may be no more than 10 minutes, poster sessions are usually allowed to run for 90 minutes or more. Poster sessions are typically much more informal and interactive than research paper sessions. Furthermore, specific aspects of the research study often can be addressed and debated in greater detail. Especially for students and young investigators, poster sessions provide an excellent opportunity for presenting research findings in a relaxed and nonthreatening atmosphere and for meeting other researchers in a similar field who may offer useful advice. Such educational "networking" not only affords opportunities for mutual learning experiences but may also lead to future research collaborations with other colleagues. A representative example of a poster session that was recently presented at an ASHA convention can be found in Appendix D.

Whatever the type of proposed presentation, it must be in accordance with certain criteria used by the program review committee for it to be accepted. In a recent call for papers for its national convention, ASHA noted that it would be guided in the selection of research submissions based on the following criteria:

* Strength of theoretical/scientific rationale for research question
* Originality of research questions(s)
* Strength of research design
* Credibility of data (or data in progress)
* Integration of findings
* Overall clarity of proposal

In summary, oral communication can be an efficient, effective, and powerful means of communicating research findings. Useful convention presenter information relating to both technical papers and poster sessions can be found on ASHA's Web site: http://www.asha.org.

SUMMARY

In this chapter, we reviewed several issues to consider in reading, writing, and presenting scientific research. We began by discussing the importance of two types of critical thinking processes that allow a researcher to evaluate and communicate scientific evidence effectively. Catabolic thinking is a useful metaphor for describing the process of breaking down a problem into its separate elements or parts. On the other hand, a researcher employs anabolic thinking when the components of such information are assembled in such a way as to define a new problem for investigation. We noted that both kinds of mental operations are necessary for reading and writing research articles. We also outlined several guidelines for critically evaluating the separate sections of a research article (catabolic thinking) and for writing a good research proposal (anabolic thinking), along with the need to carefully consider certain administrative, ethical, and financial issues for a project to succeed. Several funding sources for research were briefly reviewed including institutional funds, NIH grants and contracts, and foundation and corporate grants. The importance of acquiring critical thinking skills, as reflected in good reading and writing abilities, and their importance in preparing theses, dissertations, journal articles for publication, and professional presentations was also discussed along with some useful tips for achieving these goals.

KEY TERMS

catabolic thinking
anabolic thinking
RO-1 proposal
peer review

request for proposal (RFP)
request for application (RFA)
Foundation Grants Directory
prospectus

SELF-LEARNING REVIEW

1. Among scientists, _____ _____ is a highly regarded means of exercising judgment in the search for truth.
2. Evidence for the above fact can be found in the "_____ to the _____" section of scientific journals.
3. By being critical in reading and writing research literature, we ultimately build a rational foundation for _____ making or "quasi-_____" in what is professed.
4. _____ thinking is similar to a metabolic process that entails breaking particles down into smaller parts.
5. "Digesting" the various components of a research article by critically evaluating each of its subcomponents is akin to what the authors call _____ thinking.
6. A research article questionnaire serves as a tool for investigating a(n) _____.
7. A process that entails building up or assembling complex structures from smaller elementary components is called _____.
8. The type of scientific work that culminates in a written research proposal is representative of _____ thinking.
9. A _____ should be effective in conveying what the study is about.
10. A good rule to follow in constructing titles is to include _____ words that concisely identify the variables under investigation and _____ for testing their relationships.
11. According to the APA's publication manual, a good _____ is one that is accurate, self-contained, concise and specific, nonevaluative, coherent, and readable.
12. A detailed budget section of a proposal should be provided for the _____ year and thereafter a _____ budget for each subsequent year.
13. A good budget is realistic to the degree that it (1) _____ reflects the estimated funds needed for the research study within a given time period and (2) complies with the funding _____ of the institution from which funds are sought.

14. The biographical sketches of investigators submitted with a research proposal should highlight those _____ studies, _____ investigations, or former _____ support for projects most relevant to the proposed research.

15. The _____ _____, or objectives of the study, describe what the investigation intends to accomplish.

16. The _____ and _____ section of the protocol provides a critical review of the literature. It also marshals the facts about what presently is _____ and _____ and states the case for learning _____.

17. In the methods section, you should describe in specific terms _____ you plan to use for subjects, _____ you wish to do to them, _____ it will be done, and the _____ for assessing the outcome.

18. If human subjects are to participate in an investigation, the research proposal must be evaluated and given approval by an _____ _____ _____.

19. An IRB will look carefully at the written _____ _____ that subjects will be asked to sign as well as the research _____.

20. Many colleges and universities allocate "_____ _____" for new research projects. These are called _____ research funds.

21. The appeal of an extramural grant application can be greatly enhanced by proving that the investigator is not only motivated but also _____ to complete the proposed study. _____ research awards can assist in marshaling such evidence.

22. The _____ _____ of _____ is the primary agency for supporting research in biomedical fields. To apply for such funds, Grant Application Form _____ _____ is often used.

23. Applications must be sent to the _____ _____ _____ _____ by a certain deadline date for consideration within a particular _____ period.

24. CSR assigns applications to particular _____ or divisions within NIH.

25. Research applications undergo a _____ review by one of several Integrated Review Groups or so-called _____ sections.

26. The _____ _____ for the institute makes final decisions about whether applications are funded or not funded.

27. NIH also makes efforts to stimulate and support research in various areas by issuing a _____ _____ _____ (RFP) or a _____ _____ _____ (RFA). These announcements appear in the NIH Guide for _____ and Contracts and the Federal _____.

28. An excellent resource that describes the major foundations and the kinds of projects they fund is the _____ Grant Directory maintained by the _____ _____.

29. In seeking research support from businesses and corporations, it is important that researchers be able to conduct an _____ and _____ research study. The use of _____ control procedures in the collection and analysis of data is recommended.

30. It could be argued that the primary value of thesis and dissertation research is not so much in the research _____ but in the development of the scientific _____ processes that make the outcome possible.

31. To gain approval for a thesis or dissertation project, a _____ must be written. This is a detailed outline of the _____ for research.

32. In addition to providing an action plan for the proposed research, an approved prospectus safeguards against future criticism of the research _____ by the

advisory committee, provided that the research was conducted _____ and _____ as originally proposed.

33. In addition to conforming to grammatical rules, good writing possesses the properties of _____ and _____.

34. _____ writing conveys meaning using a minimal number of words. _____ writing also possesses the added property of _____.

35. When readers of scientific articles complain of the difficulty in comprehending the content of research, the fault often lies in the _____ verbiage of the writer.

36. ASHA journals follow the recommendations offered in the style manual of the _____ _____ _____.

QUESTIONS AND EXERCISES FOR CLASSROOM DISCUSSION

1. Explain the difference between "catabolic thinking" and "anabolic thinking." Provide one clinically relevant example for each type of thinking process.
2. Provide a detailed evaluation of a journal article from a professional journal that is relevant to the field of communication sciences and disorders according to the research article questionnaire that appears in this chapter.
3. Write a research proposal using the research proposal outline included in this chapter.
4. Discuss the ethical considerations for the use of humans and animals in research.
5. Explain the difference between intramural research funds and extramural research funds.
6. Explain the general application procedure for NIH grants and contracts.
7. What are "foundation grants"? Explain the general application procedure for obtaining such grants.
8. Describe the general procedures for completing theses and dissertations?
9. Discuss the importance of "writing well." Provide an example to explain "effective writing."
10. Discuss the merits of presenting a paper at a regional/national conference of a scholarly organization.
11. What are "poster presentations"? Discuss the merits of such presentations.
12. Identify ASHA's general guidelines and criteria for the selection of papers for presentation at its national convention.

The Tables

TABLE A-1-1   The Standard Normal Distribution:
Areas Under the Standard Normal Curve from O to z for Various Values of z

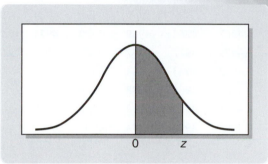

z	.00	.01	.02	.03	.04	.05	.06	.07	.08	.09
0.0	.0000	.0040	.0080	.0120	.0160	.0199	.0239	.0279	.0319	.0359
0.1	.0398	.0438	.0478	.0517	.0557	.0596	.0636	.0675	.0714	.0754
0.2	.0793	.0832	.0871	.0910	.0948	.0987	.1026	.1064	.1103	.1141
0.3	.1179	.1217	.1255	.1293	.1331	.1368	.1406	.1443	.1480	.1517
0.4	.1554	.1591	.1628	.1664	.1700	.1736	.1772	.1808	.1844	.1879
0.5	.1915	.1950	.1985	.2019	.2054	.2088	.2123	.2157	.2190	.2224
0.6	.2258	.2291	.2324	.2357	.2389	.2422	.2454	.2486	.2518	.2549
0.7	.2580	.2612	.2642	.2673	.2704	.2734	.2764	.2794	.2823	.2852
0.8	.2881	.2910	.2939	.2967	.2996	.3023	.3051	.3078	.3106	.3133
0.9	.3159	.3186	.3212	.3238	.3264	.3289	.3315	.3340	.3365	.3389
1.0	.3413	.3438	.3461	.3485	.3508	.3531	.3554	.3577	.3599	.3621
1.1	.3643	.3665	.3686	.3708	.3729	.3749	.3770	.3790	.3810	.3830
1.2	.3849	.3869	.3888	.3907	.3925	.3944	.3962	.3980	.3997	.4015
1.3	.4032	.4049	.4066	.4082	.4099	.4115	.4131	.4147	.4162	.4177
1.4	.4192	.4207	.4222	.4236	.4251	.4265	.4279	.4292	.4306	.4319
1.5	.4332	.4345	.4357	.4370	.4382	.4394	.4406	.4418	.4429	.4441
1.6	.4452	.4463	.4474	.4484	.4495	.4505	.4515	.4525	.4535	.4545

(continues)

TABLE A-1-1 (continued)

z	.00	.01	.02	.03	.04	.05	.06	.07	.08	.09
1.7	.4554	.4564	.4573	.4582	.4591	.4599	.4608	.4616	.4625	.4633
1.8	.4641	.4649	.4656	.4664	.4671	.4678	.4686	.4693	.4699	.4706
1.9	.4713	.4719	.4726	.4732	.4738	.4744	.4750	.4756	.4761	.4767
2.0	.4772	.4778	.4783	.4788	.4793	.4798	.4803	.4808	.4812	.4817
2.1	.4821	.4826	.4830	.4834	.4838	.4842	.4846	.4850	.4854	.4857
2.2	.4861	.4864	.4868	.4871	.4875	.4878	.4881	.4884	.4887	.4890
2.3	.4893	.4896	.4898	.4901	.4904	.4906	.4909	.4911	.4913	.4916
2.4	.4918	.4920	.4922	.4925	.4927	.4929	.4931	.4932	.4934	.4936
2.5	.4938	.4940	.4941	.4943	.4945	.4946	.4948	.4949	.4951	.4952
2.6	.4953	.4955	.4956	.4957	.4959	.4960	.4961	.4962	.4963	.4964
2.7	.4965	.4966	.4967	.4968	.4969	.4970	.4971	.4972	.4973	.4974
2.8	.4974	.4975	.4976	.4977	.4977	.4978	.4979	.4979	.4980	.4981
2.9	.4981	.4982	.4982	.4983	.4984	.4984	.4985	.4985	.4986	.4986
3.0	.4987	.4987	.4987	.4988	.4988	.4989	.4989	.4989	.4990	.4990
3.1	.4990	.4991	.4991	.4991	.4992	.4992	.4992	.4992	.4993	.4993
3.2	.4993	.4993	.4994	.4994	.4994	.4994	.4994	.4995	.4995	.4995
3.3	.4995	.4995	.4995	.4996	.4996	.4996	.4996	.4996	.4996	.4997
3.4	.4997	.4997	.4997	.4997	.4997	.4997	.4997	.4997	.4997	.4998
3.5	.4998	.4998	.4998	.4998	.4998	.4998	.4998	.4998	.4998	.4998
3.6	.4998	.4998	.4999	.4999	.4999	.4999	.4999	.4999	.4999	.4999
3.7	.4999	.4999	.4999	.4999	.4999	.4999	.4999	.4999	.4999	.4999
3.8	.4999	.4999	.4999	.4999	.4999	.4999	.4999	.4999	.4999	.4999
3.9	.49995	.49995	.49996	.49996	.49996	.49996	.49996	.49996	.49997	.49997
4.0	.49997									
4.5	.499997									
5.0	.4999997									

Republished with permission of Boca Raton: Chemical Rubber Company Press, adapted from *Standard Mathematical Tables,* 25th ed.,1978, p. 524; permission conveyed through Copyright Clearance Center, Inc.

TABLE A-1-2   Student's *t* Distribution

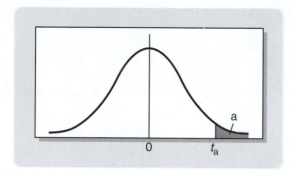

df	$t_{.005}$	$t_{.01}$	$t_{.025}$	$t_{.05}$	$t_{.10}$	$t_{.25}$
1	63.657	31.821	12.706	6.314	3.078	1.000
2	9.925	6.965	4.303	2.920	1.886	0.816
3	5.841	4.541	3.182	2.353	1.638	.765
4	4.604	3.747	2.776	2.132	1.533	.741
5	4.032	3.365	2.571	2.015	1.476	0.727
6	3.707	3.143	2.447	1.943	1.440	.718
7	3.499	2.998	2.365	1.895	1.415	.711
8	3.355	2.896	2.306	1.860	1.397	.706
9	3.250	2.821	2.262	1.833	1.383	.703
10	3.169	2.764	2.228	1.812	1.372	0.700
11	3.106	2.718	2.201	1.796	1.363	.697
12	3.055	2.681	2.179	1.782	1.356	.695
13	3.012	2.650	2.160	1.771	1.350	.694
14	2.977	2.624	2.145	1.761	1.345	.692
15	2.947	2.602	2.131	1.753	1.341	0.691
16	2.921	2.583	2.120	1.746	1.337	.690
17	2.898	2.567	2.110	1.740	1.333	.689
18	2.878	2.552	2.101	1.734	1.330	.688
19	2.861	2.539	2.093	1.729	1.328	.688
20	2.845	2.528	2.086	1.725	1.325	0.687
21	2.831	2.518	2.080	1.721	1.323	.686
22	2.819	2.508	2.074	1.717	1.321	.686
23	2.807	2.500	2.069	1.714	1.319	.685
24	2.797	2.492	2.064	1.711	1.318	.685
25	2.787	2.485	2.060	1.708	1.316	0.684
26	2.779	2.479	2.056	1.706	1.315	.684
27	2.771	2.473	2.052	1.703	1.314	.684
28	2.763	2.467	2.048	1.701	1.313	.683
29	2.756	2.462	2.045	1.699	1.311	.683
Large	2.576	2.326	1.960	1.645	1.282	.674

TABLE A-1-3 The Chi-Square Distribution

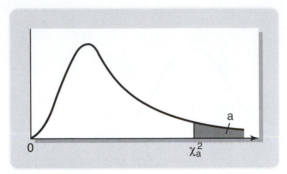

df	$\chi^2_{.995}$	$\chi^2_{.99}$	$\chi^2_{.975}$	$\chi^2_{.95}$	$\chi^2_{.90}$	$\chi^2_{.10}$	$\chi^2_{.05}$	$\chi^2_{.025}$	$\chi^2_{.01}$	$\chi^2_{.005}$
1	—	—	0.001	0.004	0.016	2.706	3.841	5.024	6.635	7.879
2	0.010	0.020	0.051	0.103	0.211	4.605	5.991	7.378	9.210	10.597
3	0.072	0.115	0.216	0.352	0.584	6.251	7.815	9.348	11.345	12.838
4	0.207	0.297	0.484	0.711	1.064	7.779	9.488	11.143	13.277	14.860
5	0.412	0.554	0.831	1.145	1.610	9.236	11.071	12.833	15.086	16.750
6	0.676	0.872	1.237	1.635	2.204	10.645	12.592	14.449	16.812	18.548
7	0.989	1.239	1.690	2.167	2.833	12.017	14.067	16.013	18.475	20.278
8	1.334	1.646	2.180	2.733	3.490	13.362	15.507	17.535	20.090	21.955
9	1.735	2.088	2.700	3.325	4.168	14.684	16.919	19.023	21.666	23.589
10	2.156	2.558	3.247	3.940	4.865	15.987	18.307	20.483	23.209	25.188
11	2.603	3.053	3.816	4.575	5.578	17.275	19.675	21.920	24.725	26.757
12	3.074	3.571	4.404	5.226	6.304	18.549	21.026	23.337	26.217	28.299
13	3.565	4.107	5.009	5.892	7.042	19.812	22.362	24.736	27.688	29.819
14	4.075	4.660	5.629	6.571	7.790	21.064	23.685	26.119	29.141	31.319
15	4.601	5.229	6.262	7.261	8.547	22.307	24.996	27.488	30.578	32.801
16	5.142	5.812	6.908	7.962	9.312	23.542	26.296	28.845	32.000	34.267
17	5.697	6.408	7.564	8.672	10.085	24.769	27.587	30.191	33.409	35.718
18	6.265	7.015	8.231	9.390	10.865	25.989	28.869	31.526	34.805	37.156
19	6.844	7.633	8.907	10.117	11.651	27.204	30.144	32.852	36.191	38.582
20	7.434	8.260	9.591	10.851	12.443	28.412	31.410	34.170	37.566	39.997
21	8.034	8.897	10.283	11.591	13.240	26.615	32.671	35.479	38.932	41.401
22	8.643	9.542	10.982	12.338	14.042	30.813	33.924	36.781	40.289	42.796
23	9.260	10.196	11.689	13.091	14.848	32.007	35.172	38.076	41.638	44.181
24	9.886	10.856	12.401	13.848	15.659	33.196	36.415	39.364	42.980	45.559
25	10.520	11.524	13.120	14.611	16.473	34.382	37.652	40.646	44.314	46.928
26	11.160	12.198	13.844	15.379	17.292	35.563	38.885	41.923	45.642	48.290
27	11.808	12.879	14.573	16.151	18.114	36.741	40.113	43.194	46.963	49.645

(continues)

TABLE A-1-3   (continued)

df	$\chi^2_{.995}$	$\chi^2_{.99}$	$\chi^2_{.975}$	$\chi^2_{.95}$	$\chi^2_{.90}$	$\chi^2_{.10}$	$\chi^2_{.05}$	$\chi^2_{.025}$	$\chi^2_{.01}$	$\chi^2_{.005}$
28	12.461	13.565	15.308	16.928	18.939	37.916	41.337	44.461	48.278	50.993
29	13.121	14.257	16.047	17.708	19.768	39.087	42.557	45.722	49.588	52.336
30	13.787	14.954	16.791	18.493	20.599	40.256	43.773	46.979	50.892	53.672
40	20.707	22.164	24.433	26.509	29.051	51.805	55.758	59.342	63.691	66.766
50	27.991	29.707	32.357	34.764	37.689	63.167	67.505	71.420	76.154	79.490
60	35.534	37.485	40.482	43.188	46.459	74.397	79.082	83.298	88.379	91.952
70	43.275	45.442	48.758	51.739	55.329	85.527	90.531	95.023	100.425	104.215
80	51.172	53.540	57.153	60.391	64.278	96.578	101.879	106.629	112.329	116.321
90	59.196	61.754	65.647	69.126	73.291	107.565	113.145	118.136	124.116	128.299
100	67.328	70.065	74.222	77.929	82.358	118.498	124.342	129.561	135.807	140.169

TABLE A-1-4   The F Distribution: Values of $F_{.05}$

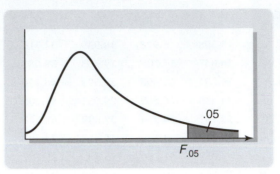

Degrees of Freedom of the Numerator

df_1/df_2	1	2	3	4	5	6	7	8	9
1	161.4	199.5	215.7	224.6	230.2	234.0	236.8	238.9	240.5
2	18.51	19.00	19.16	19.25	19.30	19.33	19.35	19.37	19.38
3	10.13	9.55	9.28	9.12	9.01	8.94	8.89	8.85	8.81
4	7.71	6.94	6.59	6.39	6.26	6.16	6.09	6.04	6.00
5	6.61	5.79	5.41	5.19	5.05	4.95	4.88	4.82	4.77
6	5.99	5.14	4.76	4.53	4.39	4.28	4.21	4.15	4.10
7	5.59	4.74	4.35	4.12	3.97	3.87	3.79	3.73	3.68
8	5.32	4.46	4.07	3.84	3.69	3.58	3.50	3.44	3.39
9	5.12	4.26	3.86	3.63	3.48	3.37	3.29	3.23	3.18
10	4.96	4.10	3.71	3.48	3.33	3.22	3.14	3.07	3.02
11	4.84	3.98	3.59	3.36	3.20	3.09	3.01	2.95	2.90
12	4.75	3.89	3.49	3.26	3.11	3.00	2.91	2.85	2.80
13	4.67	3.81	3.41	3.18	3.03	2.92	2.83	2.77	2.71
14	4.60	3.74	3.34	3.11	2.96	2.85	2.76	2.70	2.65
15	4.54	3.68	3.29	3.06	2.90	2.79	2.71	2.64	2.59
16	4.49	3.63	3.24	3.01	2.85	2.74	2.66	2.59	2.54
17	4.45	3.59	3.20	2.96	2.81	2.70	2.61	2.55	2.49
18	4.41	3.55	3.16	2.93	2.77	2.66	2.58	2.51	2.46
19	4.38	3.52	3.13	2.90	2.74	2.63	2.54	2.48	2.42
20	4.35	3.49	3.10	2.87	2.71	2.60	2.51	2.45	2.39
21	4.32	3.47	3.07	2.84	2.68	2.57	2.49	2.42	2.37
22	4.30	3.44	3.05	2.82	2.66	2.55	2.46	2.40	2.34
23	4.28	3.42	3.03	2.80	2.64	2.53	2.44	2.37	2.32
24	4.26	3.40	3.01	2.78	2.62	2.51	2.42	2.36	2.30
25	4.24	3.39	2.99	2.76	2.60	2.49	2.40	2.34	2.28
26	4.23	3.37	2.98	2.74	2.59	2.47	2.39	2.32	2.27
27	4.21	3.35	2.96	2.73	2.57	2.46	2.37	2.31	2.25
28	4.20	3.34	2.95	2.71	2.56	2.45	2.36	2.29	2.24
29	4.18	3.33	2.93	2.70	2.55	2.43	2.35	2.28	2.22
30	4.17	3.32	2.92	2.69	2.53	2.42	2.33	2.27	2.21
40	4.08	3.23	2.84	2.61	2.45	2.34	2.25	2.18	2.12
60	4.00	3.15	2.76	2.53	2.37	2.25	2.17	2.10	2.04
120	3.92	3.07	2.68	2.45	2.29	2.17	2.09	2.02	1.96
∞	3.84	3.00	2.60	2.37	2.21	2.10	2.01	1.94	1.88

(left margin) Degrees of Freedom of the Denominator

Degrees of Freedom of the Numerator

10	12	15	20	24	30	40	60	120	∞
241.9	243.9	245.9	248.0	249.1	250.1	251.1	252.2	253.3	254.3
19.40	19.41	19.43	19.45	19.45	19.46	19.47	19.48	19.49	19.50
8.79	8.74	8.70	8.66	8.64	8.62	8.59	8.57	8.55	8.53
5.96	5.91	5.86	5.80	5.77	5.75	5.72	5.69	5.66	5.03
4.74	4.68	4.62	4.56	4.53	4.50	4.46	4.43	4.40	4.36
4.06	4.00	3.94	3.87	3.84	3.81	3.77	3.74	3.70	3.67
3.64	3.57	3.51	3.44	3.41	3.38	3.34	3.30	3.27	3.23
3.35	3.28	3.22	3.15	3.12	3.08	3.04	3.01	2.97	2.93
3.14	3.07	3.01	2.94	2.90	2.88	2.83	2.79	2.75	2.71
2.98	2.91	2.85	2.77	2.74	2.70	2.66	2.62	2.58	2.54
2.85	2.79	2.72	2.65	2.61	2.57	2.53	2.49	2.45	2.40
2.75	2.69	2.62	2.54	2.51	2.47	2.43	2.38	2.34	2.30
2.67	2.60	2.53	2.46	2.42	2.38	2.34	2.30	2.25	2.21
2.60	2.53	2.46	2.39	2.35	2.31	2.27	2.22	2.18	2.13
2.54	2.48	2.40	2.33	2.29	2.25	2.20	2.16	2.11	2.07
2.49	2.42	2.35	2.28	2.24	2.19	2.15	2.11	2.06	2.01
2.45	2.38	2.31	2.23	2.19	2.15	2.10	2.06	2.01	1.96
2.41	2.34	2.27	2.19	2.15	2.11	2.06	2.02	1.97	1.92
2.38	2.31	2.23	2.16	2.11	2.07	2.03	1.98	1.93	1.88
2.35	2.28	2.20	2.12	2.08	2.04	1.99	1.95	1.90	1.84
2.32	2.25	2.18	2.10	2.05	2.01	1.96	1.92	1.87	1.81
2.30	2.23	2.15	2.07	2.03	1.98	1.94	1.89	1.84	1.78
2.27	2.20	2.13	2.05	2.01	1.96	1.91	1.86	1.81	1.76
2.25	2.18	2.11	2.03	1.98	1.94	1.89	1.84	1.79	1.73
2.24	2.16	2.09	2.01	1.96	1.92	1.87	1.82	1.77	1.71
2.22	2.15	2.07	1.99	1.95	1.90	1.85	1.80	1.75	1.69
2.20	2.13	2.06	1.97	1.93	1.88	1.84	1.79	1.73	1.67
2.19	2.12	2.04	1.96	1.91	1.87	1.82	1.77	1.71	1.65
2.18	2.10	2.03	1.94	1.90	1.85	1.81	1.75	1.70	1.64
2.16	2.09	2.01	1.93	1.89	1.84	1.79	1.74	1.68	1.62
2.08	2.00	1.92	1.84	1.79	1.74	1.69	1.64	1.58	1.51
1.99	1.92	1.84	1.75	1.70	1.65	1.59	1.53	1.47	1.39
1.91	1.83	1.75	1.66	1.61	1.55	1.50	1.43	1.35	1.25
1.83	1.75	1.67	1.57	1.52	1.46	1.39	1.32	1.22	1.00

(*continues*)

TABLE A-1-4   (Continued) The *F* Distribution: Values of $F_{.025}$

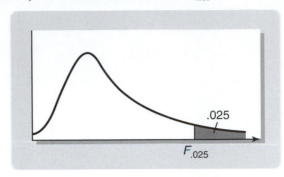

.025

$F_{.025}$

Degrees of Freedom of the Numerator

df_1/df_2	1	2	3	4	5	6	7	8	9
1	647.8	799.5	864.2	899.6	921.8	937.1	948.2	956.7	963.3
2	38.51	39.00	39.17	39.25	39.30	39.33	39.36	30.37	39.39
3	17.44	16.04	15.44	15.10	14.88	14.73	14.62	14.54	14.47
4	12.22	10.65	9.98	9.60	9.36	9.20	9.07	8.98	8.90
5	10.01	8.43	7.76	7.39	7.15	6.98	6.85	6.76	6.68
6	8.81	7.26	6.60	6.23	5.99	5.82	5.70	5.60	5.52
7	8.07	6.54	5.89	5.52	5.29	5.12	4.99	4.90	4.82
8	7.57	6.06	5.42	5.05	4.82	4.65	4.53	4.43	4.36
9	7.21	5.71	5.08	4.72	4.48	4.32	4.20	4.10	4.03
10	6.94	5.46	4.83	4.47	4.24	4.07	3.95	3.85	3.78
11	6.72	5.26	4.63	4.28	4.04	3.88	3.76	3.66	3.59
12	6.55	5.10	4.47	4.12	3.89	3.73	3.61	3.51	3.44
13	6.41	4.97	4.35	4.00	3.77	3.60	3.48	3.39	3.31
14	6.30	4.86	4.24	3.89	3.66	3.50	3.38	3.29	3.21
15	6.20	4.77	4.15	3.80	3.58	3.41	3.29	3.20	3.12
16	6.12	4.69	4.08	3.73	3.50	3.34	3.22	3.12	3.05
17	6.04	4.62	4.01	3.66	3.44	3.28	3.16	3.06	2.98
18	5.98	4.56	3.95	3.61	3.38	3.22	3.10	3.01	2.93
19	8.92	4.51	3.90	3.56	3.33	3.17	3.05	2.96	2.88
20	5.87	4.46	3.86	3.51	3.29	3.13	3.01	2.91	2.84
21	5.83	4.42	3.82	3.48	3.25	3.09	2.97	2.87	2.80
22	5.79	4.38	3.78	3.44	3.22	3.05	2.93	2.84	2.76
23	5.75	4.35	3.75	3.41	3.18	3.02	2.90	2.81	2.73
24	5.72	4.32	3.72	3.38	3.15	2.99	2.87	2.78	2.70
25	5.69	4.29	3.69	3.35	3.13	2.97	2.85	2.75	2.68
26	5.66	4.27	3.67	3.33	3.10	2.94	2.82	2.73	2.65
27	5.63	4.24	3.65	3.31	3.08	2.92	2.80	2.71	2.63
28	5.61	4.22	3.63	3.29	3.06	2.90	2.78	2.69	2.61
29	5.59	4.20	3.61	3.27	3.04	2.88	2.76	2.67	2.59
30	5.57	4.18	3.59	3.25	3.03	2.87	2.75	2.65	2.57
40	5.42	4.05	3.46	3.13	2.90	2.74	2.62	2.53	2.45
60	5.29	3.93	3.34	3.01	2.79	2.63	2.51	2.41	2.33
120	5.15	3.80	3.23	2.89	2.67	2.52	2.39	2.30	2.22
∞	5.02	3.69	3.12	2.79	2.57	2.41	2.29	2.19	2.11

Degrees of Freedom of the Denominator

Degrees of Freedom of the Numerator

10	12	15	20	24	30	40	60	120	∞
968.6	976.7	984.9	993.1	997.2	1001	1006	1010	1014	1018
39.40	39.41	39.43	39.45	39.46	39.46	39.47	39.48	39.49	39.50
14.42	14.34	14.25	14.17	14.12	14.08	14.04	13.99	13.95	13.90
8.84	8.75	8.66	8.56	8.51	8.46	8.41	8.36	8.31	8.26
6.62	6.52	6.43	6.33	6.28	6.23	6.18	6.12	6.07	6.02
5.46	5.37	5.27	5.17	5.12	5.07	5.01	4.96	4.90	4.85
4.76	4.67	4.57	4.47	4.42	4.36	4.31	4.25	4.20	4.14
4.30	4.20	4.10	4.00	3.95	3.89	3.84	3.78	3.73	3.67
3.96	3.87	3.77	3.67	3.61	3.56	3.51	3.45	3.39	3.33
3.72	3.62	3.52	3.42	3.37	3.31	3.26	3.20	3.14	3.08
3.53	3.43	3.33	3.23	3.17	3.12	3.06	3.00	2.94	2.88
3.37	3.28	3.18	3.07	3.02	2.96	2.91	2.85	2.79	2.72
3.25	3.15	3.05	2.95	2.89	2.84	2.78	2.72	2.66	2.60
3.15	3.05	2.95	2.84	2.79	2.73	2.67	2.61	2.55	2.49
3.06	2.96	2.86	2.76	2.70	2.64	2.59	2.52	2.46	2.40
2.99	2.89	2.79	2.68	2.63	2.57	2.51	2.45	2.38	2.32
2.92	2.82	2.72	2.62	2.56	2.50	2.44	2.38	2.32	2.25
2.87	2.77	2.67	2.56	2.50	2.44	2.38	2.32	2.26	2.19
2.82	2.72	2.62	2.51	2.45	2.39	2.33	2.27	2.20	2.13
2.77	2.68	2.57	2.46	2.41	2.35	2.29	2.22	2.16	2.09
2.73	2.64	2.53	2.42	2.37	2.31	2.25	2.18	2.11	2.04
2.70	2.60	2.50	2.39	2.33	2.27	2.21	2.14	2.08	2.00
2.67	2.57	2.47	2.36	2.30	2.24	2.18	2.11	2.04	1.97
2.64	2.54	2.44	2.33	2.27	2.21	2.15	2.08	2.01	1.94
2.61	2.51	2.41	2.30	2.24	2.18	2.12	2.05	1.98	1.91
2.59	2.49	2.39	2.28	2.22	2.16	2.09	2.03	1.95	1.88
2.57	2.47	2.36	2.25	2.19	2.13	2.07	2.00	1.93	1.85
2.55	2.45	2.34	2.23	2.17	2.11	2.05	1.98	1.91	1.83
2.53	2.43	2.32	2.21	2.15	2.09	2.03	1.96	1.89	1.81
2.51	2.41	2.31	2.20	2.14	2.07	2.01	1.94	1.87	1.79
2.39	2.29	2.18	2.07	2.01	1.94	1.88	1.80	1.72	1.64
2.27	2.17	2.06	1.94	1.88	1.82	1.74	1.67	1.58	1.48
2.16	2.05	1.94	1.82	1.76	1.69	1.61	1.53	1.43	1.31
2.05	1.94	1.83	1.71	1.64	1.57	1.48	1.39	1.27	1.00

(continues)

TABLE A-1-4 (continued) The *F* Distribution: Values of $F_{.01}$

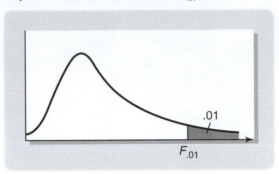

Degrees of Freedom of the Numerator

df_1/df_2	1	2	3	4	5	6	7	8	9
1	4052	4999.5	5403	5625	5764	5859	5928	5981	6022
2	98.50	99.00	99.17	99.25	99.30	99.33	99.36	99.37	99.39
3	34.12	30.82	29.46	28.71	28.24	27.91	27.67	27.49	27.35
4	21.20	18.00	16.69	15.98	15.52	15.21	14.98	14.80	14.66
5	16.26	13.27	12.06	11.39	10.97	10.67	10.46	10.29	10.16
6	13.75	10.92	9.78	9.15	8.75	8.47	8.26	8.10	7.98
7	12.25	9.55	8.45	7.85	7.46	7.19	6.99	6.84	6.72
8	11.26	8.65	7.59	7.01	6.63	6.37	6.18	6.03	5.91
9	10.56	8.02	6.99	6.42	6.06	5.80	5.61	5.47	5.35
10	10.04	7.56	6.55	5.99	5.64	5.39	5.20	5.06	4.94
11	9.65	7.21	6.22	5.67	5.32	5.07	4.89	4.74	4.63
12	9.33	6.93	5.95	5.41	5.06	4.82	4.64	4.50	4.39
13	9.07	6.70	5.74	5.21	4.86	4.62	4.44	4.30	4.19
14	8.86	6.51	5.56	5.04	4.69	4.46	4.28	4.14	4.03
15	8.58	6.36	5.42	4.89	4.56	4.32	4.14	4.00	3.89
16	8.53	6.23	5.29	4.77	4.44	4.20	4.03	3.89	3.78
17	8.40	6.11	5.18	4.67	4.34	4.10	3.93	3.79	3.68
18	8.29	6.01	5.09	4.58	4.25	4.01	3.84	3.71	3.60
19	8.18	5.93	5.01	4.50	4.17	3.94	3.77	3.63	3.52
20	8.10	5.85	4.94	4.43	4.10	3.87	3.70	3.56	3.46
21	8.02	5.78	4.87	4.37	4.04	3.81	3.64	3.51	3.40
22	7.95	5.72	4.82	4.31	3.99	3.76	3.59	3.45	3.35
23	7.88	5.66	4.76	4.26	3.94	3.71	3.54	3.41	3.30
24	7.82	5.61	4.72	4.22	3.90	3.67	3.50	3.36	3.26
25	7.77	5.57	4.68	4.18	3.85	3.63	3.46	3.32	3.22
26	7.72	5.53	4.64	4.14	3.82	3.59	3.42	3.29	3.18
27	7.68	5.49	4.60	4.11	3.78	3.56	3.39	3.26	3.15
28	7.64	5.45	4.57	4.07	3.75	3.53	3.36	3.23	3.12
29	7.60	5.42	4.54	4.04	3.73	3.50	3.33	3.20	3.09
30	7.56	5.39	4.51	4.02	3.70	3.47	3.30	3.17	3.07
40	7.31	5.18	4.31	3.83	3.51	3.29	3.12	2.99	2.89
60	7.08	4.98	4.13	3.65	3.34	3.12	2.95	2.82	2.72
120	6.85	4.79	3.95	3.48	3.17	2.96	2.79	2.66	2.56
∞	6.63	4.61	3.78	3.32	3.02	2.80	2.64	2.51	2.41

Degrees of Freedom of the Denominator

Degrees of Freedom of the Numerator

10	12	15	20	24	30	40	60	120	∞
6056	6106	6157	6209	6235	6261	6287	6313	6339	6366
99.40	99.42	99.43	99.45	99.46	99.47	99.47	99.48	99.49	99.50
27.23	27.05	26.87	26.69	26.60	26.50	26.41	26.32	26.22	26.13
14.55	14.37	14.20	14.02	13.93	13.84	13.75	13.65	13.56	13.46
10.05	9.89	9.72	9.55	9.47	9.38	9.29	9.20	9.11	9.02
7.87	7.72	7.56	7.40	7.31	7.23	7.14	7.06	6.97	6.88
6.62	6.47	6.31	6.16	6.07	5.99	5.91	5.82	5.74	5.65
5.81	5.67	5.52	5.36	5.28	5.20	5.12	5.03	4.95	4.86
5.26	5.11	4.96	4.81	4.73	4.65	4.57	4.48	4.40	4.31
4.85	4.71	4.56	4.41	4.33	4.25	4.17	4.08	4.00	3.91
4.54	4.40	4.25	4.10	4.02	3.94	3.86	3.78	3.69	3.60
4.30	4.16	4.01	3.86	3.78	3.70	3.62	3.54	3.45	3.36
4.10	3.96	3.82	3.66	3.59	3.51	3.43	3.34	3.25	3.17
3.94	3.80	3.66	3.51	3.43	3.35	3.27	3.18	3.09	3.00
3.80	3.67	3.52	3.37	3.29	3.21	3.13	3.05	2.96	2.87
3.69	3.55	3.41	3.26	3.18	3.10	3.02	2.93	2.84	2.75
3.59	3.46	3.31	3.16	3.08	3.00	2.92	2.83	2.75	2.65
3.51	3.37	3.23	3.08	3.00	2.92	2.84	2.75	2.66	2.57
3.43	3.30	3.15	3.00	2.92	2.84	2.76	2.67	2.58	2.49
3.37	3.23	3.09	2.94	2.86	2.78	2.69	2.61	2.52	2.42
3.31	3.17	3.03	2.88	2.80	2.72	2.64	2.55	2.46	2.36
3.26	3.12	2.98	2.83	2.75	2.67	2.58	2.50	2.40	2.31
3.21	3.07	2.93	2.78	2.70	2.62	2.54	2.45	2.35	2.26
3.17	3.03	2.89	2.74	2.66	2.58	2.49	2.40	2.31	2.21
3.13	2.99	2.85	2.70	2.62	2.54	2.45	2.36	2.27	2.17
3.09	2.96	2.81	2.66	2.58	2.50	2.42	2.33	2.23	2.13
3.06	2.93	2.78	2.63	2.55	2.47	2.38	2.29	2.20	2.10
3.03	2.90	2.75	2.60	2.52	2.44	2.35	2.26	2.17	2.06
3.00	2.87	2.73	2.57	2.49	2.41	2.33	2.23	2.14	2.03
2.98	2.84	2.70	2.55	2.47	2.39	2.30	2.21	2.11	2.01
2.80	2.66	2.52	2.37	2.29	2.20	2.11	2.02	1.92	1.80
2.63	2.50	2.35	2.20	2.12	2.03	1.94	1.84	1.73	1.60
2.47	2.34	2.19	2.03	1.95	1.86	1.76	1.66	1.53	1.38
2.32	2.18	2.04	1.88	1.79	1.70	1.59	1.47	1.32	1.00

TABLE A-1-5 Critical Values for the Wilcoxon Signed-Rank Test for $n = 5$ to 50

One-Sided	Two-Sided	$n=5$	$n=6$	$n=7$	$n=8$	$n=9$	$n=10$	$n=11$	$n=12$	$n=13$	$n=14$	$n=15$	$n=16$
$\alpha = .05$	$\alpha = .10$	1	2	4	6	8	11	14	17	21	26	30	36
$\alpha = .025$	$\alpha = .05$		1	2	4	6	8	11	14	17	21	25	30
$\alpha = .01$	$\alpha = .02$			0	2	3	5	7	10	13	16	20	24
$\alpha = .005$	$\alpha = .01$				0	2	3	5	7	10	13	16	19

One-Sided	Two-Sided	$n=17$	$n=18$	$n=19$	$n=20$	$n=21$	$n=22$	$n=23$	$n=24$	$n=25$	$n=26$	$n=27$	$n=28$
$\alpha = .05$	$\alpha = .10$	41	47	54	60	68	75	83	92	101	110	120	130
$\alpha = .025$	$\alpha = .05$	35	40	46	52	59	66	73	81	90	98	107	117
$\alpha = .01$	$\alpha = .02$	28	33	38	43	49	56	62	69	77	85	93	102
$\alpha = .005$	$\alpha = .01$	23	28	32	37	43	49	55	61	68	76	84	92

One-Sided	Two-Sided	$n=29$	$n=30$	$n=31$	$n=32$	$n=33$	$n=34$	$n=35$	$n=36$	$n=37$	$n=38$	$n=39$
$\alpha = .05$	$\alpha = .10$	141	152	163	175	188	201	214	228	242	256	271
$\alpha = .025$	$\alpha = .05$	127	137	148	159	171	183	195	208	222	235	250
$\alpha = .01$	$\alpha = .02$	111	120	130	141	151	162	174	186	198	211	224
$\alpha = .005$	$\alpha = .01$	100	109	118	128	138	149	160	171	183	195	208

One-Sided	Two-Sided	$n=40$	$n=41$	$n=42$	$n=43$	$n=44$	$n=45$	$n=46$	$n=47$	$n=48$	$n=49$	$n=50$
$\alpha = .05$	$\alpha = .10$	287	303	319	336	353	371	389	408	427	446	466
$\alpha = .025$	$\alpha = .05$	264	279	295	311	327	344	361	379	397	415	434
$\alpha = .01$	$\alpha = .02$	238	252	267	281	297	313	329	345	362	380	398
$\alpha = .005$	$\alpha = .01$	221	234	248	262	277	292	307	323	339	356	373

From Wilcoxon, F., and R. A. Wilcox, *Some Rapid Approximate Statistical Procedures*, (1964), p. 28. Pearl River, NY: Lederle Laboratories of the American Cyanamid Company. Courtesy of American Cyanamid Company, Philadelphia, Pennsylvania.

TABLE A-1-6   Critical Values for a Mann-Whitney Test[a]

Critical values for a one-tailed test at $\alpha = .01$ (lightface type) and $\alpha = .005$ (boldface type) and for two-tailed test at $\alpha = .02$ (lightface type) and $\alpha = .01$ (boldface type)

n_1/n_2	1	2	3	4	5	6	7	8	9	10	11	12	13	14	15	16	17	18	19	20
1	—b	—	—	—	—	—	—	—	—	—	—	—	—	—	—	—	—	—	—	—
2	—	—	—	—	—	—	—	—	—	—	—	—	0	0	0	0	0	0	1	1
													—	—	—	—	—	—	**0**	**0**
3	—	—	—	—	—	—	0	0	1	1	1	2	2	2	3	3	4	4	4	5
							—	—	**0**	**0**	**0**	**1**	**1**	**1**	**2**	**2**	**2**	**2**	**3**	**3**
4	—	—	—	—	0	1	1	2	3	3	4	5	5	6	7	7	8	9	9	10
					—	**0**	**0**	**1**	**1**	**2**	**2**	**3**	**3**	**4**	**5**	**5**	**6**	**6**	**7**	**8**
5	—	—	—	0	1	2	3	4	5	6	7	8	9	10	11	12	13	14	15	16
				—	**0**	**1**	**1**	**2**	**3**	**4**	**5**	**6**	**7**	**7**	**8**	**9**	**10**	**11**	**12**	**13**
6	—	—	—	1	2	3	4	6	7	8	9	11	12	13	15	16	18	19	20	22
				0	**1**	**2**	**3**	**4**	**5**	**6**	**7**	**9**	**10**	**11**	**12**	**13**	**15**	**16**	**17**	**18**
7	—	—	0	1	3	4	6	7	9	11	12	14	16	17	19	21	23	24	26	28
		—	**1**	**3**	**4**	**6**	**7**	**9**	**10**	**12**	**13**	**15**	**16**	**18**	**19**	**21**	**22**	**24**
8	—	—	0	2	4	6	7	9	11	13	15	17	20	22	24	26	28	30	32	34
		—	**1**	**2**	**4**	**6**	**7**	**9**	**11**	**13**	**15**	**17**	**18**	**20**	**22**	**24**	**26**	**28**	**30**
9	—	—	1	3	5	7	9	11	14	16	18	21	23	26	28	31	33	36	38	40
		0	**1**	**3**	**5**	**7**	**9**	**11**	**13**	**16**	**18**	**20**	**22**	**24**	**27**	**29**	**31**	**33**	**36**
10	—	—	1	3	6	8	11	13	16	19	22	24	27	30	33	36	38	41	44	47
		0	**2**	**4**	**6**	**9**	**11**	**13**	**16**	**18**	**21**	**24**	**26**	**29**	**31**	**34**	**37**	**39**	**42**
11	—	—	1	4	7	9	12	15	18	22	25	28	31	34	37	41	44	47	50	53
		0	**2**	**5**	**7**	**10**	**13**	**16**	**18**	**21**	**24**	**27**	**30**	**33**	**36**	**39**	**42**	**45**	**48**
12	—	—	2	5	8	11	14	17	21	24	28	31	35	38	42	46	49	53	56	60
		1	**3**	**6**	**9**	**12**	**15**	**18**	**21**	**24**	**27**	**31**	**34**	**37**	**41**	**44**	**47**	**51**	**54**
13	—	0	2	5	9	12	16	20	23	27	31	35	39	43	47	51	55	59	63	67
	—	**1**	**3**	**7**	**10**	**13**	**17**	**20**	**24**	**27**	**31**	**34**	**38**	**42**	**45**	**49**	**53**	**56**	**60**
14	—	0	2	6	10	13	17	22	26	30	34	38	43	47	51	56	60	65	69	73
	—	**1**	**4**	**7**	**11**	**15**	**18**	**22**	**26**	**30**	**34**	**38**	**42**	**46**	**50**	**54**	**58**	**63**	**67**
15	—	0	3	7	11	15	19	24	28	33	37	42	47	51	56	61	66	70	75	80
	—	**2**	**5**	**8**	**12**	**16**	**20**	**24**	**29**	**33**	**37**	**42**	**46**	**51**	**55**	**60**	**64**	**69**	**73**
16	—	0	3	7	12	16	21	26	31	36	41	46	51	56	61	66	71	76	82	87
	—	**2**	**5**	**9**	**13**	**18**	**22**	**27**	**31**	**36**	**41**	**45**	**50**	**55**	**60**	**65**	**70**	**74**	**79**
17	—	0	4	8	13	18	23	28	33	38	44	49	55	60	66	71	77	82	88	93
	—	**2**	**6**	**10**	**15**	**19**	**24**	**29**	**34**	**39**	**44**	**49**	**54**	**60**	**65**	**70**	**75**	**81**	**86**
18	—	0	4	9	14	19	24	30	36	41	47	53	59	65	70	76	82	88	94	100
	—	**2**	**6**	**11**	**16**	**21**	**26**	**31**	**37**	**42**	**47**	**53**	**58**	**64**	**70**	**75**	**81**	**87**	**92**
19	—	1	4	9	15	20	26	32	38	44	50	56	63	69	75	82	88	94	101	107
	0	**3**	**7**	**12**	**17**	**22**	**28**	**33**	**39**	**45**	**51**	**56**	**63**	**69**	**74**	**81**	**87**	**93**	**99**
20	—	1	5	10	16	22	28	34	40	47	53	60	67	73	80	87	93	100	107	114
	0	**3**	**8**	**13**	**18**	**24**	**30**	**36**	**42**	**48**	**54**	**60**	**67**	**73**	**79**	**86**	**92**	**99**	**105**

[a] To be significant for any given n_1 and n_2 observed U must be *equal to* or *less than* the value shown in the table.

[b] Dashes in the body of the table indicate that no decision is possible at the stated level of significance.

(continues)

TABLE A-1-6   (continued)

Critical values for a one-tailed test at α = .05 (lightface type) and α = .025 (boldface type) and for two-tailed test at α = .10 (lightface type) and α = .05 (boldface type).

n_1/n_2	1	2	3	4	5	6	7	8	9	10	11	12	13	14	15	16	17	18	19	20
1	—	—	—	—	—	—	—	—	—	—	—	—	—	—	—	—	—	—	0	0
																			—	—
2	—	—	—	—	0	0	0	1	1	1	1	2	2	2	3	3	3	4	4	4
	—	—	—	—	—	—	—	**0**	**0**	**0**	**0**	**1**	**1**	**1**	**1**	**1**	**2**	**2**	**2**	**2**
3	—	—	0	0	1	2	2	3	3	4	5	5	6	7	7	8	9	9	10	11
	—	—	—	—	**0**	**1**	**1**	**2**	**2**	**3**	**3**	**4**	**4**	**5**	**5**	**6**	**6**	**7**	**7**	**8**
4	—	—	0	1	2	3	4	5	6	7	8	9	10	11	12	14	15	16	17	18
	—	—	—	**0**	**1**	**2**	**3**	**4**	**4**	**5**	**6**	**7**	**8**	**9**	**10**	**11**	**11**	**12**	**13**	**13**
5	—	0	1	2	4	5	6	8	9	11	12	13	15	16	18	19	20	22	23	25
	—	—	**0**	**1**	**2**	**3**	**5**	**6**	**7**	**8**	**9**	**11**	**12**	**13**	**14**	**15**	**17**	**18**	**19**	**20**
6	—	0	2	3	5	7	8	10	12	14	16	17	19	21	23	25	26	28	30	32
	—	—	**1**	**2**	**3**	**5**	**6**	**8**	**10**	**11**	**13**	**14**	**16**	**17**	**19**	**21**	**22**	**24**	**25**	**27**
7	—	0	2	4	6	8	11	13	15	17	19	21	24	26	28	30	33	35	37	39
	—	—	**1**	**3**	**5**	**6**	**8**	**10**	**12**	**14**	**16**	**18**	**20**	**22**	**24**	**26**	**28**	**30**	**32**	**34**
8	—	1	3	5	8	10	13	15	18	20	23	26	28	31	33	36	39	41	44	47
	—	**0**	**2**	**4**	**6**	**8**	**10**	**13**	**15**	**17**	**19**	**22**	**24**	**26**	**29**	**31**	**34**	**36**	**38**	**41**
9	—	1	3	6	9	12	15	18	21	24	27	30	33	36	39	42	45	48	51	54
	—	**0**	**2**	**4**	**7**	**10**	**12**	**15**	**17**	**20**	**23**	**26**	**28**	**31**	**34**	**37**	**39**	**42**	**45**	**48**
10	—	1	4	7	11	14	17	20	24	27	31	34	37	41	44	48	51	55	58	62
	—	**0**	**3**	**5**	**8**	**11**	**14**	**17**	**20**	**23**	**26**	**29**	**33**	**36**	**39**	**42**	**45**	**48**	**52**	**55**
11	—	1	5	8	12	16	19	23	27	31	34	38	42	46	50	54	57	61	65	69
	—	**0**	**3**	**6**	**9**	**13**	**16**	**19**	**23**	**26**	**30**	**33**	**37**	**40**	**44**	**47**	**51**	**55**	**58**	**62**
12	—	2	5	9	13	17	21	26	30	34	38	42	47	51	55	60	64	68	72	77
	—	**1**	**4**	**7**	**11**	**14**	**18**	**22**	**26**	**29**	**33**	**37**	**41**	**45**	**49**	**53**	**57**	**61**	**65**	**69**
13	—	2	6	10	15	19	24	28	33	37	42	47	51	56	61	65	70	75	80	84
	—	**1**	**4**	**8**	**12**	**16**	**20**	**24**	**28**	**33**	**37**	**41**	**45**	**50**	**54**	**59**	**63**	**67**	**72**	**76**
14	—	2	7	11	16	21	26	31	36	41	46	51	56	61	66	71	77	82	87	92
	—	**1**	**5**	**9**	**13**	**17**	**22**	**26**	**31**	**36**	**40**	**45**	**50**	**55**	**59**	**64**	**67**	**74**	**78**	**83**
15	—	3	7	12	18	23	28	33	39	44	50	55	61	66	72	77	83	88	94	100
	—	**1**	**5**	**10**	**14**	**19**	**24**	**29**	**34**	**39**	**44**	**49**	**54**	**59**	**64**	**70**	**75**	**80**	**85**	**90**
16	—	3	8	14	19	25	30	36	42	48	54	60	65	71	77	83	89	95	101	107
	—	**1**	**6**	**11**	**15**	**21**	**26**	**31**	**37**	**42**	**47**	**53**	**59**	**64**	**70**	**75**	**81**	**86**	**92**	**98**
17	—	3	9	15	20	26	33	39	45	51	57	64	70	77	83	89	96	102	109	115
	—	**2**	**6**	**11**	**17**	**22**	**28**	**34**	**39**	**45**	**51**	**57**	**63**	**67**	**75**	**81**	**87**	**93**	**99**	**105**
18	—	4	9	16	22	28	35	41	48	55	61	68	75	82	88	95	102	109	116	123
	—	**2**	**7**	**12**	**18**	**24**	**30**	**36**	**42**	**48**	**55**	**61**	**67**	**74**	**80**	**86**	**93**	**99**	**106**	**112**
19	0	4	10	17	23	30	37	44	51	58	65	72	80	87	94	101	109	116	123	130
	—	**2**	**7**	**13**	**19**	**25**	**32**	**38**	**45**	**52**	**58**	**65**	**72**	**78**	**85**	**92**	**99**	**106**	**113**	**119**
20	0	4	11	18	25	32	39	47	54	62	69	77	84	92	100	107	115	123	130	138
	—	**2**	**8**	**13**	**20**	**27**	**34**	**41**	**48**	**55**	**62**	**69**	**76**	**83**	**90**	**98**	**105**	**112**	**119**	**127**

From Kirk, R., *Introductory Statistics*, pp. 423-424. Copyright © 1978 by Wadsworth, Inc. Reprinted by permission of Brooks/Cole Publishing Company, Monterey, California 93940.

Some Statistical Applications and Questions (Q) (Adapted from Published Literature)

In this appendix, we use selected data values from the published articles of well-respected journals such as the *Journal of Speech and Hearing Disorders*, the *Journal of Speech and Hearing Research*, and the *American Journal of Epidemiology* to illustrate **step-by-step calculation procedures** of several statistical methods. By doing so, we hope that readers will become familiar with some statistical techniques commonly used in the field of communication disorders. The exercises are intended to demonstrate the application and relevance of statistics to "real" problems encountered in the clinic or laboratory. A step-by-step approach to calculation is taken in order to clarify the meaning of concepts, identify the information needed to solve a set of problems, and minimize a heavy mathematical infrastructure. In some cases, n has been reduced or actual data values from various studies have been rounded to the nearest integer value to facilitate calculation.

CORRELATION COEFFICIENT, LINEAR REGRESSION, AND *t* TEST

(1) "Conversations With Children Who Are Language Impaired: Asking Questions," by J. R. Johnson, et al., October 1993, *Journal of Speech and Hearing Research, 36,* 973–978.

Samples of conversational language were elicited with a standardized interview protocol from 24 children, half with specific language impairment (SLI), half with normally developing language (LN). 12 LN children were compared to the other 12 SLI children by mean length of utterance (MLU), the CYCLE (Curtiss Yamada Comprehensive Language Evaluation, Curtiss and Yamada, 1988) score, and total number of child utterances (TCU). The results are shown in the table below.

Description of Individual Subjects

Group	ID	MLU	CYCLE	TCU
SLI	1	1.9	0	232
	2	3.2	64	220
	3	3.3	37	246
	4	3.5	54	234
	5	3.9	12	131
	6	4.0	30	185
	7	4.6	27	157
	8	4.9	62	236
	9	4.9	56	193
	10	5.0	65	148
	11	5.2	70	188
	12	5.6	36	222
LN	1	2.9	12	106
	2	3.2	30	185
	3	3.3	63	189
	4	3.6	54	178
	5	3.6	18	134
	6	4.2	38	162
	7	4.5	51	197
	8	4.6	59	186
	9	4.7	49	269
	10	4.8	66	165
	11	5.1	49	162
	12	5.9	64	202

Correlation Coefficient r
(a) Find the correlation coefficient between MLU and CYCLE for both groups. Interpret the result.

Linear Regression
(b) Would it be suitable to use a linear regression model to predict TCU from MLU for SLU group? If so, find an equation of a regression line. If not, explain why.

t test
(c) Do MLU and CYCLE differ significantly between the two groups?

Solutions

(a) You may use the raw score method to calculate the correlation coefficient *r* directly from raw scores.

Step (1). Look up the raw score formula and determine what information you need to have to use it.

Formula
Let X be MLU scores and Y be CYCLE scores.

$$r_{XY} = \frac{N(\sum XY) - (\sum X)(\sum Y)}{\sqrt{[N\sum X^2 - (\sum X)^2][N\sum Y^2 - (\sum Y)^2]}}$$

Step (2). Set up a table with headings for all information you need for the formula and enter the score on X and Y.

ID	X	X²	Y	Y²	XY
1	2.9	8.41	12	144	34.8
2	3.2	10.24	30	900	96
3	3.3	10.89	63	3969	207.9
4	3.6	12.96	54	2916	194.4
5	3.6	12.96	18	324	64.8
6	4.2	17.64	38	1444	159.6
7	4.5	20.25	51	2601	229.5
8	4.6	21.16	59	3481	271.4
9	4.7	22.09	49	2401	230.3
10	4.8	23.04	66	4356	316.8
11	5.1	26.01	49	2401	249.9
12	5.9	34.81	64	4096	377.6
	+)	+)	+)	+)	+)
	$\sum X = 50.4$	$\sum X^2 = 220.46$	$\sum Y = 553$	$\sum Y^2 = 29033$	$\sum XY = 2433$

Step (3). At the bottom of the table make a row to enter in the sum of each column. You will get $\sum X = 50.4$

$$\Sigma X^2 = 220.46$$

$$\Sigma Y = 553$$

$$\Sigma Y^2 = 29033$$

$$\Sigma XY = 2433$$

Step (4).   Calculate the correlation coefficient by substituting information in the formula and solving for r_{XY}.

$$r_{XY} = \frac{12(2433) - (50.4)(553)}{\sqrt{[12(220.46) - (50.4)^2][12(29033) - (553)^2]}}$$

$$= \frac{1324.8}{\sqrt{(105.36)(42587)}}$$

$$= \frac{1324.8}{2118.25}$$

$$= .625$$

Among LN students, there exists a reasonably strong positive correlation between MLU scores and CYCLE scores.

Using the same steps, we could derive the following information for the SLI group (verify them).

$$\Sigma X = 50 \qquad \Sigma Y = 513 \qquad \Sigma XY = 2275.7$$
$$\Sigma X^2 = 220.78 \qquad \Sigma Y^2 = 27555 \qquad r_{XY} = .5223$$

Again, there is a reasonably strong positive relationship between MLU scores and CYCLE scores.

(b) First, we draw a scatter diagram to determine if there exists a linear relationship between MLU(X) and TCU(Y).

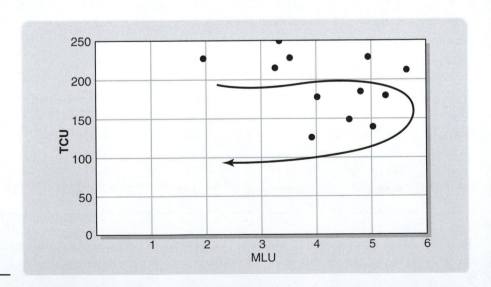

FIGURE 1.

A scatter diagram describing TCU and MLU scores

The presence of an outlier may possibly change the nature of the relationship between two variables, especially if the sample size is very small. The researcher must decide whether or not to delete the case from consideration. If the case is not deleted, then we can use the following three methods to find the shape $b_{Y \cdot X}$ and the y-intercept a.

Formula

(1) Given $Cov(X,Y)$ = covariance of X and Y
$\qquad S_x^2$ = variance of X

Use the formula

$$b_{Y \cdot X} = \frac{Cov(X,Y)}{S_X^2}$$

(2) Given r_{XY} = correlation between X and Y
$\qquad S_X$ = standard deviation of X
$\qquad S_Y$ = standard deviation of Y

Use the formula

$$b_{Y \cdot X} = \frac{(r_{XY}) \cdot (S_Y)}{S_X}$$

(3) Given n = number of subjects
$\qquad X$ = raw score on X
$\qquad Y$ = raw score on Y

Use the formula

$$b_{Y \cdot X} = \frac{n(\sum X \cdot Y) - (\sum X)(\sum Y)}{n(\sum X^2) - (\sum X)^2}$$

Let us use formula (3) to find the slope $b_{Y \cdot X}$. Since we predict TCU score (Y) from MLU score (X), we make a table with headings for all information you need for the formula. For SLI, we have:

ID	X	X²	Y	XY
1	1.9	3.61	232	440.8
2	3.2	10.24	220	704.0
3	3.3	10.89	246	811.8
4	3.5	12.25	234	819
5	3.9	15.21	131	510.9
6	4.0	16.00	185	740
7	4.6	21.16	157	722.2
8	4.9	24.01	236	1156.4
9	4.9	24.01	193	945.7
10	5.0	25.00	148	740
11	5.2	27.04	188	977.6
12	5.6	31.36	222	1243.2
	+)	+)	+)	+)
	$\sum X = 50$	$\sum X^2 = 220.78$	$\sum Y = 2392$	$\sum XY = 9811.6$

Calculate the slope by substituting all numerical values into the formula and solving for b_{YX}.

$$b_{YX} = \frac{12 \cdot (9811.6) - (50)(2392)}{12 \cdot (220.78) - (50)^2}$$

$$= \frac{-1860.8}{149.36}$$

$$= -12.458$$

The y-intercept a can be given by:

$$a = \bar{Y} - b_{y \cdot x} \cdot \bar{X}$$

$$= \left(\frac{2392}{12}\right) - (-12.458) \cdot \left(\frac{50}{12}\right)$$

$$= 199.333 - (-51.908)$$

$$= 251.241$$

The regression line (with outlier?) is given by:

$$\hat{Y} = -12.458x + 251.241$$

Using the formula for correlation coefficient gives $r_{XY} = -.345$ (verify).
If we delete the outlierpoint (3.9,131), then we would have (verify)

$$b_{YX} = -14.144, \ a = 264.821, \ r_{xy} = -.472$$

It is important to note that the outlier should be carefully studied and it should be decided whether or not to exclude it from consideration by the researcher on the basis of the nature of the study.

(c) First, we would compare MLU scores between the two groups. An independent t test would be applied to detect a difference. As a prerequisite of an independent t test, we must apply an F test to determine the homogeneity of two variances. For the SLI group, the mean MLU score is calculated as

$$\bar{X}_{SLI} = \frac{\sum X}{n} = \frac{50}{12} = 4.17$$

Also, the variance of the MLU score is given by:

$$S^2_{SLI} = \frac{n \cdot (\sum X^2) - (\sum X)^2}{n \cdot (n-1)} = \frac{12 \cdot (220.78) - (50)^2}{12 \cdot 11} = \frac{149.36}{132} = 1.13$$

For the LN group, the mean MLU score is:

$$\bar{X}_{LN} = \frac{\sum X}{n} = \frac{50.4}{12} = 4.2$$

the variance of the MLU scores is derived through the formula as follows:

$$S^2_{LN} = \frac{n \cdot (\sum X^2) - (\sum X)^2}{n \cdot (n-1)} = \frac{12 \cdot (220.46) - (50.4)^2}{12 \cdot 11} = \frac{105.36}{132} = .80$$

In summary, we may write:

SLI $\bar{X} = 4.17,$ $S^2 = 1.13,$ $n = 12.$
LN $\bar{X} = 4.2,$ $S^2 = .80,$ $n = 12.$

Step (1).   Apply an *F*-test to determine the homogeneity of two variances.

$$F = \frac{1.13}{.80} = 1.41 \text{ with d.f.} = (11, 11)$$

$F(.05) = 2.82 > 1.41$, therefore the *p*-value is greater than .05. Hence the two distributions of the groups SLI and LN are homogeneous.

Step (2).   Calculate an observed *t* value and conclude from it.

$$H_0: \mu_{SLI} = \mu_{LN} \text{ or } \mu_{SLI} - \mu_{LN} = 0$$
$$H_a: \mu_{SLI} \neq \mu_{LN} \text{ or } \mu_{SLI} - \mu_{LN} \neq 0$$

Formula for a homogeneous t-value

$$t = \frac{(\bar{X}_1 - \bar{X}_2) - (\mu_1 - \mu_2)}{\sqrt{\frac{1}{n_1} + \frac{1}{n_2}} \cdot \sqrt{\frac{(n_1 - 1) \cdot S_1^2 + (n_2 - 1) \cdot S_2^2}{n_1 + n_2 - 2}}}$$

with *d.f.* = $n_1 + n_2 - 2$
where $(\mu_1 - \mu_2)$ represents a testing population mean difference, i.e., the value on the right side of H_0 and H_a is the value.

$$t = \frac{(4.17 - 4.2) - 0}{\sqrt{\frac{1}{12} + \frac{1}{12}} \cdot \sqrt{\frac{(12 - 1) \cdot 1.13 + (12 - 1) \cdot 80}{12 + 12 - 2}}}$$
$$= \frac{-.03}{(.408) \cdot (.982)}$$
$$= -.0749$$

$t = -0.749$ with *d.f.* = 22 (compared to $t(.025) = 2.074$) has *p*-value exceeding .05, therefore, MLU did not differ significantly between the two groups.
For CYCLE scores, readers should verify the following results:

SLI	$\bar{X} = 42.75$,	$S^2 = 511.29$,	$n = 12$
LN	$\bar{X} = 46.08$,	$S^2 = 322.63$,	$n = 12$

Your $F(.05) = \dfrac{511.21}{322.63} = 1.58$ was less than the table *F*, therefore, we fail to reject $H_0: \sigma^2_{SLI} = \sigma^2_{LN}$.

Hence, the two groups are homogeneous. Next, we apply a homogeneous *t*-test to determine the following hypotheses:

$$H_0: \mu_{SLI} = \mu_{LN} \text{ or } \mu_{SLI} - \mu_{LN} = 0$$
$$H_a: \mu_{SLI} \neq \mu_{LN} \text{ or } \mu_{SLI} - \mu_{LN} \neq 0$$

$$\text{Your } t = \frac{(42.75 - 46.08) - 0}{\sqrt{\frac{1}{12} + \frac{1}{12}} \cdot \sqrt{\frac{(12 - 1) \cdot 511.29 + (12 - 1) \cdot 322.63}{12 + 12 - 2}}}$$
$$= \frac{-3.33}{(.408) \cdot (20.90)}$$
$$= -.39 \text{ with } d.f. = 22$$

observed $t = -.39$ has p-value exceeding .05; therefore, the CYCLE did not differ significantly between the two groups.

PROBABILITY AND CHI-SQUARE TEST OF INDEPENDENCE

(2) "Otitis Media and Language Development at One Year of Age," by I. F. Wallace, et al., August 1988, *Journal of Speech and Hearing Disorders, 53,* 245–251.

Part I

The effect of otitis media on emerging language was examined in a group of one year olds. Based on pneumatic otoscopy, two groups were selected from the larger cohort of 65 babies. Using otoscopy records, 15 babies (9 high-risk infants and 6 healthy full-term infants) who had normal ratings in both ears at 80% or more of their visits to the LIFE program were designated as otitis free. Another 12 babies (9 high-risk infants and 3 healthy full-term infants) demonstrating bilaterally positive otoscopy results for 30% or more of their first-year visits were designated as otitis positive. Some of the demographic and perinatal data are given in Table 1 below for the 27 studied infants.

TABLE 1 Perinatal and Demographic Characteristics of Studied Children

Characteristic	Otitis Positive ($n = 12$)	Otitis Free ($n = 15$)
Birthweight		
M	1782.1	2292.7
SD	878.0	1049.0
Gestational age		
M	33.8	35.9
SD	4.1	4.6
Maternal age		
M	27.4	23.3
SD	5.3	5.5
Race		
Black	6	10
Hispanic	5	5
White	1	0

Part II

Based on tympanometric data on 63 LIFE patients, the study was conducted for both otoscopic and tympanometric evaluations at each visit between 40 weeks and 6 months of age post term. A 3-point rating scale (i.e., clear, suspicious, positive) was used to categorize the tympanometric findings from each ear. Table 2 summarizes the results of their analysis for ears where tympanometric and otoscopic examinations were completed on the same day.

TABLE 2 Ratings of Middle Ear Status Using Otoscopy and Tympanogram

	Otoscopy		
Tympanogram	Clear	Suspect	Positive
Normal	160	31	7
Suspect	18	13	8
Positive	6	6	8

Probability

(a) Using tympanometric results as indicative of disease status, find sensitivity, specificity, predictive value positive, and predicitive value negative.

Chi-square Test of Independence

(b) Does agreement between the two measures occur? (Is there any independent relationship between them?)

Solutions

(a) Two rates that are often useful in the evaluation of a diagnostic test are the *sensitivity* rate and the *specificity* rate.

Sensitivity = Prob test result is positive given that the person carries a disease

$$= \frac{\text{Number of true positives}}{\text{Number of true positives} + \text{Number of false negatives}}$$

Specificity = Prob test result is negative given that the person does not carry a disease

$$= \frac{\text{Number of true negatives}}{\text{Number of true negatives} + \text{Number of false positives}}$$

Table 2 may be illustrated as:

	Otoscopy (Test Result)		
Tympanogram (Disease status)	Clear (Negatives)	Suspect	Positive (Positives)
Normal (Negatives)	160 (True Negatives)	31	7 (False Positives)
Suspect	18	13	8
Positive (Positives)	6 (False Negatives)	6	8 (True Positives)

$$\text{Sensitivity} = \frac{8}{8+6} = \frac{8}{14} \text{ or } 57.1\%$$

$$\text{Specificity} = \frac{160}{160+7} = \frac{160}{167} \text{ or } 95.8\%$$

Because no diagnostic or screening test is perfect, it is impossible to increase both rates of the sensitivity and specificity of a test simultaneously. Clinicians must make a decision which rate should be maximized depending on the relative costs of obtaining a false positive result and the cost of a false negative result.

Another useful set of rates (in determining the accuracy of a diagnostic test) are called *Predictive Value Positive* and *Predictive Value Negative*. They can be calculated as:

Predictive Value Positive = Prob. (a person carries a disease given that test result is positive)

$$= \frac{\text{Number of true positives}}{\text{Number of true positives} + \text{Number of false positives}}$$

Predictive Value Negative = Prob. (a person does not carry a disease given that test result is negative)

$$= \frac{\text{Number of true negatives}}{\text{Number of true negatives} + \text{Number of false negatives}}$$

In our example,

$$\text{Predictive value positive} = \frac{8}{7+8} = \frac{8}{15} \text{ or } 53.3\%$$

$$\text{Predictive value negative} = \frac{160}{160+6} = \frac{160}{166} \text{ or } 96.4\%$$

(b) First, we must specify the null and alternative hypotheses.

H_0: Tympanogram and otoscopy are independent (no agreement exists between the two measures).

H_a: Tympanogram and otoscopy are dependent. (Some agreement exists between the two measures).

Compute the chi-square statistic following these steps:

Step (1). Set up a chi-square table as follows:

| | | Otoscopy | | |
Tympanogram	Clear	Suspect	Positive	Row Total
Normal	160	31	7	198
Suspect	18	13	8	39
Positive	6	6	8	20
Column Total	184	50	23	257

Step (2). Compute the expected frequency (*E*) for each cell. The formula for *E* is given by

$$\frac{(\text{The frequency of the row which the cell is in}) \cdot (\text{The frequency of the column which the cell is in})}{\text{Grand total}}$$

The calculations for this example are shown below. (Note that N = Normal, S = Suspect, P = Positive, and C = Clear)

$$E_{NC} = \frac{(198) \cdot (184)}{257} = 141.76$$

$$E_{NS} = \frac{(198) \cdot (50)}{257} = 38.52$$

$$E_{NP} = \frac{(198) \cdot (23)}{257} = 17.72$$

$$E_{SC} = \frac{(39) \cdot (184)}{257} = 27.92$$

$$E_{SS} = \frac{(39) \cdot (50)}{257} = 7.59$$

$$E_{SP} = \frac{(39) \cdot (23)}{257} = 3.49$$

$$E_{PC} = \frac{(20) \cdot (184)}{257} = 14.32$$

$$E_{PS} = \frac{(20) \cdot (50)}{257} = 3.89$$

$$E_{PP} = \frac{(20) \cdot (23)}{257} = 1.79$$

Step (3). Construct a contingency table shown below and enter the frequencies into O, E, $(O - E)^2$, and $\dfrac{(O-E)^2}{E}$ where O = the observed frequency.

	O	E	$(O - E)$	$(O - E)^2$	$\dfrac{(O-E)^2}{E}$
NC	160	141.76	18.24	332.70	2.35
NS	31	38.52	−7.52	56.55	1.47
NP	7	17.72	−10.72	114.92	6.49
SC	18	27.92	−9.92	98.41	3.52
SS	13	7.59	5.41	29.27	3.86
SP	8	3.49	4.51	20.34	5.83
PC	6	14.32	−8.32	69.22	4.83
PS	6	3.89	2.11	4.45	1.14
PP	8	1.79	6.21	38.56	21.54

Step (4). Examine the following and decide how to proceed.

(a) If $d.f. = 1$, then Yates' correction for continuity is applied. (The method is explained in Chapter 12 of the text.)

(b) If $d.f. > 1$, then proceed with the computations.
For our example, $d.f. = (\text{row} - 1) \cdot (\text{column} - 1) = (3 - 1) \cdot (3 - 1) = 4$, which is greater than 1, therefore, we will calculate our observed chi-square value, denoted by χ^2_{obs}, through the following formula:

$$\chi^2_{obs} = \sum \frac{(O-E)^2}{E} = \text{a total sum of } \frac{(O-E)^2}{E}$$

$\chi^2_{obs} = 2.35 + 1.47 + 6.49 + 3.52 + 3.86 + 5.83 + 4.83 + 1.14 + 21.54 = 51.03$
with $d.f. = 4$.

Step (5).   Find the critical value of χ^2 denoted by χ^2 crit(α, *d.f.*), and conclude it. Let us set up $\alpha = .05$ with *d.f.* $= 4$, we get χ^2 crit(.05, 4) $= 9.488$

If $\chi^2_{obs} \geq \chi^2$ crit(α, *d.f.*), then we reject H_0
If $\chi^2_{obs} < \chi^2$ crit(α, *d.f.*), then we do not reject H_0

For our example, since $\chi^2_{obs} = 51.03 > \chi^2$ crit(.05, 4) $= 9.488$, we must reject H_0 (accept H_a). Hence, tympanogram and otoscopy measures are dependent (or related to each other) at 5% level of significance.

TIME SERIES ANALYSIS

(3) "From Pronoun Reversals to Correct Pronoun Usage: A Case Study of a Normally Developing Child" by N. B. Schiff-Myers, November 1983, *Journal of Speech and Hearing Disorders*, 48, 394–402.

A total of 1386 intelligible utterances were transcribed from audiotapes. Approximately 27% of these contained first- and second-person pronouns. An additional 480 utterances with pronouns were collected using hand-written notes. There were developmental changes during the three observed periods, namely Time 1 (21 months), Time 2 (23 months), and Time 3 (25 months). Proportions of pronoun confusion and imitated utterances at different ages and linguistic levels are summarized in the Table.

Proportion of Pronoun Confusion and Imitated Utterances in a Normal Child's Speech at Different Ages and Linguistic Levels

	(TUT) Total Number of Utterance Types	% of Imitated Utterances	% of Pronoun Confusion	MLU (Mean Length of Utterance)
Time 1 (21 months)	246	21	59	2.69
Time 2 (23 months)	418	9	26	3.82
Time 3 (25 months)	307	3	3	4.7

(a) Which statistical method would be suitable if you wish to predict TUT scores at a specified time period such as Time 4 (27 months) and Time 5 (29 months)?

(b) Perform the method you chose to predict TUT scores at Time 4 and Time 5.

Solution

(a) We frequently encounter the situation in which data become available in a time-ordered sequence. Analysis of this kind of data set involves two main purposes such as (1) description of the generating mechanism in building up a mathematical model, and (2) using the mathematical model (based on available data) to forecast a future value at a specified time period. The body of statistical methodology available for accomplishing these objectives is referred to as "time series analysis."

The mathematical derivation of a suitable time series model for a particular set of data requires sophisticated knowledge of mathematics, especially calculus, and can be a very frustrating task. It generally consists of three major components as follows:

(1) The selection of a tentative model

(2) Estimation of the model parameters

(3) Testing for adequacy of fit

The most complex stage is the last component because the validity of forecasting procedures heavily depends on the historical (or past) trend; that is, we often predict the future value based on the assumption that the future trends behave like the past. But in the behavioral and clinical sciences, this assumption is rarely warranted for an extended time horizon; therefore, the particular model gears toward the Bayesian distribution which updates new forecast values (posterior distribution) whenever new data becomes available (data distribution). A set of historical data is referred to as a prior distribution.

For our example, *a time series analysis for a single-subject design* is the most suitable model to predict the future TUT scores, since data are continuous and to be updated whenever new data emerge.

First, we must present the formula for time series as model. It is written as:

$$\hat{Y}_{t+1} = \mu + \varnothing(Y_t - \mu)$$

where $\hat{Y}_{t+1}$ (read "Y hat sub $t + 1$") = the future value at time $t + 1$.

Y_t = the actual observed value at time t.

$\mu = \bar{Y}$ = Sample mean (from 1 to t)

$$= \frac{\sum\limits_{i=1}^{t} Y_i}{n}$$

$\varnothing$ (read "phi")" = the autocorrelation coefficient

$$= \frac{\sum\limits_{i=1}^{t-1}(Y_t - \mu)(Y_{t+1} - \mu)}{\sum\limits_{i=1}^{t-1}(Y_t - \mu)^2}$$

The time series model may be considered as a regression model on a continuous basis; therefore, $\varnothing$ may be interpreted as the rate of change from one time to another and Y as the Y-intercept. The table TUT data gives:

$Y_1 = 246,$ $Y_2 = 418,$ $Y_3 = 307.$

$t = 3,$ $\mu = Y = \dfrac{246 + 418 + 307}{3} = 323.67$

Therefore,

$$= \frac{(246 - 323.67) \cdot (418 - 323.67) + (418 - 323.67) \cdot (307 - 323.67)}{(246 - 323.67)^2 + (418 - 323.67)^2}$$

$$= \frac{(-77.67) \cdot (94.33) + (94.33) \cdot (-16.67)}{(-77.67)^2 + (94.33)^2}$$

$$= \frac{-7326.61 + (1572.48)}{14930.78}$$

$$= \frac{-8899.09}{14930.78}$$

$$= -5.96$$

The equation of time series model for this particular set of data is

$$\hat{Y}_{t+1} = 323.67 - .596\,(Y_t - 323.67)$$

(b) Using the equation $\hat{Y}_{t+1} = 323.67 - .596(Y_t - 323.67)$ we could predict TUT score at time 4. It gives:

$$\hat{Y}_4 = 323.67 - .596\,(307 - 323.67)$$
$$= 333.61$$

The predictive TUT score at time 4 (on the basis of three previous times) is 333.61. Time series analysis also allows us to forecast the value of two time periods ahead from present. The procedure is very similar to the one for forecasting the first future value. Symbolically, we write $\hat{Y}_{t+2}$ describing the predictive value at $(t + 2)^{\text{th}}$ time period, then we have

$$\hat{Y}_{t+2} = \mu + \varnothing(\hat{Y}_{t+1} - \mu)$$

Alternatively, it is possible to express $\hat{Y}_{t+2}$ entirely in terms of μ, $\varnothing$, and the available observed values. Substituting the expression for $\hat{Y}_{t+1}$ into the equation above gives

$$\hat{Y}_{t+2} = \mu + \varnothing[\mu + \varnothing(Y_t - \mu) - \mu]$$
$$= \mu + \varnothing^2(Y_t - \mu)$$

So, the predictive value of TUT at time 5 given that $t = 3$ is expressed as

$$\hat{Y}_5 = \mu + \varnothing(\hat{Y}_3 - \mu)$$
$$= 323.67 + (-.596)^2[307 - 323.67]$$
$$= 317.75$$

Therefore, the predictive TUT score at time 5 is 317.75.

THE MANN-WHITNEY U TEST

(4) "F2 Transitions During Sound/Syllable Repetitions of Children Who Stutter and Predictions of Stuttering Chronicity," by J. S. Yaruss and E. G. Contour, October 1993, *Journal of Speech and Hearing Research, 36*, 883–896.

Subjects were 13 children who stutter, divided into two groups based on their predicted risk of continuing to stutter as measured by the SPI (Stuttering Prediction Instrument). The high-risk group consisted of 7 boys with a mean age of 50.57 months with a standard deviation of 10.95 months, and the low-risk group consisted of 5 boys and 1 girl with a mean age of 48.50 months with a standard deviation of 12.18 months. The table summarizes the children's reported ages at the time of onset of stuttering and their ages at the time of the videotaping session as well as their diagnostic evaluation.

Solution
First, we may wish to check if the *t* test's assumptions, such as normality and equal variances, are violated. Since sample sizes of both groups are fairly small, it may be reasonable to assume that the normality assumption was violated. Hence, we would apply the nonparametric version of the independent *t* test called the Mann-Whitney *U* test. The purpose of this test is to determine if two independent groups were drawn from two same populations. The calculation of this statistic is very simple.

The steps for conducting the Mann-Whitney *U* test are presented here. (We would show such steps in (i)).

Subjects' Ages on the Stuttering Severity Instrument and SPI

Subject Group and Number	Reported Age at Onset of Stuttering (Months)	Age at Audio/ Video Taping (Months)	Age at Diagnostic Evaluation (Months)
High-risk			
1	28	34	36
2	24	47	51
3	28	48	46
4	42	48	48
5	42	50	50
6	43	57	59
7	30	70	72
Mean	33.86	50.57	51.71
(SD)	8.13	10.95	11.27
Low-risk			
1	29	36	41
2	30	36	42
3	29	41	44
4	48	57	62
5	41	58	54
6	57	63	65
Mean	39.00	48.50	51.33
(SD)	11.74	12.18	10.54

(a) Determine whether or not there were significant differences between the high-risk and low-risk groups in terms of (i) age at the time of videotaping, (ii) age at the time of diagnostic evaluation, and (iii) reported age at the onset of stuttering.

Step (1).   State two hypotheses:

$H_0: \mu_H = \mu_L$
$H_a: \mu_H \neq \mu_L$

where H = High-risk,   and L = Low-risk.

Step (2).   Compute the U statistic

(i) First, we arrange the data by rank order from lowest to highest (see below), noting the group membership:

Score	24	28	28	29	29	30	30	41	42	42	43	48	51
Group	H	H	H	L	L	H	L	L	H	H	H	L	L
Rank	1	2.5	2.5	4.5	4.5	6.5	6.5	8	9.5	9.5	11	12	13

If two or more scores are tied for the same rank, average the ranks and assign the average rank to two or more scores.

(ii) Next we calculate the sum of the ranks for each group. Designate the larger sum of ranks as T_L.

$$\text{Group H (High-risk)} = 1 + 2.5 + 2.5 + 6.5 + 9.5 + 9.5 + 11 = 42.5$$

(iii) Group L (Low-risk) $= 4.5 + 4.5 + 6.5 + 8 + 12 + 13 = 48.5$

$$T_L = 48.5, \text{ since } 48.5 > 42.5$$

(iv) Compute U_1 and U_2 using the following formulas. The value of the Mann-Whitney U statistic is whichever is the smaller.

Formula:

$$U_1 = n_L \cdot n_S + \frac{n_L \cdot (n_S + 1)}{2} - T_L$$
$$U_2 = n_L \cdot (n_S) - U_1$$

where n_L = number of subjects in group with larger sum of ranks.
n_S = number of subjects in group with smaller sum of ranks.
T_L = larger sum of ranks.

For our example, we have:

$$n_L = 6 \cdot n_S = 7, \ T_L = 48.5$$

$$U_1 = (6) \cdot (7) + \frac{6 \cdot (6+1)}{2} - 48.5$$

$$= 42 + 21 - 48.5 = 14.5$$

$$U_2 = (6) \cdot (7) - 14.5$$

$$= 42 - 14.5$$

$$= 27.5$$

Therefore, U_1 (14.5) is the value of the Mann-Whitney U statistic.

Step (3).   Determine whether or not to reject H_0. To find the critical U value, consult Appendix A-1-6, which lists critical values for interpreting the Mann-Whitney U statistic. The table shows a critical value of 6 at $\alpha = .05$ with $df = (6, 7)$. Because the observed U value of 14.5 is greater than 6, H_0 will be retained.

LATIN SQUARE DESIGN AND RANDOMIZED BLOCKED ANOVA

(5) "Effects of Temporal Alterations on Speech Intelligibility in Parkinsonian Dysarthria," by V. L. Hammen, et al., April 1994, *Journal of Speech and Hearing Research, 37,* 244–253.

The effect of two types of temporal alterations, paced and synthetic, on the intelligibility of parkinsonian dysarthic speech was investigated. Six speakers with idiopathic Parkinson's disease served as subjects. Paced temporal alterations were created by slowing each speaker to 60% of his/her habitual speaking rate. The synthetic alterations were created by modifying the habitual rate speech samples using digital signal processing. Three types of synthetic alterations were examined: paused altered, speech duration altered, and the combination of both.

A total of 150 sentence files were created during the signal processing phase of the project, (5 sentences × 5 conditions [2 unmodified and 3 synthetic temporal alterations] × 6 peakers). A 5 × 5 Latin square (listeners × sentences) was created for each subject, with the five conditions counterbalanced under the rows and columns of the square. The Latin square table is shown below.

    (a) Explain the advantages of the Latin square design briefly.
    (b) Using Latin squares design, test the hypothesis that there is no significant differences among the five treatments.

Solution

(a) The advantage of this design is that a reduced number of listeners are required to obtain measures of intelligibility. Because each listener is presented a different sentence for each condition, the problem of listener familiarity confounding the intelligibility measure is avoided. This design eliminates determining the reliability of the listeners using correlation methods. Therefore, relative homogeneity of the variables assigned to the row and columns is assumed.

(b) The table below presents mean percentage intelligibility under five treatments. The form of the F statistic for testing treatment effects in a Latin square design may be obtained by substituting degrees of freedom into the general expression for the F statistic.

	Judges				
	1	**2**	**3**	**4**	**5**
Subject					
1	83(A)	88(B)	84(C)	81(D)	91(E)
2	83(B)	80(C)	50(D)	70(E)	81(A)
3	48(C)	54(D)	57(E)	54(A)	67(B)
4	21(D)	14(E)	14(A)	26(B)	26(C)
5	5(E)	3(A)	16(B)	6(C)	4(D)

Notice that each score is a function of three possible influences: subjects, judges, and treatment condition (five levels: A = habitual rate, B = paced habitual rates, C = pausal alteration, D = speech duration alteration, and E = combined alteration). Therefore, a full model for the data may be written as:

$$Y_{ijk} = \mu + \alpha_j + \beta_k + \Pi_i + E_{ijk}.$$

where Y_{ijk} represents the score on the dependent variable for the ith subject at the jth level of treatment and kth level of judges, μ is the grand mean parameter, α_j is the treatment effect parameter, β_k is the judge effect parameter, Π_i is the subject effect parameter, and E_{ijk} is the error term.

Since the Latin square model is strictly a main-effects model, it has no interaction effects. As previously mentioned, the null hypothesis may be written as:

$$H_0: \alpha_A = \alpha_B = \alpha_C = \alpha_D = \alpha_E$$

that is to say, every α_j becomes zero when H_0 is true. Consequently, it gives

$$Y_{ijk} = \mu + \beta_k + \Pi_i + E_{ijk}.$$

In summary, we can construct the mixed-effects RBANOVA (randomized blocked ANOVA) table to calculate the sum of squares (SS), degrees of freedom (d.f.), the mean squares (MS), and an F statistic.

Judge Levels Subjects	1	2	3	4	5	Row Totals
1	83	88	84	81	91	427
2	83	80	50	70	81	364
3	48	54	57	54	67	280
4	21	14	14	26	26	101
5	5	3	16	6	4	34
Column Totals	240	239	221	237	269	1206
$k = 5$ levels,	$n = 5$ subjects					

Step (1). Square the grand total and divide by $(n) \cdot (k)$, denoted by $\{1\}$.

$$\{1\} = \frac{(1206)^2}{25} = 58{,}177.44$$

Step (2). Sum the squared row totals and divide by the number of treatment levels (k), denoted by $\{2\}$.

$$\{2\} = \frac{(427)^2 + (364)^2 + (280)^2 + (101)^2 + (34)^2}{5}$$
$$= 80{,}916.4$$

Step (3). Sum the square column totals and divide by the number of subjects (n), denoted by $\{3\}$.

$$\{3\} = \frac{(240)^2 + (239)^2 + (221)^2 + (237)^2 + (269)^2}{5}$$
$$= 58{,}418.4$$

Step (4). Square each individual score and find the sum of the squared scores, denoted by $\{4\}$.

$$\{4\} = (83)^2 + (88)^2 + (84)^2 + (81)^2 + (91)^2 + (83)^2 + (80)^2 + (50)^2 + (70)^2 +$$
$$(81)^2 + (48)^2 + (54)^2 + (57)^2 + (54)^2 + (67)^2 + (21)^2 + (14)^2 + (14)^2 +$$
$$(26)^2 + (26)^2 + (5)^2 + (3)^2 + (16)^2 + (6)^2 + (4)^2 = 82{,}182$$

Step (5). Compute the sum of squares total (SS total), sum of squares for judges (SS judges), sum of squares for subjects (SS subjects), and sum of squares for residual (SS residual).

$$SS \text{ total} = \{4\} - \{1\} = 82{,}182 - 58{,}177.44 = 24{,}004.56$$

$$SS \text{ judges} = \{3\} - \{1\} = 58{,}418.4 - 58{,}177.44 = 240.46$$

$$SS \text{ subjects} = \{2\} - \{1\} = 80{,}916.4 - 58{,}177.44 = 22{,}738.96$$

$$SS \text{ residual} = SS \text{ total} - SS \text{ judges} - SS \text{ subjects}$$
$$= 24{,}004.56 - 240.46 - 22{,}738.96$$
$$= 1025.14$$

Step (6). Calculate the degrees of freedom for treatments, subjects, residuals, and total. The full model has one μ parameter, $(j - 1)$ independent α parameters, $(k - 1)$ independent β parameters, and $(i - 1)$ independent Π parameters.

$$d.f. \text{ full} = \text{Total } d.f. - (j - i) - (k - 1) - (i - 1)$$
$$= \{(5)(5) - 1\} - (5 - 1) - (5 - 1) - (5 - 1) = 12$$

which is equal to the degrees of freedom of the denominator.

The restricted model has one μ parameter, $(k - 1)$ independent β parameters, and $(i - 1)$ independent parameters.

Thus, $d.f. \text{ restricted} = \{(5)(5) - 1\} - (5 - 1) - (5 - 1) = 16.$

The difference $(d.f. \text{ full})$ and $(d.f. \text{ restricted})$ gives the degrees of freedom of the numerator, namely $16 - 12 = 4$.

Step (7). Calculate the F score for testing treatment effects in a Latin square design.

$$F = \frac{SS \text{ treatment}/4}{SS \text{ residual}/12}$$

where $SS \text{ treatment} = (i) \cdot \sum_{j=1}^{5} (\bar{Y}_{\cdot j\cdot} - \bar{Y}\ldots)^2$

$i = 5$ subjects, $\bar{Y}_{\cdot j\cdot} = $ the mean value of each level

$\bar{Y}\ldots = $ grand total mean

$$= \frac{1206}{25} = 48.24$$

$\bar{Y}_{\cdot 1\cdot} = 47, \quad \bar{Y}_{\cdot 2\cdot} = 56, \quad \bar{Y}_{\cdot 3\cdot} = 48.8, \quad \bar{Y}_{\cdot 4\cdot} = 42, \text{ and } \bar{Y}_{\cdot 5\cdot} = 47.4$

$SS \text{ treatment} = 5 \cdot [(47 - 48.24)^2 + (56 - 48.24)^2 + (48.8 - 48.24)^2 + (42 - 48.24)^2$
$+ (47.4 - 48.24)^2] = 508.56$

$$F_{obs} = \frac{508.56/4}{1025.14/12} = \frac{127.14}{85.43}$$
$$= 1.49$$

Step (8). Under the decision rule, decide whether or not we reject H_0.

F_{crit} for treatment
$F_{crit} (.05, 4.12){:}3{,}26 > F_{obs} = 1.49$

Therefore, we do not reject H_0. At 5% level of significance, the five treatments have equal effects on intelligibility scores.

ANALYSIS OF COVARIANCE AND SPEARMAN CORRELATION COEFFICIENT

(6) "Duration of Sound Prolongation and Sound/Syllable Repetition in Children Who Stutter: Preliminary Observations," by P. M. Zebrowski, April 1994, *Journal of Speech and Hearing Research, 37,* 254–263.

The purpose of the study was to measure rate of sound/syllable repetitions (stutterings) per second in the conversational speech of school-age children who stutter. Nine randomly selected subjects were assigned to one of three treatment groups to reduce the rate of repetitions: A, B, and C. Suppose each subject was given a pretest to determine their severity levels prior to assignment. After the treatments, a posttest was administered and the data in the table below were collected. Note that the pretest is labeled as X, and the posttest as Y. For the purpose of calculation illustration, we intentionally work with a very small (hypothetical) size. If this were a real study, then the sample size would be much larger.

Treatment	A		B		C	
	X	Y	X	Y	X	Y
	2	1	5	3	3	3
	3	2	4	6	7	5
	4	3	6	6	5	4
Mean	3	2	5	5	5	4
SD	1	1	1	1.73	2	1
Variance	1	1	1	3	4	1

(a) What type of statistical analysis is the most suitable to test the null hypothesis, namely, that there is no treatment effect on the rate of repetition of sound/syllable per second? Explain why.

(b) Using the statistical analysis, test the null hypothesis.

Solution

(a) The analysis of covariance (ANCOVA) is a better way (than ANOVA) to determine individual differences among subjects under the treatment, which is gathered prior to the treatment (called the covariant) and is highly correlated with the outcome measure (called the posttest). One of the advantages over ANOVA is that we could remove the portion of variance from the posttest which is accounted for by the systematic differences among subjects (covariant). This results in decreasing the residual term which is in the denominator of the F ratio. When it is decreased, the size of the F statistics increases, all other things being equal. In short, the ANCOVA is designed for research questions such as "Are the observed differences due to chance, or do they reflect population differences?"

The ANCOVA would be more powerful than ANOVA if the following assumptions are met:

1. Independence of each score for pre and post.
2. Normality of pre and post distributions.
3. Homogeneity of variances for pre and post distributions.
4. Linearity: for each treatment, the regression of the post variable (Y) on the covariant (X) is linear in each group. If this assumption is not met, then the ANCOVA should not be used. You can "eyeball" the relationship between X and Y.

5. Homogeneity of regression slopes: the slopes of all groups are equal. It can be again verified by "eyeballing" their similarity across groups. If this assumption is violated, then the ANCOVA should not be used.

6. Independence of covariant and treatments: the scores on the covariant must not be affected by treatments. If this assumption is violated, then the ANCOVA should not be used.

(b) The information pertinent to the ANCOVA may be summarized in an ANCOVA table shown below. This section guides you through the step-by-step methods to fill in the ANCOVA table.

ANCOVA Table

Source	Sum of Squares (SS)	Degrees of Freedom (d.f.)	Mean Squares (MS)	F_{OBS} (F)
(Treatment) adj				
(Within) adj				
(Covariant) adj.				
Total				

Step (1).   Calculate the adjusted sums of squares (SS treat) adj., (SS within) adj., (SS total) adj., and the sum of squares for the covariant, denoted by SS cov. In order to find them, we must calculate (SS treat), (SS within), and (SS total). The steps for calculating the various types of sums of squares is quite tedious and time-consuming work, therefore, we make three treatment tables to derive such outcomes.

Treatment A

X_A	X_A^2	Y_A	Y_A^2	$(X_A \cdot Y_A)$
2	4	1	1	2
3	9	2	4	6
4	16	3	9	12
9	29	6	14	20
ΣX_A	ΣX_A^2	ΣY_A	ΣY_A^2	$\Sigma X_A \cdot Y_A$

Treatment B

X_B	X_B^2	Y_B	Y_B^2	$(X_B \cdot Y_B)$
5	25	3	9	15
4	16	6	36	24
6	36	6	36	36
15	77	15	81	75
ΣX_B	ΣX_B^2	ΣY_B	ΣY_B^2	$\Sigma X_B Y_B$

Treatment C

X_C	X_C^2	Y_C	Y_C^2	$(X_C \cdot Y_C)$
3	9	3	9	9
7	49	5	25	35
5	25	4	16	20
15	83	12	50	64
ΣX_C	ΣX_C^2	ΣY_C	ΣY_C^2	$\Sigma X_C Y_C$

Step (2). Find the square of the sum of the squared covariants between the groups, denoted by $(SS\, X_{between})^2$

$$(SS\, X_{between})^2 = (\Sigma X_A)^2 + (\Sigma X_B)^2 + (\Sigma X_C)^2$$
$$= (9)^2 + (15)^2 + (15)^2$$
$$= 531$$

Step (3). Square the sum of the squared postscores between the group, denoted by $(SS\, Y_{between})^2$

$$(SS\, Y_{between})^2 = (\Sigma Y_A)^2 + (\Sigma Y_B)^2 + (\Sigma Y_C)^2$$
$$= 6^2 + (15)^2 + (12)^2$$
$$= 405$$

Step (4). Find the cross product of the sum of X and the sum of Y, for each group, denoted by $(SS\, XY_{between})$.

$$(SS\, XY_{between}) = (\Sigma X_A) \cdot (\Sigma Y_A) + (\Sigma X_B) \cdot (\Sigma Y_B) + (\Sigma X_C) \cdot \Sigma Y_C)$$
$$= (9 \cdot 6) + (15 \cdot 15) + (15 \cdot 12)$$
$$= 459$$

Step (5). Find the total sum of X, $(SS\, X_{total})$, and the total sum of Y, $(SS\, Y_{total})$.

$$(SS\, X_{total}) = (\Sigma X_A) + (\Sigma X_B) + (\Sigma X_C)$$
$$= 9 + 15 + 15 = 39$$
$$(SS\, Y_{total}) = (\Sigma Y_A) + (\Sigma Y_B) + (\Sigma Y_C)$$
$$= 6 + 15 + 12 = 33$$

Step (6). Find the total of the cross product of X and Y (denoted by $SS\, XY_{total}$), the total of the squared X's (denoted by $SS\, X_{total}^2$), and the total of the squared Y's (denoted by $SS\, Y_{total}^2$).

$$(SS\, XY_{total}) = (\Sigma X_A Y_A) + (\Sigma X_B Y_B) + (\Sigma X_C Y_C)$$
$$= 20 + 75 + 64$$
$$= 159$$

$$(SS\,X^2_{total}) = (\Sigma X^2_A) + (\Sigma X^2_B) + (\Sigma X^2_C)$$

$$= 29 + 77 + 83$$

$$= 189$$

$$(SS\,Y^2_{total}) = (\Sigma Y^2_A) + (\Sigma Y^2_B) + (\Sigma Y^2_C)$$

$$= 14 + 81 + 50 = 145$$

Step (7).   Using the values we derived in Step (6), find $(SSSY_{total})$, $(SSSX_{total})$, $(SSSY_{within})$, and $(SSSX_{within})$.

$$(S\,SS\,Y_{total}) = (SS\,Y^2_{total}) - \frac{(SSY_{total})^2}{N}$$

$$= 145 - \frac{(33)^2}{n_A + n_B + n_C}$$

$$= 145 - \frac{1089}{9}$$

$$= 145 - 121$$

$$= 24$$

where $n_A = 3$, $n_B = 3$, $n_C = 3$, and $N = 3 + 3 + 3 = 9$

$$(S\,SS\,X_{total}) = (SS\,X^2_{total}) - \frac{(SSX_{total})^2}{N}$$

$$= 189 - \frac{(39)^2}{9}$$

$$= 189 - 169$$

$$= 20$$

$$(S\,SS\,Y_{within}) = (SS\,Y^2_{total}) - \frac{(SSY_{between})^2}{n}$$

$$= 145 - \frac{405}{3}$$

$$= 145 - 135$$

$$= 10$$

$$(S\,SS\,X_{within}) = (SS\,X^2_{total}) - \frac{(SSX_{between})^2}{n}$$

$$= 189 - \frac{531}{3}$$

$$= 189 - 177$$

$$= 12$$

Step (8).   Find the two sums of cross products (SCPtotal) and (SCPwithin), which will be used to find the adjusted sums of squares.

$$(SCP_{total}) = (SS\,XY_{total}) - \frac{(SSX_{total}) \cdot (SSY_{total})}{N}$$

$$= 159 - \frac{(39) \cdot (33)}{9}$$

$$= 159 - 143$$

$$= 16$$

$$(SCP_{within}) = (SS\,XY_{total}) - \frac{(SS\,XY_{between})}{n}$$

$$= 159 - \frac{459}{3}$$

$$= 159 - 153$$

$$= 6$$

Step (9). Using the values from Step (8), find $[(S\,SS_{total})adj.]$, $[(S\,SS_{treatment})\,adj.]$, and $[(S\,SS_{within})\,adj.]$.

$$[(SSS_{total})\,adj.] = [(S\,SS\,Y_{total})adj.] - \frac{(SCP_{total})^2}{S\,SS\,X_{total}}$$

$$= 24 - \frac{(16)^2}{20}$$

$$= 11.2$$

$$[(S\,SS_{within})\,adj.] = [(S\,SS\,Y_{within})adj.] - \frac{(SCP_{within})^2}{S\,SS\,X_{within}}$$

$$= 10 - \frac{(6)^2}{12}$$

$$= 7$$

$$[(S\,SS_{treatment})\,adj.] = [(S\,SS\,Y_{total})\,adj.] - [(S\,SS\,Y_{within})\,adj.]$$

$$= 11.2 - 7$$

$$= 4.2$$

Step (10). Find the sum of squares for the covariant, denoted by (SS_{cov}).

$$(SS_{cov}) = (S\,SS\,Y_{within}) - [(S\,SS\,Y_{within})\,adj.]$$

$$= 10 - 7$$

$$= 3$$

Step (11). Find degrees of freedom for the treatment $(d.f._{treatment})$, within groups $(d.f._{within})$, and the covariant $(d.f._{cov})$.

$$d.f._{treatment} = (\text{total number of groups}) - 1$$

$$= 3 - 1$$

$$= 2$$

$$d.f._{within} = [(\text{total number of groups}) \cdot (\text{one less than the number of subjects in each group})] - 1$$

$$= [(3) \cdot (3 - 1)] - 1$$

$$= 6 - 1$$

$$= 5$$

$$d.f._{\text{total}} = N - 1$$
$$= 9 - 1$$
$$= 8$$

$$d.f._{\text{cov}} = d.f._{\text{total}} - d.f._{\text{treatment}} - d.f._{\text{within}}$$
$$= 8 - 5 - 2$$
$$= 1$$

Step (12).   Calculate the mean squares for the treatment ($MS_{\text{treatment}}$), within groups (MS_{within}), and the covariant (MS_{cov}).

$$MS_{\text{treatment}} = \frac{(S\,SS_{\text{within}})\text{adj}}{d.f._{\text{treatment}}}$$
$$= \frac{4.2}{2}$$
$$= 2.1$$

$$MS_{\text{within}} = \frac{(S\,SS_{\text{within}})\text{adj}}{d.f._{\text{within}}}$$
$$= \frac{7}{5}$$
$$= 1.4$$

$$MS_{\text{cov}} = \frac{(SS_{\text{cov}})\,\text{adj}}{d.f._{\text{cov}}}$$
$$= \frac{3}{1}$$
$$= 3$$

Step (13).   Calculate F_{obs} for the treatment and for the covariant.

$$F_{\text{obs}}(\text{treatment}) = \frac{MS_{\text{treatment}}}{MS_{\text{within}}}$$
$$= \frac{2.1}{4}$$
$$= 1.5$$

$$F_{\text{obs}}(\text{covariant}) = \frac{MS_{\text{cov}}}{MS_{\text{within}}}$$
$$= \frac{3}{1.4}$$
$$= 2.14$$

Step (14).   Enter all values into the ANCOVA table:

Source	Sum of Squares	D.F.	MS	F_{OBS}
Treatment	4.2	2	2.1	1.5
Within	7	5	1.4	
Covariant	3	1	3	2.14
Total	14.2	8		

Step (15).   Using the decision rule to decide whether or not we reject the null hypothesis.

$$F_{crit} (.05, 2, 5) = 5.79 > F_{obs} = 1.5$$

We do not reject H_0

$$F_{crit} (.05, 1, 5) = 6.61 > F_{obs} = 2.14$$

We do not reject H_0

Therefore, there is neither treatment effects nor covariant effects on the rate of repetition of sound/syllable per second.

(c) The table shown below describes the mean age and interval since onset (the length of time the children had exhibited stuttering problems) for 11 children who stutter in the same study. Using correlational analysis, determine whether or not age was significantly correlated with interval since onset.

Mean Age and Interval Since Onset for 11 Children Who Stutter

ID		Age (Yr: Mos)	Interval (Mos)
Subject	1	5.5	42
	2	5.7	39
	3	6.5	54
	4	6.8	21
	5	7.8	28
	6	8.3	63
	7	10.6	103
	8	11.0	67
	9	11.2	98
	10	11.3	65
	11	11.5	78

Solution

Spearman rank-order correlation coefficient (r_s) is the suitable correlational analysis to answer the question since this nonparametric analysis could possibly avoid violating assumptions of normality and homogeneity of variance. The following steps would lead you to the derivation of r_s

Step (1). Convert the scores on ages (X) to ranks. Do the same for the scores on interval (Y).

ID	Age (Yrs: MOS)	Rank of X (X_R)	Interval (MOS)	Rank of Y (Y_R)
1	5.5	1(the lowest)	42	4
2	5.7	2	39	3
3	6.5	3	54	5
4	6.8	4	21	1
5	7.8	5	28	2
6	8.3	6	63	6
7	10.6	7	103	11
8	11.0	8	67	8
9	11.2	9	98	10
10	11.3	10	65	7
11	11.5	11(the highest)	78	9

A rank of "1" is given to the lowest score, "2" to the next lowest score, and so on. The highest rank assigned must be the same value as the number of subjects in the sample. If two scores are tied for the same rank, average the ranks and assign the average rank to both scores.

Step (2). Derive derivation scores of the rank of X and Y.

ID	X_R	$\bar{X}_R$	X	X^2	Y_R	$\bar{Y}_R$	Y	Y^2	XY
1	1	6	-5	25	4	6	-2	4	10
2	2	6	-4	16	3	6	-3	9	12
3	3	6	-3	9	5	6	-1	1	3
4	4	6	-2	4	1	6	-5	25	10
5	5	6	-1	1	2	6	-4	16	4
6	6	6	0	0	6	6	0	0	0
7	7	6	1	1	11	6	5	25	5
8	8	6	2	4	8	6	2	4	4
9	9	6	3	9	10	6	4	16	12
10	10	6	4	16	7	6	1	1	4
11	11	6	5	25	9	6	3	9	15

$$\bar{X}_R = 6 \qquad \Sigma X^2 = 110 \qquad \bar{Y}_R = 6 \quad \Sigma Y^2 = 110 \qquad \Sigma XY = 79$$

where $X = X_R - \bar{X}_R$ and $Y = Y_R - \bar{Y}_R$.

Step (3). Calculate the covariance (Cov (X, Y) and the standard deviations of X and Y (S_X and S_Y) which are needed in the formula of the Spearman rank correlation coefficient r_{XY}.

$$\text{Cov}(X, Y) = \frac{\Sigma XY}{N-1} = \frac{79}{10} = 7.9$$

$$S_X = \sqrt{\frac{\Sigma X^2}{N-1}} = \sqrt{\frac{110}{10}} = \sqrt{11} = 3.32$$

$$S_Y = \sqrt{\frac{\Sigma X^2}{N-1}} = \sqrt{\frac{110}{10}} = \sqrt{11} = 3.32$$

$$r_{XY} = \frac{\text{Cov}(X, Y)}{(S_X) \cdot (S_Y)} = \frac{7.9}{(3.32) \cdot (3.32)} = .717$$

As expected, age was significantly correlated with the length of time the children had exhibited stuttering problems.

KRUSKAL-WALLIS ANALYSIS OF VARIANCE

(7) "The Operant Manipulation of Vocal Pitch in Normal Speakers," by J. C. Moore and A. Holbrook, 1971, *Journal of Speech and Hearing Research, 14,* 283–290.

A device consisting of variable electronic filters and voice-actuated relays was used to raise or lower the vocal pitch of four normal-speaking subjects by the differential reinforcement of selected frequencies emitted by them during oral reading. The sequence of investigation with each subject was to measure the habitual pitch level (*HPL*), to adjust the filters to a higher or lower range called conditioning pitch level (*CPL*), and to establish the baseline responding rate at *CPL*. A fixed interval (*FI*) reinforcement schedule was alternated with a fixed ratio (*FR*) reinforcement schedule. Extinction trials (*EXT*) separated the four experimental conditions, with reinstatement by continuous reinforcement (*CR*) preceding each new condition. The results of changes in modal fundamental frequency of subjects during experimental conditions for four participants were summarized in the table below:

Subjects	1	2	3	4
HPL	250	182	222	125
CPL	180	260	160	180
CR	200	240	175	175
FR	175	235	160	150
FI	180	250	175	160
EXT	255	200	195	120

Compute a Kruskal-Wallis one-way ANOVA on the data above to determine if there is a significant difference among the four subjects or not. Use $\alpha = .05$.

Solution

Step (1).   State the null (H_0) and alternative (H_a) hypotheses.

H_0: The four subjects are identical.

H_a: At least one subject differs from the others with respect to means or medians.

Step (2).   Verify the assumptions.

1. *Independence:* the data values are randomly assigned to respective groups independently.
2. *Minimum number of subjects:* the individual sample sizes are each at least 5.
3. *Shape of distribution:* the groups have identical shapes or are symmetric.

Step (3). Calculate the test statistic K. First we construct a data summary table for each subject and regardless of group membership rank (R) the scores from lowest to highest. If two or more scores are equal, then average the ranks and assign the average to each member of the tie.

Subject	1		2		3		4	
	Score	Rank	Score	Rank	Score	Rank	Score	Rank
	250	21.5	182	14	222	18	125	2
	180	12	260	24	160	5	180	12
	200	16.5	240	20	175	8.5	175	8.5
	175	8.5	235	19	160	5	150	3
	180	12	250	21.5	175	8.5	160	5
	255	23	200	16.5	195	15	120	1
Sums		93.5		115		60		31.5

Secondly, we calculate the mean square of the sum of ranks for each group, denoted by MS.

$$
\begin{aligned}
MS &= \sum_{i=1}^{J} \frac{R_i^2}{n_i} \\
&= \frac{(93.5)^2}{6} + \frac{(115)^2}{6} + \frac{(60)^2}{6} + \frac{(31.5)^2}{6} \\
&= 1457.04 + 2204.17 + 600 + 165.38 \\
&= 4426.59
\end{aligned}
$$

Lastly, we calculate the K statistic and conclude it under the decision rule such that

(i) Reject H_0 if $K > \chi^2 (\alpha, J - 1)$ where J = total number of groups.
(ii) Do not reject H_0 if $K \leq \chi^2 (\alpha, J - 1)$.

$$
K = \frac{12}{N(N+1)} \cdot (MS) - 3 \cdot (N+1)
$$

where N = total sample size. We now would be able to derive the observed K statistic and critical χ^2 value.

Given: $N = 6 + 6 + 6 + 6 = 24$ scores
$\quad\quad J = 4$ groups (or 4 participants)
$\quad\quad MS = 4426.59$

$$
K = \frac{12}{24 \cdot (24+1)} \cdot (4426.59) - 3 \cdot (24+1)
$$

$$
= 88.53 - 75
$$

$$
= 13.53
$$

$$
\chi^2_{.05, 3} = 7.815 < 13.53
$$

Therefore, we reject H_0; that is, the observed differences are significant and the distributions of scores in the four subjects are not identical.

ONE-WAY AND TWO-WAY ANOVA

(8) "Predictive Values of Routine Blood Pressure Measurements in Screening for Hypertension," by B. Rosner and B. F. Polk, 1990, *American Journal of Epidemiology, 117* (4), 250–259.

An epidemiologist conducted a study to compare systolic blood pressure and diastolic blood pressure for the purpose of hypertension detection for those who have speech fluency disorders within age, race, and gender. The results are summarized in the table below.

Systolic Blood Pressure (mm Hg)

Age	Gender	White			Black		
		M	*SD*	*n*	*M*	*SD*	*n*
Young							
30–49	M	126.8	14.3	262	135.6	19.0	41
30–49	F	119.7	15.9	172	130.8	21.3	52
Old							
50–69	M	136.5	19.6	179	145.1	22.8	42
50–69	F	135.7	21.0	196	145.1	23.7	47

Diastolic Blood Pressure (mm Hg)

Age	Gender	White			Black		
		M	*SD*	*n*	*M*	*SD*	*n*
Young							
30–49	M	82.2	10.9	262	87.8	13.7	41
30–49	F	77.1	10.8	172	84.6	14.2	52
Old							
50–69	M	83.6	11.5	179	89.2	14.0	42
50–69	F	80.4	11.3	196	87.8	13.8	47

(a) What statistical test procedure can be used to test for significant differences of diastolic blood pressure levels among the four groups (young males, young females, old males, and old females) within the white race?

(b) Perform the test mentioned in (a) and conclude from it.

(c) What statistical test procedure can be used to test for significant differences of systolic blood pressure among the young group by gender by race?

(d) Perform the test mentioned in (c) and conclude from it.

Solution

(a) Whenever the means of more than two groups need to be compared, we frequently use the analysis of variance (ANOVA). For our example, we may start out by summarizing the results of the four groups as follows.

Group:

1. (Young white males)	$\bar{Y}_1 = 82.2,$	$S_1 = 10.9,$	$n_1 = 262$
2. (Young white females)	$\bar{Y}_2 = 77.1,$	$S_2 = 10.8,$	$n_2 = 172$
3. (Old white males)	$\bar{Y}_3 = 83.6,$	$S_3 = 11.5,$	$n_3 = 179$
4. (Old white females)	$\bar{Y}_4 = 80.4,$	$S_4 = 11.3,$	$n_4 = 196$

where $\bar{Y}_i$ = the sample mean and S_i = the sample standard deviation.
    Prior to ANOVA, we must determine the following assumptions.

(i) Normality
The data values within each group are normally distributed. Fortunately, the ANOVA procedures are *not very sensitive* (robust) to violation of normality assumption. As a matter of fact, the ANOVA becomes more robust (less sensitive to lack of normality) as the sample sizes increase because of the effect of the central limit theorem.

(ii) Homogeneity of variance
The variances of the data values in each group are equal. Again, the ANVOA is robust to the violation of homogeneity of variance if (i) all samples have the same or similar sizes, (ii) no sample is extremely small (less than 3), and/or (iii) the largest sample standard deviation is no more than twice as large as the smallest sample standard deviation. If any one of the three rules fail to be met, then we must use Bartlett's test for homogeneity of variance (available on SPSS, BMDP, or SAS software) to determine whether or not we should use a nonparametric version of the ANOVA such as the Kruskal-Wallis test. In summary, the following flowchart would help readers understand general procedures for comparing the means of several independent groups:

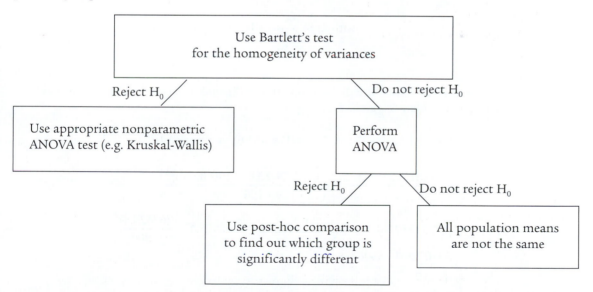

(b)   Using Bartlett's test, we could verify that the assumption of homogeneity of variance, along with the assumption of normality, has been met for the ANOVA.

Step (1).   State the null and alternative hypotheses.

$$H_0: \mu_1 = \mu_2 = \mu_3 = \mu_4 \text{ (All means are equal)}$$

H_a: Not all means are equal.

Step (2).   Calculate the between sum of squares (SS_B) and the within sum of squares (SS_W) figures.

Case (1) If the raw data are available, then:

$$SS_B = \sum_{j=1}^{J} n_j \cdot (\bar{Y}_j - \bar{Y})^2 \text{ with } d.f. = J - 1$$

$$SS_W = \sum_{j=1}^{J} \sum_{i=1}^{n} (\bar{Y}_{ij} - \bar{Y}_j)^2 \text{ with } d.f. = \sum_{j=1}^{J} (n_j - 1)$$

where n_j = sample size of the jth group.
$\quad J$ = total number of groups
$\quad Y_j$ = the sample mean of the jth group
$\quad \bar{Y}$ = the overall mean
$\quad Y_{ij}$ = the ith observed value of the jth group
Case (2) If the raw data are not available, then

$$SS_B = \left[\sum_{j=1}^{J} n_j \bar{Y}_j^2 \right] - \frac{\left(\sum_{j=1}^{J} n_j \bar{Y}_j^2 \right)}{n}$$

$$SS_W = \sum_{j=1}^{J} (n_j - 1) \cdot S_j^2$$

$$\text{with } d.f. = \sum_{j=1}^{J} (n_j - 1)$$

For our example, we must use the formula in case (2) since the raw data are not available. Now, we calculate SS_B and SS_W.

$$SS_B = [262 \cdot (182.2)^2 + 172 \cdot (77.1)^2 + 179 \cdot (83.6)^2 + 196 \cdot (80.4)^2]$$

$$- \left[\frac{\{(262 \cdot 82.2) + (172 \cdot 77.1) + (179 \cdot 83.6) + 196 \cdot (80.4)\}^2}{262 + 172 + 179 + 196} \right]$$

$$= [1770292.1 + 1022438.5 + 1251023.8 + 1266975.4] - \frac{(65520.4)^2}{809}$$

$$= 5310729.8 - 5306455.9$$

$$= 4273.9$$

$$SS_W = [(262 - 1) \cdot (10.9)^2 + (172 - 1) \cdot (10.8)^2 + (179 - 1) \cdot (11.5)^2 + (196 - 1) \cdot (11.3)^2]$$

$$= 31009.41 + 19945.44 + 23540.5 + 24899.55 = 99394.9$$

$$= 99394.9$$

Step (3). Construct the ANOVA table to calculate the *F*-ratio

Sources	SS	d.f.	$MS\left(=\dfrac{SS}{d.f.}\right)$	$F\left(=\dfrac{MS_B}{MS_W}\right)$
Between	4273.9	3	$\dfrac{4273.9}{3}=1424.63$	$F=\dfrac{1424.63}{123.47}$
Within	99394.9	805*	$\dfrac{99394.9}{85}=123.47$	$=11.54$

where *J* = 4 groups

$$MS_B = \frac{SS_B}{d.f._B} \text{ and } MS_W = \frac{SS_W}{d.f._W}$$

$$d.f._W = (262-1)+(172-1)+(179-1)+(196-1)=805$$

Step (4). Under the decision rule (at $\alpha = .05$), determine whether or not we reject H_0.
  $F_{crit}(.05, d.f. = 3, 805) = 2.60 < F_{obs} = 11.54$; therefore, we reject H_0. This tells us that the differences among the means of the four groups are not equal.

(c) The results of testing for the four younger groups are summarized in the table below.

Status (Row Effect)	Race (Column Effect)			
	White		Black	
Young males	M	126.8	M	135.6
	SD	14.3	SD	19.0
	n	262	n	41
Young females	M	119.7	M	130.8
	SD	15.9	SD	21.3
	n	172	n	52

We are interested in the effects of race and gender on systolic blood pressure. They may be independent or they may be related or interact with each other. One strategy for this problem would be to establish a two-way ANOVA model to detect the effects of race, gender, and the combination of both on systolic blood pressure. There are two important assumptions for the two-way ANOVA that must be verified.

(i) Normality
The data values within each cell are drawn from a population in which the data values are normally distributed. The two-way ANOVA is robust to the violation of this assumption.

(ii) Homogeneity of Variances
The variances of data values in the populations underlying all the cells of the design are equal. Like the one-way ANOVA assumptions, we must use Bartlett's test for the homogeneity of variances to verify this assumption. Normally, the two-way ANOVA is robust to

the violation of this assumption if (a) the cell sizes are equal, (b) no sample is extremely small (less than 3), and/or (c) the largest sample standard deviation is no more than twice as large as the smallest sample standard deviation.

Step (1).   Check all basic assumptions of a two-way ANOVA and determine whether or not we can use it.

Step (2).   If we can, then we construct the two-way ANOVA table to calculate all infromation. For our example, we would use the formula for no raw data.

Source	SS	d.f.	MS	F
Row (Gender)	$\dfrac{\sum_{i=1}^{r} Y_{i\cdot}^2}{c} - \dfrac{Y_{\cdot\cdot}^2}{rc}$	$r-1$	Row $SS/r-1$	$F_{row} = \dfrac{MS\ row}{MS\ residual}$
Column (Race)	$\dfrac{\sum_{j=1}^{c} Y_{\cdot j}^2}{r} - \dfrac{Y_{\cdot\cdot}^2}{rc}$	$c-1$	Column $SS/c-1$	$F_{column} = \dfrac{MS\ column}{MS\ residual}$
Interaction (Gender + Race)	$\left(\sum_{i=1}^{r}\sum_{j=1}^{c} \bar{Y}_{ij}^2 - \dfrac{Y_{\cdot\cdot}^2}{rc} \right)$ $-$ Row SS $-$ Column SS	$(r-1)\cdot(c-1)$	$\dfrac{\text{Interaction } SS}{(r-1)(c-1)}$	$F_{int} = \dfrac{MS\ interaction}{MS\ residual}$
Residual (Error)		$n - rc$	$\sum_{i=1}^{r}\sum_{j=1}^{c} \dfrac{(n_{ij}-1)\cdot(S_{ij}^2)}{(n-rc)\cdot n_h}$	

For the two way ANOVA model , we can state the following three hypotheses.

1. H_0: No gender effects on systolic blood pressure level after controlling   for the effects of race.

$$\text{Use } F_{row} = \frac{MS_{row}}{MS_{residual}} \text{ to test it.}$$

2. H_0: No race effects on systolic blood pressure level after controlling for the effects of gender.

$$\text{Use } F_{column} = \frac{MS_{column}}{MS_{residual}} \text{ to test it.}$$

3. H_0: No interaction effects* on systolic blood pressure level.

$$\text{Use } F_{interaction} = \frac{MS_{interaction}}{MS_{residual}} \text{ to test it.}$$

*An interaction effect between two variables is defined as one in which the effect of one variable depends on the level of the other variable. It may be stated as "Is there a differential effect of race among different gender groups?" An interaction effect is extremely important for readers to understand when you study the two-way ANOVA. If there are more than one treatment effect (for our example, they are gender and race), then we may expect to observe a differential effect of both treatment effects on individual differences. To simplify the basic concept of an interaction effect, a graphic representation is probably one of the most effective ways to present. For our example, we plot the systolic blood pressure levels on the ordinate and place the gender variable on the abscissa.

Gender	White	Black
Male (M)	126.8	135.6
Female (F)	119.7	130.8

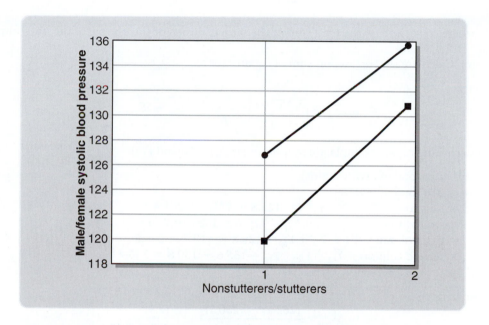

To determine whether or not there is an interaction, you must see the pattern for each pair of lines. If the lines intersect at a point, then we could say that there exists a differential effect. Otherwise, there is no differential effect between the two independent variables. For our example, since there is no intersection point, an individual difference is not significantly affected by the interaction effect of gender and race. Actual calculations would verify this fact.

4. Residual (or Error) represents simply a measure of the amount of variability within the individual samples.

Before we calculate the sum of squares, we need to define some notations as follows:

(a) Calculate ROW SS (or SS_{row})

$$SS_{row} = \frac{\sum_{i=1}^{r} Y_{i\cdot}^2}{c} - \frac{Y_{\cdot\cdot}^2}{rc}$$

where $c =$ the total number of columns

r = the total number of rows

$$Y_{i\cdot} = \sum_{j=1}^{c} \bar{Y}_{ij} = \text{the total sum of the sample means of the } j\text{th column of the } i\text{th group.}$$

$$Y_{\cdot\cdot} = \sum_{i=1}^{r}\sum_{j=1}^{c} \bar{Y}_{ij} = \text{the total sum of the sample means of the } i\text{th row and } j\text{th column.}$$

(b) Calculate Column SS (or SS_{column})

$$SS_{\text{column}} = \frac{\displaystyle\sum_{j=1}^{c} Y_{\cdot j}^2}{r} - \frac{Y_{\cdot\cdot}^2}{rc}$$

where $Y_{\cdot j} = \displaystyle\sum_{i=1}^{r} \bar{Y}_{ij} = \text{the total sum of the sample means of the } i\text{th row of the } j\text{th group.}$

(c) Calculate the Interaction sum of squares (or $SS_{\text{interaction}}$)

$$SS_{\text{interaction}} = \left(\sum_{i=1}^{r}\sum_{j=1}^{c} \bar{Y}_{ij}^2 \right) - \frac{Y_{\cdot\cdot}^2}{rc} - SS_{\text{row}} - SS_{\text{column}}$$

Returning to our example, we first need c, r, $(Y_{i\cdot})$, $(Y_{\cdot j})$, and $(Y_{\cdot\cdot})$.

c = 2 (a total of two columns)
r = 2 (a total of two rows)
i = first row = $\bar{Y}_{1\cdot} = \bar{Y}_{11} + \bar{Y}_{12} = 126.8 + 135.6 = 262.4$
i = second row = $\bar{Y}_{2\cdot} = \bar{Y}_{21} + \bar{Y}_{22} = 119.7 + 130.8 = 250.5$
j = first column = $\bar{Y}_{\cdot 1} = \bar{Y}_{11} + \bar{Y}_{21} = 126.8 + 119.7 = 246.5$
j = second column = $\bar{Y}_{\cdot 2} = \bar{Y}_{12} + \bar{Y}_{22} = 135.6 + 130.8 = 266.4$
$\bar{Y}_{\cdot\cdot} = \bar{Y}_{11} + \bar{Y}_{12} + \bar{Y}_{21} + \bar{Y}_{22} = 512.9$

We now have:

$$SS_{\text{row}} = \frac{(262.4)^2 + (250.5)^2}{2} - \frac{(512.9)^2}{2\cdot 2}$$

$$= 35.402$$

$$d.f._{\text{row}} = 2 - 1 = 1$$

$$MS_{\text{row}} = \frac{35.402}{1} = 35.402$$

$$SS_{\text{column}} = \frac{(246.5)^2 + (266.4)^2}{2} - \frac{(512.9)^2}{2\cdot 2}$$

$$= 99.002$$

$$d.f._{\text{column}} = 2 - 1 = 1$$

$$MS_{column} = \frac{99.002}{1} = 99.002$$

$$SS_{interaction} = [(126.8)^2 + (135.6)^2 + (119.7)^2 + (130.8)^2] - \frac{(512.9)^2}{2 \cdot 2}$$
$$- 35.402 - 99.002$$

$$(SS_{row})(SS_{column})$$

$$= 1.323$$

$$d.f._{interaction} = (2-1) \cdot (2-1) = 1$$

$$MS_{interaction} = \frac{1.323}{1} = 1.323$$

Next, we would calculate the mean square of residuals, denoted by $MS_{residual}$. To do so, we need the value of n_b.

$$\frac{1}{n_b} = \left[\frac{\left(\frac{1}{262} + \frac{1}{41} + \frac{1}{172} + \frac{1}{52} \right)}{4} \right]$$

$$= .0133$$

$$n_b = \frac{1}{.0133} = 75.188$$

Thus,

$$MS_{residual} = \frac{[261 \cdot (14.3)^2 + 40 \cdot (19.0)^2 + 171 \cdot (15.9)^2 + 51 \cdot (21.3)^2]}{[(242 + 41 + 172 + 52) - 4] \cdot (75.188)}$$
$$= 3.25$$

$$d.f._{residual} = (262 + 41 + 172 + 52) - 4 = 523$$

Lastly, we must test the following null hypotheses as we previously stated.

Question 1 Are there any gender effects on systolic blood pressure level after controlling for the effects of race?

H_0: Not significant
H_a: Significant

Calculate an F_{row} ratio.

$$F_{row} = \frac{MS_{row}}{MS_{residual}} = \frac{35.402}{3.25} = 10.89 > F_{crit}(.05, 1.523) = 3.84$$

Hence, we reject H_0; that is, the effects of gender are significant at $\alpha = 5\%$.

Question 2 Are there any race effects on systolic blood pressure level after controlling for the effects of gender?

H_0: Not significant
H_a: Significant

Calcuate an F_{column} ratio.

$$F_{column} = \frac{MS_{column}}{MS_{residual}} = \frac{99.002}{3.25} = 30.46 > F_{crit}(.05, 1.523) = 3.84$$

Hence, we reject H_0; that is, the effects of race is significant.

Question 3 Are there any interaction effects on systolic blood pressure level?

H_0: Not significant
H_a: Significant

Calculate an $F_{interaction}$ ratio.

$$F_{interaction} = \frac{MS_{interaction}}{MS_{residual}} = \frac{1.323}{3.25} = 0.407 > F_{crit}(.05, 1.523) = 3.84$$

Hence we do not reject H_0; that is, the interaction effect is not significant.
    These results computed above are displayed in the table below.

Two-Way ANOVA for Systolic Blood Pressure

Sources	SS	d.f.	MS	F-statistics	Decision
Gender	35.402	1	35.402	10.89	Significant
Race	99.002	1	99.002	30.46	Significant
Interaction	1.323	1	1.323	0.407	Not significant
Residuals		523	3.41		

When we interpret the results of a two-way ANOVA, we start out with the interaction effect. If it is not significant, then we must go back to find out which main effect (or possibly both) causes the individual differences. If it is significant, then we concentrate on that and interpret the significant main effects later, if at all, in light of the interaction.
    For our own example, it implies that the differences in systolic blood pressure level by race are as significant as the differences by gender independently. But the differences are not caused by the combination of the two effects.

MULTIPLE REGRESSION

(9) "Duration of Sound Prolongation and Sound/Syllable Repetition in Children Who Stutter: Preliminary Observations," by P. M. Zebrowski, April 1994, *Journal of Speech and Hearing Research, 37,* 254–263.

The purpose of this study was to measure the duration of sound prolongations and sound/syllable repetitions (stuttering) in the conversational speech of school-age children

who stutter. The correlation coefficients (R) between age (A), the duration of sound prolongations (SP), and the duration of sound/syllable repetitions (SSR) was summarized in the
table below.

Correlations ($N = 14$)	Age (A)	Sound Prolongations (SP)	Sound/Syllable Repetitions (SSR)
A	1.00		
SP	.36	1.00	
SSR	−.14	.05	1.00
Means:	8.2	706	724
Standard Deviations:	2.4	296	145

$r_{A,SP} = .36, r_{A, SSR} = -.14,$ and $r_{SP, SSR} = .05$

(a) With this information above, predict the SSR score of an incoming child whose age is
9.5 years old and whose SP score is 720.
(b) Find the multiple correlation coefficient (R^2) and test the significance of it at $\alpha = 5\%$.
(c) Find the standardized partial regression coefficients (β beta) and determine which of
the independent variables is the best predictor of SSR.

Solution

(a) There are three primary reasons why many researchers want to use multiple regression
analysis. They are as follows:

(i) By establishing the functional relationship between one dependent variable (Y) and
a group of two or more independent variables (X1, X2, . . . , XK), it will tell you how
each of two or more independent variables (X's) predicts the dependent variable (Y).
(ii) If you have no prior knowledge or empirical evidence for choosing a group of predictor variables, the multiple regression analysis would help you find which variables are associated most with a particular dependent variable.
(iii) A researcher may wish to test a theory to see if the sample data support the theory. Suppose the theory suggests that SSR score is influenced not only by age, but
also by SP score. A multiple regression analysis can be used to determine whether
or not SP score would add anything to the prediction of SSR score beyond what
can be predicted from age.

The idea behind multiple regression analysis is very similar to that of simple linear
regression. In simple linear regression, we predict one variable (Y) from another variable (X).
In multiple regression analysis, we would have two or more variables ($X_1, X_2, \ldots, X_K$) to predict one variable. Symbolically, a general equation for multiple regression analysis is given by

$$\hat{Y} = b_0 + b_1 X_1 + b_2 X_2 + \ldots + b_K X_K$$

where

$$\hat{Y} = \text{predictive value of } Y$$
$$b_0 = y\text{-intercept}$$
$$(b_1 \ldots, b_K) = \text{partial regression coefficients.}$$

$$(X_1, \ldots, X_K) = \text{independent variables.}$$

The set of the partial regression coefficients tells us how strong each X (the predictor) is associated with Y (predicted score).

In simple linear regression, r^2 gives a measure of the proportion of variance in Y which is predictable from X. The multiple correlation coefficient (R) can be squared (R^2) to measure the proportion of variance in Y which is predictable from several X's.

The reader must be aware of the complexities of calculating partial regression coefficients of multiple regression analysis that has more than two independent variables. When there are three or more independent variables, the mathematical deviation of a set of partial regression coefficients becomes increasingly abstract and difficult; therefore, the authors have decided to illustrate such calculations of b's only to a multiple regression with two independent variables. (Any statistical software package would calculate partial regression coefficients).

So now imagine that we have one dependent variable (Y) and two predictor variables (X_1, X_2), and we wish to graph them in three-dimensional space. The graph looks like the lines where the adjoining walls come together. The line which extends from the floor to the ceiling is the Y axis.

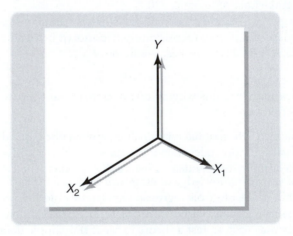

To plot sample data points, we simply take a set of values (Y, X_1, X_2) for each individual in a data set, locate them on their respective axes, and then find the point in space where those values meet. Repeating this process until all subjects are plotted, result in a collection of points suspended in space representing the data.

The multiple regression equation is the best-fit plane, not a line, through our swarm of points. The best-fit plane represents the predicted values at Y for a linear combination of X_1 and X_2. So whenever you wish to predict the value of Y, you can locate the point on the plane where X_1 and X_2 meet and then find the corresponding value of Y. This Y is the predictive value of Y, denoted by $\hat{Y}$. The y-intercept of the multiple regression, denoted by b_0, is the point on the Y axis where the regression plane intersects that axis. At this point, X_1 and X_2 are both equal to 0, therefore,

$$b_0 = \bar{Y} - b_1\bar{X}_1 - b_2\bar{X}_2$$

The partial regression coefficients give the relationship between Y and (X_1, X_2) for our example. The partial correlation coefficient b_1 represents the association between Y and X_1

while X_2 is constant; b_2 represents the association between Y and X_2 while X_1 is constant. The formulas for b_1 and b_2 are given by:

$$b_1 = \left[\frac{r_{YX1} - (r_{YX2}) \cdot (r_{X1X2})}{1 - r_{X1X2}^2}\right] \cdot \left(\frac{SY}{SX_1}\right)$$

$$b_2 = \left[\frac{r_{YX2} - (r_{YX1}) \cdot (r_{X1X2})}{1 - r_{X1X2}^2}\right] \cdot \left(\frac{SY}{SX_2}\right)$$

where:

r_{YX1} = correlation between Y and X_1

r_{YX2} = correlation between Y and X_2

r_{X1X2} = correlation between X_1 and X_2

S_{X1} = standard deviation of X_1

S_{X2} = standard deviation of X_2

S_Y = standard deviation of Y

b_1 = partial regression coefficient of X_1

b_2 = partial regression coefficient of X_2

For our example, we could find the multiple regression equation describing Y (SSR) for a linear combination of X_1 (Age) and X_2 (SP).

$$\bar{Y} = b_0 + b_1 X_1 + b_2 X_2$$

Step (1).   Find b_1 and b_2.

b_1 = partial regression coefficient of Age

$$= \left[\frac{r_{SSR, Age} - (r_{SSR, SP}) \cdot (r_{Age, SP})}{1 - r_{Age, SP}^2}\right] \cdot \left(\frac{S_{SSR}}{S_{Age}}\right)$$

$$= \left[\frac{(-.14) - (.05) \cdot (.36)}{1 - (.36)^2}\right] \cdot \left(\frac{145}{2.4}\right)$$

$$= \left(\frac{-.158}{.8704}\right) \cdot (60.417)$$

$$= -10.967$$

b_2 = partial regression coefficient of SP

$$= \left[\frac{r_{SSR, SP} - (r_{SSR, Age}) \cdot (r_{SP, Age})}{1 - r_{SP, Age}^2}\right] \cdot \left(\frac{S_{SSR}}{S_{SP}}\right)$$

$$= \left[\frac{(.05) - (-.14) \cdot (.36)}{1 - (.36)^2}\right] \cdot \left(\frac{145}{296}\right)$$

$$= \left(\frac{.1004}{.8704}\right) \cdot (.490) = .0565$$

Step (2). Find the y-intercept b

$$b_0 = \bar{Y}_{SSR} - (b_{Age} \cdot \bar{X}_{Age}) - (b_{SP} \cdot \bar{X}_{SP})$$

Given:

$$\bar{Y}_{SSR} = \text{the sample mean of } SSR = 724$$

$$b_{Age} = -10.967$$

$$\bar{X}_{Age} = \text{the sample mean of } Age = 8.2$$

$$b_{SP} = .0565$$

$$\bar{X}_{SP} = \text{the sample mean of } SP = 706$$

Hence, $b_0 = 724 - (-10.967) \cdot (8.2) - (.0565) \cdot (706)$

$$= 774.040$$

Step (3). Compute the value of $\hat{Y}$ using the multiple regression formula.
Recall that the incoming child is 9.5 years old and has 720 on SP.

$\bar{Y} = $ the best predictive *SSR* score given that he/she is 9.5 years old and has 720 on *SP*.

$$\bar{Y} = 774.04 + (-10.967) \cdot (9.5) + (.0565) \cdot (720)$$

$$= 710.534$$

(b) R^2 is a measure of the proportion of variance in Y (*SSR*) accounted for by X_1 (*Age*) and X_2 (*SP*). The value of R^2 can be calculated through the formula below.

$$R^2 = \frac{r_{YX_1}^2 + r_{YX_2}^2 - 2(r_{YX_1})(r_{YX_2})(r_{X_1 X_2})}{1 - r_{X_1 X_2}^2}$$

or for our example,

$$R^2 = \frac{r_{SSR, Age}^2 + r_{SSR, SP}^2 - 2(r_{SSR, Age})(r_{SSR, SP})(r_{Age, SP})}{1 - r_{Age, SP}^2}$$

$$= \frac{(-.14)^2 + (.05)^2 - 2(-.14) \cdot (.05)(.36)}{1 - (.36)^2}$$

$$= \frac{.02714}{.8704}$$

$$= .0312 \text{ or } 3.12\%$$

This tells us that approximately 3.12% of the variance in *SSR* score can be accounted for by the linear combination of *Age* and *SP* score.

Next, we will test the significance of R^2

Step (1).   State the null and alternative hypotheses.

H_0: $R^2 = 0$ (Not significant)
H_a: $R^2 \neq 0$ (Significant)

Step (2).   Calculate the observed F (F_{obs})

$$F_{obs} = \frac{R^2/K}{(1-R)^2/(N-K-1)}$$

with *d.f.* = numerator K, denominator $N - K - 1$

Where R^2 = square of multiple correlation coefficient
     K = number of independent variables
     N = number of subjects

For our example it gives:

$$F_{obs} = \frac{(.0312)/2}{(1-.0312)/(14-2-1)}$$

with *d.f.* = numerator 2, denominator 11

$$= \frac{.0156}{.9688/11}$$
$$= .177$$

Step (3).   Find the critical value of F (F_{crit}) and conclude from it under the decision rule. Since $F_{obs} = .177 < F_{crit}$ (.05, 2, 11) = 3.98, we do not therefore reject H_0 and conclude that there is no significant association between *SSR* scores and the combination of *Age* and *SP* scores.
(c) If the researcher wishes to determine which of the predictors (independent variables) are the best predictors of Y, then we would have to examine the partial regression coefficients in relation to each other; that is to say, we must calculate the standardized regression coefficients, denoted by the Greek letter β (beta), to determine the strength of associations between Y and each X.

Step (1).   Calculate $\hat{\beta}_{Age}$ and $\hat{\beta}_{SP}$

$$\hat{\beta}_{Age} = b_{Age} \cdot \frac{S_{Age}}{S_{SSR}}$$
$$= (-10.967) \cdot \frac{2.4}{145}$$
$$= -.182$$

$$\hat{\beta}_{SP} = b_{SP} \cdot \frac{S_{SP}}{S_{SSR}}$$
$$= (.0565) \cdot \frac{296}{145}$$
$$= .115$$

Step (2).   Take the absolute values of $\hat{\beta}_{Age}$ and $\hat{\beta}_{SP}$

$$|\hat{\beta}_{Age}| = |-.182| = .182$$

$$|\hat{\beta}_{SP}| = |.115| = .115$$

This indicates that *Age* is a slightly better predictor of *SSR* than *SP* is.

Calculation of the Power of a Statistical Test

Ideally, one wants to avoid (or at least minimize) making both Type I and Type II errors at the same time. Unfortunately, the two errors always work against one another. That is to say, if one tires to decrease α (Type I error), one is likely increase β (Type II error), and vice versa. In most cases, researchers pay more attention to a Type II error, because it is β that determines the power of a statistical test, denoted by $(1 - \beta)$.

The power represents the probability of rejecting a false null hypothesis correctly; that is, it is the ability of a statistical test to detect a difference between the mean under H_0 and the mean under H_1 when it exists. For example, researchers might suspect that the mean IQ score of a certain group of children is 105. Knowing the population mean score (μ) under the null hypothesis is 100, and the standard deviation (σ) is 15, the alternative mean is 105 for $n = 36$.

How do we calculate the power of this test? The following steps are necessary.

Step (1). State H_0 and H_1.

$H_0 : \mu_0 = 100$
$H_1 : \mu_1 = 105$

Step (2). Draw a diagram of two sampling distributions.

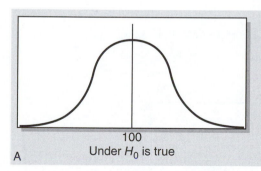

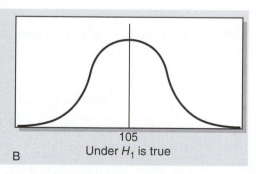

A   100
Under H_0 is true

B   105
Under H_1 is true

Step (3). Set up α (say, .05) and drop a line down through Z_{critical} to meet Figure B. The point at which this line meets the abscissa in Figure B is referred to as μ_M. Identify the "rejection areas" for both diagrams by drawing a dash line.

465

Figure A. H₀ is true

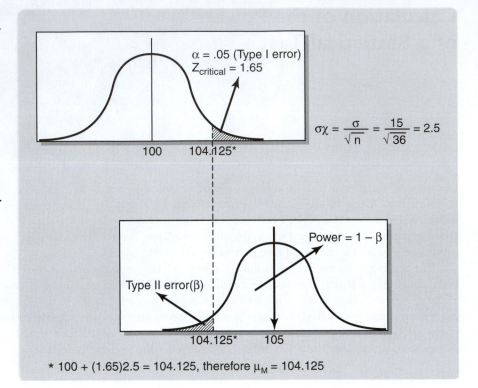

$$\sigma\chi = \frac{\sigma}{\sqrt{n}} = \frac{15}{\sqrt{36}} = 2.5$$

Figure B. H₁ is true

* 100 + (1.65)2.5 = 104.125, therefore μ_M = 104.125

Step (4). Calculate β and power.

Under Figure B, Z is calculated as

$$Z = \frac{104.125 - 105}{2.5} = -.35$$

Therefore, the probability of β is calculated as 50% − 13.68% = 36.32%.

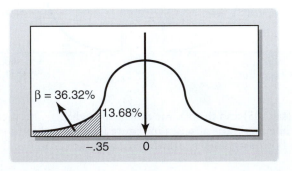

Hence, the power of the test is given by:

$$100\% - 36.32\% = 63.68\%$$

This means that given a specific alternative hypothesis, researchers will correctly reject a false null hypothesis about 63.68% of the time.

It is extremely important to do what you can to increase the power of a test. The following are some factors that influence power.

(i) Sample size (n): The power of a statistical test increases as the sample size increases, because increasing the sample size decreases the variability in the sampling distribution, which eventually increases power.

(ii) Significance level (α): As α increases, the power of a statistical test also increases, because the ability to detect a difference when it exists becomes better if you use a less credible level of significance.

(iii) Standard deviation (s or σ): The power of a statistical test increases if the standard deviation (s or σ) decreases.

In summary, the following decision table may be useful for understanding types of errors and power.

	H_0 is true	H_0 is false
Do not reject H_0	Correct decision ($1 - \alpha$)	Type II error (β)
Reject H_0	Type I error (α)	Correct decision power ($1 - \beta$)

Evidence-Based Medicine: Calculations of Various Probabilities with Nomogram

Evidence-based medicine (EBM) is the conscientious, explicit, and judicious use of current best evidence in making clinical decisions about the care of individual clients. The practice of EBM integrates individual clinical expertise with the best available external clinical evidence from systematic research. One of the clinical techniques, developed by the Oxford Centre for Evidence-Based Medicine, is the likelihood ratio nomogram. It calculates the posttest probability (posterior probability) for both positive and negative test results, by means of graphing that is based on pretest probability (prior probability), sensitivity, and specificity.

Let us now illustrate the necessary steps in calculating the posttest probability in the context of our example. (Readers should refer to Table 9-5 in Chapter 9 for calculation of several probabilities in determining the accuracy of a screening test.)

Step (1). Calculate the pretest probability for a positive test (prevalence) and a negative test.

$$P(D^+) = \text{Pretest probability for a positive test} = \frac{118 + 12}{1000} = .13$$

$$P(D^-) = \text{Pretest probability for a negative test} = \frac{113 + 757}{1000} = .87$$

Step (2). Calculate sensitivity, specificity, LR^+, and LR^-.

$$Sensitivity = P(T^+ \mid D^+) = \frac{118}{130} = .908$$

$$Specificity = P(T^- \mid D^-) = \frac{757}{870} = .87$$

$$LR^+ = \frac{Sensitivity}{1 - Specificity} = \frac{.908}{1 - .87} = 6.98$$

and

$$LR^- = \frac{1 - Sensitivity}{Specificity} = \frac{1 - .908}{.87} = .106$$

Step (3). Calculate pretest odds for a positive test (denoted by *PreOdds*(+)) and a negative test (denoted by *PreOdds*(−)).

$$PreOdds(+) = \frac{P(D^+)}{1 - P(D^+)} = \frac{.13}{1 - .13} = .15$$

$$PreOdds(-) = \frac{P(D^-)}{1 - P(D^-)} = \frac{.87}{1 - .87} = .6.69$$

Step (4). Calculate posttest odds for a positive test (denoted by *PostOdds*(+)) and a negative test (denoted by *PostOdds*(−)).

$$\text{Posttest odds } (+) = PreOdds\ (+) \cdot LR^+ = .15 \cdot 6.98 = 1.05$$

$$\text{Posttest odds } (-) = PreOdds\ (-) \cdot LR^- = 6.69 \cdot .106 = .71$$

Step (5). Calculate posttest probability for a positive test (denoted by *PostProb*(+)) and a negative test (denoted by *PostProb*(−)).

$$PostProb(+) = \frac{PostOdds(+)}{1 + PostOdds(+)} = \frac{1.05}{1 + 1.05} = .51$$

$$PostProb(-) = \frac{PostOdds(-)}{1 + PostOdds(-)} = \frac{.71}{1 + .71} = .42$$

Hence, (.13, .51) and (.87, .42) would be plotted on a nomogram curve. (See the following Nomogram table.).

Alternatively, instead of doing all of the above calculations, we could simply graph the posttest probability in relation to the pretest probability. Referring to our example, a value of the pretest probability or prevalence, (.13) would be plotted along the horizontal axis (*x* axis) and a value of the posttest probability (.51) would be plotted along the vertical axis (*y* axis). Similarly, we can write (.87, .42) for a negative test, where the first value represents the pretest probability and the second value represents the posttest probability. Applying the likelihood nomogram in making clinical decisions, we can answer the following three questions with respect to the levels of evidence and grades of recommendation established by EBM.

1. Are the results of the given diagnostic information valid?
2. Are the valid results of the diagnostic study important?
3. Can we apply this valid, important evidence about a diagnostic test in caring for your clients or a larger general target population?

Pretest Probability
This is the prevalence rate of a certain disorder, denoted by $P(D^+)$. It is calculated as

$$P(D^+) = \frac{\text{Number of disorders}}{\text{Total number of clients examined}}$$

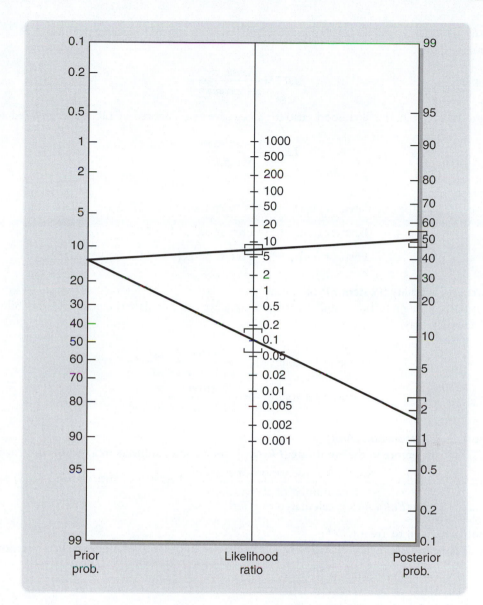

Prior prob. | Likelihood ratio | Posterior prob.

Pretest Odds

It is a ratio of events to nonevents. For instance, pretest odds for a positive test are calculated as $\dfrac{P(D^+)}{P(D^-)}$ and for a negative test, pretest odds are given by $\dfrac{P(D^-)}{P(D^+)}$.

Likelihood Ratio

This is the likelihood that a given test result would be expected in a client with the target disorder compared to the likelihood that the same test result would be expected in a client without that disorder. The likelihood ratio for a positive test, denoted by LR^+, is calculated as

$$LR^+ = \frac{Sensitivity}{1 - Specitivity}$$

By the same token, the likelihood ratio for a negative test, denoted by LR^-, is calculated as

$$LR^- = \frac{1 - Sensitivity}{Specificity}$$

Posttest Odds

These odds can be calculated as Posttest Odds = Pretest Odds · LR. More specifically,

$$\text{Posttest odds } (+) = \text{Pretest odds } (+) \cdot LR^+$$

$$\text{Posttest odds } (-) = \text{Pretest odds } (-) \cdot LR^-$$

Posttest Probability (Posterior Probability)

By updating the pretest probability with new data, we can calculate the posttest probability. It is calculated as

$$\text{Posttest probability } (+) = \frac{\text{Posttest Odds } (+)}{1 + \text{Posttest odds } (+)}$$

$$\text{Posttest probability } (-) = \frac{\text{Posttest Odds } (-)}{1 + \text{Posttest odds } (-)}$$

Absolute Risk Reduction (ARR)

ARR is the difference in the event rate (*ER*, the proportion of subjects in a group wherein an event is observed, i.e., $\frac{\text{Number of observations of an event}}{\text{Total number of observations}}$) between a control group (*CER*) and a treated group (*EER*). *ARR* is calculated as $|CER - EER|$.

Number Needed to Treat (NNT)

This is the number of subjects who need to be treated in order to prevent one bad outcome. It is the inverse of *ARR*; that is, $NNT = \frac{1}{ARR}$.

Sample Calculation of ARR and NNT

In a randomized clinical trial study, the effects of two treatment approaches for clients with a particular voice disorder was evaluated. 10.5% of the clients were randomly assigned to a control group and 4.4% of the clients were randomly assigned to the experimental group. Calculate *ARR* and *NNT* for the study.

Solution

$$ARR = |CER - EER| = |10.5\% - 4.4\%| = 6.1\%$$

$$NNT = \frac{1}{ARR} = \frac{1}{6.1\%} = \frac{1}{.061} = 16.4 \text{ or } 17$$

Therefore, we need to treat 17 clients with the experimental therapy to prevent one from developing the voice disorder.

The purpose of this section was to introduce some common performance measures of the likelihood nomogram, show how to use and compute the pretest and posttest probabilities, and give some intuitive understanding of the method. More mathematically inclined readers are encouraged to select one or more of the books on the subject in the bibliography for further reading.

Measures of Disorder/Disease Occurrence

Descriptive Studies

According to our view, studies can be best classified based on the degree to which they explain the causal relations among variables. In achieving this goal, the weakest of the lot are *descriptive studies*, or those intended to observe, illustrate, record, classify, or by other means attempt to clarify the distinctive features of research variables. The methods of description include surveys, case histories, clinical reports, prevalence/incidence studies, and field studies. Such studies often result in a better understanding of phenomena as they exist *in the here and now*, thereby establishing the conditions for later scientific work when questions as to the relationship among variables might arise.

Prevalence/Incidence

Measures of disorder occurrence describe either the pool of actual existing cases, or the occurrence of new cases. *Prevalence* is defined as the proportion of the target population who carry a particular disorder (under discussion) at one specific point in time, whereas *incidence* is defined as the frequency of disorder occurrence of new cases during a time period. Each subject is categorized into two states, namely disorder (D^+) or normal (D^-). The prevalence, in this framework, is the proportion of the given population that is in D^+ at a specific time. The incidence describes the rate of flow from D^- to D^+.

The magnitude of prevalence always depends on incidence, because a greater rate of occurrence of new cases will be likely to increase the number of actual existing cases. We will now present the formulas for two specific measures of disorder occurrence. The first one is a prevalence measure, and the second is an incidence measure.

Prevalence

Prevalence, denoted by P, is calculated as follows:

$$P = \frac{\text{Number of subjects carrying the disorder at a specific time}}{\text{Size of a target population at that point in time}}$$

or symbolically,

$$P = \frac{D^+}{N}$$

A $(1 - \alpha)$ confidence interval for P is given as

$$P \pm \left| Z_{\frac{\alpha}{2}} \right| \cdot \sqrt{\frac{P \cdot (1 - P)}{N}}$$

Example: Adapted From the Article, "Epidemiology of Stuttering in the Community Across the Entire Life Span," by A. Craig, et al December 2002, *Journal of Speech, Language, and Hearing Research, 45*, 1097–1105.

The authors of the article conducted an extensive study ($N = 12,131$) to investigate the number and age of the persons living in their household who stuttered (prevalence) of respondents of a telephone interview. Contingent upon the households' permissions, a series of corroborative questions were asked and permission was requested to record the speech of the person who stutters. Confirmation of stuttering was based on (1) a positive detection of stuttering from the taped phone conversation and (2) an affirmative answer to at least one of the corroborative questions supporting the diagnosis. The following table summarizes the results of their study.

Age (yrs)	SC	PSC	# Makes	Total N
2–5	10	10	389	720
6–10	13	18	465	902
11–20	10	32	1006	1881
21–50	42	71	2607	5405
Over 50	12	45	1556	3207
All ages	87	176	6023	12,131

Where SC = stuttering cases, PSC = prior stuttering cases

Find the prevalence (P) and its 95% confidence interval for the age 2–5 category.

Age 2–5

$$P = \frac{10}{720} = .014 \text{ or } 1.4\%$$

95% C.I. for P

$$.014 \pm \left| Z_{\frac{.05}{2}} \right| \cdot \sqrt{\frac{.014 \cdot (1 - .014)}{720}}$$
$$= .014 \pm 1.96 \cdot (.00438)$$
$$= (.0054, .0226)$$

Incidence

The basic measure of disorder occurrence, "incidence rate," denoted by I, is calculated as follows:

$$I = \frac{\text{Number of disorder cases that occur in a population during a period of time}}{\text{Sum for each subject in the population of the length of time at risk of having the disorder}}$$

or, symbolically,

$$I = \frac{A}{R}$$

where A represents the quantity in the numerator

    R represents the quantity in the denominator and is often referred to as "risk time"

    A $(1 - \alpha)$ confidence interval for I is given as

$$I \pm \left| Z_{\frac{\alpha}{2}} \right| \cdot \sqrt{\frac{I}{R}}$$

Note: The basic probability model for incidence rates is called the *Poisson distribution*. The confidence interval is based on the normal approximation of the Poisson distribution.

Hypothetically, in the table in our example, 25 were found to be confirmed stuttering cases among subjects aged 6–10 in 2002. The number of risk time was 38,287 for subjects in that age group. Find the incidence rate I and the 95% confidence interval for I.

With the symbolic notations used here $A = 25$ and $R = 38{,}287$. Hence,

$$I = \frac{25}{38{,}287} = .000653$$

The 95% confidence interval is computed as

$$= .000653 \pm \left| Z_{\frac{.05}{2}} \right| \cdot \sqrt{\frac{.000653}{38287}}$$

$$= .000653 \pm 1.96 \cdot (.0001306)$$

$$= .000653 \pm .000256$$

$$= (.000397, \ .000909)$$

The Relationship Between Prevalence (P) and Incidence Rate (I)

As we noted earlier, prevalence is dependent on the incidence rate and the duration of a particular disorder. This association can be expressed as follows:

$$\frac{P}{1 - P} = I \cdot B$$

where B denotes average duration of the disorder.

The denominator of the fraction that appears on the left-hand side of the equation above represents the part of the population that is free from the disorder. It is included in the formula because only those who are free from the disorder are at risk of getting it. Therefore, in case of rare disorders, $(1 - P)$ will get closer to 1; that is, P is very small. Then the formula will be revised as simply $P = I \cdot B$.

Flowchart for Classical Statistical Approach versus Bayesian Statistical Approach in Hypothesis Testing

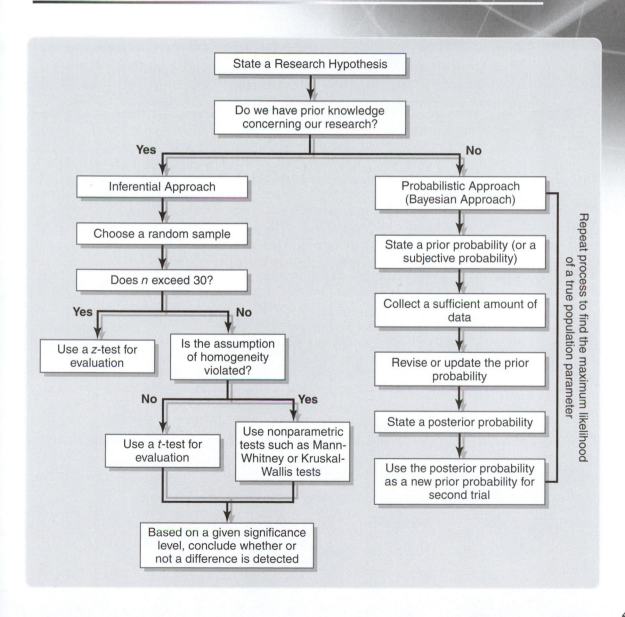

State a Research Hypothesis

Do we have prior knowledge concerning our research?

Yes / **No**

Inferential Approach

Probabilistic Approach (Bayesian Approach)

Choose a random sample

State a prior probability (or a subjective probability)

Does *n* exceed 30?

Yes / **No**

Collect a sufficient amount of data

Use a *z*-test for evaluation

Is the assumption of homogeneity violated?

Revise or update the prior probability

No / **Yes**

State a posterior probability

Use a *t*-test for evaluation

Use nonparametric tests such as Mann-Whitney or Kruskal-Wallis tests

Use the posterior probability as a new prior probability for second trial

Repeat process to find the maximum likelihood of a true population parameter

Based on a given significance level, conclude whether or not a difference is detected

Partial Listing of Scholastic and Professional Journals Relevant to the Field of Communication Sciences and Disorders

A.A.C., Augmentative and Alternative Communication
A.S.H.A., Journal of the American Speech-Language-Hearing Association
Academic Therapy
Acta Oto-Laryngologica
Advances in Speech-Language Pathology
Alzheimer's Disease and Associated Disorders
American Annals of the Deaf
American Journal of Audiology
American Journal of Mental Deficiency
American Journal of Mental Retardation
American Journal of Otolaryngology
American Journal of Otology
American Journal of Speech-Language Pathology
Annals of Dyslexia
Annals of Neurology
Annals of Otology, Rhinology, Laryngology
Annual Review of Language Acquisition
Aphasiology
Applied Linguistics
Applied Psycholinguistics
Archives of Otolaryngology
Archives of Otolaryngology—Head and Neck Surgery
Audecibel
Audiological Medicine
Audiology: A Journal of Auditory Communication
Auris, Nasus, Larynx
Australian Journal of Human Communication Disorders

Behavior Research and Therapy
Brain and Cognition
Brain and Language
Brain Impairment
Brain Injury
British Journal of Audiology
British Journal of Disorders of Communication

Child Language Teaching and Therapy
Cleft Palate Bulletin
Cleft Palate Journal
Cleft Palate—Craniofacial Journal
Clinical Linguistics & Phonetics
Clinics in Communication Disorders
Cognitive Neuropsychology
Cognitive Rehabilitation

D.S.H. Abstracts
Developmental Medicine & Child Neurology
Dysphagia

Ear and Hearing
European Journal of Disorders of Communication
Exceptional Children

Folia Phoniatrica
Folia Phoniatrica et Logopaedica

Health Communication
Hearing Journal
Hearing Rehabilitation Quarterly
Human Communication
Human Communication Canada

Index to Speech, Language & Hearing Journal Titles, 1954–78
Intervention in School and Clinic

Journal of Auditory Research
Journal of Autism and Developmental Disorders
Journal of Child Language
Journal of Childhood Communication Disorders
Journal of Cognitive Neuroscience
Journal of Cognitive Rehabilitation
Journal of Communication Disorders
Journal of Computer Users in Speech and Hearing
Journal of Fluency Disorders
Journal of Head Trauma Rehabilitation
Journal of Learning Disabilities
Journal of Motor Behavior
Journal of Multilingual Communication Disorders
Journal of Negative Results in Speech and Audio Sciences
Journal of Rehabilitation of the Deaf
Journal of Special Education
Journal of Speech and Hearing Research
Journal of Speech-Language Pathology and Audiology
Journal of the Academy of Rehabilitative Audiology

Journal of the Acoustical Society of America
Journal of the American Academy of Audiology
Journal of the American Audiology Society
Journal of the American Auditory Society
Journal of the American Deafness and Rehabilitation Association
Journal of Voice

Language and Cognitive Processes
Language and Intercultural Communication
Language and Language Behavior Abstracts
Language, Speech and Hearing Services in Schools
Language Testing
Laryngoscope
Learning Disability Quarterly
Linguistics and Language Behavior Abstracts

Memory & Cognition
Mind & Language

Newsounds

Otolaryngology—Head and Neck Surgery

Perspectives in Education and Deafness
Perspectives on Dyslexia
Phonetica

R.A.S.E., Remedial and Special Education
Reading and Writing
Rehabilitation Literature
Remedial and Special Education

Seminars in Hearing
Seminars in Speech and Language
Sign Language Studies
Specific Learning Disabilities Gazette
Studies in Communication Sciences

Topics in Early Childhood Special Education
Topics in Language Disorders

Volta Review
Volta Voices

Evidence-Based Practice Reference Analysis Worksheet

Reprinted with permission from the Department of Communicative Disorders and Sciences, Wichita State University.[*]

Wichita State University
Evidence-Based Practice Reference Analysis Worksheet[1]

Check one: ☐ Assessment article   ☐ Intervention article

Reference:

_____

_____

Purpose Statement:

_____

_____

Participants:

a. Level of evidence: _____ (see descriptors on page 3)

b. Number of participants: Total #: _____   Total #/group: _____

c. Participant selection: (age, gender, disorder-type, native language, etc.):

_____

_____

d. Quality of participant description:

1	2	3	4	5
can't replicate		may be able to replicate		replicable
lacks sign. info		mostly complete info		all info present

Comments: _____

Method:

a. Evaluation tools:

_____

_____

[1]Based on American Academy for Cerebral Palsy and Developmental Medicine, 2002; ASHA, 2002; Ashford, 2002; Law, 2000; Technical Report: Evidence-Based Practice in Communication Disorders (RSAC, 2003)

*Note: The Department of Communicative Disorders and Sciences, Wichita State University, would like to acknowledge that this document is always a work in progress and that many individuals at WSU had input in its development.

Quality of evaluation tools:

1	2	3	4	5
seems inappropriate		appropriate		appropriate
no rationale		no rationale		rationale for use

Comments: _____

b. Procedures:

_____

_____

c. Time period: _____

d. Reliability/validity/control of bias:

1	2	3	4	5
no controls		some control		controls used
inadequate		minimally adequate		adequate

Comments: _____

e. Outcome measures/Dependent variables:

_____

_____

Quality of Outcome Measures/DVs:

1	2	3	4	5
seems inappropriate		appropriate		appropriate
no rationale		no rationale		rationale for use

Comments: _____

Results:

a. Significant findings/Strong effect sizes:

_____

_____

b. Means and standard deviations

_____

c. Other findings

_____

_____

d. Interpretation of results:

1	2	3	4	5
interpretation		some extension of		data related
beyond data		interpretation beyond data		tied to past research

Comments: _____

Overall comments:

Credibility of Source:

1	2	3	4	5
source unknown		trade journal or		peer-reviewed
self-published/reported		edited publication		professional journal

Comments: _____

Feasibility of use in a clinical setting:

1	2	3	4	5
unlikely		possible, with some modifications		highly likely

Comments: _____

Ideas for future research:

Levels of Evidence:

Level		May use when:
1	Large randomized controlled trials	Identified population matches client seen and clinical setting
2	Small randomized controlled trials; repeated randomized single-case designs	Identified population matches clients seen and clinical setting; Identified case matches client seen and clinical setting
3	Non-randomized study with control group(s); single-case design using alternating treatments or multiple baseline methods	Identified population matches clients seen and clinical setting; Identified case matches client seen and clinical setting
4	Case control study	Identified case matches client seen and clinical setting
5	Data from basic research with theoretical implications for clinical services	No evidence is available from aforementioned levels
6	Opinion of clinical expert	No evidence is available from aforementioned levels

Meta-Analysis Review

Check one: ☐ Assessment article   ☐ Intervention article

Reference:
_____

_____

Purpose Statement:
_____

_____

Number of Studies: _____

1	2	3	4	5
seems inappropriate		appropriate		appropriate

Comments: _____

Time Range for Inclusion: _____

| 1 | 2 | 3 | 4 | 5 |

seems inappropriate   appropriate   appropriate

Comments: _____

Types of Designs Included: Check all applicable: ☐ Large randomised controlled trials ☐ Small randomized controlled trials ☐ Repeated randomized single-case designs ☐ Non-randomized study with control group(s) ☐ Single-case design using alternating treatments or multiple baseline methods ☐ Case control study ☐ Case reports

| 1 | 2 | 3 | 4 | 5 |

seems inappropriate   appropriate   appropriate

Comments: _____

Criteria for Inclusion in Meta-Analysis:

_____

Comments: _____

Variables Studied:

_____

Comments: _____

Main Points/Strategies Found to be Effective:

_____

Comments: _____

Effect Size: _____

Comments: _____

Interpretation of results:

| 1 | 2 | 3 | 4 | 5 |

interpretation   some extension of   data related
beyond data   interpretation beyond data tied to past research

Comments: _____

Credibility of source:

| 1 | 2 | 3 | 4 | 5 |

source unknown   trade journal or   peer-reviewed
self-published/reported edited publication professional journal

Comments: _____

NIH Grant Application Form Example

Form Approved Through 09/30/2007

OMB No. 0925-0001

Department of Health and Human Services
Public Health Services

Grant Application

Do not exceed character length restrictions indicated.

LEAVE BLANK—FOR PHS USE ONLY.		
Type	Activity	Number
Review Group		Formerly
Council/Board (Month, Year)		Date Received

1. TITLE OF PROJECT *(Do not exceed 81 characters, including spaces and punctuation.)*

Vocabulary Expansion in Severe MR

2. RESPONSE TO SPECIFIC REQUEST FOR APPLICATIONS OR PROGRAM ANNOUNCEMENT OR SOLICITATION ☒ NO ☐ YES
(If "Yes," state number and title)
Number: _____ Title: _____

3. PRINCIPAL INVESTIGATOR/PROGRAM DIRECTOR | New Investigator ☒ No ☐ Yes

3a. NAME (Last, first, middle)	3b. DEGREE(S)	3h. eRA Commons User Name
Krista M. Wilkinson	BA MA PhD.	

3c. POSITION TITLE
Assistant Professor

3d. MAILING ADDRESS *(Street, city, state, zip code)*
Emerson College
120 Boylston St.
Boston MA
02116

3e. DEPARTMENT, SERVICE, LABORATORY, OR EQUIVALENT
Communication Sciences & Disorders

3f. MAJOR SUBDIVISION

3g. TELEPHONE AND FAX *(Area code, number and extension)*
TEL: (617) 824- FAX: (617) 824-

E-MAIL ADDRESS:

4. HUMAN SUBJECTS RESEARCH
☐ No ☒ Yes

4b. Human Subjects Assurance No.

4c. Clinical Trial ☒ No ☐ Yes
4d. NIH-defined Phase III Clinical Trial ☒ No ☐ Yes

4a. Research Exempt ☒ No ☐ Yes
If "Yes," Exemption No. _____

5. VERTEBRATE ANIMALS ☒ No ☐ Yes
5a. If "Yes," IACUC approval Date
5b. Animal welfare assurance no.

6. DATES OF PROPOSED PERIOD OF SUPPORT *(month, day, year—MM/DD/YY)*

From	Through
6/1/02	4/31/03

7. COSTS REQUESTED FOR INITIAL BUDGET PERIOD

7a. Direct Costs ($)	7b. Total Costs ($)
$	$

8. COSTS REQUESTED FOR PROPOSED PERIOD OF SUPPORT

8a. Direct Costs ($)	8b. Total Costs ($)
$	$

9. APPLICANT ORGANIZATION
Name
Address   Emerson College
120 Boylston St.
Boston MA
02116

10. TYPE OF ORGANIZATION
Public: → ☐ Federal ☐ State ☐ Local
Private: → ☒ Private Nonprofit
For-profit: → ☐ General ☐ Small Business
☐ Woman-owned ☐ Socially and Economically Disadvantaged

11. ENTITY IDENTIFICATION NUMBER
TIN:
DUNS NO. _____ Cong. District _____

12. ADMINISTRATIVE OFFICIAL TO BE NOTIFIED IF AWARD IS MADE
Name
Title   Vice President for Academic Affairs
Address   Emerson College
120 Boylston St.
Boston MA
02116
Tel: (617) 824- FAX: (617) 824-
E-Mail:

13. OFFICIAL SIGNING FOR APPLICANT ORGANIZATION
Name
Title   Vice President for Academic Affairs
Address   Emerson College
120 Boylston St.
Boston MA
02116
Tel: (617) 824- FAX: (617) 824-
E-Mail:

14. PRINCIPAL INVESTIGATOR/PROGRAM DIRECTOR ASSURANCE: I certify that the statements herein are true, complete and accurate to the best of my knowledge. I am aware that any false, fictitious, or fraudulent statements or claims may subject me to criminal, civil, or administrative penalties. I agree to accept responsibility for the scientific conduct of the project and to provide the required progress reports if a grant is awarded as a result of this application.

SIGNATURE OF PI/PD NAMED IN 3a.
(In ink. "Per" signature not acceptable.)
DATE

15. APPLICANT ORGANIZATION CERTIFICATION AND ACCEPTANCE: I certify that the statements herein are true, complete and accurate to the best of my knowledge, and accept the obligation to comply with Public Health Services terms and conditions if a grant is awarded as a result of this application. I am aware that any false, fictitious, or fraudulent statements or claims may subject me to criminal, civil, or administrative penalties.

SIGNATURE OF OFFICIAL NAMED IN 13.
(In ink. "Per" signature not acceptable.)
DATE

Example of a Poster Session Presentation (Reprinted with permission of Krista M. Wilkinson)

Use of Mutual Exclusivity and/or N3C for Word Learning by Second Language Learners

Krista M. Wilkinson, Ph.D.
Neha Shah, BA.
Emerson College
Communication Sciences & Disorders

Poster presented at the annual conference of the
American Speech-Language-Hearing Association,
2003, Chicago IL

• This research was supported by R29 HD 35107 from the National Institute of Child Health.

• Thanks to all the children, families, and staff at Lexicare Children's Center for their time and enthusiasm for this project.

• Thanks to Aranya Albert, Kristen Lombard, and Sharon Wang for data collection.

Abstract

A common observation is that during early word learning, children appear to adhere to one or both of two assumptions: (a) that new labels do not refer to already-labeled items, but instead (b) that they refer to unlabeled items. These two assumptions have been called *Mutual Exclusivity* (ME) and *Novel-Name, Nameless-Category* (N3C), respectively. Yet the experience of children learning a second language is not wholly consistent with these assumptions, because known items commonly do have more than one label. Do second language learners demonstrate ME/N3C? Does exposure to new word-referent relations through ME/N3C result in actual word learning? In this poster, we evaluated whether children learning first and second languages adhered to these assumptions, and how well the assumptions led to actual word learning in familiar or unfamiliar languages.

Background: Early word learning

One well-documented phenomenon of early language is the remarkable rate of vocabulary expansion. Infants at the outset of lexical development learn an average of three new words a week; older toddler and preschool-aged children seem to learn multiple new words daily (e.g., Bates, Dale, & Thal, 1995). One candidate process for explaining this rapid vocabulary acquisition is "fast mapping" (Carey & Bartlett, 1978). Fast mapping refers to children's ability to sketch partial maps of a word's meaning even after brief and oftentimes incidental exposure (Rice, 1989).

One commonly used task for studying or eliciting fast mapping is illustrated in Figure 1, along with a conceptualization of children's possible responses. The child is presented with three items. Two are familiar, already-labeled items, and one is unknown to the child. What does the child do if he hears a novel, unfamiliar label?

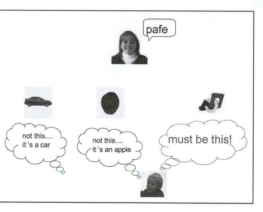

What supports children's fast mapping? It has been proposed that children learn general strategies for "disambiguating" or figuring out word meaning (Merriman & Bowman, 1989) that then lead to fast mapping itself. For instance, one proposal is that during the second year of life, children learn that new words most likely do not refer to already-labeled items. Under this proposal, the child's selection of a novel item upon hearing the word "pafe" reflects his assumption that a novel label does not refer to the car or apple picture. This assumption has been called "mutual exclusivity" of word meaning (ME; Markman, 1989). A slightly different proposal argues that children assume that novel labels refer to unnamed referents. On this assumption, the child hearing the word "pafe" will actively seek an unnamed referent to match to this label. This assumption has been called "novel name – nameless category" (N3C; Golinkoff, Mervis, & Hirsh-Pasek, 1994).

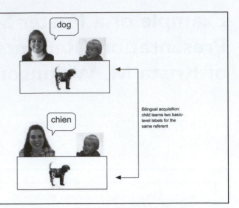

dog

chien

Bilingual acquisition: child learns two basic-level labels for the same referent

Research Question #1

Both the ME and the N3C assumptions derive from children's general experience with the way words work. In monolingual speakers, these assumptions are relatively accurate. However, Figure 2 illustrates that the experiences of children learning a second language are not necessarily consistent with either assumption. In contrast to ME, objects regularly are assigned more than one basic-level name; one in the first language, another in the second language. In contrast to N3C, novel labels in a second language often refer to objects that already have names in the first language.

Because the experiences of children learning two languages are not necessarily consistent with the ME/N3C assumptions, it seems reasonable to ask: Are the two assumptions demonstrated as reliably in second language learners as in monolingual learners?

Research Question #2

The interest in fast mapping (and its underlying ME/N3C assumptions) derives from the proposal that it provides at least one mechanism supporting actual vocabulary learning (e.g., Markman, 1989; Golinkoff et al., 1994). Yet little research has actually examined if, indeed, presence of ME/N3C leads to effective and efficient word learning. From the standpoint of second language learning, the issue is also complicated by features of the task not necessarily related to the child's semantic capabilities. A child who is dominant in one language and then begins to learn a second must attune her ear to an unfamiliar phonological system (phonemic inventory and phonotactic rules), one that oftentimes includes distinctions not made in the native tongue.

To what extent does the challenge of learning words in a relatively unfamiliar phonological system affect actual word learning outcomes after ME/N3C experiences?

- Subject information
  - Six participants in each of 3 groups
  - language status obtained from family interview & score on PPVT (in English)
  - Group information on the next panel

- Research environment/approach:
  - computer presented stimuli
  - computer recorded responses
  - general feedback provided ("you're working so hard ")

- Data analysis:
  - performance on ME/N3C trials compared for groups
  - performance on tests for learning compared across groups and across two instruction protocols
  - order or protocols alternated randomly across participants

Subjects

Group	CA (mos)	PPVT (mos)
ESL	49 [a] (40-58)	31** [c] (25-40)
BIL	50 [a] (45-58)	52 [b] (36-72)
ENG	48 [a] (40-57)	52 [b] (40-64)

** = all ESL participants scored at least 10 months below chronological age on age-equivalent of PPVT (administered in English)

[a] = statistical analysis confirmed that the three groups did not differ on this measure

[b] = statistical analysis confirmed that BIL and ENG groups did not differ on this measure

[c] = statistical analysis confirmed that ESL group was significantly lower on this measure than the other two groups

This study used procedures developed in previous research that examined the relative efficacy of two approaches to teaching two novel word-referent relations. The previous research consistently demonstrated that one procedure (*successive introduction*) resulted in significantly more reliable learning of two new words than the other (*concurrent introduction*). The procedures included two phases, each of which addressed a the research question:

- Instructional/exposure phase: During this phase, the child is asked to demonstrate behavior consistent with ME/N3C; selecting a novel item when presented with a novel label. This phase probes Research Question #1.

- Testing phase: During this phase, the child is asked to demonstrate how well s/he has learned the relations between each of two new words and its referent. This phase probes Research Question #2.

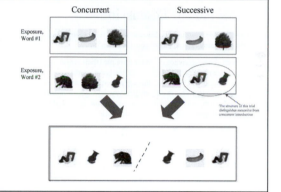

Results

• Instructional/exposure phase : During this phase, the child is asked to demonstrate behavior consistent with ME/N3C; selecting a novel item when presented with a novel label. This phase probes Research Question #1.

    • Participants in all groups showed virtually error-free performance on the 24 instruction trials.
        • ESL: 99% accurate on concurrent, 97% accurate on successive introduction
        • BIL: 100% accurate on concurrent, 99% accurate on successive introduction
        • ENG: 97% accurate on concurrent, 96% accurate on successive introduction

• Testing phase : During this phase, the child is asked to demonstrate how well s/he has learned the relations between each of two new words and its referent. This phase probes Research Question #2.

    • As illustrated in Figure 4, both BIL and ENG children performed well on learning tests irrespective of procedure. ESL children performed equally well as their peers when tested under successive introduction conditions, but significantly worse under concurrent introduction.

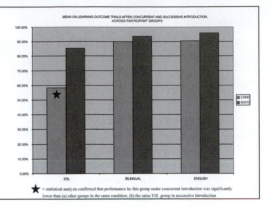

MEAN ON LEARNING OUTCOME TRIALS AFTER CONCURRENT AND SUCCESSIVE INTRODUCTION, ACROSS PARTICIPANT GROUPS

★ = statistical analysis confirmed that performance by this group under concurrent introduction was significantly lower than (a) other groups in the same condition, (b) the same ESL group in successive introduction

Discussion

• Are the two assumptions demonstrated as reliably in second language learners as in monolingual learners?

Yes. The experience of having multiple labels for single exemplars does not interfere with the basic lexical assumptions of ME/N3C, that are presumed to underlie fast mapping. This is demonstrated by the highly accurate performances of all children, including those in the ESL and BIL groups, on the 24 exposure trials.

• To what extent does the challenge of learning words from a relatively unfamiliar phonological system affect actual word learning outcomes after ME/N3C experiences?

Although ME/N3C are clearly operating in the ESL learners, acquisition of maps (fast or otherwise) on the basis of these assumptions was not necessarily independent of other factors, in this case, phonological and instructional factors. This is demonstrated by the observation that ESL children acquiring words in a language with a relatively unfamiliar phonological structure required the support available in the successive introduction procedure. With that support, they learned equally well as their peers who were learning words from their native language.

Answers to Self-Learning Reviews

Chapter 1. History and Philosophy of Science

1. explain; predict; control
2. animistic; deities
3. quantifiable or mathematical; Empirical; theories
4. causal; variables
5. theoretical; relations
6. science; valid; reliable
7. research; statistical
8. verb; noun
9. means; ends
10. hypothesis; conditions
11. interconnected; causally
12. laws; probability; error
13. Logical; inductive; deductive
14. form; content
15. empiricism
16. objective; speculative
17. operationism; concepts; constructs
18. Variables
19. operationally
20. independent; dependent
21. hypothesis; controlled
22. Inductive; deductive
23. idols; cave; culture
24. operational; measurement
25. empirical; parsimonious; heuristic; questions; acceptable
26. Qualitative; multiple; triangulation
27. theories
28. eclectic; technician
29. literacy; content; shortcomings
30. efficacy; NOMS; outcome
31. functional communication measures
32. validity; reliability
33. clinical scientist; scientific method
34. code; ethics; competence; effectiveness
35. scientific perspective

Chapter 2. Getting Started: Basic Concepts of Research

1. describe; hypothesized; means
2. variables
3. Descriptive; classify; categorize
4. variables; association
5. correlated
6. causal relations
7. between-group; within-group
8. control
9. independent; dependent
10. extensive; intensive; subjects/participants
11. reliability; replication
12. qualitative
13. ethnographic
14. qualitative; viewpoint
15. spoken; written; discourse
16. measurements
17. assignment; manipulation; control
18. Quasi
19. randomization; true
20. constructed; matching; confounding
21. randomization; matching; equivalence
22. ex post facto
23. circularity
24. coefficient
25. scientific; thinking; action
26. blueprint
27. introduction
28. internal; external; generalizable
29. Descriptive; Inferential; sample; population
30. sample; true
31. probability; confidence
32. presenting; explaining; hypotheses; Interpretation
33. subjects/participants; harm

Chapter 3. Selecting a Research Problem

1. descriptive; categorize; classify
2. diagnostic criteria
3. question; rationale; feasibility
4. interpret; understand; predict
5. Federal Register; NIH
6. NIDCD, or National Institute of Deafness and other Communicative Disorders
7. frequency; citations
8. trivial; consequential
9. question; hypothesis; testable
10. criterion of testability
11. protection; IRB, or institutional review board; compliance
12. risk; benefit; informed; consent

Chapter 4. Reviewing Literature and Stating Research Problems

1. research question; hypothesis
2. null; rejected
3. $\mu_X = \mu_Y$; $\mu_X \neq \mu_Y$
4. $\mu_X > \mu_Y$; $\mu_X < \mu_Y$
5. rejection; statistical testing
6. Type I; Type II
7. Type I; false positive; type II; false negative
8. alpha; beta
9. rejected; $< .05$; $< .01$
10. before
11. not yet proved; inconclusive
12. null hypothesis
13. false positive; convicting; innocent
14. false negative; convict; guilty
15. Bayesian Method
16. probabilities; prior; data; posterior
17. prior
18. probability
19. prior; posterior
20. paradigm
21. data; hypothesis; theory
22. groups; individual
23. systematic replication

Chapter 5. Sampling Theory and Methods

1. population; causal inference; elements
2. parameter; statistic
3. target population; sampling error; chance
4. random assignment
5. ideal; actual
6. internally valid inference; externally valid inference
7. equal chance; selected; 50/20,000 or .0025 or .25%
8. sampling frame; targeted
9. Systematic
10. sampling interval; N/n; 20; 1; 4,000; random; 20th
11. Periodicity
12. Stratified; strata
13. Cluster
14. probability proportionate to size; PPS; number of clusters selected; cluster size/population size; elements selected per cluster/cluster size
15. .03 or 3%
16. sampling error; homogenous
17. Consecutive; limited; stringent; reduce; generality
18. Response rate; validity
19. Convenience
20. purposive; unrepresentative
21. Snowballing

22. matching
23. rank ordering; matched pairs; randomly
24. differences
25. independent; levels; randomly; randomized block
26. a priori
27. ex post facto
28. Errors in sampling; chance
29. inclusion criteria; exclusion criteria; bias
30. pilot study; methodological
31. Bernoulli; indefinitely
32. homogenous; smaller; heterogeneous; larger
33. precision; sample statistic
34. effect size
35. 10; 20; 30; 30; 15

Chapter 6. Controlling, Measuring, and Recording Variables

1. independent; phenomenon; dependent; independent
2. systematic variance; between-group variance
3. directionality
4. controlled experimental studies
5. organismic
6. systematic variance; error variance; $\dfrac{V_b}{V_e}$
7. errors; fluctuations
8. Within-group
9. systematic errors
10. constancy; measurements; subject responses; testing
11. Intraobserver; Interobserver
12. counterbalancing
13. Order effects
14. eliminate; elimination
15. constancy; conditions
16. homogenous
17. Analysis; covariance
18. double-blind investigation
19. sensitive; specific
20. Ceiling effects; sensitive; floor effect; insensitive
21. systematic; unsystematic; $\dfrac{\text{True Score}}{\text{True Score} + \text{Error Score}}$
22. Test-retest; alternate-forms
23. split-half reliability estimate; .86
24. dichotomous; continuous; averages; inter-item correlations
25. stability; accuracy
26. $\dfrac{\text{\# of agreements}}{\text{Total \# of cases}}$

27. kappa (k); $\dfrac{0-c}{1-c}$ or $\dfrac{\text{Observed} - \text{Chance}}{1 - \text{Chance}}$

28. Content; sampling validity
29. Criterion; predictive; theoretical construct; concurrent; valid
30. Construct
31. convergence; discriminant
32. dichotomous; ranked or ordinal
33. response latency
34. Total response duration
35. amplitude-intensity

Chapter 7. Causal Inferences and Threats to Their Validity

1. association; correlation
2. coefficient of correlation
3. -1; $+1$
4. -1; 0
5. spurious association
6. effect; directionality
7. correlation
8. agreement; X; Y; difference; X; not Y
9. temporal precedence; sufficient; X; Y
10. Internal; variations
11. confounding effect
12. within-subjects or repeated measures; between-subjects
13. Proactive history; Retroactive history
14. Maturation
15. Sleeper effects
16. Practice effects
17. counterbalancing; carryover; equally
18. instrumentation
19. calibration; maintenance
20. Statistical regression
21. selection bias; differential attrition; compensatory rivalry; resentful demoralization; experimenter bias or Rosenthal effect
22. Selection bias
23. Differential attrition; mortality
24. Compensatory rivalry
25. Resentful demoralization
26. Experimenter; Rosenthal
27. External; subject; Hawthorne
28. good
29. perverse
30. pretest; sample; measurement; treatment
31. Pretest sensitization
32. Sample
33. Measurement

34. treatment
35. null; between; within; treatment
36. I; null; II; null
37. Construct validity

Chapter 8. Experimental Designs

1. manipulation; elimination; statistical
2. True; random assignment; independent variables; independent variables
3. Quasi-experiments; random assignment
4. Pre-experimental; pseudo
5. Pretest-posttest control; t; null hypothesis; $\mu_1 = \mu_2$; difference, or gain
6. treated; control; systematic influence; random fluctuation; between-group; B_v/W_v
7. analysis of covariance, or ANCOVA; covariates
8. probability; equal; independent variables
9. random assignment; extraneous preexisting; pretesting; sensitize; repeated measurement
10. Solomon four group; interaction; factorial design; main effects; interaction effect
11. large; four; time
12. ANOVAR; analysis of variance
13. factorial; treatment; level
14. random assignment
15. efficiency; effectiveness; efficiency; effectiveness
16. randomized controlled; confounding
17. selection; blinding; treatment; likelihood; chance
18. completely randomized
19. randomized block; primary
20. within-subject; homogeneous
21. parallel group
22. repeated measures; within-subject
23. statistical precision
24. carryover effects; order effects
25. washout
26. preceding; period
27. counterbalancing; crossover; randomized; treatment
28. Latin square
29. split-plot
30. nonequivalent; nonrandom; pretested; unpaired t test
31. dependent variable; time series; baseline
32. sleeper; sensitization
33. multiple time-series; spurious
34. experimental; responding, or baseline; treated behavior, or dependent variable; visual; statistical
35. A-B; A-B-A
36. withdrawal; replication
37. alternating treatment; different; randomly; multiple-treatment
38. Multitreatment interference
39. reversal

40. Multiple-baseline; true experiment; withdrawal; efficacy; independent
41. changing criterion; step-wise
42. single-subject
43. experimenter
44. within; baseline; treatment; 80–90; 15
45. before; adjacent
46. last data; first data; adjacent
47. first; last; smaller; larger; positive (or negative); negative (or positive)
48. Trend; accelerating; decelerating; zero
49. replication; robust
50. true; one-group posttest design
51. one-group pretest-posttest; pretest; pretest sensitization; interaction
52. static-group

Chapter 9. Nonexperimental Research Methods

1. hypothesis; test; hypothesis
2. case series
3. cross-sectional; longitudinal
4. cohort; case-control; risk factors
5. current; future status; rare
6. present; past; faster; economically; existing
7. presumed cause; presumed effect; case-control; presumed effect; presumed cause
8. prospective cohort; rare; after; bias; prospective cohort
9. incidence rate; new; prevalence rate; existing
10. causal-comparative; ex post facto
11. Temporal precedence
12. between-group; correlational
13. multiple regression; predictor; criterion
14. describing; multivariate analysis
15. unit of analysis; units; representative; how
16. representativeness; potential response rate
17. 50; 60; 70
18. variables; distribution; longitudinal
19. Trend
20. cohort; trend
21. Prevalence; at risk; Incidence; new; at risk
22. Incidence; prevalence
23. questionnaires; interviews; administration; recording
24. cost
25. double-barreled; loaded; leading
26. Open-ended; Closed-ended
27. Likert scale; range; variation
28. structure; design; contingency questions
29. Location; Contact; Completion; Total response
30. Guttman; cumulative
31. Thurstone; factor; reduce
32. personal; telephone; schedule

33. structured; unstructured
34. gold standard; true positive; false positive; true negative; false negative
35. Test sensitivity; test specificity
36. Predictive value positive; predictive value negative
37. prevalence; false positive

Chapter 10. Qualitative Research Methods

1. logical positivist position; phenomena
2. meaning
3. what; intensity; how many times
4. subjective; interpreting
5. observation; observing; field
6. naturalistic
7. complete-number; insider perspective
8. active-member
9. peripheral-member; insider's
10. undisguised (or overt); disguised (covert); obtrusive
11. disguise
12. validity; minimal; debriefing
13. Ethnography
14. emic; etic
15. behavior; artifacts; speech
16. ethnographic record
17. research interview; methodic; dynamic; critical
18. degree of structure; style; content
19. unstructured; open-ended
20. semi-structured; semi-structured; broader; in-depth
21. Grounded; grounded
22. inductive; interview; categorizes
23. Theoretical; pertinent
24. Phenomenology
25. case study
26. discourse; constructing; express; convey
27. Conversational; talk-in-interaction
28. Content; texts
29. recording units; physical; syntactical; referential; propositional; thematic
30. frequency; direction; intensity; space
31. manifest; latent
32. deciding; borrowing; developing
33. cover; included; semantic
34. quasi-statistical; template; editing; immersion/crystallization; comprehending; synthesizing; theorizing; recontextualizing
35. intercoder reliability; two
36. Intracoder reliability; same; kappa
37. credibility; confirmability; meaning-in-context; recurrent; saturation; transferability
38. Methods triangulation; Triangulation of sources; Analyst triangulation
39. lamination

Chapter 11. Analyzing Data Descriptive Statistics

1. descriptive; inferential; Descriptive
2. Frequency; categories; order
3. nominal; dichotomous; presence; absence
4. classifies; mutually exclusive
5. ordinal; ranking; ordering
6. bar graph; ordinate; abscissa
7. order; mutually exclusive; amount
8. equal; zero
9. ratio; absolute
10. dichotomous; discrete; continuous
11. frequency; class intervals; tally
12. class intervals; detail
13. divide; range
14. relative; frequency; sample; 100
15. histogram; bar; equal
16. frequency polygon; midpoints
17. bell; left; right; center
18. negatively; left; high; low
19. positively; right; low; high
20. center; dispersion; central tendency; variability
21. mean; median; mode
22. symmetrical; central tendency; interval; quantitative
23. middle; $(N + 1)/2$ OR $(n + 1)/2$
24. limit; cumulative; class interval
25. median; asymmetrical; unknown
26. mode; lowest; highest
27. tie; twice; nominal
28. unimodal; bimodal; nominal; central tendency
29. law of errors; normally; bell
30. homogeneous; variability
31. difference; fluctuations
32. deviation; mean
33. more; mean deviation
34. $\dfrac{\sum\left(X-\mu\right)^{2}}{N}$; σ^{2}
35. dispersion; square root
36. position; mean distance; mean
37. normal distribution; shape
38. 68.26; 95.44; 99.74
39. dispersion; percentile rank
40. 55
41. 25; varied
42. Pearsonian; $\dfrac{3(\bar{X} - M_{d})}{S}$; 1.2; positively
43. z; standard deviation

44. at; below; percentage
45. symmetrical; 100
46. 28.98; 87.4
47. criterion; predictor
48. mutually dependent; related
49. r; linear; two; 0.8; 0.4
50. variability; predicted
51. slope; Y-intercept; predicted
52. logistic; probability; dichotomous

Chapter 12. Analyzing Data: Inferential Statistics

1. probability
2. prognosis
3. Bernoulli; probable; long
4. 50; increases
5. frequentist; a posteriori
6. parameters; statistics
7. alpha; greater
8. Bayes
9. standard; mean; deviation; measurement
10. variability; variability; future
11. population; $\sigma/\sqrt{n}$
12. probability; systematic
13. 102
14. single; population
15. two; direction
16. one; less; two; variance
17. t; 30
18. rejected; greater than; 1.96
19. $\dfrac{\bar{X} - \mu}{SE}$
20. $S/\sqrt{n}$
21. freedom; $n - 1$
22. α; rejecting; true
23. β; retaining; false
24. I; power
25. unpaired
26. $n_1 + n_2 - 2$
27. paired; $n - 1$
28. matched; pairing
29. within; repeated
30. difference; standard deviations; pairs

31. homogeneity; interval; ratio; normal; randomness
32. nonparametric
33. chi; χ^2; expected
34. categorical; independent; fit
35. paired
36. 95%
37. unpaired; medians
38. I
39. between; within
40. interaction
41. Scheffe's; Tukey
42. increases; power
43. within; systematic
44. before
45. χ^2
46. ANOVA; *U*
47. meta-analysis
48. one
49. group
50. intercorrelations; factors
51. Minitab
52. coding
53. SPSS
54. JMP
55. Reject; .01; null

Chapter 13. Reading, Writing, and Presenting Research

1. critical thinking
2. letters; editor
3. decision; faith
4. Catabolic
5. catabolic
6. investigation
7. anabolism
8. anabolic
9. title
10. key; conditions
11. abstract
12. first; summary
13. truly; guidelines
14. pilot; completed; grant
15. specific aims
16. background; significance; known; unknown; more
17. who; what; how; means
18. institutional review board
19. consent form; protocol
20. seed money; intramural

21. competent; Intramural
22. National Institutes; Health; PHS 398
23. Center for Scientific Review; review
24. institutes
25. peer, study
26. advisory council
27. Request for Proposal; Request for Application; Grants; Register
28. Foundation; Foundation Center
29. independent; impartial; blinding
30. outcome; thinking
31. prospectus; plan
32. protocol; carefully; competently
33. efficiently; effectiveness
34. Efficient; Effective; clarity
35. obscure
36. American Psychological Association

A posteriori conclusion: A conclusion drawn from inductive reasoning based on actual facts or research outcomes.

A-B design: The most basic of the small-N (time series) designs in which observations are made over a period of time to establish a baseline (A) for the subsequent comparison of retest data. Next, a treatment (B) is introduced (independent variable) and changes in the dependant variable are noted.

A-B-A design: A type of small-N design in which a baseline condition is first established, followed by a treatment condition, and then finally by the withdrawal of the treatment condition (return to baseline).

A-B-A-B design: The most commonly used of the small-N designs. First, a baseline phase is established. Second, treatment is introduced. Third, treatment is withdrawn. Fourth, treatment is introduced again to assess its reliability. A variation of this design involves substituting an independent variable in the final B condition that is different than the first B condition.

Abscissa: The horizontal axis of a graph.

Alternating treatment design: Two treatments, A and B, are alternated randomly as they are applied to a single subject. The results are examined to determine whether one of the treatments is more effective than the other treatment.

Amplitude (intensity): Amount or level of a quality as it is perceived or judged to exist by an observer, or an acoustic measurement whose psychoacoustic correlate is loudness.

Anabolic thinking: A thinking process that entails building up or assembling complex structures from more elementary components.

Analysis of covariance (ANCOVA): One of the parametric ANOVA designs that allows for the statistical adjustment of data values of a dependant variable in accord with known quantities of one or more unwanted variables that the investigator might wish to control.

Analysis of variance (ANOVA): A method for analyzing population variances of two or more groups in order to make inferences about the population.

ANOVAR designs: Designs that entail the comparison of two or more groups and involve the use of ANOVA statistical techniques.

Applied behavior analysis: Aimed at the precise analysis, control, or modification of behavior, typically within the framework of single-subject research.

Applied research: Scientific research that focuses on solutions to problems that have immediate application.

Arithmetic average: Sum of all values, divided by the number of values.

Autocorrelation: A problem involving serial dependency in a temporally ordered sequence of data points.

Balanced Latin square: Similar to a Latin square, except all treatments precede and follow each other only once, thereby minimizing order effects.

Bar graph: A graph or chart that portrays the frequencies or relative frequencies of responses.

Bartlett test (or Levene's test): Frequently used to determine whether the assumption of *homogeneity of variance among groups* is met, thereby allowing for the use of any parametric ANOVA.

Baseline: The measured rate of responding prior to introducing an intervention or treatment.

BASIC: One of the most widely-used computer languages for classroom instruction. It stands for Beginner's All-Purpose Symbolic Instruction Code.

Basic research: Research that might have no presently identifiable application but is done simply to advance knowledge for its own sake.

Bayesian method: A mathematical basis for determining the degree to which a prior belief corresponds with the actual facts of subsequent observations. Statistically, a formula for computing the conditional probability of one event $P(A|B)$ from the conditional probability of another event, $P(B|A)$.

Behaviorism: Goal is to improve *observation, prediction,* and *control* of behavior rather than to uncover or explain through hypothesis testing the factors that underlie its occurrence.

Bernoulli theorem: States that the relative frequency of an observed event will approximate its probable frequency of future occurrence if observed over an indefinitely long series of trials.

Between-group variance: The amount of variation between means due to a systematic treatment effect. Also known as "systematic experimental variance."

Between-subjects design: The comparison of groups that have been treated differently on some independent variable.

Bimodal: A distribution that has two modes.

Biomedical Computer Programs P-Series (BMDP): An advanced statistical software package that is especially suitable for many medical and biological applications.

Bivariate: The relationship between two variables.

Blocking: Matched random assignment procedure in which ranked and segregated subjects are matched into pairs (blocks) so that each pair member has approximately the same score on the variable to be matched. Then, paired members are randomly assigned to the conditions of the experiment.

Bonferroni *t* procedure: A method for making a priori pair-wise comparisons of group means; used in cases in which the researcher wishes to increase the power of the test. Also called the Dunn multiple comparison procedure.

Carryover effects: When the effects of two or more treatments are being compared within the same group of subjects, the sequence in which the treatments are presented might confound interpreting the results.

Case series: Three or more cases in a case report.

Case study: A single individual or a few individuals sharing similar characteristics are studied and the findings reported.

Case-control study: Subjects are selected at the outset based on whether they have or do not have a particular disorder or disease of interest. Cases are then compared based on their previous exposure to factors thought related to their current status.

Catabolic thinking: A type of critical thinking process in which the various parts of a complex problem or structure, such as a research article, are broken down for evaluation of each component.

Categorical data: Data that can only be classified according to the characteristics of an observation.

Causal-comparative study: The dependent variable has already occurred so that its relationship to other variables can only be studied *ex post facto,* "after the fact" of such an occurrence.

Ceiling effects: When scores on a test pile up at the high end of a distribution because the test is too easy or the dependent variable is too sensitive to the treatment employed.

Celeration line: A straight line that most closely approximates the majority of the data points in a series.

Central limit theorem: In general, this theorem states that sample means tend to be normally distributed provided that the size of the sample is sufficiently large.

Central tendency: Measures that reflect the average size of a frequency distribution such as the mean, median, or mode.

Changing criterion design: A variation of the small-*n* designs. First, a series of behavioral criteria are established. A treatment plan is then introduced and its effectiveness is judged based on the extent to which the response level of the target behavior matches the present criteria.

Class intervals: Intervals of the same numerical size within a frequency table that are used for grouping a distribution of scores.

Classical approach: When testing hypotheses at a level of significance α, we reject the null hypothesis if an absolute value of the observed value is greater than α, and we fail to reject the null hypothesis if an absolute value of the observed value is less than or equal to α.

Closed-ended question: Participants choose from a list of preselected answers on a written questionnaire or during an interview.

Cluster sampling: A multistage sampling procedure in which smaller samples are selected from larger units or clusters. Often used to assure balanced, geographical representation of a population.

Code book: A sheet containing precoded response categories that is often used by qualitative researchers for assigning a range of numbers to the variables of interest.

Codes: Shorthand devices for labeling or marking the units of text as they relate meaningfully to categories of variables under investigation (concepts, themes, constructs).

Coefficient of correlation: A coefficient that indicates the strength of a relationship between X and Y.

Coefficient of variation: The ratio of the mean to the standard deviation.

Cohort studies: Individuals who lack a disorder or disease are followed over a period of time while examining factors thought to influence the development of a disorder or disease.

Cohort survey studies: Studies of the *same* people from one time period to the next.

Compensatory rivalry: Unwanted competition between the groups of an experiment that can inadvertently emerge to confound the interpretation of a treatment effect.

Completely randomized design: A design that places no restrictions on how participants are allocated to the study groups as long as they meet the inclusion criteria.

Concurrent validity: The results from a new test must agree with those of existing tests that are presumed to be valid.

Conditions: Controlled circumstances under which a research hypothesis can be tested or evaluated.

Confidence interval: The statistical means of estimating (with confidence) the interval that contains the population parameter.

Confounding effect: The consequence of an extraneous variable that produces an unwanted influence on the dependent variable.

Construct validity: The degree to which a particular test or measuring instrument actually measures the theoretical construct under investigation.

Constructed control group: Matching group members based on common variables so that any subse-

quent positive between-group differences could be confidently attributed to your program.

Constructs: Concepts refined to such a degree as to serve as premises for theories.

Content validity: The extent to which a particular test or measurement is judged to be representative of the behavior or skills it is designed to assess.

Contingency question: Questions that allow respondents to skip from one question to the next as appropriate.

Contingency table: A two-dimensional table used to illustrate the frequencies of responses for two or more nominal or quantitative variables in various combinations.

Continuous variables: Observations that can potentially take on any value including fractional units of measurement along some line segment or interval.

Control group: The group of subjects to whom the independent variable is not assigned or applied.

Controlled experimental studies: Designs that involve the active and systematic manipulation of one or more independent variables.

Convenience sampling: Sometimes called "on-the-street" or "opportunistic sampling," it is a technique commonly used by the media to poll attitudes or opinions about current events.

Convergence evidence: Strong intercorrelations among the various test items, thereby providing evidence that they are all measuring a single construct.

Conversational analysis: An account of "talk-in-interaction."

Correlated variable: When the measure of one variable is said to predict the measure of a second variable, the variables are said to be *correlated*.

Correlation: The statistical method that describes the relationship between two or more variables.

Correlation coefficient: A measure used to denote a range of relations among variables where $+1$ expresses a perfect positive correlation and -1 a perfect negative correlation.

Counterbalancing: A method that controls for the effects of one condition preceding another by "balancing" the order in which they are administered to subjects, so that each subject is exposed to each condition an equal number of times.

Covariates: Secondary variables that are predicted to have an influence on the test or evaluation.

Criterion of testability: Determination of whether or not the question or hypothesis is testable.

Criterion variable: The performance variable (Y) that is estimated from another *predictor variable* (X). Also called the outcome or dependent variable.

Critical values for the t distribution: Table values used to determine the probability that a t score as large as or larger than the value obtained might have resulted as the consequence of chance.

Cronbach's alpha: Method for evaluating the internal consistency of a test. More appropriate for continuous data.

Cross-sectional design: The sample data is collected at a particular point (cross-section) in time for purposes of describing variables and their patterns of distribution.

Crossover design: An experimental design in which each group of subjects receives both the control and experimental treatments. This is accomplished by alternating the sequence of treatments administered.

Data probability: An intermediate mathematical probability of new sample data prior to deriving a posterior probability.

Debriefing: Disclosing to the subjects the purpose of the research in which they were asked to participate, after they are done.

Deception: There are at least two types of deception in research practice. The first type, *deception by commission,* occurs as a result of actively misrepresenting the purpose of the research or the procedures to be used, lying about the identity of the researcher, or falsely promising some gain to the participants. The second type, *deception by omission,* entails a passive form of deceit. In such a case, the researcher may fail to tell subjects that they are being studied or that their behavior may be recorded in a clandestine manner.

Deduction: A logical thought process that begins with a general premise or law presumed to be true that is then used to explain a specific observation.

Degrees of freedom: The number of scores in a distribution that are allowed to vary (remain free). In a single sample, this index number is expressed as the number of scores minus one: denoted by $n - 1$.

Dependent variable: The consequence or effect caused by assigning or manipulating the independent variable.

Descriptive question: Asks about the objective or empirical features of objects or events without regard to their interrelationship.

Descriptive statistics: Measures such as percentages, averages, and standard deviations used to summarize, condense, and organize data into a more convenient form.

Deviation: The difference between each data value in a distribution and the mean.

Dichotomous qualitative variables: Variable that has only two outcomes, e.g., male\female, yes\no, normal\abnormal.

Difference question: A question that entails comparison of between-group differences in a search for causal explanations.

Difference scores (gain scores): The difference between the pretest and posttest in the experimental condition to be compared to the difference between the pretest and posttest in the control condition for each subject.

Differential attrition: Subjects may terminate their participation in an experiment for reasons other than that implied by the more ominous term.

Directionality problem: The inability of an investigator to determine which of two variables causes a change in the other.

Discourse analysis: Studies that are concerned with the analysis of spoken and written text messages used to convey meaning or to perform particular social functions such as asking or answering questions, accusing or complementing others, justifying actions, etc.

Discrete variable: Values of observations that can potentially assume or constitute a sequence of isolated or separated points along a number line represented by integers.

Discriminant analysis: A statistical method for determining which dependent variables among a set of such variables are most responsible for discriminating among groups.

Discriminant evidence: Evidence used to establish the case that test items normally considered to be unrelated to the construct in question are, indeed, unrelated to it.

Disguised participant: By concealing one's identity, the researcher is able to observe behavior and derive conclusions without impeding or distorting the outcome due to subject reactivity.

Distribution free: Distributions that are free of assumptions about the shape of the underlying population distribution and that employ nonparametric tests.

Doctrine of empiricism: The doctrine that states nothing can be said to exist until it is actually *observed* to exist to some degree.

Double-barreled question: Contain two queries that are impossible to untangle with respect to the intended answer.

Double-blind investigation: *Both* the judges and the subjects would be kept blind as to the type of treatments (drug or placebo) being used as well as to the results that might be anticipated.

Eclectic approach: A research rationale that emphasizes flexibility and innovation in behavioral management applicable to the clinical environment wherein the needs of diverse individuals must be addressed.

Ecological validity: Whether treatment developed in a research setting may be difficult to apply within an educational or clinical context.

Effect size: The measure of the degree to which the phenomenon is present in the population, or the degree to which the null hypothesis is false. An index of the magnitude of the effect of the independent variable; the degree to which the phenomenon of interest exists in the population.

Elements: People, objects, events, organizations, etc. that make up a population.

Emic perspective: Based on the way the members of a group see their world given their particular culture.

Errors in sampling: The degree to which a sample variable differs from the same variable as found in the population due to random or chance factors alone.

Errors of measurement: A source of uncontrolled variation of the dependent variable that can arise from inaccuracy or inconsistency of methods of data collection.

Ethnographic record: May take a variety of forms including tabulations of observed behavior, verbatim transcriptions of interviews or conversations, audio or video recordings, notes based on memory, archival material such as clinic files, journal articles, newspapers or magazines, etc. These and many other materials may be used to establish the reliability and validity of the researcher's conclusions.

Ethnography: Studies that seek to document the customs, social patterns, and rule-governed behavior of a culture or group of individuals.

Etic perspective: An objective view or "outsider's framework" in order to make sense of one's own observations and derive theory based on a scientific explanation of reality.

Ex post facto studies: Studies that lack purposeful experimental manipulation of an independent variable and that search for past causes of an observed phenomenon.

Exclusion criteria: Criteria that will effectively eliminate unwanted individuals with the type of characteristics (e.g., certain psychological or physical impairments) that might bias a sample.

Expected frequency: Probability estimate (or theoretical frequency) for a cell of a contingency table.

Experimental analysis of behavior: (*See* Applied behavior analysis.)

Experimenter bias (Rosenthal effect): Conscious or unconscious bias held by an experimenter that can influence the outcome of a study.

External validity: The degree to which the results of a study can be generalized to a population from which a sample was drawn.

Externally valid inference: An inference that can be generalized from the sample to the finite population and, hopefully, to the infinite population as well.

Extraneous variables: Factors unrelated to the treatment of interest.

F **distribution:** A distribution that can be used to test the equality of two or more population variances.

Face validity: Validity based merely on the surface appearance of things.

Factor analysis: A statistical method for organizing data so that existing relationships among numerous variables can be more readily identified and comprehended. This is accomplished by reducing a large number of observations into a small number of key indicators of underlying constructs.

Factor loadings: Final step of factor analysis to determine the degree to which the measure correlates with a certain factor.

Factorial design: Any design in which more than one treatment factor is investigated.

Factors: Measures that are found to be correlated.

False negative conclusion: A negative test result when the person actually has the disorder or disease in question.

False positive conclusion: A positive test result when the person actually does not have the disorder or disease in question.

Floor effects: When the majority of scores fall near the lower limit of a distribution, indicating that the test may be too difficult or perhaps the dependent variable is insensitive to the experimental treatment.

Fluctuations in the conditions of testing: Uncontrolled variations that might unduly influence the outcome of an experiment.

Foundation Grants Directory: Resource that describes the goals and objectives of major foundations and the kinds of projects they fund. Maintained by a national organization called the *Foundation Center*.

Frequency polygon: A line graph used to plot the frequencies of scores falling into the particular class intervals of a grouped frequency table.

Friedman two-way analysis of variance by ranks: A nonparametric test especially useful for randomized block designs in which a block consists of three or more repeated measures obtained from the same subject.

Gain scores: (*See* Difference scores.)

Gold standard: The standard against which the merit of new tests can be judged.

Good subject effect: Subjects who try hard to perform in accordance with what they believe are the expectations of the experimenter.

Goodness-of-fit: A type of chi-square test that deals with questions pertaining to whether distributions of scores fall equally into certain categories.

Grounded theory: Studies that focus on the symbolic interactions among people and how they use

symbols, such as language, to interpret or "make sense" of their experiences over time.

Guttman scale: Has ordinal properties like the Likert scale but can be used in cumulative scaling of statements of increasing intensity.

Heterogeneous: Members of a population that have diverse characteristics.

Histograms: Much like bar charts in their visual appearance, except the data are partitioned along the abscissa (horizontal or *x* axis) so as to fall within several equal class intervals.

History effect: Types of subject variation due to historical influences that may alter the validity of a study. Consists of proactive history and retroactive history.

Homogeneity: A statistical assumption that the standard deviation of the dependent variable within two or more groups is the same regardless of the level of the independent variable administered; i.e., the two populations have equal variances. The validity of this assumption is important in the use of ANOVA and regression techniques.

Homogeneity of variance: Variances between or among the groups of an experiment are relatively equal.

Homogeneous samples: Experiments in which the samples employed have similar characteristics.

Hypothesis testing: The scientific means of investigating problems under controlled, empirical conditions. Statistically, this entails determining whether a probability estimate of a population parameter is justifiable based on the research findings.

Incidence rate: Number of new cases.

Inclusion criteria: Criteria that specify the age, gender, clinical characteristics, etc. of subjects.

Independence: The method used to determine whether two characteristics are related.

Independent variable: A variable that is manipulated or assigned to determine its influence on the dependent variable. Also known as the antecedent condition or cause.

Induction: A form of reasoning wherein a general theory or set of laws is ultimately derived from specific observations or individual cases.

Inferential statistics: A type of statistics that allow an investigator to generalize results from a particular sample to the population from which the sample was drawn.

Informed consent: Approval from a prospective research subject showing that he/she understands the background, significance, purpose, and methods of the project as well as all risks/benefits involved in participating.

Institutional review board: A group of diverse individuals charged with reviewing research proposals of investigators and their compliance with regulations for protecting the rights of human and animal subjects.

Instrumentation effect: Changes in the accuracy or precision of measuring devices or human observations.

Interaction effect: The joint effect of two independent variables—how the two treatments combine or interact to influence certain outcomes.

Intercoder reliability: The researcher's internal consistency.

Intercorrelations: A list that shows the results of correlating each test item with all other test items.

Internal consistency reliability: Shown to be measuring the same attribute.

Internal validity: Causal inferences are justified based on observed changes in a dependent variable in response to systematic variations in an independent variable.

Internally valid inference: Inference in which the characteristic being studied in a particular sample can be generalized because it accurately represents the phenomenon of interest.

Interobserver reliability: The consistency of judgments between two or more observers based on measurements or ratings made at the same point in time.

Interval scale: Possesses the properties of a nominal and ordinal scale. In addition, data values are distributed at equal intervals along a continuous number line but the line contains no meaningful zero.

Interval/ratio data: Data that should be quantifiable on a numerical scale when common arithmetic is appropriate.

Interview schedule: Contains explicit instructions to guide the interviewer in asking respondents a list of questions designed to obtain complete and honest answers. Such a schedule also contains instructions and reminders for the interviewer to facilitate this process.

Intraobserver reliability: The degree of internal consistency of an individual observer with her or himself in administering tests or experimental procedures and in measuring and assessing the results.

JMP: The statistical software package used in the behavioral, social, and natural sciences to perform more complex statistical/probabilistic designs.

Kappa formula: A statistical method for determining the interobserver or intraobserver agreement for nominal measures.

Kruskal-Wallis one-way analysis of variance by ranks (KWANOVA): A nonparametric version of the one-way ANOVA and an extension of the Mann-Whitney U test; it is useful for deciding whether the distribution of scores in the populations underlying each group are identical. Like other nonparametric tests, ranks are substituted in order to represent the dependant variable.

Kuder and Richardson's formula 20: Method for evaluating the internal consistency of a test. More appropriate for dichotomous test items.

Lamination: Cross-checking the interpretation of multiple assessors of the findings of a qualitative study.

Latin square design: A repeated measures design in which the presentation of conditions is counterbalanced so that each occurs in each sequential position of a block.

Law of errors: The majority of repeated measurements made on the same subject *normally* cluster about the center of a distribution to form a bell-shaped curve with progressively fewer values dispersed symmetrically toward the tail ends on the left and right of center.

Leading question: Tends to guide or channel an answer in a particular direction.

Likert scale: Respondents are asked to express their degree of agreement or disagreement on a numerical scale, e.g., 1 = very mild, 2 = mild, 3 = moderate, 4 = severe, 5 = very severe.

Linear regression: A statistical method that predicts the best estimated value of a dependent variable from an independent variable when a linear relationship between two variables exists.

Linear relationship: A relationship between two variables that can be depicted by a straight line drawn through a number of given points when a scatterplot of the two variables is constructed.

Loaded question: Question that contains emotionally charged language.

Logical positivist position: Begins with a definite set of questions or hypotheses that, through the use of explicit and sustained systematic methods, are intended to discover the characteristics, interrelatedness, or causes of phenomena.

Logistic regression: Useful in estimating the probability that an event will occur when the independent variables in an experiment include both quantitative and qualitative measures and the criterion or outcome variable is dichotomous.

Longitudinal study: Repeated observations are made over an extended period of time.

Longitudinal survey designs: Survey studies that collect information over an extended period of time.

Main effect: The average effect of an independent variable across levels of the dependent variable.

Mann-Whitney *U* test: A highly useful nonparametric test analog of the unpaired *t* test for two independent samples that is concerned with determining the equality of medians rather than means.

Matched random assignment: A sampling technique that combines matching and random assignment of subjects to groups.

Matching: A control procedure designed to restrict the degree to which subjects in different groups are allowed to differ by pairing them according to particular characteristics.

Maturation effect: Internal biological or psychological changes within subjects that may occur over a span of time resulting in performance variations unrelated to the treatment of interest.

Mean: The arithmetic average value.

Mean squared deviation from the mean: The numerical value that is found by squaring each deviation from the mean and summing these squared deviation scores.

Measurement error: Difference between the hypothetical test score and the observed test score.

Measurement restrictions: Restrictions in which the measure selected to represent a dependent variable is not truly representative of the phenomenon that the experimenter wants to assess.

Measures of central tendency: Descriptive statistics used to derive averages, means, and so on .

Measures of variability: Descriptive statistics used to show the way in which individual scores are dispersed around measures of central tendency.

Median: The mid-score value in a distribution of scores.

Meta-analysis: Statistically combining the results from two or more independent studies.

Method of agreement: *If X occurs then Y occurs.* In other words, when the presumed cause is present the effect should be present also.

Method of association: The method that merely describes the relationship (correlation) among two or more events without reference to causation.

Method of constancy: Method for controlling inconsistencies in an experiment including measurements, subject responses during the repeated performance of the same task, the conditions of testing, and so on.

Method of constant stimuli: The method that requires that several comparison stimuli be randomly paired with a fixed standard.

Method of counterbalancing: Method for reducing order effects.

Method of difference: Two effects are typically examined: one of these preceded by the presumed cause and the other when the presumed cause is absent.

Method of elimination: Removing extraneous variables from the experiment.

MINITAB: A statistical software package appropriate for an introduction to computerized statistical analysis techniques. Data values can be stored and displayed in columns and rows like a spreadsheet.

Mode: The most frequently occurring value.

Multiple baseline design: Small-*N* designs that involve the application of a treatment to different baselines at different times. Appropriate for the analysis of a treatment influence across different subjects, behaviors, and settings.

Multiple regression: Regression techniques for determining the relationship between one independent variable and two or more independent variables.

Multiple time-series design: $O_1 O_2 O_3 O_4 X O_5 O_6 O_7 O_8$

Multitrait-multimethod matrix: A statistical means of examining the validity of a test according to the degree that it is measuring what it is intended to measure as opposed to something else.

Multitreatment interference effects: The influence of one treatment on another in cases in which the same subject is exposed to each of them. More specifically, it is possible for preceding treatments to make successive treatments more or less effective.

Multivariate: Three or more variables.

Multivariate analysis of variance (MANOVA): A statistical technique designed for problems in which there is more than one dependent variable under investigation. Two or more different measures of approximately the same characteristic (related variables) are taken, and a question is asked regarding the degree to which these dependent variables serve to separate two or more groups.

Mutually dependent: An observed change in one variable appears to be associated with a concomitant change in another.

n: The size of the sample.

N: The size of the population.

Negatively skewed distribution: A distribution in which the tail points to the left (negative) side of the curve, signifying that the proportion of high scores in the distribution is greater than that of low scores.

Negativistic or perverse subject effect: Subjects who may be hostile toward a particular research project and attempt to undermine what they perceive its goals to be by their dishonest or uncooperative behavior.

Nominal data: Observations that can only be named and counted.

Nominal scale: A scale of measurement in which data can only be named or counted and where numbers are used solely for purposes of classification or labeling.

Nomogram: A means for converting pretest probabilities into posttest probabilities for certain diagnostic outcomes using likelihood ratios (LRs).

Nonequivalent comparison group design: Entails the use of at least two nonrandom comparison groups both of whom are pretested prior to treatment. Subsequently, the groups are posttested to examine between-group differences.

Nonexperimental research: An investigation in which causal relations definitely cannot be established.

Nonmanipulated variables: Variables that are not controllable by a researcher but preexist as states or conditions within the participants of a study.

Nonparametric statistics: Statistical methods that do not depend on a knowledge of the population distribution or its parameters. Such techniques are well suited for situations in which the population distributions are skewed or unknown, especially when the sample size is small.

Nonrandom sampling: Sampling techniques in which the probability for subject selection is unknown.

Nonsignificant: Findings from statistical testing that could have resulted from chance (accidental) factors unknown to the researcher.

Nonsignificant difference: A statistical result that should be interpreted to mean "not yet proved" or "inconclusive."

Normal distribution curve: Bell shaped with data points symmetrically distributed along a horizontal line to the left and right of center.

Normality: The population distribution is normal.

Null hypothesis: A statement of statistical equality (no relationship between two or more variables), denoted as H_0.

Observed frequencies: The actual counts recorded in one cell of a contingency table.

Occam's razor: A parsimonious theory that contains the fewest noncontradictory explanations is preferable.

One-group posttest design: Also known as the *one-shot case study,* it involves studying the presumed effect of an independent variable in a single group of subjects by administering a posttest after some intervention(s).

One-group pretest-posttest design: This preexperimental design allows for the comparison of pretest and posttest data subsequent to treatment. However, because no control group is used, there is inadequate control for internal and external validity.

One-tailed test: "Less stringent" than a two-tailed test because a smaller amount of variance between mean scores is needed to be considered a significant finding.

One-way ANOVA: The simplest of the ANOVA designs involving the analysis of a single factor.

Open-ended question: Ask respondents to answer questions in their own words.

Operant (instrumental) conditioning: A class of behavior (defined as operant) whose acquisition and rate of emission is dependant on its consequences (reinforcing stimuli).

Operationism: A doctrine that emphasizes the importance of defining the quantitative meaning of theoretical terms in accordance with specified measurements or observations.

Order effects: Interactions arising from one treatment variable preceding another.

Ordinal scale: Possesses the properties of a nominal scale. In addition, data can be arranged in order or ranked, but quantitative differences between data values (how much larger or smaller one value is from another) cannot be determined.

Ordinate: The vertical axis of a graph.

Organismic variables: Relatively stable physical or psychological characteristics that are not subject to active experimental manipulation (e.g., age, sex, height, weight, auditory/visual acuity).

***p*-value:** The probability (actual probability) that a test statistic in a hypothesis test is at least as extreme as the value obtained.

Paired *t* test: The *t* test for paired observations.

Pairing-design: A study that involves dependent, correlated, or related samples.

Parallel group design: Experiments that generally employ at least two randomly assigned independent groups of participants, each of whom receive only one of the treatments (independent variables) under investigation.

Parameter: A number or quantity used to describe characteristics of a population.

Pearson product-moment correlation: Computes a parametric correlation coefficient, reflecting the association between two variables measured on a continuous scale.

Pearsonian measure of skewness: The median is generally located about two-thirds of the distance from the mode to the mean in moderately skewed frequency distribution. It also calculates the degree of skewness of a given frequency distribution, i.e., it determines whether it is normal, positively skewed, or negatively skewed.

Peer reviews: Working scientists reviewing proposals in the research field of their own expertise.

Percentile ranks: Simply a number on a particular measurement scale at or below which a given percentage of the remaining distribution of scores can be found.

Period effects: Effects of time variations on an investigation.

Periodicity: The elements in the list are arranged in a cyclical manner or particular pattern that might bias the outcome.

Phenomology: Studies that aim to understand how people attribute meaning to events and interactions with others during the course of daily living.

Pie diagram: Graphical method for representing the proportion of a data set falling into certain categories in the form of a circle containing wedges.

Pilot study: A preliminary study useful in planning and rehearsing the steps involved in a more extensive research project.

Planned (or a priori) comparison procedures: Procedures in which an investigator wishes to accomplish the analysis of a limited number of pairwise comparisons in lieu of performing a more comprehensive and time-consuming ANOVA.

Point estimate: A sample proportion, denoted by p, is calculated by dividing the observed values (x) from the sample by the size of the sample (n), i.e., $p = x/n$.

Polyotomous qualitative variables: Variables that have more than two levels of assignment.

Population: All of the subjects within a well defined group to whom the research findings are applied. An all-inclusive data set about which a conclusion or causal inference is drawn.

Positively skewed distribution: The tail points to the right (positive) side because the frequency of low scores greatly outnumbers that of high scores in the distribution.

Posterior probability: The conditional probability calculated by using Bayes' rule. It represents the predictive value of a positive test or a negative test.

Posttest-only control group design: The most basic version of the true experimental designs. Given the assumption that randomization has effectively balanced extraneous between-group differences, only a post test is given following treatment to avoid the potential sensitizing influence of a pretest on performance.

Power analysis: Method for estimating both the size of a sample needed for a research study and the probability for committing a type II error.

Power of the test: The probability of rejecting a false null hypothesis, i.e., the probability of reaching a correct decision.

Practice effect: (*See* Testing effect.)

Predictive validity: The degree to which a particular measure or procedure is able to accurately predict some other variable or performance outcome.

Predictive value negative (PV⁻): The probability that a person does not carry a disorder or disease, given that the test result is negative.

Predictive value positive (PV⁺): The probability that a person carries a disorder or disease, given that the test result is positive.

Predictor variable: The variable (X) that is used to predict performance on another *criterion variable* (Y). Also called the independent variable.

Preexperimental design: Studies that fail to meet at least two of the three criteria necessary for a true experiment. Essential goal is to explore or describe new phenomena rather than to explain their causes.

Pretest sensitization: Threats to external validity resulting from certain biasing influences involving subjects' attitudes, expectations, or perceptions about their role in a particular experiment.

Pretest-posttest control group design: The most commonly used of the true experimental designs. Two groups of subjects are randomly assigned to either an experimental condition where treatment (X) is administered or to a control condition where no treatment is given.

Prevalence rate: Number of existing cases.

Prevalence/incidence survey designs: A statistical measure descriptive of the proportion of the people in a population surveyed or examined that have a disorder or disease.

Prior probability: The unconditional probability used in the numerator of Bayes' rule. It represents the prevalence of a disease prior to performing an actual diagnostic test.

Proactive history: Preexisting differences due to learned or inherent abilities that subjects might bring to an investigation.

Probability: The relative degree of certainty versus uncertainty about a particular research outcome. Statistically, a ratio reflecting long-run percentages for the generality of observed results.

Probability proportionate to size (PPS) sampling: A method for assuring that each element within a cluster has an equal chance for selection, regardless of cluster size.

Prognosis: A prediction of the outcome of a proposed course of treatment for a given case.

Prospective cohort study: The cohort is selected using *current information* about the people comprising it who are then tracked forward in time to determine their future status.

Prospectus: A detailed outline of the plan for research.

Pseudoexperiments: Investigations are essentially limited to describing outcomes because appropriate statistical comparisons cannot be performed on the results of preexperimental studies.

***P*-value approach:** In hypothesis testing, we report the conclusion by determining the significance of the test results based on a *p*-value.

Qualitative methods: Strategies that emphasize non-numerical data collection methods such as observations, interviews, etc. When numbers are used, typically they are intended to code, classify, or simply represent the presence or absence of the quality under study.

Quantitative methods: The collection of numerical measures of behavior under controlled conditions that can be subjected to statistical analysis.

Quasi-experimental research experimental design: Designs that are used when true experimentation is impractical or impossible to perform. Typically, subjects are assigned to groups on the basis of preexisting conditions or circumstances.

r: (*See* Correlation coefficient.)

Random assignment: An effort to establish equivalent groups by randomly assigning subjects from the available subject pool to various treatments or conditions.

Random errors: Errors due to unknown causes of variation.

Random selection: Involves drawing observations from a population defined as all members of any well-defined class of people, events, or objects in such a way that each observation has an equal chance of being represented.

Randomized block design: Allows for an analysis of particular subject attributes on a dependent variable. In addition to a single attribute, various combinations of attributes (e.g., gender, age, intelligence, socioeconomic status) can be blocked, analyzed, and interpreted using this approach.

Randomized controlled trials (RCTs): Designs that entail randomization to allow for a valid interpretation of the influence of the independent variable by controlling for confounding variables.

Randomized-blocks analysis of variance (RBANOVA): Used for determining whether the differences between two or more groups may be due to chance or to systematic differences among the groups. It is especially appropriate for within-subject designs in which repeated measures of the same subject are made.

Randomness: Chance variation.

Range: The difference between the lowest and highest value in a distribution.

Ratio scale: The most powerful of the numerical measurement scales. Possesses the properties of all others.

Rationale: Underlying reason for asking the question in the first place.

Recording units: These often serve as the focus for content analysis in research studies: physical units, syntactical units, referential units, propositional units, thematic units.

Regression analysis: A statistical means of determining the nature of the relationship between two variables based on estimating or predicting the value of one from the other.

Regression equation: Calculates what is called "the best fit" of the data points of the X and Y variables as they are scattered about a regression line.

Regression line: The best-fitted straight line through a joint distribution that represents predicted values of the dependent variable for each value of the independent variable.

Related: When an observed change in one variable appears to be associated with a concomitant change in another.

Relationship question: Asks about the degree to which an observed phenomenon may change in association with other variables (e.g., age, gender, cognitive ability).

Relative frequency distribution: Shows the percentage of scores that fall within each class interval. This can be determined by dividing the frequency of scores falling within each interval by the size of the sample (n) and multiplying the result by 100.

Repeated measures design: Each participant is exposed to all the treatments administered in an experiment according to a randomly assigned sequence and the effects of these treatments are compared within each individual.

Representativeness of the sample: The selection of participants should yield units of analysis that are appropriate for answering the questions asked.

Request for Application (RFA): A research grant awarded by the National Institutes of Health (NIH) to conduct research created by an investigator.

Request for Proposal (RFP): A research grant awarded to conduct research as determined by the NIH.

Research hypothesis: A problem statement derived from theoretical reasoning, prior data, or both used for predicting associative or causal relations among variables, denoted as H_1.

Research process: A problem-solving process that involves the following steps: identifying a problem that leads to an idea for a research question or hypothesis, developing a research design appropriate for investigating for the question or hypothesis, collecting data and analyzing results pertinent to the question or hypothesis, and interpreting the results in a manner that refines understanding and leads to new questions.

Resentful demoralization: A confounding factor associated with an outcome just opposite to that of compensatory rivalry can occur when some subjects in an experiment perceive that other subjects, as compared to themselves, are receiving a more favorable treatment.

Response duration: Expressed as a proportion (percentage) of time spent in emitting a particular behavior during a defined period.

Response frequency: The total number of response units observed to occur or measured per unit of time (rate).

Response latency: How long it takes for a response to occur following some specified event.

Response rate: The proportion of subjects willing to participate of those selected.

Retroactive history: Change-producing environmental events, tangential to the purposes of an experiment, that intervene between two observations or measurements.

Retrospective cohort study: Study based on past records where the outcome is already known. From such historical records, individuals are selected for the study of factors that might explain their present status.

Reversal design: Baseline measures are first recorded prior to a treatment. An intervention is then introduced that is followed in the next phase by a therapeutic reversal in intervention.

Revised version of the *t* test: An alternative method to accomplish the analysis of a limited number of pairwise comparison in lieu of performing a more comprehensive and time-consuming ANOVA. Instead of using the pooled standard deviation, the error mean squared standard deviation is used.

Risk factor: Factor believed to be related to the occurrence of certain disorders or diseases.

Risk tolerance: The percent chance of error that the conclusions may be incorrect.

Risk/benefit ratio: The potential for harm or injury versus the possible benefits in an investigation.

Robust: Generality of a treatment effect under different conditions and with different people.

RO-1 proposal: The most common of research application to the National Institutes of Health (NIH) that is self-initiated by an investigator.

Sample: A collection of some of the elements drawn from a population.

Sample restrictions: The degree that a sample of subjects truly reflects the behaviors, physical and mental attributes, socioeconomic status, motivation, level of skill, etc. of the target population to whom we wish to extrapolate our findings.

Sampling distribution of the mean of size *n*: The mean of all possible sample means from the original population.

Sampling error: The difference between the measures collected for a randomly selected sample and the population it is believed to represent. More specifically, sampling error can be defined as the expected amount of variance owing to *chance* alone rather than to *systematic* influences.

Sampling frame: A full listing of all subjects in a targeted population that one wishes to sample.

Sampling interval: The standard distance between the elements in a list.

Sampling validity: (*See* Content validity.)

Scheffe's method: One of the post hoc multiple comparison methods to determine which specific group means among the various comparisons are significantly different from others. It is highly useful when the sample sizes among the comparison groups are unequal.

Scientific method: Certain systematic thinking and action processes involving the control and measurement of variables that lead to valid and reliable answers to questions.

Selection bias: Preexisting factors may preclude or interfere with the establishment of equivalent groups so that it cannot be assumed that the operative influences or treatments in an experiment differ systematically only with respect to the independent variable.

Sensitive test: The proportion of people who test positive on a screening test to those people with a disorder or disease.

Serendipity: The process of accidentally discovering valuable information while exploring an unrelated problem.

Significance level: The probability selected for rejecting the null hypothesis. Conventionally, the cutoff value between results attributed to chance and results attributed to a systematic influence is set at either $p < .05$ or $p < .01$.

Significant result: A statistically reliable result.

Simple linear regression: Concerns the degree to which Y (the dependent or criterion variable) can be predicted from X (the independent or predictor variable).

Simple random sampling: A technique in which each member of a population has a chance of being selected for a sample equal to that of every other member of the population.

Single-group design: Hypothesis testing that involves the one-sample case.

Skewed: Asymmetrical distributions.

Sleeper effect: A change in a dependent variable due to a treatment effect that is not immediately observable but tends to become increasingly observable over a span of time.

Slope (b): The general magnitude or rate of change of a linear regression line which describes how two variables go together.

Snowballing: One or more identified participants can be asked to identify others in the population as prospective candidates for study.

Soloman four-group design: A design that attempts to control for certain interaction effects between a pretest and independent variable and their combined influence on a dependent variable.

Spearman rank correlation (Rho): A nonparametric analog of the Pearson product-moment correlation computed on two variables with ranked scores.

Spearman-Brown Prophecy formula: An adjustment formula of the split-half reliability estimate that is used to calculate the reliability coefficient for the entire test.

Specific test: The ratio of people who test negative on a screening test to those people without the disorder or disease.

Split-half reliability estimate: Reliability method specifically designed to determine the internal consistency of the items within a test by splitting the items on a test in half with the odd-numbered items constituting one half of the test and the even-numbered comprising the other half.

Split-plot design: A design that evolved from agricultural investigations that incorporates both within-subject and between-design elements in the statistical analysis of treatment effects.

Spurious association: A false relationship.

Standard deviation: The square root of variance, denoted by σ or s.

Standard error of the mean: An estimate of the expected deviation of sample means from the true population mean as a result of chance or measurement errors.

Static-group comparison: A type of preexperimental design in which the performance of two groups is compared, one group receiving treatment and the other not receiving treatment. No effort is made to pretest subjects, nor randomly assign subjects to groups.

Statistic: A number derived by counting or measuring sample observations drawn from a population that is used in estimating a population parameter.

Statistical control methods: (*See* Analysis of covariance (ANCOVA).)

Statistical equality: No significant between-group difference.

Statistical Package for the Social Sciences (SPSS): One of the most widely used packages for statistical analysis, designed for educational, social, and behavioral science research.

Statistical regression: The tendency for extreme scores in a data set, on repeated testing, to move toward the average score of a distribution.

Stratified sampling: A technique in which random samples are drawn from defined subgroups (strata) of a population to assure adequate representation of members within each subgroup.

Structured interview: Incorporates closed-ended questions.

Student *t* test: Where a *t* test is actually a ratio in which the numerator is the difference between two means.

Subject bias (Hawthorne effect): Changes in performance in subjects' performance when they believe that they have attracted the attention of significant others or have been "singled out" for observation.

Systematic error: When the same error is made consistently throughout the entire process of measurement.

Systematic sampling: A parsimonious way of drawing a sample from a large population when a membership list is available. A sampling interval size such as every tenth name on a list may be used to define the sampling frame.

Systematic variance (between-group variance): Systematic differences between the scores of two or more groups resulting from the assignment or active manipulation of the independent variable.

***t* distribution:** A bell shaped distribution usally associated with small sample size ($n < 30$). The basis for the so-called Student *t* test used in null hypothesis testing.

***t* test:** To be used for evaluating the null hypothesis when the population standard deviation (σ) is unknown, and when the sample size is small ($n \leq 30$).

Table area: The percentage of a *z* distribution such that the *z* score falls between 0 and some specific positive value.

Tally: The number of observations that fall within each class interval.

Target population: The population to which the investigator wishes to generalize.

Tchebysheff's theorem: States that, for any data set, at least $100 \cdot (1 - \dfrac{1}{K^2})\%$ are lying within K standard deviations of the mean, where $K > 1$.

Temporal precedence: The "cause" must precede the "effect."

Test sensitivity: The probability that the test result is positive given that the person has the disorder or disease.

Test specificity: The probability that the test result is negative given that the person does not have the disorder or disease.

Testing effect: The facilitative influence of previous testing on performance measures, accruing as the result of familiarity, practice, or learning with repeated exposure to the same or similar test.

Test-retest reliability: The extent to which a certain test or measuring procedure yields consistent findings when repeatedly administered to the same subjects.

Texts: Any type of message designed for communicating information including the content of spoken and written narratives, films, videotapes, photographs, music, artistic productions, etc.

Theoretical sampling: Designed to build from and add to the findings that emerge from an interview in order to construct as many categories as possible as these relate to a wide range of pertinent areas.

Theory: A systematic structure of thought for guiding scientific inquiry and for organizing new facts as they emerge.

Third variable problem: An investigator concludes that there is a causal linkage between two variables when the true cause(s) is quite distinct from the variables under investigation.

Thurstone scale: Designed to have equal-appearing intervals between response items, yet it is seldom employed in present-day survey research because of the great difficulty and energy required in developing the items associated with its use.

Time-series analysis: A statistical method that involves the analysis of a sequence of measurements taken on a response that tends to vary over time.

Time-series design: Repeated measures of a dependent variable are made before and after administering an independent variable.

Treatment period: The time during which each intervention is administered.

Treatment restrictions: Restrictions on the ability of an investigator to generalize research findings based on the selection of an independent variable that was inappropriate given the purpose of the experiment.

Trend charts: Used to illustrate frequencies or percentages of change in a data set arranged in a temporal or developmental order.

Trend survey studies: Used to evaluate one or more attributes in a population by sampling such attributes over an extended time period.

Triangulation: The means of enhancing the value of theory by using multiple methods and perspectives to investigate the truth of its tenets.

True experimental design: Distinguished from other designs on the basis of one or more of the following factors: random assignment of subjects to at least two groups, use of a control group, and active manipulation of an independent variable.

True test score: One that should result as the consequence of repeated sampling over a very long series of trials under ideal conditions using a perfect test instrument.

Tukey's method: One of the post hoc multiple comparison methods to determine which specific groups' means among the various comparisons are significantly different from others. It is highly useful when the sample sizes among comparison groups are equal.

Two-tailed test: Selected when the direction of the difference cannot be predicted on the basis of preexisting knowledge.

Type I error (alpha): Rejecting a null hypothesis when it is true. Results in a false-positive conclusion.

Type II error (beta): Retaining a null hypothesis when it is false. Results in a false-negative conclusion.

Undisguised participant: Makes no effort to conceal an intention of observing the group for the purpose of collecting data.

Ungrouped data: Raw, uncategorized data.

Unimodal: A distribution having one mode.

Units of analysis: Part of a population of individuals that are the *ones* under study.

Univariate: Having a single variable.

Unstructured interview: Incorporating open-ended questions.

Unsystematic error: Errors resulting from random fluctuations in observed test scores due to factors unknown to the investigator or beyond his or her control.

Variability: The degree of fluctuation in a population of scores when sampled.

Variables: The factors described by constructs that are capable of assuming different values.

Variance (σ^2): A measure of the dispersion in a distribution of observations in a population or sample, i.e., the mean of the squared deviation from the mean.

Visual (graphical) analysis: The most commonly used method for determining the efficacy of treatment in single-subject research.

Washout period: Time interval interposed between successive treatments so as to allow for the dissipation of treatment effects.

Wilcoxon matched-pairs signed-ranks test: A commonly used nonparametric analog of the paired t test that utilizes information about both the magnitude and direction of differences for pairs of scores.

Within-group variance: The degree of error variance that may involve both sampling errors and measurement errors.

Within-subjects design: Involves a comparison within the same subjects under circumstances in which they were exposed to two or more treatment conditions.

Y intercept: The value of a dependent variable when not influenced by an independent variable.

Yates' correction for continuity: The chi-square formula exclusively designed for degrees of freedom = 1. The correction deals with the inconsistency between the theoretical chi-square distribution and the actual distribution having 1 degree of freedom. This is accomplished by subtracting 0.5 from the numerator of each term in the chi-square test prior to squaring the term.

z distribution: A bell-shaped distribution, usually associated with a large sample size ($n > 30$). Also termed the standard normal distribution where the mean = 0 and the standard deviation = 1.

z score: The amount of deviation of a score (X) from the mean of the distribution divided by the standard deviation.

z test: The test for examining the significance of differences between the means based on the z distribution.

Adams, M. R., Freeman, F. J., & Conture, E. G. (1984). Laryngeal dynamics of stutterers. In R. F. Curlee and W. H. Perkins (Eds.), *Nature and treatment of stuttering: New directions*. San Diego: College-Hill Press.

Adler, P. A., & Adler, P. (1987). *Membership roles in field research*. Newbury Park, CA: Sage.

Adler, P. A., & Adler, P. (1998). Observational techniques. In Norman Denzin and Yvonna Lincoln (Eds.), *Collecting and interpreting qualitative materials*. Thousand Oaks, CA: Sage.

Agar, M. (1986). *Speaking of ethnography*. Beverly Hills, CA: Sage.

Alley, M. (1987). *The craft of scientific writing*. Englewood Cliffs, NJ: Prentice-Hall.

Almor, A., Kempler, D., MacDonald, M., Andersen, E., & Tyler, L. (1999). Why do Alzheimer patients have difficulty with pronouns? Working memory, semantics, and reference in comprehension and production in Alzheimer's disease. *Brain and Language, 67*, 202–227.

Altheide, D. L., & Johnson, J. M. (1998). Criteria for assessing interpretative validity in qualitative research. In Norman Denzin and Yvonna Lincoln (Eds.), *Collecting and interpreting qualitative materials*. Thousand Oaks, CA: Sage.

Altman, D. G., Schulz, K. F., Moher, D., Egger, M., Davidoff, F., Elbourne, D., et al. (2001). The revised CONSORT statement for reporting the randomized trials: explanation and elaboration. *The CONSORT Group, Ann Intern Med, 2001: 134*: 663–694.

American Educational Research Association, American Psychological Association, & National Council on Measurement in Education. (1999). *Standards for educational and psychological testing*. Washington, DC: Author.

American Psychological Association (1992). Ethical principles of psychologists and code of conduct. *American Psychologist, 47*, 1597–1611.

Anastasi, A. (1988). *Psychological testing* (6th ed.). New York: McGraw-Hill.

Andrews, B., Guitar, B., & Howie, P. (1980). Meta-analysis of the effects of stuttering treatment. *Journal of Speech and Hearing Disorders, 45*, 287–307.

Apel, K. (1999). Checks and balances: Keeping the science in our profession. *Language, Speech, and Hearing Services in Schools, 30*, 98–107.

Apel, K., & Self, T. (2003). The marriage of research and clinical service. *ASHA Leader, 8* (16), 6–7.

Aram, D. M. (1991). Comments on specific language impairment as a clinical category. *Language, Speech, and Hearing Services in Schools, 22*, 66–87.

Aram, D., Scott, D., Shaywitz, S. E., Fletcher, J. M., & Francis, D. J. (1994). Project II. Emergence of reading disability in children with early language impairments. NIH-NICHD Program Project: 5P0l HD21888-07. Project Leader: D. Aram, Emerson College, Boston, MA.

Arellano-Galdames, F. J. (1972). Some ethical problems in research on human subjects. Unpublished doctoral dissertation, University of New Mexico, Albuquerque.

Armstrong, J. S. (1980). Unintelligible management research and academic prestige. *Interfaces, 10*, 80.

Armstrong, L., & MacDonald, A. (2000). Aiding chronic written expression difficulties: A case study. *Aphasiology, 14*, 93–108.

Attanasio, J. S. (1994). Inferential statistics and treatment efficacy studies in communication disorders. *Journal of Speech and Hearing Research, 37*, 755–759.

Babbie, E. (1990). *Survey research methods*. Belmont, CA: Wadsworth.

Baer, D. M. (1975). In the beginning there was a response. In E. Ramp & G. Semb (Eds.), *Behavior analysis: Areas of research and application*. Englewood Cliffs, NJ: Prentice-Hall.

Baird, F. (2000). *Philosophic classics, Vol. III*. New York: Prentice Hall.

Bakan, D. (1966). The test of significance in psychological research. *Psychological Bulletin, 66*, 423–437.

Bales, R. (1950). *Interaction process analysis*. Cambridge, MA: Addison Wesley.

Barresi, B. (1996). *Proper name recall in older and younger adults: The contributions of word uniqueness and strategies*. Unpublished doctoral dissertation, Emerson College, Boston, Massachusetts.

Bayes, T. (1763). Essay towards solving a problem in the doctrine of chances. *Philosophical transactions. Royal Society London, 53*, 370–418. (Reprinted in *Biometrika (1958), 45*, 293–315).

Berelson, B. (1952). *Content analysis in communication research*. Glencoe, IL: Free Press.

Bishop, D. V. M., Carlyon, R. P., Deeks, J. M., & Bishop, S. J. (1999). Auditory temporal processing impairment: Neither necessary nor sufficient for causing language impairment in children. *Journal of Speech, Language, and Hearing Research 42*, 1295–1310.

Bloodstein, O. (1987). *A handbook on stuttering*. Chicago: National Easter Seal Society.

Bloom, M., & Fischer, J. (1982). *Evaluating practice: Guidelines for the accountable professional*. Englewood Cliffs, NJ: Prentice-Hall.

Blumer, H. (1969). *Symbolic interactionism*. Englewood Cliffs, NJ: Prentice-Hall.

Boyle, J. S. (1994). Styles of ethnography. In J. M. Morse (Ed.), *Critical issues in qualitative research*, Thousand Oaks, CA: Sage.

Brady, J. V. (1958). Ulcers in executive monkeys. *Scientific American, 199*, 95–100.

Brinton, B., & Fujiki, M. (2003). Blending quantitative and qualitative methods in language research and intervention. *American Journal Speech-Language Pathology, 12*, 165–171.

Brown, W. H., Odom, S. L., & Holcombe, A. (1996). Observational assessment of young children's social behavior with peers. *Early Childhood Research Quarterly, 11*, 19–40.

Browner, W. S., Newman, T. B., Cummings, S. R., & Hulley, S. B. (1988). Getting ready to estimate sample size: Hypotheses and underlying principles. In S. B. Hulley & S. R. Cummings (Eds.), *Designing clinical research*. Baltimore: Williams & Wilkins.

Brutten, G. J. (1975). Typography, assessment and behavior change strategies. In J. Eisenson (Ed.), *Stuttering: A second symposium*. New York: Harper & Row.

Campbell, D. T. (1969). Reforms as experiments. *American Psychologist, 24*, 409–429.

Campbell, D. T. (1984). Can we be scientific in applied social science? In R.F. Conner, D. G. Altman, & C. Jackson (Eds.), *Evaluation studies: Review annual*, Newbury Park, CA: Sage.

Campbell, D. T. & Fiske, D. W. (1959). Convergent and discriminant validation by the multitrait-multimethod matrix. *Psychological Bulletin, 56*, 81–105.

Campbell, D. T. & Stanley, J. C. (1963). Experimental and quasi-experimental designs for research on teaching. In N. L. Gage (Ed.), *Handbook of research on teaching*: Chicago: Rand McNally.

Campbell, D. T., & Stanley, J. C. (1966). *Experimental and quasi-experimental designs for research*. Chicago: Rand McNally.

Cannon, W. B. (1945). *The way of an investigation*. New York: W.W. Norton.

Carter, J. A., Murira, G. M., Ross, A. J., Mungàla, V., & Newton, C. R. (2003). Speech and language sequelae of severe malaria in Kenyan children. *Brain Injury, 17*, 217–240.

Carver, R. P. (1983). The case against statistical significance testing. In P. Hauser-Cram & F. C. Martin (Eds.), *Essays on educational research: Methodology, testing and application*. Cambridge, MA: Harvard Education Review, Reprint No. 16.

Caswell, E. (2004). The latest and best research at your finger tips—literally. *ASHA Leader, 9*, 4–5, 21.

Catts, H. W., Fey, M. E., Tomblin, J. G., & Zhang, X. (2002). A longitudinal investigation of reading outcomes in children with language impairments. *Journal of Speech, Language, and Hearing Disorders, 45*, 1142–1157.

Chadwick, B. A., Bahr, H. M., & Albrecht, S. L. (1984). *Social science research methods*. Englewood Cliffs, NJ: Prentice-Hall.

Chambless, D. L., & Hollon, S. D. (1998). Defining empirically supported therapies. *Journal of Consulting and Clinical Psychology, 66*, 7–18.

Champion, T. B., Katz, L., Muldrow, R., & Dail, R. (1999). Storytelling and storymaking in an urban preschool classroom: Building bridges from home to school culture. *Topics in Language Disorders, 19*, 52–67.

Child, D. (1990). The essentials of factor analysis (2nd ed.). London: Cassell Academic.

Clark, Heather. (2003). Neuromuscular treatments for speech and swallowing: A tutorial. *American Journal of Speech-Language Pathology, 12*, 400–415.

Cochran, W. G. (1965). The planning of observational studies of human populations. *Journal of the Royal Statistical Society, 128*, 234–265.

Cochran, W. G. (1977). *Sampling techniques* (3rd ed.), New York: Wiley.

Cohen, J. (1977). *Statistical power analysis for the behavioral sciences* (Rev. ed.). New York: Academic Press.

Cohen, J. (1988). *Statistical power analysis for the behavioral sciences* (2nd ed.), Hillsdale, NJ: Lawrence Erlbaum.

Cohen, R. (2003). A passion for learning. *ASHA leader, 8, 2*, 17–18.

Colaizzi, P. (1978). *Psychological research as the phenomenologist views it. Existential phenomenological alternatives for psychology*. Oxford: Oxford University Press.

Cole, P. (1979). The evolving case-control study. *Journal of Chronic Diseases, 32*, 15–34.

Colton, T. (1974). *Statistics in medicine*. Boston: Little, Brown.

Cook, T. D., & Campbell, D. T. (1979). *Quasi-experimentation*. Chicago: Rand McNally.

Cooper, H. M., & Lemke, K. M. (1991). On the role of meta-analysis in personality and social psychology. *Personality and Social Psychology Bulletin, 17*, 245–251.

Cornett, R. O. (1967). Cued speech. *American Annals of the Deaf, 112*, 3–13.

Coyle, A. (1995). Discourse analysis. In G. M. Breakwell, S. Hammond & C. Fife-Schaw (Eds.), *Research methods in psychology*. Thousands Oaks, CA: Sage.

Crabtree, B. F., & Miller, W. L. (Eds.). (1992). *Doing qualitative research*. Newbury Park, CA: Sage.

Craig, A., Hancock, K., Tran, Y., Craig, M., & Peters, K. (2002). Epidemiology of stuttering in the community across the entire life span. *Journal of Speech, Language, and Hearing Research, 45*, 1097–1105.

Creaghead, N. A. (1999). Evaluating language intervention approaches: Contrasting perspectives. *Language, Speech, and Hearing Services in Schools, 30*, 415–416.

Creswell, J. W. (2003). *Research design: Qualitative, quantitative, and mixed methods approaches*. Thousand Oaks, CA: Sage.

Crichton, M. (1975). Medical obfuscation: Structure and function. *New England Journal of Medicine, 293*, 1257.

Cronbach, L. J. (1951). Coefficient alpha and the internal structure of tests. *Psychometrika, 16*, 297–334.

Cronbach, L. J. (1971). Test validation. In R. L. Thorndike (Ed.), *Educational measurement*. Washington, DC: American Council on Education.

Crosbie, J. (1993). Interrupted time-series analysis with brief single-subject data. *Journal of Consulting and Clinical Psychology, 61*, 966–974.

Culatta, B., Kovarsky, D., Theadore, G., Franklin, A. & Timler, B. (2003). Quantitative and qualitative documentation of early literacy instruction. *American Journal of Speech-Language Pathology, 12*, 172–188.

Cureton, E. E. (1951). Validity. In E. F. Lindquist (Ed.), *Educational measurement*. Washington, DC: American Council on Education.

Damico, J. S., & Simmons-Mackie, N. N. (2003). Qualitative research and speech-language pathology: A tutorial for the clinical realm. *American Journal of Speech-Language Pathology, 12*, 131–143.

Davis, A. (1995). The experimental method in psychology. In G. Breakwell, S. Hammond, & C. Fife-Schaw (Eds.), *Research methods in psychology*. Thousand Oaks, CA: Sage.

Dember, W. N., & Jenkins, J. J. (1970). *General psychology: Modeling behavior and experience*. Englewood Cliffs, NJ: Prentice-Hall.

Denzin, N. K., & Lincoln, Y. S. (Eds). (1998). *Collecting and interpreting qualitative methods*. Thousand Oaks, CA: Sage.

Depoy E., & Gitlin, L. N. (1994). *Introduction to research*. Saint Louis: Mosby.

Dewey, J. (1922). *Human nature and conduct*. New York: Holt, Rinehart and Winston.

Dillman, D. A. (1978). *Mail and telephone surveys: The total design method*. New York: Wiley.

Dollaghan, C. (2004). Evidence-based practice: Myths and realities. *ASHA Leader, 9*, 4.

Driscoll, D. A., Spinner, N. B., Budarf, M. L., McDonald-McGinn, D. M., Zackal, E. H., Goldberg, R. B., Shprintzen, R. J., Saal, R. M., Zonana, J., Jones, M. C., Mascarello, J. T., & Emanuel, B. S. (1992). Deletions and microdeletion of 22q11.2 in velo-cardio-facial syndrome. *American Journal of Medical Genetics, 44*, 261–268.

Duchan, J. F. (2002). What do you know about the history of speech-language pathology? And why it is important. *ASHA leader, 7*, 4.

Dunn, L. M., & Dunn, L. M. (1981). *Peabody picture vocabulary test* (Revised). Circle Pines, MN: American Guidance Service.

Erler, S. F., & Garstecki, D. C. (2002). Hearing loss- and hearing aid-related stigmas: Perceptions of women with age-normal hearing. *American Journal of Audiology, 11,* 83–91.

Eysenck, H. L. (1983). Special review [review of M. L. Smith, G. V. Glass, & T. I. Miller, *The benefits of psychotherapy*]. *Behavior Research and Therapy, 21,* 315–320.

Fey, M. E., & Johnson, B. W. (1998). Research to practice (and back again) in speech-language intervention. *Topics in Language Disorders, 18,* 23–24.

Filstead, W. J. (Ed.). (1970). *Qualitative methodology: Firsthand involvement with the social world.* Chicago: Markam.

Franke, R. H., & Kaul, J. D. (1978). The Hawthorne experiments: First statistical interpretation. *American Sociological Review, 43,* 623–643.

Frattali, C. (2004, April 13). Developing evidence-based practice guidelines. *ASHA Leader,* 13–14.

Frattali, C. M. (1998). Outcomes measurement: Definitions, dimensions, and perspectives. In C. M. Frattali (Ed.), *Measuring outcomes in speech-language pathology.* New York: Thieme.

Fry, D. B. (1979). *The physics of speech.* Cambridge: Cambridge University Press.

Gay, L. R. (1995). *Education research: Competencies for analysis and application* (5th ed.). Upper Saddle River, NJ: Merrill/Prentice Hall.

Gelfand, D. M., & Hartmann, D. P. (1984). *Child behavior analysis and therapy.* New York: Pergamon Press.

Glaser, B. G., & Strauss, A. L. (1967). *The discovery of grounded theory: Strategies for qualitative research.* Chicago: Aldine.

Glass, G. V. (1977). Integrating findings: The meta-analysis of research. *Review of Research in Education, 5,* 351–379.

Glesne, C., & Peshkin, A. (1992). *Becoming qualitative researchers: An introduction.* White Plains, NY: Longman.

Globerman, J. (1995). The unencumbered child: Family reputations and responsibilities in the care of relatives with Alzheimer's disease. *Family Process, 34,* 67–99.

Goddard, R., & Villanova, P. (1996). Designing surveys and questionnaires for research. In F. T. Leong & J. T. Austin (Eds.), *The psychology research handbook.* Thousand Oaks, CA: Sage.

Goldberg, R. B., Motzkin, B., Marion, R., Scambler, P. J., & Shprintzen, R. J. (1993). Velocardiofacial syndrome: A review of 120 patients. *American Journal of Medical Genetics, 45,* 313–319.

Goldstein, H. (1990). The future of language science: A plea for language intervention research. *ASHA Reports, 20,* 41–50.

Gorsuch, R. L. (1983). *Factor analysis.* Hillsdale, NJ: Lawrence Erlbaum Associates.

Gray, S. (2003). Word-learning by preschoolers with specific language impairment: What predicts success? *Journal of Speech, Language, and Hearing Research, 46,* 56–67.

Hammer, C. S. & Weiss, A. L. (1999). Guiding language development: How African American mothers and their infants structure play interaction. *Journal of Speech, Language, Hearing Research, 42,* 1219–1233.

Hammersley, M. (1992). *What's wrong with ethnography? Methodological explorations.* London: Routledge.

Harris, M. (1979). *Cultural materialism: The struggle for a science of culture.* New York: Random House.

Hays, W. L. (1973). *Statistics for the social sciences* (2nd ed.). New York: Holt, Rinehart & Winston.

Herson, M., & Barlow, D. H. (1976). *Single case experimental designs: Strategies for studying behavior change in the individual.* New York: Pergamon Press.

Hewitt, L. E. (2000). Does it matter what your client thinks? The role of theory in intervention: Response to Kamhi. *Language, Speech, and Hearing Services in Schools, 31,* 186–193.

Holland, A. L. (1998). Some guidelines for bridging the research practice gap in adult neurogenic communication disorders. *Topics in Language Disorders, 18,* 49–57.

Hoover, K. R. (1976). *The elements of social scientific thinking.* New York: St. Martin's Press.

Hulley, S. B., Gove, S., Browner, W. S., & Cummings, S. R. (1988). Choosing the study subjects: Specification and sampling. In S. B. Hulley & S. R. Cummings (Eds.), *Designing clinical research.* Baltimore: Williams & Wilkins.

Hwa-Froelick, D. A., & Westby, C. E. (2003). Framework of education: Perspective of Southeast Asian parents and Head Start staff. *Language, Speech, and Hearing Services in the Schools, 34,* 299–319.

Jacobs, Glen. (Ed.). (1970). *The participant observer.* New York: George Braziller.

Jaeger, R. M. (1984). *Sampling in education and the social sciences.* New York: Longman.

James, W. (1890). *The principles of psychology. 2 vols.* New York: Henry Holt.

Jenicek, M. (1999). *Clinical case reporting in evidence-based medicine.* Woburn, MA: Butterworth-Heinemann.

Jerger, J. (1963). Viewpoint. *Journal of Speech and Hearing Research, 6,* 301.

Jerger, J., Burney, P., Maulden, L., & Crump, B. (1993). Predicting hearing loss from the acoustic reflex. In B. Alford & S. Jerger (Eds.), *Clinical audiology: The Jerger perspective.* San Diego: Singular Publishing Group.

Johnson, M. B., & Ottenbacher, K. J. (1991). Trendline influence on visual analysis of single subject data. *Internal Disabilities Studies, 13,* 55–59.

Johnston, J. (1983). What is language intervention? The role of theory. In J. Miller, D. Yoder, & R. Schiefelbusch (Eds.), *Contemporary issues in language intervention,* ASHA Reports, *12,* 52–57. Rockville, MD: American Speech-Language-Hearing Association.

Jourard, S. M. (1968). *Disclosing man to himself.* New York: Van Nostrand Reinhold.

Justice, L. M., & Fey, M. E. (2004). Evidence-based practice in schools. *ASHA Leader, 9,* 17, 32.

Kaku, M., & Thompson, J. (1995). *Beyond Einstein.* New York: Anchor.

Kamhi, A. G. (1993). Some problems with the marriage between theory and clinical practice. *Language, Speech, and Hearing Services in Schools, 24,* 56–60.

Kamhi, A. G. (1999). To use or not to use: Factors that influence the selection of new treatment approaches. *Language, Speech, and Hearing Services in Schools, 30,* 92–97.

Kant, I. (1965). *Critique of pure reason* (N. K. Smith, Trans.). New York, St. Martin's Press.

Kaplan, E., Goodglass, H., & Weintraub, S. (1983). *Boston naming test.* Philadelphia: Lea Fibiger.

Kaplan, R. M., & Saccuzzo, D. P. (1997). *Psychological testing: Principles, applications, and issues.* Pacific Grove, CA: Brooks/Cole.

Katz, R. C., Hallowell, B., Code, C., Armstrong, E., Roberts, P., Pound, C., & Katz, L. (2000). A multinational comparison of aphasia management practices. *International Journal of Language & Communication Disorders, 35,* 303–304.

Kazdin, A. E. (1978). *History of behavior modification.* Baltimore: University Park Press.

Kazdin, A. E. (1982). *Single-case research designs: Methods for clinical and applied settings.* New York: Oxford University Press.

Kent, R. D., & Read, C. (1992). *The acoustic analysis of speech.* San Diego, CA: Singular.

Keppel, G., Saufley, W. H., & Tokunaga, H. (1992). *Introduction to design and analysis: A student's handbook*. New York: W.H. Freeman.

Kerlinger, F. N. (1967). *Foundations of behavioral research*. New York: Holt, Rinehart & Winston.

Kerlinger, F. N. (1973). *Foundations of behavioral research* (2nd ed.). New York: Holt, Rinehart & Winston.

Kerlinger, F. N. (1986). *Foundations of behavioral research* (3rd ed.). New York: Holt, Rinehart & Winston.

Kidder, L. H. (1981). *Seliltiz. Wrightsman, & Cook's research methods in social relations*. New York: Holt, Rinehart & Winston.

Kimmel, A. J. (1988). *Ethics and values in applied social research*. Beverly Hills, CA: Sage.

Kirk, J., & Miller, M. L. (1986). *Reliability and validity in qualitative research*. Beverly Hills, CA: Sage.

Kish, L. (1965). *Survey sampling*. New York: Wiley.

Klee, T., Carson, D. K., Gavin, W. J., Hall, L., Kent, A., & Reece, S. (1998). Concurrent and predictive validity of an early language screening program. *Journal of Speech, Language, and Hearing Research, 41*, 627–641.

Klee, T., Pearce, K., & Carson, D. K. (2000). Improving the positive predictive value of screening for developmental language disorder. *Journal of Speech, Language, and Hearing Research, 43*, 821–833.

Knapp, R. G., & Miller, M. C. (1992). *Clinical epidemiology and biostatistics*. Baltimore: Williams and Wilkins.

Krasner, L. (1971). Behavior therapy. *Annual Review of Psychology, 22*, 483–532.

Kratochwill, T. R., & Levin, J. R. (1978). What time-series designs may have to offer educational researchers. *Contemporary Educational Psychology, 3*, 273–329.

Krippendorff, K. (1980). *Content analysis. An introduction to its methodology*. Newbury Park, CA: Sage.

Kuder, G. & Richardson, M. (1937). The theory of the estimation of test reliability. *Psychometrika, 2,* 151–160.

Kuster, J. (2003). Don't forget the library. *ASHA leader, 8*, 2, 18.

Lass, N. J., Ruscello, D. M., Pannbacker, M. D., Middleton, G. F., Schmitt, J. F., & Scheuerle, J. F. (1995). Career selection and satisfaction in the professions, *ASHA, 37*, 48–51.

Leahy, M. M. (2004). Analyzing therapeutic discourse. *Language, Speech and Hearing Services in Schools, 35*, 70–81.

Leininger, M. (1994). Evaluation criteria and critique of qualitative research studies. In C. M. Morse (Ed.), *Critical issues in qualitative research methods*. Thousand Oaks, CA: Sage.

Liebert, R. M., & Liebert, L. L. (1995). *Science and behavior: An introduction to methods of psychological research*. Englewood Cliffs, NJ: Prentice-Hall.

Liebow, E. (1967). *Tally's corner: A study of street corner Negro men*. Boston: Little, Brown.

Lincoln, Y., & Guba, E. (1985). *Naturalistic inquiry*. Beverly Hills, CA: Sage.

Lindlof, T. R. & Taylor, B. C. (2002). *Qualitative research methods*. Thousand Oaks, CA: Sage.

Logemann, J. A. (2000a). From the president: Are clinicians and researchers different? *The ASHA Leader, 5*(8), 2.

Logemann, J. A. (2000b). From the president: What is evidence-based practice and why should we care? *The ASHA Leader, 5*(5), 3.

Maxwell, D. L., & Satake, E. (1993). *Applications of Bayesian statistics to the diagnosis of stuttering*. Anaheim, CA: American Speech-Language-Hearing Association.

McCracken, G. (1988). *The long interview*. Newbury Park, CA: Sage.

McCready, W. (1996). Applying sampling procedures. In *The Psychology Research Handbook*, F. B. Leong & J. A., (Eds.), Thousand Oaks, CA: Sage.

McGuigan, F. J. (1993). *Experimental psychology. Methods of research*. Englewood Cliffs, NJ: Prentice-Hall.

Meline, T. & Paradiso, T. (2003). Evidence-based practice in schools: Evaluating research and reducing barriers. *Language, Speech, and Hearing Services in Schools, 34*, 273–283.

Melton, A. W. (1962). Editorial. *Journal of Experimental Psychology, 64*, 553–557.

Menyuk, P., & Looney, P. (1972). Relationships among components of grammar in language disorder. *Journal of Speech and Hearing Research, 15*, 395–406.

Merriam, S. B. (1995). What can you tell from an N of 1? Issues of validity and reliability in qualitative research. *PAACE: Journal of Lifelong Learning, 4*, 54–60. (Pennsylvania Association for Adult and Continuing Education.)

Merton, R. K. (1959). Notes on problem-finding in sociology. In R. K. Merton, L. Broom, & L. Conttrell, Jr. (Eds.), *Sociology today: Problems and prospects*. New York: Basic Books.

Messick, S. (1988). Validity. In R.L. Linn (Ed.), *Educational measurement*. New York: Macmillan.

Milgram, S. (1977). *Subject reaction. The neglected factor in the ethics of experimentation*. Hastings Center Report, October 1977.

Mishler, E. G. (1983). Meaning in context: Is there any other kind? In P. Hauser-Cram & F. C. Martin (Eds.), *Essays on educational research: Methodology, testing and application*. Cambridge, MA: Harvard Educational Review, Reprint No. 16.

Monette, D. R., Sullivan, T. J., & DeJong, C. R. (1998). *Applied social research*. Fort Worth, TX: Harcourt Brace.

Morrison, D. E., & Henkel, R. E. (1970). Significance tests in behavioral research: Skeptical conclusions and beyond. In D. E. Morrison & R. E. Henkel (Eds.), *The significance test controversy: A reader*. Chicago: Aldine.

Morse, J. M. and Field, P. A. (1995). *Qualitative methods for health professionals*. Thousand Oaks, CA: Sage.

Mullen, R. (2003). *ASHA's National Outcomes Measurement System (NOMS). Outcomes of Research Evidence-Based Practice*. 13th Annual NIDCD-Sponsored Research Symposium.

Mustain, W. (2003). ASHA's code of ethics modified to address research ethics. *The ASHA Leader, 8*, 28.

Neuman, W. L. (2000). *Social research methods: Qualitative and quantitative approaches*. Needham Heights, MA: Allyn and Bacon.

Nicholls, G. H., & Ling, D. (1982). Cued speech and the reception of spoken language. *Journal of Speech and Hearing Research, 25*, 262–269.

Noldus, L. P. (1991). The observer: A software system for collection and analysis of observational data. *Behavior Research Methods, Instruments, & Computers, 23*, 415–429.

Nye, C., & Turner, I. (1990). Summarizing articulation disorder treatment effects: A meta-analysis. In L. B. Olswang, C. K. Thompson, S. F. Warren, & N. J. Minghetti, (Eds.), *Treatment efficacy research in communication disorders*. Rockville, MD: American Speech-Language-Hearing Foundation.

Onslow, M., & Packman, A. (1997). Control of children's stuttering with response-contingent time-out: Behavioral, perceptual, and acoustic data. *Journal of Speech, Language, and Hearing Research, 40*, 121–133.

Orne, M. T. (1959). The nature of hypnosis: Artifact and essence. *Journal of Abnormal and Social Psychology, 58*, 277–299.

Ortman A., & Hertwig, R. (1997). Is deception acceptable? *American Psychologist, 52*, 746–747.

Ottenbacher, K. J. (1992). Analysis of data in idiographic research: Issues and methods. *American Journal of Physical Medicine and Rehabilitation, 71*, 202–208.

Ottenbacher, K. J. (1993). Interrater agreement of visual analysis in single-subject, decisions: Quantitative review and analysis. *American Journal of Mental Retardation, 98,* 135–142.

Panagos, J. M., & Prelock, P. A. (1982). Phonological constraints on the sentence productions of language-disordered children. *Journal of Speech and Hearing Research, 25,* 171–177.

Parsonson, B. S., & Baer, M. M. (1986). Reliability and accuracy of visually analyzing graphed data from single-subject designs. *American Journal of Occupational Therapy, 40,* 464–469.

Patton, M. Q. (2002). *Qualitative research & evaluation methods.* Thousand Oaks, CA: Sage.

Peach, R. K. (2004). From the editor. *American Journal of Speech-Language Pathology, 13,* 2.

Pedhazur, E. J., & Schmelkin, L. P. (1991). *Measurement, design, and analysis: An integrated approach.* Hillsdale, NJ: Lawrence Erlbaum Associates.

Peters, W. S. (1987). *Counting for something: Statistical principles and personalities.* New York: Springer-Verlag.

Peterson-Falzone, S. J., Hardin-Jones, M. A., & Karnell, M. P. (2001). *Cleft palate speech.* St. Louis, MO: Mosby.

Piaget, J. (1932). *The language and thought of the child.* New York: Harcourt, Brace.

Pillimer, D. B., & Light, R. J. (1980). Synthesizing outcomes: How to use research evidence from many studies. *Harvard Education Review, 50,* 176–195.

Pirsig, R. M. (1974). *Zen and the art of motorcycle maintenance.* New York: Bantam.

Poincare, H. (1913). *The foundations of science.* New York: Science Press.

Polit, D. F., Beck, C. T., & Hungler, B. P. (2001). *Essentials of nursing research.* Philadelphia: Lippincott.

Popper, K. R. (1968). *The logic of scientific discovery.* London: Hutchinson.

Potter, J. (1996). Discourse analysis and constructionist approaches: Theoretical background. In L. Richardson (Ed.), *A handbook for qualitative methods for social psychologists and other social scientists.* Leicester: British Psychological Society.

Potter, J., & Wetherall, M. (1987). *Discourse and social psychology: Beyond attitudes and behavior.* London: Sage.

Pratt, S. R., Heintzelman, A. T., & Deming, S. E. (1993). The efficacy of using the IBM speech viewer vowel accuracy module to treat young children with hearing impairment. *Journal of Speech and Hearing Research, 36,* 1063–1974.

Prizant, B. M. (1992). Childhood autism rating scale (review). In J. Conoley & J. Kramer (Eds.), *Mental measurements yearbook.* Lincoln, NE: Buros Institute, University of Nebraska-Lincoln.

Ramhoj, P., & de Oliveira, E. (1991). A phenomenological hermeneutic access to research of the old age area. *Scandinavian Journal of Caring Science, 5,* 238–249.

Ray, M. A. (1994). The richness of phenomenology: Philosophic, theoretic, and methodologic concerns. In J. M. Morse (Ed.), *Critical issues in qualitative research methods.* Thousand Oaks, CA: Sage.

Reeder, F. (1989). *Conceptual foundations of science and key phenomenological concepts.* Monograph, Wayne State University, College of Nursing.

Rescorla, L. (1989). The language development survey: A screening tool for delayed language in toddlers. *Journal of Speech and Hearing Disorders, 54,* 587–599.

Richards, T. J., & Richards, L. (1998). Using computers in qualitative research. In N. K. Denzin & Y. S. Lincoln (Eds.), *Collecting and interpreting qualitative materials.* Thousand Oaks, CA: Sage.

Riley, G. D. (1972). A stuttering severity instrument for children and adults. *Journal of Speech and Hearing Disorders, 37,* 314–320.

Riley, G. D. (1986). *Stuttering severity instrument for children and adults* (Revised). Austin, TX: Proed.

Robey, R. (2004). Evidence-based practice: Levels of evidence. *ASHA Leader, 9,* 5.

Robey, R. R., Schultz, M. C., Crawford, A. B., & Sinner, C. A. (1999). Single-subject clinical-outcome research: Designs, data, effect sizes, and analyses. *Aphasiology, 13,* 445–473.

Rodriquez, B. L., & Olswang, L. G. (2003). Mexican-American and Anglo-American mothers' beliefs and values about child rearing, education, and language impairment. *American Journal of Speech-Language Pathology, 12,* 452–462.

Rosenberg, K. M., & Daly, H. B. (1993). *Foundations of behavioral research.* Fort Worth, TX: Harcourt Brace.

Rosenfeld, R. M., Goldsmith, A. J., Tetlus, L., & Balzano, A. (1997). Quality of life for children with otitis media. *Archives of Otolaryngology, Head and Neck Surgery, 123,* 1049–1054.

Rosenthal, R., & Jacobson, L. (1968). *Pygmalion in the classroom: Teacher expectation and pupils' intellectual development.* New York: Holt, Rinehart & Winston.

Rosnow, R. D. L., & Rosnow, M. (1995). *Writing papers in psychology* (3rd ed.). Pacific Grove, CA: Brooks/Cole.

Rosnow, R.R., & Rosenthal, R. (1996). *Beginning behavioral research.* Englewood Cliffs, NJ: Prentice-Hall.

Ruiz, Nadeen. (1995). The social construction of ability and disability. *Journal of Learning Disabilities, 28,* 478.

Russell, B. (1948). *Human knowledge.* New York: Simon & Schuster.

Rutter, M. (1989). Attention deficit disorder/hyperkinetic syndrome: Conceptual and research issues regarding diagnosis and classification. In T. Sagvolden & T. Archer (Eds.), *Attention deficit disorder: Clinical and basic research.* Hillsdale, NJ: Lawrence Erlbaum.

Rvachew, S. (1994). Speech perception training can facilitate sound production learning. *Journal of Speech and Hearing Research, 37,* 347–357.

Sachs, H. S., Berrier, J., Reitman, D., Ancora-Berk, V. A., & Chalmers, T. C. (1987). Meta-analysis of randomized controlled trials. *New England Journal of Medicine, 316,* 450–455.

Sacks, H. (1992). *Lectures on conversation* (2 volumes republished as one volume). Oxford: Blackwell.

Sacks, O. (2000). Brilliant light. In D. Quammen (Ed.), *The best American science and nature writing.* Boston-New York: Houghton Mifflin Co.

Schlesselman, J. J., & Stolley, P. D. (1982). *Case-control studies: Design, conduct, analysis.* New York/Oxford: Oxford University Press.

Schloss, P. J., & Smith, M. A. (1999). *Conducting research.* Upper Saddle River, NJ: Merrill.

Schopler, E., Reichler, R., & Renner, B. (1988). *The childhood autism rating scale.* Los Angeles: Western Psychological Services.

Shaffir, W. B., & Stebbins, R. A. (Eds.). (1991). *Experiencing fieldwork: An inside view of qualitative research.* Newbury Park, CA: Sage.

Sharpe, T. & Koperwas, J. (2003). *Behavior and sequential analyses: Principles and practice.* Thousand Oaks, CA: Sage.

Sharpley, C. F. (1986). Fallability in the visual assessment of behavioral intervention: Time-series statistics to analyze time-series data. *Behavior Change, 3,* 26–33.

Shaughnessy, J. J., & Zechmeister, E. B. (1994). *Research methods in psychology.* New York: McGraw-Hill.

Shavelson, R. J. (1988). *Statistical reasoning for the behavioral sciences* (2nd ed.). Boston: Allyn and Bacon.

Shprintzen, R. J., Goldberg, R. B., Lewin, M., Sidoti, E., Berkman, M., Argamaso, R., & Young, D. (1978). A new syndrome involving cleft palate, cardiac anomalies, typical facies, and learning disabilities: Velo-cardio-facial syndrome. *Cleft Palate Journal 15,* 56–62.

Shriberg, L. D., Kwiatkowski, J., & Gruber, F. A. (1994). Developmental phonological disorders II: Short-term speech-sound normalization. *Journal of Speech and Hearing Research, 37,* 1127–1150.

Sidman, M. (1960). *Tactics of scientific research*. New York: Basic Books.

Siegel, S. (1956). *Nonparametric statistics for the behavioral sciences*. New York: McGraw-Hill.

Silverman, I. (1977). *The human subject in the psychological laboratory*. New York: Pergamon Press.

Simmons-Mackie, N., Code, C., Armstrong, E., Stiegler, L., & Elman, R. (2002). What is aphasia? Results of an international survey. *Aphasiology, 16,* 837–848.

Simmons-Mackie, N., & Damico, J. (2003). Contributions of qualitative research to the knowledge base of normal communication. *American Journal of Speech-Language Pathology, 12,* 144–154.

Siu, R.H. (1957). *The Tao of science*. Cambridge, MA: M.I.T. Press.

Skinner, B. F. (1956). A case study in scientific method. *American Psychologist, 11,* 221–233.

Spector, P. E. (1992). *Summated rating scale construction*. Newbury Park, CA: Sage.

Spradley, J. P. (1980). *Participant observation*. New York: Holt, Reinhart, & Winston.

SPSS Reference Guide (1990). Chicago: SPSS Inc.

Stern, P. N. (1980). Grounded theory methodology: Its uses and processes. *Image, 12,* 20–23.

Steven, S. S. (1960). *Handbook of experimental psychology* (3rd edition). New York: Wiley.

Steven, S. S. (1968). Measurements, statistics, and schematics. *Science, 161,* 849–856.

Strauss, A., & Corbin, J. (1998). *Basics of qualitative research*. Thousand Oaks, CA: Sage.

Sudman, S., & Bradburn, N. M. (1982). *Asking questions: A practical guide to questionnaire design*. San Francisco: Jossey-Bass.

Tallal, P., Hirsch, L. S., Realpe-Bonila, T., Miller, S., Brzustowicz, L. M., Bartlett, C., & Flax, J. F. (2001). Familial aggregation in specific language impairment. *Journal of Speech, Language, and Hearing Research, 44,* 1172–1182.

Tapp, J., & Walden, T. (1993). PROCODER; a professional take control, coding, and analysis system for behavioral research using videotape. *Behavior Research Methods, Instruments, and Computers, 25,* 53–56.

Tapp, J., Wehby, J., & Ellis, D. (1995). A multiple option observation system for experimental studies (M.O.O.S.E.S). *Behavior Research Methods, Instruments and Computers, 27,* 15–21.

Tawney, J. W., & Gast, D. L. (1984). *Single subject research in special education*. Columbus, OH: Charles Merrill.

Tetnowski, J. A., & Damico, J. S. (2001). A demonstration of the advantages of qualitative methodologies in stuttering research. *Journal of Fluency Disorders, 26,* 17–42.

Tetnowski, J. A., & Franklin, T. C. (2003). Qualitative research: Implications for description and assessment. *American Journal of Speech-Language Pathology, 12,* 155–164.

Tharpe, A. M., Fino-Szumski, M. S., & Bess, F. H. (2001). Survey of hearing aid fitting practices for children with multiple impairments. *American Journal of Audiology, 10,* 32–40.

Thayer, N., & Dodd, B. (1996). Auditory processing and phonologic disorders. *Audiology, 35,* 37–44.

Thorndike, E. L. (1938). The law of effect. *Psychological Review, 45,* 204–205.

Thorton, B. S. (1999). *Plagues of the mind: The new epidemic of false knowledge*. Wilmington, DE: ISI Books.

Thurstone, L. L. (1947). *Multiple factor analysis*. Chicago: University of Chicago Press.

Todman, J. B. & Dugard, P. (2001). *Single-case and Small-n Experimental Designs: A Practical Guide to Randomization Tests*. Mahwah, NJ: Erlbaum.

Van Riper, C. (1971). *The nature of stuttering*. Englewood Cliffs, NJ: Prentice-Hall.

Van Riper, C. (1982). *The nature of stuttering*. (2nd ed.). Englewood Cliffs, NJ: Prentice-Hall.

Wakefield, J. C. (1995). When an irresistible epistemology meets an immovable ontology. *Social Work Research, 19,* 9–17.

Wallace, S. R. (1965). Criteria for what? *American Psychologist, 20,* 411–417.

Wambaugh, J., & Bain, B. (2002). Make research methods an integral part of your clinical practice. *The ASHA Leader, 7,* 9–11

Watson, J. B. (1924). *Behaviorism*. New York: Norton.

Wechsler, D. (1991). *Wechsler Intelligence Scale for Children* (3rd ed.). San Antonio, TX: Psychological Corporation.

Weismer, S. E., Murray-Branch, J., & Miller, J. F. (1993). The influence of prosodic and gestural cues on novel word acquisition by children with specific language impairment. *Journal of Speech and Hearing Research, 36,* 1037–1050.

Werner, O., & Schoepfle, G. M. (1987a). *Systematic fieldwork: Vol. 1. Foundations of ethnography and interviewing*. Newbury Park, CA: Sage.

Wiig, E., Secord, W., & Semel, E. (1992). *Clinical evaluation of language fundamentals—preschool*. San Antonio, TX: Psychological Corporation/Harcourt Brace Jovanovich.

Wilcox, M. J., Hadley, P. A., & Bacon, C. K. (1998). Linking science and practice in management of childhood language disorders: Models and problem-solving strategies. *Topics in Language Disorders, 18,* 10–22.

Wilson, H. S. (1989). The craft of qualitative analysis. In H. S. Wilson (Ed.), *Research in nursing* (2nd ed.) Menlo Park CA: Addison-Wesley.

Wolery, M., & Harris, S. R. (1982). Interpreting results of single-subject research designs. *Physical Therapy, 62,* 445–452.

Wolery, M., & Ezell, H. K. (1993). Subject descriptions in single-subject research. *Journal of Learning Disabilities, 26,* 642–647.

Wolf, F. M. (1986). *Meta-analysis. Quantitative methods for research synthesis*. Beverly Hills, CA: Sage.

World Health Organization. (1980). *International classification of impairments, disabilities, and handicaps*: Geneva.

Yorkston, K. M., Klasner, E. R., & Swanson, K. M. (2001). Communication in context: A qualitative study of the experiences of individuals with multiple sclerosis. *American Journal of Speech-Language Pathology, 10,* 126–137.

Young, M. A. (1993). Supplementing tests of statistical significance: Variation accounted for. *Journal of Speech and Hearing Research, 36,* 644–656.

Young, M. A. (1994). Evaluating differences between stuttering and nonstuttering speakers: The group difference design. *Journal of Speech and Hearing Research, 37,* 522–534.

Zebrowski, P. M. (1994). Duration of sound prolongations and sound syllable repetition in children who stutter: Preliminary observations. *Journal of Speech and Hearing Research, 37,* 254–263.

INDEX

A

A-B-A-B design, 188–89, 189f, 201
A-B-A design, 188, 188f
A-B design, 187–88, 187f, 201
A-B experiments, mini, 192
ABRs (auditory brainstem responses), latency measures of, 137, 138f
Abscissa (*x* axis), 282, 286
  in graphical analysis, 196, 197f
Absolute risk reduction (ARR), 472–73
Abstract
  computerized database of, 56
    search strategies for, 56–57
  of professional presentations, 56, 402
  in research article, 37, 38t
    catabolic evaluation of, 385f
  in research proposal, 387–88
Abstract language, verbal intelligence and, 130
Abstract thinking, origin of, 2
Academy of Neurologic Communication Disorders and Sciences (ANCDS), evidence-based practice guidelines, 10
Acceleration, in graphical analysis, 198, 198f
Accessory behaviors, with stuttering, 114
Accountability, in research protocol, 390
Accuracy
  of diagnostic tests, 233–34, 234t
    measures of, 234–35, 237
  of estimations, 129t, 130
  of judgments, stability versus, 124–25, 126t
  of measurements, 119–26. *See also* Reliability
  of measuring instruments, 119, 121
  of predictions, 129–30, 129t
  of tests, 128. *See also* Validity
Acoustic reflex measurements
  amplitude-intensity, 140, 141f
  hearing threshold levels and, 118–19
Acoustic stimuli, cochlear neuron discharges with, 136–37, 136f
Acoustic tumors, 137, 141f
Action plan, for theses, 399–400
Active-member researcher role, in participant observation, 249–50
Adaptation effect, in stuttering, 286
Advisors, for theses, 399–400
Advisory committee/council
  for animal studies, 390
  for grant applications, 395
  for human studies. *See* Institutional Review Boards (IRBs)
  for theses, 400
AERA. *See* American Educational Research Association (AERA)

Agreement, method of, in causality determination, 150
AJA (American Journal of Audiology), 53–54, 59, 481
AJSLP (American Journal of Speech-Language Pathology), 53–54, 59, 481
ALC (audition and lip reading), cued speech and, 352–53, 353t
Allied Health Literature, Cumulative Index to, 58
Alpha error. *See* Type I error
Alternate-form reliability, 121–22, 121t, 123t
Alternating treatment design, 190–91, 190f
Alternative hypothesis, 78, 82
  p-value approach and, 354, 355f
  in rank-order tests, 340, 342
  in single-group design, 323–25, 326f–327f, 328t
  in two-sample cases, 329–30
    dependent, 333–36, 336f
    independent, 330, 332–33, 333f
Alzheimer's disease, caregiver interviews, 256–57
Ambiguity
  in nonexperimental research, 35, 118
  of research problems, 76
  in writing, 401
American Educational Research Association (AERA)
  Code of Ethics, 65
  on measurement, 119, 128
American Journal of Audiology (AJA), 53–54, 59, 481
American Journal of Speech-Language Pathology (AJSLP), 53–54, 59, 481
American Psychological Association (APA)
  Code of Ethics, 65–66, 251–52
  on measurement, 119, 128
  publication manual, 401
  reference style, 391, 393
American Sociological Association (ASA), Code of Ethics, 65
American Speech-Language-Hearing Association (ASHA)
  Code of Ethics, 16–18, 66
  evidence-based practice support, 9–10, 12
  guidelines for human or animal research, 390, 391f
  journals published by, 53–54, 481
  merit evaluations, xxiii
  presentation proposal guidelines, 402–3
  research collaboration commitment, 13
  sampling members of, 88, 93–95, 96t
  scholarly publishing program of, 54–55
  Web site, 56, 396
American Speech-Language-Hearing Foundation (ASHF), funding applications, 396, 398
Americans with disabilities, 60
Amplitude-intensity, of response, 139–40, 141f
Anabolic thinking, in writing research, 387–99
  funding requests, 393–99, 395f